2000 Red Book:

Report of the Committee on Infectious Diseases

Twenty-fifth Edition

Author: Committee on Infectious Diseases
American Academy of Pediatrics

Larry K. Pickering, MD, FAAP, Editor

Georges Peter, MD, FAAP, Emeritus Editor

Carol J. Baker, MD, FAAP, Associate Editor
Michael A. Gerber, MD, FAAP, Associate Editor
Noni E. MacDonald, MD, FAAP, Associate Editor

Walter A. Orenstein, MD
Centers for Disease Control and Prevention, Liaison

Peter Patriarca, MD
Food and Drug Administration, Liaison

American Academy of Pediatrics
141 Northwest Point Blvd
Elk Grove Village, IL 60009-0927

Suggested Citation: American Academy of Pediatrics. [chapter title]. In: Pickering LK, ed. *2000 Red Book: Report of the Committee on Infectious Diseases.* 25th ed. Elk Grove Village, IL: American Academy of Pediatrics; 2000:[page number]

25th Edition
1st Edition–1938
2nd Edition – 1939
3rd Edition – 1940
4th Edition – 1942
5th Edition – 1943
6th Edition – 1944
7th Edition – 1945
8th Edition – 1947
9th Edition – 1951
10th Edition – 1952
11th Edition – 1955
12th Edition – 1957
13th Edition – 1961
14th Edition – 1964
15th Edition – 1966
16th Edition – 1970
16th Edition Revised – 1971
17th Edition – 1974
18th Edition – 1977
19th Edition – 1982
20th Edition – 1986
21st Edition – 1988
22nd Edition – 1991
23rd Edition – 1994
24th Edition – 1997

ISSN No. 1080-0131
ISBN No. 1-58110-038-8 hardcover
1-58110-039-6 softcover
MA0001

Quantity prices on request. Address all inquiries to:
American Academy of Pediatrics
PO Box 927, 141 Northwest Point Blvd
Elk Grove Village, IL 60009-0927

or Phone:
1-888-227-1770 Publications

The recommendations in this publication do not indicate an exclusive course of treatment or serve as a standard of medical care. Variations, taking into account individual circumstances, may be appropriate.

Committee on Infectious Diseases 1997–2000

Jon S. Abramson, MD, FAAP, Chairperson 1999–2000
Neal A. Halsey, MD, FAAP, Chairperson, 1995–1999

Carol J. Baker, MD, FAAP
P. Joan Chesney, MD, FAAP
Margaret C. Fisher, MD, FAAP
Michael A. Gerber, MD, FAAP
S. Michael Marcy, MD, FAAP
H. Cody Meissner, MD, FAAP
Dennis L. Murray, MD, FAAP
Gary D. Overturf, MD, FAAP
Charles G. Prober, MD, FAAP
Margaret B. Rennels, MD, FAAP
Thomas N. Saari, MD, FAAP
Leonard B. Weiner, MD, FAAP
Richard J. Whitley, MD, FAAP
Ram Yogev, MD, FAAP

Larry K. Pickering, MD, FAAP, Ex-Officio, *Red Book* Editor
Georges Peter, MD, FAAP, Ex-Officio, Emeritus *Red Book* Editor

Liaison Representatives

Anthony Hirsch, MD, FAAP, AAP Pediatric Practice Action Group
Richard F. Jacobs, MD, American Thoracic Society
Gilles Delage, MD, Canadian Paediatric Society
Noni E. MacDonald, MD, FAAP, Canadian Paediatric Society
Scott Dowell, MD, MPH, Centers for Disease Control and Prevention
Walter A. Orenstein, MD, FAAP, Centers for Disease Control and Prevention
Benjamin Schwartz, MD, Centers for Disease Control and Prevention
Peter A. Patriarca, MD, Food and Drug Administration
N. Regina Rabinovich, MD, National Institutes of Health
Robert F. Breiman, MD, National Vaccine Program Office
Martin G. Myers, MD, National Vaccine Program Office

Consultants to the Editors

John S. Finlayson, PhD
Edgar O. Ledbetter, MD, FAAP
Morven S. Edwards, MD, FAAP
Peter J. Hotez, MD, PhD
George H. McCracken, Jr, MD
Catherine M. Wilfert, MD, FAAP

Collaborators

On behalf of the American Academy of Pediatrics, the Committee gratefully acknowledges the invaluable assistance provided by the following individuals who served as contributors and reviewers in the preparation of this edition of the *Red Book.* Their expertise, critical review, and cooperation are essential in the Committee's continuing review and revisions of its recommendations for the management, control, and prevention of infectious diseases in children.

Every attempt has been made to recognize all those who contributed to this edition of the *Red Book*; the Academy regrets any omissions that may have occurred.

Penny M. Adcock, MD, Centers for Disease Control and Prevention, Atlanta, GA
David G. Addiss, MD, Centers for Disease Control and Prevention, Atlanta, GA
Mercedes Albuerne, MD, Food and Drug Administration, Bethesda, MD
Miriam J. Alter, PhD, Centers for Disease Control and Prevention, Atlanta, GA
Larry J. Anderson, MD, Centers for Disease Control and Prevention, Atlanta, GA
Frederick J. Angulo, MD, Centers for Disease Control and Prevention, Atlanta, GA
Juan Arciniega, DSc, Food and Drug Administration, Bethesda, MD
Paul Arguin, Centers for Disease Control and Prevention, Atlanta, GA
Jane Ellen Aronson, DO, Winthrop Pediatric Specialty Center, Mineola, NY
David Asher, MD, Food and Drug Administration, Bethesda, MD
David A. Ashford, DVM, MPH, DSc, Centers for Disease Control and Prevention, Atlanta, GA
C.D. Atreya, PhD, Food and Drug Administration, Bethesda, MD
Sophie J. Balk, MD, Albert Einstein College of Medicine, Bronx, NY
Leslie Ball, MD, Food and Drug Administration, Bethesda, MD
Sharon Balter, MD, Centers for Disease Control and Prevention, Atlanta, GA
Robert S. Baltimore, MD, Yale University School of Medicine, New Haven, CT
Lawrence Barat, MD, Centers for Disease Control and Prevention, Atlanta, GA
Michael Beach, PhD, Centers for Disease Control and Prevention, Atlanta, GA
Judy Beeler, MD, Food and Drug Administration, Bethesda, MD
Ermias Belay, MD, Centers for Disease Control and Prevention, Atlanta, GA
Beth Bell, MD, Centers for Disease Control and Prevention, Atlanta, GA
David M. Bell, MD, Centers for Disease Control and Prevention, Atlanta, GA
Thomas A. Bell,† MD, MPH, Cowlitz County Health Department, Longview, WA
Stuart M. Berman, MD, Centers for Disease Control and Prevention, Atlanta, GA
Richard E. Besser, MD, Centers for Disease Control and Prevention, Atlanta, GA
Kristine M. Bisgard, MD, Centers for Disease Control and Prevention, Atlanta, GA
David Blair, PhD, James Cook University of North Queensland, Australia

† Deceased

Martin J. Blaser, MD, Vanderbilt University School of Medicine, Nashville, TN
Peter B. Bloland, MD, Centers for Disease Control and Prevention, Atlanta, GA
Ann Bolger, MD, University of California, Riverside, CA
Robert Bortolussi, MD, Dalhousie University, Halifax NS, Canada
Michael Brennan, PhD, Food and Drug Administration, Bethesda, MD
Joseph S. Bresee, MD, Centers for Disease Control and Prevention, Atlanta, GA
Thomas Breuer, MD, MS, Centers for Disease Control and Prevention, Atlanta, GA
Marc Bulterys, MD, PhD, Centers for Disease Control and Prevention, Atlanta, GA
Drusilla Burns, PhD, Food and Drug Administration, Bethesda, MD
Jane L. Burns, MD, University of Washington, Seattle, WA
Bill Cameron, MD, Ottawa General Hospital, Ottawa, Ontario, Canada
Kathryn Carbone, MD, Food and Drug Administration, Bethesda, MD
Martin Cetron, MD, Centers for Disease Control and Prevention, Atlanta, GA
Mary E. Chamberland, MD, MPH, Centers for Disease Control and Prevention, Atlanta, GA
Bob Chen, MD, Centers for Disease Control and Prevention, Atlanta, GA
James Childs, MD, Centers for Disease Control and Prevention, Atlanta, GA
John C. Christenson, MD, University of Utah School of Medicine, Salt Lake City, UT
Thomas G. Cleary, MD, University of Texas Medical School, Houston, TX
Susan Cookson, MD, Centers for Disease Control and Prevention, Atlanta, GA
Ralph L. Cordell, PhD, Centers for Disease Control and Prevention, Atlanta, GA
Edward Cox, MD, Food and Drug Administration, Bethesda, MD
Nancy J. Cox, PhD, Centers for Disease Control and Prevention, Atlanta, GA
Adnan S. Dajani, MD, Children's Hospital of Michigan, Detroit, MI
Nicholas A. Daniels, MD, MPH, Centers for Disease Control and Prevention, Atlanta, GA
Jeffrey P. Davis, MD, Bureau of Public Health, Madison, WI
Carolyn Deal, PhD, Food and Drug Administration, Bethesda, MD
David T. Dennis, MD, Centers for Disease Control and Prevention, Fort Collins, CO
Vance Dietz, MD, Centers for Disease Control and Prevention, Atlanta, GA
Leigh G. Donowitz, MD, University of Virginia School of Medicine, Charlottesville, VA
D. Peter Drotman, MD, MPH, Centers for Disease Control and Prevention, Atlanta, GA
Lawrence F. Eichenfield, MD, Children's Hospital, San Diego, CA
Karen Elkins, PhD, Food and Drug Administration, Bethesda, MD
Joanne E. Embree, MD, FRCPC, University of Manitoba, Winnipeg, Manitoba, Canada
Joseph J. Esposito, PhD, Centers for Disease Control and Prevention, Atlanta, GA
Karen Farizo, MD, Food and Drug Administration, Bethesda, MD
Ronald A. Feinstein, MD, University of Alabama at Birmingham School of Medicine, Birmingham, AL
Stephen Feinstone, MD, Food and Drug Administration, Bethesda, MD

Theresa Finn, PhD, Food and Drug Administration, Bethesda, MD
Patricia M. Flynn, MD, St. Jude Children's Research Hospital, Memphis, TN
E. Lee Ford-Jones, MD, The Hospital for Sick Children, Toronto, Ontario, Canada
Ellen C. Frank, RPh, Food and Drug Administration, Bethesda, MD
Barbara L. Frankowski, MD, MPH, University of Vermont, Burlington, VT
Frazier W. Frantz, MD, Naval Medical Center, Portsmouth, VA
Carl Frasch, PhD, Food and Drug Administration, Bethesda, MD
Cindy R. Friedman, MD, Centers for Disease Control and Prevention, Atlanta, GA
Lawrence M. Gartner, MD, University of Chicago, Chicago, IL
Lillian Gavnlovich, MD, Food and Drug Administration, Bethesda, MD
Francis Gigliotti, University of Rochester School of Medicine and Dentistry, Rochester, NY
Roger Glass, MD, Centers for Disease Control and Prevention, Atlanta, GA
Hana Golding, PhD, Food and Drug Administration, Bethesda, MD
Donald Goldmann, MD, Harvard Medical School, Boston, MA
David P. Greenberg, MD, Children's Hospital of Pittsburgh, Pittsburgh, PA
Samuel L. Groseclose, DVM, MPH, Centers for Disease Control and Prevention, Atlanta, GA
Dalya Guris, MD, MPH, Centers for Disease Control and Prevention, Atlanta, GA
Laura T. Gutman, MD, Duke University Medical Center, Durham, NC
Rana Hajjeh, MD, Centers for Disease Control and Prevention, Atlanta, GA
Caroline Breese Hall, MD, University of Rochester School of Medicine, Rochester, NY
Holli Hamilton, MD, Food and Drug Administration, Bethesda, MD
Craig Hedburg, PhD, Minnesota Department of Health, Minneapolis, MN
Barbara L. Herwaldt, MD, MPH, Centers for Disease Control and Prevention, Atlanta, GA
David R. Hill, MD, DTM&H, University of Connecticut School of Medicine, Farmington, CT
Robert Hopkins, MD, Food and Drug Administration, Bethesda, MD
Margaret Hostetter, MD, Yale Child Health Research Center, New Haven, CT
Robert R. Jacobson, MD, PhD, Gillis W. Long Hansens Disease Center, Carville, LA
William R. Jarvis, MD, Centers for Disease Control and Prevention, Atlanta, GA
Jerri Ann Jenista, MD, Independent Consultant, Ann Arbor, MI
John Jereb, MD, Centers for Disease Control and Prevention, Atlanta, GA
Richard B. Johnston, Jr, MD, University of Colorado School of Medicine, Denver, CO
Dennis D. Juranek, MD, Centers for Disease Control and Prevention, Atlanta, GA
Patrick Kachur, MD, Centers for Disease Control and Prevention, Atlanta, GA
Gerardo Kaplan, PhD, Food and Drug Administration, Bethesda, MD
Sheldon L. Kaplan, MD, Baylor College of Medicine, Houston, TX
Richard Kenney, MD, Food and Drug Administration, Bethesda, MD
Rima Khabbaz, MD, Centers for Disease Control and Prevention, Atlanta, GA
Ali S. Khan, MD, Centers for Disease Control and Prevention, Atlanta, GA

Mark Kline, MD, Baylor College of Medicine, Houston, TX
Steve Kohl, University of California, San Francisco, CA
Emilia H. Koumans, MD, Centers for Disease Control and Prevention, Atlanta, GA
Peter J. Krause, MD, University of Connecticut School of Medicine, Hartford, CT
Philip Krause, MD, Food and Drug Administration, Bethesda, MD
Mary Lambert, MN, RN, CS, CNAA, Centers for Disease Control and Prevention, Atlanta, GA
Philip LaRussa, MD, Columbia University, New York, NY
Howard Lederman, MD, PhD, Johns Hopkins University School of Medicine, Baltimore, MD
Brad Leissa, MD, Food and Drug Administration, Bethesda, MD
Nicole LeSaux, MD, Children's Hospital of Eastern Ontario, Ottawa, Ontario Canada
Roland A. Levandowski, MD, Food and Drug Administration, Bethesda, MD
Matthew E. Levison, MD, Allegheny University of Health Sciences, MCP/Hahnemann School of Medicine, Philadelphia, PA
Andrew Lewis, Jr, MD, Food and Drug Administration, Bethesda, MD
Jay M. Lieberman, MD, Miller Children's Hospital, Long Beach, CA
Jairam Lingappa, MD, PhD, Centers for Disease Control and Prevention, Atlanta, GA
John R. Livengood, MD, Centers for Disease Control and Prevention, Atlanta, GA
Mark Lobato, MD, Centers for Disease Control and Prevention, Atlanta, GA
Hans O. Lobel, MD, Centers for Disease Control and Prevention, Atlanta, GA
Sarah S. Long, MD, Allegheny University of Health Sciences, Philadelphia, PA
G. Marshall Lyon, III, MD, Centers for Disease Control and Prevention, Atlanta, GA
William R. MacKenzie, MD, Centers for Disease Control and Prevention, Atlanta, GA
Mamodikoe Makhene, MD, MPH, Food and Drug Administration, Bethesda, MD
Susan A. Maloney, MD, MHS, Centers for Disease Control and Prevention, Atlanta, GA
Edgar K. Marcuse, MD, University of Washington, Seattle, WA
Harold S. Margolis, MD, Centers for Disease Control and Prevention, Atlanta, GA
Lewis Markoff, MD, Food and Drug Administration, Bethesda, MD
Eric Mast, MD, Centers for Disease Control and Prevention, Atlanta, GA
David O. Matson, MD, PhD, Center for Pediatric Research, Norfolk, VA
Anne E. McCarthy, MD, FRCPC, DTM&H, University of Ottawa, Ottawa General Hospital, Ottawa, Ontario, Canada
Michael M. McNeil, MD, Centers for Disease Control and Prevention, Atlanta, GA
Paul Mead, MD, Centers for Disease Control and Prevention, Atlanta, GA
Bruce Meade, MD, PhD, Food and Drug Administration, Bethesda, MD
Andrea Meyerhoff, MD, Food and Drug Administration, Bethesda, MD
John F. Modlin, MD, Dartmouth Medical School, Lebanon, NH
Lynne M. Mofenson, MD, National Institute of Child Health and Human Development at the National Institute of Health, Bethesda, MD

Nasim Moledina, MD, Food and Drug Administration, Bethesda, MD
John S. Moran, MD, MPH, Centers for Disease Control and Prevention, Atlanta, GA
Juliette Morgan, MD, Centers for Disease Control and Prevention, Atlanta, GA
Stephen A. Morse, MD, Centers for Disease Control and Prevention, Atlanta, GA
M. Dianne Murphy, MD, Food and Drug Administration, Bethesda, MD
Trudy V. Murphy, MD, Centers for Disease Control and Prevention, Atlanta, GA
Hira Nakhasi, PhD, Food and Drug Administration, Bethesda, MD
James P. Nataro, MD, PhD, University of Maryland School of Medicine, Baltimore, MD
Thomas R. Navin, MD, Centers for Disease Control and Prevention, Atlanta, GA
Soraya Nouri, MD, St. Louis University, St. Louis, MO
Thomas B. Nutman, MD, National Institute of Health, Laboratory of Parasitic Diseases, Bethesda, MD
Sonja J. Olsen, PhD, MS, MA, Centers for Disease Control and Prevention, Atlanta, GA
James G. Olson, MD, Centers for Disease Control and Prevention, Atlanta, GA
Christopher D. Paddock, MD, Centers for Disease Control and Prevention, Atlanta, GA
Mark Pallansch, PhD, Centers for Disease Control and Prevention, Atlanta, GA
Adelisa L. Panlilio, MD, Centers for Disease Control and Prevention, Atlanta, GA
Mark Papania, MD, MPH, Centers for Disease Control and Prevention, Atlanta, GA
Jan Paradise, MD, Boston University School of Medicine, Boston, MA
Monica E. Parise, MD, Centers for Disease Control and Prevention, Atlanta, GA
Sue Partridge, MD, Centers for Disease Control and Prevention, Atlanta, GA
Andrew T. Pavia, MD, University of Utah, Salt Lake City, UT
Philip E. Pellett, Centers for Disease Control and Prevention, Atlanta, GA
Bradley A. Perkins, MD, Centers for Disease Control and Prevention, Atlanta, GA
C.J. Peters, MD, Centers for Disease Control and Prevention, Atlanta, GA
Douglas R. Pratt, MD, Food and Drug Administration, Bethesda, MD
D. Rebecca Prevots, PhD, MPH, Centers for Disease Control and Prevention, Atlanta, GA
Alexander Rakowsky, MD, Food and Drug Administration, Bethesda, MD
Mobeen H. Rathore, MD, University of Florida Health Science Center, Jacksonville, FL
Susan Reef, MD, Centers for Disease Control and Prevention, Atlanta, GA
Russell Regnery, PhD, Centers for Disease Control and Prevention, Atlanta, GA
Frank Richards, MD, Centers for Disease Control and Prevention, Atlanta, GA
Lance Rodewald, MD, Centers for Disease Control and Prevention, Atlanta, GA
James P. Rosen, MD, University of Connecticut, West Hartford, CT
Nancy A. Rosenstein, MD, Centers for Disease Control and Prevention, Atlanta, GA
Lorry G. Rubin, MD, Schneider Children's Hospital, New Hyde Park, NY
Trenton Ruebush, Centers for Disease Control and Prevention, Atlanta, GA

Charles Rupprecht, MD, PhD, Centers for Disease Control and Prevention, Atlanta, GA
Lindy Samson, MD, Children's Hospital of Eastern Ontario, Ottawa, Ontario Canada
Pablo J. Sanchez, MD, University of Texas, Dallas, TX
Peter M. Schantz, MD, Centers for Disease Control and Prevention, Atlanta, GA
Neil L. Schechter, MD, University of Connecticut School of Medicine, Hartford, CT
George Schmid, MD, MSc, Centers for Disease Control and Prevention, Atlanta, GA
Lawrence Schonberger, MD, Centers for Disease Control and Prevention, Atlanta, GA
Anne Schuchat, MD, Centers for Disease Control and Prevention, Atlanta, GA
Joann Schulte, MD, Centers for Disease Control and Prevention, Atlanta, GA
Gordon E. Schutze, MD, University of Arkansas for Medical Sciences, Little Rock, AR
Jane Seward, MBBS, MPH, Centers for Disease Control and Prevention, Atlanta, GA
Eugene Shapiro, MD, Yale University, New Haven, CT
Stanford T. Shulman, MD, Northwestern University Medical School, Chicago, IL
Jane D. Siegel, MD, University of Texas, Dallas, TX
Robert Slinger, MD, Laboratory Centre for Disease Control, Health, Canada
Bob Snyder, MA, Centers for Disease Control and Prevention, Atlanta, GA
John D. Snyder, MD, University of California Medical Center, San Francisco, CA
Richard A. Spiegel, DVM, MPH, Centers for Disease Control and Prevention, Atlanta, GA
Mary Allen Staat, MD, MPH, Children's Hospital Medical Center, Cincinnati, OH
Jeffrey R. Starke, MD, Baylor College of Medicine, Houston, TX
Barbara W. Stechenberg, MD, Baystate Medical Center Children's Hospital, Springfield, MA
David K. Stein, MD, Johns Hopkins, Baltimore, MD
Ellen B. Steinberg, MD, Centers for Disease Control and Prevention, Atlanta, GA
Gail Stennies, MD, Centers for Disease Control and Prevention, Atlanta, GA
John A. Stewart, MD, Centers for Disease Control and Prevention, Atlanta, GA
Katherine M. Stone, MD, Centers for Disease Control and Prevention, Atlanta, GA
Raymond A. Strikas, MD, Centers for Disease Control and Prevention, Atlanta, GA
Lillian Sung, MD, Children's Hospital of Eastern Ontario, Ottawa, Ontario, Canada
Douglas S. Swanson, MD, The Children's Mercy Hospital, Kansas City, MO
David Swerdlow, MD, Centers for Disease Control and Prevention, Atlanta, GA
Howard L. Taras, MD, University of California, San Diego, CA
James Kennedy Todd, MD, The Children's Hospital, Denver, CO
Paul Turkeltaub, MD, Food and Drug Administration, Bethesda, MD
Thomas J. Van Gilder, MD, Centers for Disease Control and Prevention, Atlanta, GA
Willie Vann, PhD, Food and Drug Administration, Bethesda, MD

Govinda Visvesvara, MD, Centers for Disease Control and Prevention, Atlanta, GA
Charles Vitek, MD, MPH, Centers for Disease Control and Prevention, Atlanta, GA
Ellen R. Wald, MD, University of Pittsburgh School of Medicine, Pittsburgh, PA
Richard J. Wallace, Jr, MD, University of Texas Health Center at Tyler, Tyler, TX
Elaine E.L. Wang, MD, University of Toronto, Toronto, Ontario, Canada
Diane W. Wara, MD, University of California, San Francisco, CA
John Ward, MD, Centers for Disease Control and Prevention, Atlanta, GA
John C. Watson, MD, MPH, Centers for Disease Control and Prevention, Atlanta, GA
Jerry Weir, PhD, Food and Drug Administration, Bethesda, MD
A. Clinton White, MD, Baylor College of Medicine, Houston, TX
Cynthia G. Whitney, MD, MPH, Centers for Disease Control and Prevention, Atlanta, GA
Walter R. Wilson, MD, Mayo Medical School, Rochester, MN
Christopher W. Woods, Centers for Disease Control and Prevention, Atlanta, GA
Kimberly Workowski, MD, Centers for Disease Control and Prevention, Atlanta, GA
Edward J. Young, MD, VA Medical Center, Houston, TX
Paul N. Zenker, MD, MPH, Ramsey Clinic, St Paul, MN
Moritz M. Ziegler, MD, Children's Hospital of Boston, Boston, MA

Committee on Infectious Diseases, 1998–1999

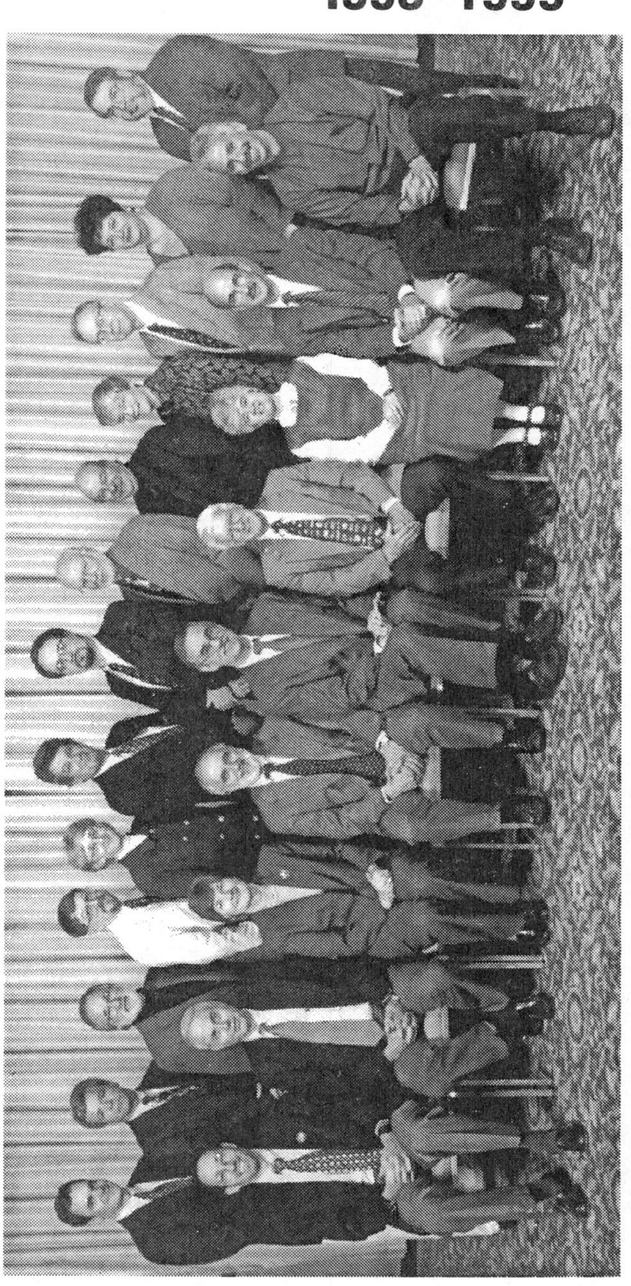

Front row: Walter A. Orenstein, Georges Peter, Carol J. Baker, Neal A. Halsey, Larry K. Pickering, Edgar O. Ledbetter, Noni E. MacDonald, Michael A. Gerber, Jon S. Abramson

Second row: Scott F. Dowell, Charles G. Prober, Leonard B. Weiner, Dennis L. Murray, P. Joan Chesney, S. Michael Marcy, Richard F. Jacobs, Richard J. Whitley, Anthony Hirsch, Margaret C. Fisher, Gary D. Overturf, N. Regina Rabinovich, Thomas N. Saari

Not pictured: Margaret B. Rennels, H. Cody Meissner, Gilles Delage, Peter A. Patriarca, Martin G. Myers, Steve Kohl, Ram Yogev, Ben Schwartz, Robert Breiman

Dedication

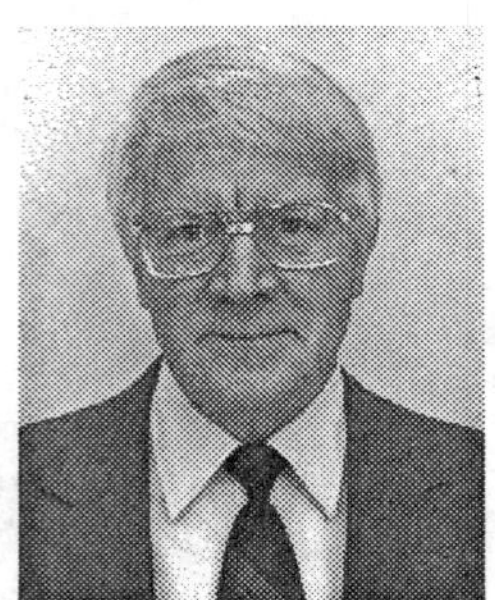

This edition of the *Red Book* is dedicated to Edgar O. Ledbetter, MD, FAAP, who served as the Director of the Department of Maternal, Child and Adolescent Health (now the Department of Committees and Sections) at the American Academy of Pediatrics (AAP) from 1988 through 1998. During those 10 years, Ed provided outstanding leadership for the AAP in a broad range of programs while his department provided administrative support to many AAP committees. His expertise and vast experience in general pediatrics, pediatric infectious diseases, medical ethics, and human relations were invaluable to the Committee on Infectious Diseases (the *Red Book* Committee). The *Red Book* Committee received special attention and guidance because of those interests.

Ed's perspective was always highly valued. His advice and guidance helped the *Red Book* Committee deal with complex issues, especially the process of developing new policies or modifying existing policies that had an impact on other areas of pediatric practice. All of us benefited enormously from his leadership. The *Red Book* Committee, the AAP, and children everywhere will be forever indebted to him for his strong commitment to child health.

Preface

The Committee on Infectious Diseases is dedicated to providing practitioners with the most current and accurate information available. Because the practice of pediatric infectious diseases is changing rapidly and because of the emergence of new infectious diseases, the ability to obtain information quickly is paramount. Although the *Red Book* is updated every 3 years, it is important that practitioners who care for children read *Pediatrics* and *AAP News,* where interim updates will be provided. The American Academy of *Pediatrics* (AAP) and other organizations have developed systems that allow electronic access to information that is pertinent to the health care of children. Policy statements of the AAP that support information in the *Red Book* can now be accessed electronically through the AAP Web site (http://www.aap.org).

The Committee on Infectious Diseases relies on information and advice from many experts as evidenced by the lengthy list of contributors. We are especially indebted to the many contributors from other AAP committees, the Centers for Disease Control and Prevention, the Food and Drug Administration, the National Institutes of Health, the Canadian Paediatric Society, the World Health Organization, and many other organizations that have made this edition possible. In addition, many suggestions made by individual AAP members to improve the presentation of information on specific issues have been taken into account under the able leadership of Larry K. Pickering, MD, Editor, and Associate Editors Carol J. Baker, MD, Michael A. Gerber, MD, and Noni E. MacDonald, MD. We also are indebted to Georges Peter, MD, previous Editor of the *Red Book* for the past 5 editions, who provided invaluable assistance with this edition.

As noted in previous editions of the *Red Book,* some omissions and errors are inevitable in a book of this type. We hope that AAP members will continue to assist the Committee actively by suggesting specific ways to improve the quality of future editions.

Jon S. Abramson, MD, FAAP
Chairperson, Committee on Infectious Diseases

Introduction

The Committee on Infectious Diseases (COID) of the American Academy of Pediatrics (AAP) is responsible for developing and revising guidelines of the AAP for control of infectious diseases in children. At intervals of approximately 3 years, the Committee issues the *Red Book: Report of the Committee on Infectious Diseases,* which contains a composite summary of current AAP recommendations concerning infectious diseases in and immunizations for infants, children, and adolescents. These recommendations represent a consensus of opinions developed by members of the Committee in conjunction with liaison representatives from the Centers for Disease Control and Prevention (CDC), the Food and Drug Administration (FDA), the National Institutes of Health, the National Vaccine Program, the Canadian Paediatric Society, *Red Book* consultants, and numerous collaborators. This edition is based on information available as of January 2000.

Unanswered scientific questions, the complexity of medical practice, the explosion of new information, and inevitable differences of opinion among experts result in inherent limitations of the *Red Book.* In the context of these limitations, the Committee endeavors to provide current, relevant, and defensible recommendations for the prevention and management of infectious diseases in infants, children, and adolescents. In some cases, other committees and experts may differ in their interpretation of data and resulting recommendations. In some instances, no single recommendation can be made because several options for management are equally acceptable.

In making recommendations in the *Red Book,* the Committee acknowledges these differences in viewpoints by judicious use of the phrases "most experts recommend..." and "some experts recommend..." Both phrases indicate valid recommendations, but the first signifies more support among experts, and the second, less support. Hence "some experts recommend..." indicates a minority view that is based on data and/or experience and is sufficiently valid to warrant consideration.

Inevitably in clinical practice, questions arise that cannot be answered on the basis of currently available data. In such cases, the Committee attempts to provide guidelines and information that in conjunction with clinical judgment will facilitate well-reasoned decisions. We appreciate the questions, different perspectives, and alternative recommendations that we have received, and encourage any suggestions or correspondence that will improve future editions of the *Red Book.* Through this process, the Committee seeks to provide a practical and authoritative guide for physicians and other health care professionals in their care of children.

To aid physicians and other health care professionals in assimilating current changes in the recommendations in the *Red Book,* a list of major changes has been compiled (see Summary of Major Changes, p xxiii). However, this listing does not include many changes of lesser importance, and health care professionals should consult individual chapters and sections of the book for further guidelines. In addition, new information inevitably begins to outdate some recommendations in the *Red Book,* even in the year of its publication, and necessitates that health care professionals remain informed of new developments and resulting changes in recommendations. Between editions, the AAP publishes new recommendations from the Committee in *Pediatrics, AAP News,* and on the AAP Web site (http://www.aap.org). In this edition, we have provided Web site addresses throughout the text to enable early access to new information.

When using antimicrobial agents, physicians should review the package inserts (product labels) prepared by manufacturers, particularly for information concerning contraindications and adverse reactions. No attempt has been made in the *Red Book* to provide this information, since it is readily available in the *Physicians' Desk Reference* and in package inserts (product labels). As in previous editions, recommended dosage schedules for antimicrobial agents are given (see Section 4, Antimicrobial Agents and Related Therapy). Recommendations in the *Red Book* for drug dosages may differ from those of the manufacturer in the package insert. Physicians also should be familiar with information in the package insert for vaccines and immune globulins as well as recommendations of other committees (see Sources of Vaccine Information, p 2).

This book could not have been prepared without the dedicated professional and administrative competence of Edgar O. Ledbetter, MD, past Director of the Department of Maternal, Child and Adolescent Health (now the Department of Committees and Sections) at the AAP. The AAP staff has been invaluable in their committed work and contributions, particularly Hope Hurley, Manager, who served as the administrative director for the Committee and coordinated the preparation of the *Red Book;* Claudia Appeldorn, Medical Copy Editor; Barbara Scotese, Senior Medical Copy Editor; Rachael Hagan, Department Assistant; and Joann Kim, MD, consultant to the AAP. Special thanks are given to Linda Merhige and Anne Wright, secretaries to the Editor, for their work, patience, and support. Walter Orenstein, MD, and Peter Patriarca, MD, of the CDC and FDA, respectively, devoted a great deal of time and effort in providing input from their organizations. I am especially indebted to the Associate Editors, Carol Baker, MD, Michael Gerber, MD, and Noni MacDonald, MD, for their expertise, tireless work, and immense contributions in their editorial and Committee work. Neal Halsey, MD (past COID Chairperson), and Georges Peter, MD (Editor of the past five editions), provided constant support and advice. Members of the Committee contributed countless hours and deserve appropriate recognition for their dedication, revisions, and reviews. As a Committee, we particularly appreciate the guidance and dedication of the current Committee Chairperson, Jon Abramson, MD, whose knowledge, dedication, insight, and leadership are reflected in the quality and productivity of the Committee's work.

These individuals are only a few of the many contributors whose professional work and commitment have been essential in the Committee's preparation of the *Red Book.*

Larry K Pickering, MD
Editor

Table of Contents

SECTION 2
RECOMMENDATIONS FOR CARE OF CHILDREN IN SPECIAL CIRCUMSTANCES

SECTION 3
SUMMARIES OF INFECTIOUS DISEASES

SECTION 4
ANTIMICROBIAL AGENTS AND RELATED THERAPY

SECTION 5
ANTIMICROBIAL PROPHYLAXIS 729

APPENDICES

Summary of Major Changes in the 2000 *Red Book*

Major changes in recommendations and information concerning pediatric infectious diseases and immunizations since publication of the 1997 *Red Book* are listed here to aid physicians and other health care professionals in implementing these changes in their practices. Because the *Red Book* is divided into 5 major sections plus the appendices, the summary of the changes are grouped accordingly. In addition, on February 17, 2000, the Food and Drug Administration (FDA) approved a license application for pneumococcal 7-valent conjugate vaccine for active immunization of infants and toddlers against invasive disease caused by *Streptococcus pneumoniae* due to capsular serotypes included in the vaccine, beginning at 2 months of age. Information about recommendations for use of this vaccine will be published in *Pediatrics* and is available at http://www.aap.org/.

The *Visual Red Book on* **CD-ROM** contains more than 640 photographs and source data related to clinical and laboratory manifestations of many infectious diseases. This material will assist pediatricians, family practitioners, nurse practitioners, and other health care professionals caring for children to more expeditiously diagnose and manage these infections. Many of the disease manifestations depicted are now less frequently seen because of the availability and routine use of immunizations in infants, children, and adolescents.

SECTION 1. ACTIVE AND PASSIVE IMMUNIZATION

1. **Prologue.** A table of the baseline 20th century annual morbidity, the 1998 morbidity and percentage decrease in 9 diseases with vaccines recommended before 1990 for universal use in children in the United States is given (Table 1.1, p 2).
2. **Sources of Vaccine Information.** Information in this section has been updated to include Web sites and fax and telephone numbers where additional information can be obtained (p 2).
3. **Informing Patients and Parents.** A table outlining the use of Vaccine Information Statements has been added (Table 1.2, p 5).
4. **Scheduling Immunizations.** The year 2000 schedule (Figure 1.1, p 22) for recommended childhood immunizations is given. Changes reflected in this schedule are reviewed in detail in the disease-specific chapters and include exclusive use of acellular pertussis vaccines, an all-inactivated poliovirus (IPV) vaccine schedule, special considerations for the use of hepatitis B vaccine products, and routine use of hepatitis A vaccine in some states and regions. The footnotes in the schedule provide further guidelines. This schedule is revised and published in January of each year in *Pediatrics* and is available at http://www.aap.org/.

5. **Thimerosal Content of Some Vaccines and Immune Globulin (IG) Preparations** (p 36). Information about thimerosal content of vaccines and IG preparations is provided.
6. **Indications for the Use of Immune Globulin Intravenous (IGIV)** (Table 1.6, p 45). A table providing the recommendations of the FDA and National Institutes of Health (NIH) for use of IGIV has been added.
7. **Immunocompromised Children** (p 56). This section (titled in previous editions, "Immunodeficient and Immunosuppressed Children") has been expanded to include recommendations for immunization of children and adolescents with primary and secondary immune deficiencies.
8. **New Chapters and Sections**
   - Risk Communication (p 5)
   - Managing Injection Pain (p 19)
   - Vaccine Safety Datalink (VSD) Project (p 32)
   - Parental Misconceptions About Immunizations (p 39)

SECTION 2. RECOMMENDATIONS FOR CARE OF CHILDREN IN SPECIAL CIRCUMSTANCES

9. **School Health.** Recommendations published by the AAP in 1999 for prevention of transmission of human immunodeficiency virus (HIV) and other bloodborne pathogens in the athletic setting are included in this chapter as well as in the HIV chapter (p 325).
10. **Sexually Transmitted Diseases (STDs) in Adolescents and Children** (p 138). This chapter has undergone extensive revision to include the 1998 Centers for Disease Control and Prevention (CDC) *Guidelines for Treatment of Sexually Transmitted Diseases.* Tables and text have been added regarding criteria for adolescents considered at increased risk for contracting an STD, implications of commonly encountered STDs for diagnosing and reporting sexual abuse of infants and prepubescent children, testing children and adolescents for STDs when sexual abuse is suspected or has occurred, and tables giving recommended prophylaxis after sexual victimization of preadolescent children and adolescents has occurred.
11. **New Chapters and Sections**
    - Chemical-Biological Terrorism (p 83)
    - Blood Safety – Reducing the Risk of Transfusion-Transmitted Infections (p 88)
    - Pet Visitation (p 136)
    - Infection Control in Physicians' Offices (p 137)

SECTION 3. SUMMARIES OF INFECTIOUS DISEASES

12. **Anthrax** (p 168). This chapter has been updated to include revised treatment options for persons infected with susceptible and resistant strains of *Bacillus anthracis* and to highlight the potential use of this organism as a bioterrorist weapon.
13. **Arbovirus** (p 170). Characteristics of the West Nile virus have been added.
14. **Bacterial Vaginosis** (p 183). Therapy for females with bacterial vaginosis has been defined by pregnancy status, and treatment options have been revised.

15. ***Chlamydia trachomatis*** (p 208). Prophylactic antibodies are no longer routinely recommended for asymptomatic infants born to mothers known to have untreated chlamydial infections. Information is given on the increased risk of developing infantile hypertrophic pyloric stenosis for infants less than 6 weeks of age who are given oral erythromycin for chlamydia, pertussis, or ureaplasma.
16. **Hepatitis A** (p 280). New data about the epidemiology of hepatitis A; information about the effectiveness of community-based hepatitis A immunization programs; and recommendations for the routine immunization of children in states, counties, and communities with elevated rates of hepatitis A virus infection are given.
17. **Hepatitis B** (p 289). Hepatitis B vaccine dosages, formulations, and immunization schedules; and schedules and vaccine formulations for immunization of premature infants have been updated. Additional information concerns the comprehensive immunization strategy of the CDC to eliminate transmission of hepatitis B in the United States.
18. **Hepatitis C** (p 302). The guidelines for preventing hepatitis C virus transmission have been revised. Interferon-α in combination with ribavirin is a new treatment option for chronic hepatitis C virus infection in adolescents and adults.
19. **Herpes Simplex Virus** (p 309). Therapeutic options for different HSV infections have been expanded to include valaciclovir, famciclovir, and penciclovir (also see Table 4.8, "Antiviral Drugs for Non-HIV Infections," p 675).
20. **Human Herpesvirus 6 (Including Roseola) and 7.** This chapter now includes herpesvirus 7.
21. **Human Immunodeficiency Virus Infection** (p 325). This chapter has been extensively revised to include the following: (1) an update of the epidemiology of HIV infections; (2) addition of a table (p 332) listing diagnostic tests for HIV infection; (3) revision of the surveillance case definition for HIV infection according to the 1999 CDC recommendations (Table 3.23, p 326); (4) updated guidelines on antiretroviral therapy (see Tables 4.9, p 678; 4.10, p 683; and 4.11, p 687), including Table 4.12 (p 692) showing considerations for changing antiretroviral therapy; (5) Web sites where current drugs and treatment recommendations can be found; and (6) guidelines for use of varicella and hepatitis A vaccines in HIV-infected children in the United States. The section entitled "Reduction of Perinatal HIV transmission" has been expanded and guidelines for postexposure prophylaxis for possible sexual or other nonoccupational exposure to HIV has been updated. Recommendations for the prevention of opportunistic infections in children with AIDS have been revised in accordance with the 1999 USPHS/IDSA *Guidelines for Prevention of Opportunistic Infections in Persons Infected With HIV.* Characteristics of antiretroviral drugs are given in tables in Section 4.
22. **Influenza** (p 351). Indications for antiviral therapy with a neuraminidase inhibitor for treatment of influenza A and B infections in adolescents and adults are provided.
23. ***Listeria monocytogenes* Infections.** Dietary recommendations for persons at high risk of listeriosis are given in Table 3.33 (p 374).

24. **Lyme Disease** (p 374). Current recommendations for the use of Lyme disease vaccine are included.
25. **Meningococcal Infections.** A change concerns the need to inform and educate college students and parents about the risk of meningococcal disease and possible benefit of immunization (p 396).
26. **Pelvic Inflammatory Disease (PID).** Recommendations for treatment of PID have been updated to be consistent with the 1998 CDC *Guidelines for Treatment of Sexually Transmitted Diseases.*
27. **Pertussis.** The list of licensed DTaP products has been expanded to include all FDA-approved preparations (Table 3.43, p 441). Only acellular pertussis vaccines given as DTaP are recommended for the pertussis immunization series in theUnited States. The association between orally administered erythromycin for treatment or prevention of pertussis in infants less than 6 weeks of age and infantile hypertrophic pyloric stenosis has been included.
28. ***Pneumocystis carinii*** (p 460). Recommendations concerning therapy and prevention have been updated and are consistent with the 1999 USPHS/ IDSA *Guidelines for Prevention of Opportunistic Infections in Persons Infected With HIV.*
29. **Poliovirus Infections.** The AAP now recommends a 4 dose all-IPV schedule for routine immunization of all infants and children in the United States (p 465).
30. **Rabies** (p 475). New information includes an update on the epidemiology of rabies and anti-rabies biologics in the United States (Table 3.48, p 477) and recommendations regarding an observation period for domestic ferrets, and the recommendation for local administration of Rabies Immune Globulin.
31. **Respiratory Syncytial Virus** (p 483). Recommendations for the use of palivizumab, a humanized mouse monoclonal antibody given intramuscularly, are included.
32. **Staphylococcal Infections** (p 514). Changes include new information about coagulase-negative staphylococci and methods of transmission of both susceptible and resistant *S aureus* and coagulase negative staphylococci. Table 3.51 (p 520) gives the recommendations for detecting and preventing spread of *S aureus* with reduced susceptibility to vancomycin. Table 3.52 (p 521) gives current antibiotic choices for bacteremia and other serious staphylococcal infections.
33. **Non-Group A or B Streptococcal and Enterococcal Infections.** A new drug combination of quinupristin/dalfopristin for treatment of vancomycin-resistant *Enterococcus faecium* is now available.
34. **Syphilis.** Table 3.57 (p 556) gives the current recommended therapy for syphilis and is consistent with the 1998 CDC *Guidelines for Treatment of Sexually Transmitted Diseases.*
35. **Tuberculosis.** The definition section of this chapter has been expanded (p 593) and the treatment section has been updated.
36. **Diseases Caused By Non-Tuberculous Mycobacteria.** The chemoprophylaxis (p 617) section has been updated to include the 1999 USPHS/IDSA *Guidelines for Prevention of Opportunistic Infections in Persons Infected With HIV.* Table 3.71 (p 616) gives current recommendations for therapy.

37. **Varicella-Zoster Infections.** New recommendations include use of the varicella vaccine following exposure, use of vaccine for outbreak control, use of the vaccine for some children infected with HIV, immunization of adults and adolescents at high risk for exposure and new data about storage and administration of varicella vaccine. The advantages and disadvantages of the various diagnostic tests for VZ infections are listed in Table 3.72 (p 627). Treatment options with famciclovir and valaciclovir have been added.
38. **New Chapters**
    - *Burkholderia* Infections (p 194)
    - *Cyclospora* (p 226)
    - Fungal Diseases (p 249)
    - Hantavirus Cardiopulmonary Syndrome (p 272)
    - Hepatitis G (p 308)
    - Human Herpesvirus 8 (p 324)
    - Prion Diseases (p 471)
    - Toxic Shock Syndrome (p 576). This chapter gives information and management guidelines for both staphylococcal and streptococcal toxic shock syndrome.

SECTION 4. ANTIMICROBIAL AGENTS AND RELATED THERAPY

39. The following tables have been updated:
    - Tables of Antibacterial Drug Doses (p 650)
    - Sexually Transmitted Diseases (Table 4.3, p 663)
    - Antiviral Drugs for Non-HIV Infections (Table 4.8, p 675)
    - Drugs for Parasitic Infections (p 693)
40. The section entitled "Antifungal Drugs for Systemic Fungal Infections" (p 668) is updated to include information about all classes of antifungal agents.
41. **New Chapters and Sections**
    - Judicious Use of Antimicrobial Agents (p 647)
    - Characteristics of Antiretroviral Drugs: Nucleoside Analogue Reverse Transcriptase Inhibitors (Table 4.9, p 678)
    - Characteristics of Antiretroviral Drugs: Nonnucleoside Reverse Transcriptase Inhibitors (Table 4.10, p 683)
    - Characteristics of Antiretroviral Drugs: Protease Inhibitors (Table 4.11, p 687)
    - Considerations for Changing Antiretroviral Therapy (Table 4.12, p 692)

SECTION 5. ANTIMICROBIAL PROPHYLAXIS

42. **Prevention of Bacterial Endocarditis** (p 735). The recommendations for prevention of bacterial endocarditis have been updated according to the most recent (1997) recommendations from the American Heart Association

APPENDICES

43. **Appendix I,** "Directory of Services" (p 743), has been updated to include fax numbers and Web sites, as well as international telephone numbers of contact organizations.

44. **Appendix VIII,** "Nationally Notifiable Infectious Diseases in the United States" (p 777), now includes cyclosporiasis, ehrlichiosis, and varicella deaths.
45. **Appendix VI,** "Potentially Contaminated Food Products" (p 770), is a new table.

No list is likely to be complete, and the designation of a change as major can be arbitrary. Therefore, physicians and other health care professionals are urged to review relevant chapters, tables, figures, and sections in the *Red Book.* In addition, since preparation of each edition involved extensive review of the entire book, a considerable amount of new information is included in many chapters and sections, and a number of new tables have been added to aid health care professionals. Throughout the *Red Book,* references to policy statements of the American Academy of Pediatrics, publications of the Advisory Committee on Immunization Practices, and Web site addresses have been provided to facilitate acquisition of source data and access to new information.

Active and Passive Immunization

PROLOGUE

The ultimate goal of immunization is eradication of disease; the immediate goal is prevention of disease in individuals or groups. To accomplish these goals, physicians must maintain timely immunization, including both active and passive immunoprophylaxis, as a high priority in the care of infants, children, adolescents, and adults. The global eradication of smallpox in 1977 and elimination of poliomyelitis from the Americas in 1991 serve as models for control of disease through immunization. Both of these accomplishments were achieved by combining an effective immunization program with intensive surveillance and effective public health control measures.

Many infectious diseases can be prevented by immunoprophylaxis. With active immunization, a person is stimulated to develop immunologic defenses against future natural exposure. With passive immunization, a person already exposed, or about to be exposed, is given preformed human or animal antibody.

In the United States, immunization has dramatically curtailed or almost eliminated diphtheria, measles, mumps, polio, rubella (congenital and acquired), tetanus, and *Haemophilus influenzae* type b disease (see Table 1.1, p 2).

Yet, because the organisms that cause these diseases persist in the United States and in other countries, immunizations need to be continued. New knowledge of immunology and molecular biology, as well as new technology such as genetic engineering, has resulted in burgeoning vaccine research and the licensing of new and improved vaccines. Population-based epidemiologic studies of new vaccines after licensing provide evaluation of adverse events temporally associated with immunization that were not detected during prelicensure clinical trials. Physicians must regularly update their knowledge about specific vaccines because information about their optimal use, safety, and efficacy continues to develop after a vaccine is licensed and because recommendations are updated regularly.

Each edition of the *Red Book* gives recommendations for immunization of children and adolescents based on the knowledge, experience, and premises at the time of publication. The recommendations represent a consensus with which reasonable physicians may at times disagree. No claim is made for infallibility, and the American Academy of Pediatrics Committee on Infectious Diseases acknowledges that individual circumstances may warrant decisions differing from the recommendations given herein.

Table 1.1. **Baseline 20th Century Annual Morbidity and 1998 Morbidity From 9 Diseases With Vaccines Recommended Before 1990 for Universal Use in Children: United States***

Disease	Baseline 20th Century Annual Morbidity	1998 Morbidity	% Decrease
Smallpox	48 164[†]	0	100
Diphtheria	175 885[‡]	1	100[§]
Pertussis	147 271[‖]	7405	95
Tetanus	1 314[¶]	41	97
Poliomyelitis (paralytic)	16 316[#]	1	100[§]
Measles	503 282[**]	100	100[§]
Mumps	152 209[††]	666	>99
Rubella	47 745[‡‡]	364	>99
Congenital rubella syndrome	823[§§]	7	>99
Haemophilus influenzae type b	20 000[‖‖]	61[¶¶]	>99

* Adapted from Impact of vaccines universally recommended for children: United States, 1990–1998. *MMWR Morb Mortal Wkly Rep.* 1999;48:243–248 and Summary of notifiable diseases, United States, 1998. *MMWR Morb Mortal Wkly Rep.* 1999;47:1–92.

† Average annual number of cases during 1900–1904.

‡ Average annual number of reported cases during 1920–1922, 3 years before vaccine development.

§ Rounded to nearest tenth.

‖ Average annual number of reported cases during 1922–1925, 4 years before vaccine development.

¶ Estimated number of cases based on reported number of deaths during 1922–1926 assuming a case-fatality rate of 90%.

\# Average annual number of reported cases during 1951–1954, 4 years before vaccine licensure.

** Average annual number of reported cases during 1958–1962, 5 years before vaccine licensure.

†† Number of reported cases in 1968, the first year reporting began and the first year after vaccine licensure.

‡‡ Average annual number of reported cases during 1966–1968, 3 years before vaccine licensure.

§§ Estimated number of cases based on seroprevalence data in the population and on the risk that women infected during a childbearing year would have a fetus with congenital rubella syndrome.

‖‖ Estimated number of cases from population-based surveillance studies before vaccine licensure in 1985.

¶¶ Excludes 194 cases of *Haemophilus influenzae* disease of unknown serotype or not type b. Represents invasive disease in children younger than 5 years of age.

SOURCES OF VACCINE INFORMATION

In addition to the *Red Book,* which is published at intervals of approximately 3 years, physicians should use the scientific literature and other sources for data or answers to specific questions encountered in practice. These sources include the following:

- ***Pediatrics.*** Statements developed by the Committee on Infectious Diseases (COID) giving updated recommendations are published in *Pediatrics* between editions of the *Red Book.* Access to policy statements also may be gained through the American Academy of Pediatrics (AAP) Web site (http://www.aap.org/).

The updated national immunization schedule is published annually in the January issue of *Pediatrics*, as well as in other sources (see Scheduling Immunizations, p 20).

- ***AAP News.*** Policy statements (or statement summaries) from the COID often are published initially in *AAP News,* the Academy's monthly newspaper, to inform its membership promptly of new recommendations.
- ***Morbidity and Mortality Weekly Report (MMWR).*** Published weekly by the Centers for Disease Control and Prevention (CDC), *MMWR* contains current vaccine recommendations, reports of specific disease activity, and changes in policy statements. Recommendations of the Advisory Committee on Immunization Practices (ACIP) of the CDC are published periodically, usually as supplements, and are posted on the CDC Web site (http://www.cdc.gov/).
- **Official package inserts (product labels).** Manufacturers provide product-specific information with each vaccine product. This information also is published in the *Physicians' Desk Reference.* The product label must be in full compliance with US Food and Drug Administration (FDA) regulations pertaining to labeling for prescription drugs, including indications and usage, dosages, routes of administration, clinical pharmacology, contraindications, and adverse reactions. The package insert lists contents of each vaccine, including preservatives, stabilizers, antibiotics, adjuvants, and suspending fluids, that may cause inflammation or elicit an allergic response. Health care professionals should be familiar with the label for each product they administer.
- ***Health Information for International Travel.*** This useful monograph is published approximately every 2 years by the CDC as a guide to requirements of the various countries for specific immunizations. It also provides information about other vaccines recommended for travel in specific areas and other information for travelers. This document can be purchased from the Superintendent of Documents, US Government Printing Office, Washington, DC 20402-9235. This information also is available on the CDC Web site (http://www.cdc.gov/). For further sources of information on international travel, see Foreign Travel (p 77).
- **CDC materials.** A CDC textbook, *Epidemiology and Prevention of Vaccine Preventable Diseases* (1999), provides detailed information on the use and administration of childhood vaccines, as well as selected ACIP statements. To obtain CDC materials, call 1-800-232-2522, fax 1-404-639-8828, or access the National Immunization Program (NIP) Web site (http://www.cdc.gov/nip/).
- ***Control of Communicable Diseases Manual.*** The American Public Health Association publishes this manual at intervals of approximately 5 years. It contains information about most infectious diseases, their worldwide occurrence, diagnostic and therapeutic information, immunizations, recommendations on isolation, and other control measures for specific diseases. The 17th edition, published in 1999, is available from the American Public Health Association, 800 I St NW, Washington, DC 20001-3710 (telephone, 202-777-APHA [202-777-2742]; Web site, http://www.apha.org).
- **Committee on Infectious Diseases.** Physicians can consult members of the COID by e-mail or letter. Specific questions may be addressed directly to the AAP.*

Printed information on immunization also can be obtained from CDC's NIP through the Web site (http://www.cdc.gov/nip/) or through the fax system by calling 1-888-CDC-FAXX (1-888-232-3299). Specific consultations can be obtained by contacting the NIP* or through e-mail (nipinfo@cdc.gov). Other resources include the FDA*; infectious disease experts at university-affiliated hospitals, medical schools, and in private practice; and regional public health departments. Information can be obtained from the latter about current epidemiology of diseases, immunization recommendations, legal requirements, public health policies, foreign travel, and nursery school, child care, and school health concerns.

INFORMING PATIENTS AND PARENTS

Parents and patients should be informed about the benefits and risks of preventive and therapeutic procedures, including immunization.

The patient, parents, and/or legal guardian should be informed about the benefits to be derived from vaccines in preventing disease in individuals and in the community and about the risks of those vaccines. Questions should be encouraged so that the information is understood.

The National Childhood Vaccine Injury Act (NCVIA) of 1986 included requirements for notifying all patients and parents about vaccine benefits and risks.

This legislation, as subsequently amended, mandates that a Vaccine Information Statement (VIS) be provided each time a vaccine covered under the National Vaccine Injury Compensation Program is administered (see Table 1.2, p 5). For vaccines not yet included in the Vaccine Injury Compensation Program (VICP), such as the Lyme disease vaccine, VISs are available but are not mandated unless the vaccine is purchased through a CDC contract (ie, the Vaccines for Children program, state immunization grants, or state purchases through CDC). Copies of the current VISs can be obtained from state and local health departments, the CDC, the American Academy of Pediatrics (AAP), and vaccine manufacturers or by calling the CDC Immunization Hotline (1-800-232-2522 in English and 1-800-232-0233 in Spanish). Persons with Internet access can obtain copies from the National Immunization Program Web site.† Copies also are available on the Immunization Action Coalition Web site‡ in English and in 16 other languages. Physicians need to ensure that the VIS provided is the current version by noting the date of publication given on the first page. The latest version can be determined by calling CDC's Immunization Hotline or accessing the National Immunization Program Web site.‡

The NCVIA requires physicians administering vaccines covered by the VICP to record the date of administration, vaccine manufacturer, lot number, and the name and business address of the provider in the patient's medical record (see Table 1.2, p 5). In addition, CDC regulations require that physicians record the VIS date *and* the date on which the VIS was provided to the patient, caregiver, and/or parent. Vaccines purchased under CDC contract have the same record-keeping requirements

* See Appendix I, Directory of Resources, p 743.

† http://www.cdc.gov/nip/publications/VIS/default.htm

‡ http://www.immunize.org

Table 1.2. Guidance in Using Vaccine Information Statements

Distribution	Documentation in the Patient's Medical Record
Must be provided each time a VICP-covered vaccine is administered*	Vaccine manufacturer, lot number, and date of administration*
Given to parent, legal guardian, or patient (nonminor)*	Name and business address of the health care professional administering the vaccine*
Must be the current version†	VIS version date and date it is provided†
Can provide (not substitute) other written materials or audiovisual aids in addition to VISs	Site (eg, deltoid area), route of administration (eg, intramuscular), and expiration date of the vaccine‡

* Required under the National Childhood Vaccine Injury Act. VICP indicates Vaccine Injury Compensation Program; VIS, Vaccine Information Statement.

† Required by Centers for Disease Control and Prevention regulations.

‡ Recommended by the American Academy of Pediatrics.

as those included in the VICP. Although the VIS distribution and vaccine record-keeping requirements do not apply to privately purchased vaccines not covered by the VICP, the AAP recommends using the VISs and following the same record-keeping practices with these vaccines. The AAP also recommends recording the site, route of administration, and vaccine expiration date after administering any vaccine (see Vaccine Safety and Contraindications, p 30).

The new VISs do not include space for the parents' or patients' signatures to indicate that they have read and understood the material. However, the health care professional has the option to obtain a signature. Whether or not a signature is obtained, the AAP recommends that physicians document in the chart that the VIS has been provided and discussed with the parent, legal representative, and/or patient.

Risk Communication

Health care professionals should anticipate that some parents will question the need for or the safety of immunizations, refuse certain vaccines, or even decide to reject all immunizations for their child. A few may have religious or philosophical objections to immunization; others want only to enter into a dialogue with their child's physician about the risks and benefits of one or more vaccines. A nonjudgmental approach to such parents is best. Ideally, health care professionals should determine in general terms what parents understand about the vaccines their children will be receiving. The nature of their concerns, their health beliefs, and what information they find credible also should be assessed.

Individuals understand and react to vaccine information based on a variety of factors, including prior experiences, attitudes, health beliefs, personal values, education, method of data presentation, perceptions of the risks of disease, perceived ability to control those risks, and their risk preference. For some who choose alternative medicine, the risk of immunization may be viewed as disproportionately great so that immunization is not perceived as beneficial. Others may dwell on sociopolitical issues, such as mandatory immunization, informed consent, and the primacy of individual rights to that of societal benefit.

Parents may be aware through the media or information from nonauthoritative Internet Web sites of controversial issues about vaccines their child is scheduled to receive. Many issues about childhood vaccines communicated by these means are presented inaccurately. When a parent initiates discussion about a vaccine controversy, the health care professional should discuss the specific concerns and provide factual information, using language appropriate for parents. Through direct dialogue with parents and the use of available resources, health care professionals can help prevent acceptance of media reports and information from nonauthoritative Internet Web sites as scientific facts.

Effective, empathetic, vaccine risk communication is essential for responding to misinformation and concerns while recognizing that risk assessment and decision making for some parents may be difficult and confusing. Some vaccines may be acceptable to the resistant parent. Their concerns should be addressed in the context of this information, using the mandated VISs (see p 5) and offering other resource materials (see Parental Misconceptions About Immunizations, p 39). Health care professionals can reinforce important points about each vaccine, including vaccine safety, and emphasize the risks encountered by unimmunized children. Parents should be advised of state laws pertaining to school or child care entry, which may require that unimmunized children stay home from school during outbreaks. Documentation of such discussions in the patient's record may help to reduce any potential liability should a vaccine-preventable disease occur in the unimmunized patient.

ACTIVE IMMUNIZATION

Active immunization involves administration of all or part of a microorganism or a modified product of that microorganism (eg, a toxoid, a purified antigen, or an antigen produced by genetic engineering) to evoke an immunologic response mimicking that of the natural infection but that usually presents little or no risk to the recipient. The immunization can result in antitoxin, anti-invasive, or neutralizing activity or other types of protective humoral or cellular response in the recipient. Some immunizing agents provide complete protection against disease for life, some provide partial protection, and some must be readministered at intervals. The effectiveness of a vaccine or toxoid is assessed by evidence of protection against the natural disease. Induction of antibodies frequently is an indirect measure of protection, but in some circumstances (eg, pertussis) the immunologic response correlated with protection is poorly understood, and serum antibody concentrations are not always predictive of protection.

Vaccines incorporating an intact infectious agent may be either live (attenuated) or killed (inactivated). Licensed vaccines are listed in Table 1.3 (p 7). Many viral vaccines contain live-attenuated virus. Although active infection (with viral replication) ensues after administration of these vaccines, little or no adverse host reaction

Table 1.3. Vaccines Licensed in the United States and Their Routes of Administration

Vaccine*	Type	Route†
Adenovirus‡	Live virus	Oral
Anthrax§	Inactivated bacteria	SC
BCG	Live bacteria	ID (preferred) or SC
Cholera	Inactivated bacteria	SC, IM, or ID
Diphtheria-tetanus (dT, DT)	Toxoids	IM
DTP	Toxoids and inactivated bacteria	IM
DTaP	Toxoids and inactivated bacterial components	IM
Hepatitis A	Inactivated viral antigen	IM
Hepatitis B	Inactivated viral antigen	IM
Hib conjugates‖	Polysaccharide-protein conjugate	IM
Hib conjugate-DTP (HbOC‖-DTP and PRP-T‖ reconstituted with DTP)	Polysaccharide-protein conjugate with toxoids and inactivated bacteria	IM
Hib conjugate-DTaP (PRP-T‖ reconstituted with DTaP)	Polysaccharide-protein conjugate with toxoids and inactivated bacterial components	IM
Hib conjugate (PRP-OMP‖)-hepatitis B	Polysaccharide-protein conjugate with inactivated virus	IM
Influenza	Inactivated virus (whole virus), viral components	IM
Japanese encephalitis	Inactivated virus	SC
Lyme disease	Inactivated protein	IM
Measles	Live virus	SC
Meningococcal	Polysaccharide	SC
MMR	Live viruses	SC
Measles-rubella	Live viruses	SC
Mumps	Live virus	SC
Pertussis§	Inactivated bacteria	IM
Plague	Inactivated bacteria	IM
Pneumococcal	Polysaccharide	IM or SC
Poliovirus		
IPV	Inactivated virus	SC
OPV	Live virus	Oral
Rabies	Inactivated virus	IM or ID¶
Rubella	Live virus	SC
Tetanus	Toxoid	IM

Table 1.3. **Vaccines Licensed in the United States and Their Routes of Administration, continued**

Vaccine*	Type	Route†
Typhoid		
Parenteral	Inactivated bacteria	SC
Parenteral	Capsular polysaccharide	SC (boosters may be ID)
Oral	Live bacteria	Oral
Varicella	Live virus	SC
Yellow fever	Live virus	SC

* BCG indicates bacillus Calmette-Guérin; DTP, diphtheria and tetanus toxoids and pertussis, adsorbed; DTaP, diphtheria and tetanus toxoids and acellular pertussis, adsorbed; Hib, *Haemophilus influenzae* type b; MMR, live measles-mumps-rubella viruses; OPV, oral poliovirus; IPV, inactivated poliovirus; dT, diphtheria and tetanus toxoids (for children 7 years of age or older and adults); and DT, diphtheria and tetanus toxoids (for children younger than 7 years of age).

† SC indicates subcutaneous; ID, intradermal; and IM, intramuscular.

‡ Available only to US Armed Forces. No longer being manufactured; existing supplies continue to be used.

§ Distributed by Bio Port Corporation, Lansing, Mich.

‖ See Table 3.10, p 267.

¶ Human diploid cell rabies vaccine for intradermal use is different in constitution and potency from the IM vaccine; it should be used for preexposure immunization only. Rabies vaccine adsorbed and RabAvert should not be given intradermally.

usually occurs. The vaccines for some viruses and most bacteria are inactivated (killed) or subunit preparations. Inactivated and subunit preparations are incapable of replicating in the host; therefore, these vaccines must contain a sufficient antigenic mass to stimulate the desired response. Maintenance of long-lasting immunity with inactivated viral or bacterial vaccines often requires periodic administration of booster doses. Inactivated vaccines may not elicit the range of immunologic response provided by live-attenuated agents. For example, an injected inactivated viral vaccine may evoke sufficient serum antibody or cell-mediated immunity but fail to evoke local antibody in the form of secretory immunoglobulin (Ig) A. Thus, mucosal protection after administration of inactivated vaccines generally is inferior to the mucosal immunity induced by live vaccines. Although systemic infection is prevented or ameliorated by the presence of serum and cellular factors, local infection or colonization with the agent can occur. However, inactivated vaccines cannot replicate in or be excreted by the vaccine recipient as infectious agents and thereby cannot adversely affect immunosuppressed hosts or their contacts.

Recommendations for dose, route, technique of administration, and schedules should be followed for predictable effective immunization. Related recommendations are critical to the success of immunization practices.

Immunizing Antigens

Physicians should be familiar with the major constituents of the products they use. The major constituents are listed in the package inserts. If a vaccine is produced by different manufacturers, some differences may exist in the active and inert ingredients contained in the various products. The major constituents of vaccines include the following:

1. ***Active immunizing antigens.*** Some vaccines consist of a single antigen that is a highly defined constituent (eg, tetanus or diphtheria toxoid); in other vaccines, the antigens are complex or less well defined (eg, live viruses or killed bacteria).
2. ***Suspending fluid.*** The suspending fluid frequently is as simple as sterile water for injection or saline, but it may be a complex tissue-culture fluid. This fluid may contain proteins or other constituents derived from the medium and biologic system in which the vaccine is produced (eg, egg antigens, gelatin, or tissue-culture–derived antigens).
3. ***Preservatives, stabilizers, and antibiotics.*** Trace amounts of chemicals (eg, mercurials, such as thimerosal (see Thimerosal content of some vaccines and immune globulin preparations, p 36) and certain antibiotics (such as neomycin or streptomycin) frequently are included to prevent bacterial growth or to stabilize the antigen. Allergic reactions may occur if the recipient is sensitive to one or more of these additives. Whenever feasible, these reactions should be anticipated by identifying known host hypersensitivity to specific vaccine components.
4. ***Adjuvants.*** An aluminum salt frequently is used to increase immunogenicity and to prolong the stimulatory effect, particularly for vaccines containing inactivated microorganisms or their products (eg, hepatitis B, diphtheria and tetanus toxoids). Investigational adjuvants are under evaluation.

Vaccine Handling and Storage

Inattention to vaccine storage conditions can contribute to vaccine failure. Certain vaccines, such as oral poliovirus (OPV) vaccine, measles, varicella, and yellow fever vaccines, are sensitive to increased temperature. Others are damaged by freezing; examples are diphtheria and tetanus toxoids and pertussis vaccines (DTaP [diphtheria and tetanus toxoids and acellular pertussis], DTP [diphtheria and tetanus toxoids and pertussis], DT [diphtheria and tetanus toxoids], and dT [diphtheria and tetanus toxoids]), inactivated poliovirus (IPV) vaccine, *Haemophilus influenzae* type b (Hib) conjugate, hepatitis A virus, hepatitis B virus, and influenza vaccines. Some products may show physical evidence of altered integrity, while others may retain their normal appearance despite a loss of potency. Therefore, all personnel responsible for handling vaccines in an office or clinic setting should be familiar with standard procedures designed to minimize the risk of vaccine failure. Recommended storage conditions for commonly used vaccines are listed in Table 1.4 (p 10). New vaccines and new formulations of currently available products may have storage requirements different from those listed in the Table. In addition, storage recommendations may be revised by the manufacturer. Revisions require approval by the US Food and Drug Administration (FDA).

Table 1.4. Recommended Storage of Commonly Used Vaccines*

Vaccine	Recommended Temperature	Duration of Stability	Normal Appearance
Diphtheria and tetanus toxoids and acellular pertussis vaccine, adsorbed (DTaP)	2°C–8°C (35°F–46°F). Do not freeze. As little as 24 hours at <2°C (<35°F) or >25°C (>77°F) may cause antigens to fall from suspension and be difficult to resuspend.	Not more than 18 mo from the time of issue from manufacturer's cold storage	Markedly turbid and whitish suspension. If product contains clumps of material that cannot be resuspended with vigorous shaking, it should NOT be used.
Diphtheria and tetanus toxoids, whole-cell pertussis vaccine adsorbed, and *Haemophilus influenzae* b conjugate vaccine (DTP-HbOC)	2°C–8°C. Do not freeze. As little as 24 hours at <2°C or >25°C may cause antigens to fall from suspension and be difficult to resuspend.	Not more than 18 mo from the time of issue from manufacturer's cold storage	Markedly turbid, white suspension. If product contains clumps of material that cannot be resuspended with vigorous shaking, it should NOT be used.
Diphtheria toxoid, adsorbed	2°C–8°C. Do not freeze.	Not more than 2 y from the time of issue from manufacturer's cold storage	Turbid and white, slightly gray, or slightly pink suspension
H influenzae b conjugate vaccine: HbOC (diphtheria CRM197 protein conjugate)	2°C–8°C. Do not freeze.	Not more than 2 y from date of issue from manufacturer's cold storage	Clear, colorless liquid
H influenzae b conjugate vaccine: PRP-D (diphtheria toxoid conjugate)	2°C–8°C. Do not freeze.	Not more than 2 y from date of issue from manufacturer's cold storage	Clear, colorless liquid
H influenzae b conjugate vaccine: PRP-OMP (meningococcal protein conjugate)	Lyophilized formulation: 2°C–8°C. Do not freeze formulation or diluent.	Not more than 2 y from date of issue from manufacturer's cold storage	
	Reconstituted formulation: 2°C–8°C. Do not freeze.	Discard reconstituted vials if not used within 24 h.	Reconstituted: after agitation, slightly opaque, white suspension

Table 1.4. Recommended Storage of Commonly Used Vaccines,* continued

Vaccine	Recommended Temperature	Duration of Stability	Normal Appearance
H influenzae b conjugate vaccine: PRP-T (tetanus toxoid conjugate)	Lyophilized formulation: 2°C–8°C. Do not freeze formulation or diluent.	Not more than 2 y from date of issue from manufacturer's cold storage	
	Reconstituted formulation: 2°C–8°C. Do not freeze.	Vaccine should be used immediately when reconstituted.	Reconstituted: clear and colorless
Hepatitis A virus vaccine, inactivated	2°C–8°C. Do not freeze. Do not use if product has been frozen.	2 y, if kept refrigerated	Opaque, white suspension
Hepatitis B virus vaccine inactivated (recombinant)	2°C–8°C. Storage outside this temperature range may reduce potency. Freezing substantially reduces potency.	2 y from date of issue from manufacturer's cold storage	After thorough agitation, a slightly opaque, white suspension
Influenza virus vaccine (subvirion)	2°C–8°C. Freezing destroys potency.	Use of vaccine is recommended only during the year for which it is manufactured; antigenic composition differs annually.	Clear, colorless liquid
Lyme disease	2°C–8°C. Do not freeze.	2 y, if kept refrigerated	With thorough agitation, suspension is turbid and white.
Measles-mumps-rubella virus (MMR) vaccine, live	Lyophilized formulation: 2°C–8°C, but may be frozen. Protect from light, which may inactivate virus.		
	Diluent: store at room temperature or refrigerated. Do not freeze.		
	Reconstituted formulation: 2°C–8°C. Protect from light, which may inactivate virus.	Discard reconstituted vials if not used within 8 hours.	Reconstituted: clear, yellow solution

Table 1.4. Recommended Storage of Commonly Used Vaccines,* continued

Vaccine	Recommended Temperature	Duration of Stability	Normal Appearance
Measles virus vaccine, live	See MMR.	See MMR.	See MMR.
Mumps virus vaccine, live	See MMR.	See MMR.	See MMR.
Rubella virus vaccine, live	See MMR.	See MMR.	See MMR.
Pneumococcal vaccine, polyvalent	2°C–8°C. Freezing destroys potency.	See expiration date on vial.	Clear, colorless, or slightly opalescent liquid.
Poliovirus vaccine, inactivated (IPV)	2°C–8°C. Do not freeze.	Not more than 1 y from date of issue	Clear, colorless suspension. Vaccine that contains particulate matter, develops turbidity, or changes color should NOT be used.
Poliovirus vaccine, live, oral (OPV)	Must be stored at <0°C (<32°F). Because of sorbitol in the vaccine, it will remain fluid at temperatures above −14°C (7°F). Refreezing the thawed product is acceptable (maximum of 10 thaw-freeze cycles) if the temperature never exceeds 8°C and the cumulative thawing time is <24 h.	Not more than 1 y from date of issue from manufacturer's cold storage	Clear solution, usually red or pink, from the phenol red (pH indicator) it contains; may be yellow if shipment was packed with dry ice. Color changes that occur during storage or thawing are unimportant, provided the solution remains clear.
Tetanus and diphtheria toxoids, adsorbed (DT and dT)	2°C–8°C. Do not freeze.	Not more than 2 y from the time of issue from manufacturer's cold storage	Markedly turbid and white suspension. If product contains clumps of material that cannot be resuspended with vigorous shaking, it should NOT be used.

Table 1.4. **Recommended Storage of Commonly Used Vaccines,* continued**

Vaccine	Recommended Temperature	Duration of Stability	Normal Appearance
Varicella virus vaccine[†]	Lyophilized formulation: keep frozen, temperature of −15°C (5*F) or colder. Protect from light. Diluent: store at room temperature or refrigerated.	Lyophilized formulation: 18 mo	Lyophilized formulation: whitish powder.
	Reconstituted formulation: use immediately; do not store.	Discard reconstituted vials if not used within 30 min.	Reconstituted formulation: clear, colorless to pale yellow liquid
	For temporary storage, unreconstituted . vaccine may be stored at 2°C–8°C for a maximum of 72 h	Discard unreconstituted vaccine if not used within 72 h (do not refreeze).	

* For recently licensed combination vaccines, see package inserts; instructions may be different from those for products listed in the Table. Also any changes in the formulation of currently available immunizing agents may alter their appearance, stability, and storage requirements. Questions about the stability of biologics subjected to potentially harmful environmental conditions should be addressed to the manufacturer of the product in question.

† For questions about stability, contact the manufacturer by calling 1-800-9-VARIVAX.

Recommendations for handling and storage of selected biologics are summarized in the package insert for each product and in a publication, *Vaccine Management,* available from the Centers for Disease Control and Prevention (CDC).* The most current information about recommended vaccine storage conditions and handling instructions can be obtained directly from manufacturers; their phone numbers are listed in the product label (package insert) and in the *Physicians' Desk Reference (PDR),* which is published yearly. The following guidelines are suggested as part of a quality control system for safe handling and storage of vaccines in an office or clinic setting.

PERSONNEL

- Designate one person as the vaccine coordinator, and assign to this person responsibility for ensuring that vaccines and other biologic products are handled in a careful, safe, and documentable manner.
- Inform all persons who will be handling vaccines about specific storage requirements and stability limitations of the products they will encounter (see Table 1.4, p 10). The details of proper storage conditions should be posted on or near each refrigerator or freezer used for vaccine storage or should be readily available.

EQUIPMENT

- Ascertain that refrigerators and freezers in which vaccines are to be stored are working properly.
- Do not connect refrigerators or freezers to an outlet with a ground-flow interrupter (GFI) or one activated by a wall switch. Use plug guards to prevent accidental dislodging of the wall plug.
- Equip each refrigerator with a thermometer located at the center of the storage compartment. This thermometer should be of the constant recording type with graphed readings or one that indicates the upper and lower extremes of temperature during the observation period ("minimum-maximum" thermometer). These thermometers provide a means of establishing whether vaccines have been exposed to potentially harmful temperatures. Placement of vaccine cold-chain monitor cards† in refrigerators can serve to detect potentially harmful elevations in temperature.
- Keep a log book in which temperature readings are systematically recorded daily and the date and time of any mechanical malfunctions or power outages are noted.
- Place in the refrigerator a tray in which all opened vials of vaccine are kept. To avoid mishaps, do not store other pharmaceuticals in the same tray.
- Equip refrigerators with several bottles of chilled water and freezers with several ice trays or ice packs to fill empty space to minimize temperature fluctuations, should a brief electrical or mechanical failure occur.

---

* Centers for Disease Control and Prevention. *Vaccine Management: Recommendations for Handling and Storage of Selected Biologicals.* Atlanta, GA: US Department of Health and Human Services, Public Health Service; January 1999

† Available from 3M Pharmaceuticals, St Paul, Minn.

PROCEDURES

- Acceptance of vaccine on receipt of shipment:
  - Ensure that the delivered product is not past the expiration date.
  - Examine the merchandise and its shipping container for any evidence of damage during transport.
  - Consider whether the interval between shipment from the supplier and arrival of the product at its destination is excessive (more than 48 hours) and whether the product has been exposed to excessive heat or cold that might alter its integrity. Review vaccine cold-chain monitor cards if included in the vaccine shipment.
  - Do not accept the shipment if reasonable suspicion exists that the delivered product may have been damaged by environmental insult or improper handling during transport.
  - Contact the vaccine supplier or manufacturer when unusual circumstances raise questions about the stability of a delivered vaccine. Store suspect vaccine under proper conditions until its viability is determined.
- Refrigerator inspection:
  - Measure the temperature of the central part of the storage compartment daily, and record this temperature in a log book. If a minimum-maximum thermometer is available, record the extremes in temperature fluctuation and reset to baseline.
  - Inspect the unit weekly for outdated vaccine and dispose of expired products appropriately.
- Routine procedures:
  - Store vaccines according to the recommended temperatures in the package insert.
  - Promptly remove expired (outdated) vaccines from the refrigerator or freezer and dispose of them appropriately at the earliest possible time to avoid accidental use.
  - Keep opened vials of vaccine in a tray so that they are readily identifiable.
  - Indicate on the label of each vaccine vial the date and time it was reconstituted or first opened.
  - Reconstitution of multiple doses of vaccine and drawing up of multiple doses of vaccine in syringes from vials before immediate use is discouraged because of possible mix-ups and the uncertainty of vaccine stability in these conditions.
  - Prefilled unit-dose syringes can prevent contamination of multidose vials and errors in labeling syringes.
  - Discard reconstituted live-virus and other vaccines if not used within the interval specified in the package insert. Examples include varicella vaccine after 30 minutes, measles-mumps-rubella (MMR) vaccine after 8 hours, and PedvaxHIB (PRP-OMP) after 24 hours (see *Haemophilus influenzae* Infections, p 262).
  - Store vaccines in the refrigerator throughout the office day.
  - Do not open more than 1 vial of a particular vaccine at a time.
  - Store vaccine only in the central storage area of the refrigerator, not on the door shelf or in peripheral areas of the unit where temperature fluctuations are greater.
  - Do not keep food in refrigerators where vaccine is stored; this practice will lead to more frequent opening of the unit and greater chance for thermal instability.

- Do not store radioactive materials in the same refrigerator in which vaccines are stored.
- Discuss with all clinic or office personnel any violation of handling protocol or any accidental storage problem (eg, electrical failure), and contact vaccine suppliers for information about the handling of the affected vaccine.

Vaccine Administration

GENERAL INSTRUCTIONS FOR PERSONS ADMINISTERING VACCINES

Personnel administering vaccines should take appropriate precautions to minimize the risk of spread of disease to or from patients. Such personnel should have evidence of immunity or be immunized against measles, mumps, rubella, varicella, hepatitis B, and influenza, as well as tetanus and diphtheria. Hands should be washed before and after each new patient contact. Gloves are not required when administering vaccines unless the health care worker has open hand lesions or will come into contact with potentially infectious body fluids. Syringes and needles must be sterile and preferably disposable. To prevent accidental needle sticks or reuse, a needle should **not** be recapped after use, and disposable needles and syringes should be discarded promptly in puncture-proof, labeled containers. Changing needles between drawing the vaccine into the syringe and injecting it into the child generally is not necessary. Different vaccines should not be mixed in the same syringe unless specifically licensed and labeled for such use.

Because of possible hypersensitivity to vaccine components, persons administering vaccines or other biologic products should be prepared to recognize and treat allergic reactions, including anaphylaxis (see Hypersensitivity Reactions to Vaccine Constituents, p 35). Facilities and personnel should be available for treating immediate hypersensitivity reactions. This recommendation does not preclude administration of vaccines in school-based or other nonclinic settings. Whenever possible, patients should be observed for an allergic reaction for 15 to 20 minutes after receiving immunization(s).

Syncope may occur after immunization, particularly in adolescents and young adults. Personnel should be aware of presyncopal manifestations and take appropriate measures to prevent injuries if weakness, dizziness, or loss of consciousness occurs. The relatively rapid onset of syncope in most cases suggests that having vaccine recipients sit or lie down for 15 minutes after immunization could avert many syncopal episodes and secondary injuries. If syncope develops, patients should be observed until they are asymptomatic.

SITE AND ROUTE OF IMMUNIZATION (ACTIVE AND PASSIVE)

Oral Vaccines. Breastfeeding does not interfere with successful immunization with OPV vaccine. If the patient immediately spits out, fails to swallow, or regurgitates OPV vaccine, the dose of OPV should be repeated. Vomiting within 10 minutes of receiving an OPV dose also is an indication for repeating the dose. If the second dose is not retained, neither dose should be counted, and the vaccine should be readministered. In the United States as of the year 2000, only IPV vaccine is recommended for the routine immunization schedule (see Poliovirus Infections, p 465).

Parenteral Vaccines.* Injectable vaccines should be administered in a site as free as possible from the risk of local neural, vascular, or tissue injury. Data in the medical literature do not warrant recommendation of a single preferred site for all injections, and many manufacturers' product recommendations allow some flexibility in the site of injection. Preferred sites for vaccines administered subcutaneously or intramuscularly include the anterolateral aspect of the upper thigh and the deltoid area of the upper arm.

Recommended routes of administration are included in the package inserts of vaccines and are listed in Table 1.3 (p 7). The recommended route is based on results of studies designed to demonstrate maximum safety and efficacy. To minimize untoward local or systemic effects and ensure optimal efficacy of the immunizing procedure, vaccines should be given by the recommended route.

For intramuscular (IM) injections, the choice of site is based on the volume of the injected material and the size of the muscle. In children younger than 1 year of age (ie, infants), the anterolateral aspect of the thigh provides the largest muscle and is the preferred site. In older children, the deltoid muscle is usually large enough for IM injection. Some physicians prefer to use the anterolateral thigh muscles for toddlers. Parents and children, however, often prefer use of the deltoid muscle for immunization at 18 months of age and older because it is associated with less pain in the affected extremity when ambulating.

Ordinarily, the upper, outer aspect of the buttocks should not be used for active immunization because the gluteal region is covered by a significant layer of subcutaneous fat and because of the possibility of damaging the sciatic nerve. However, clinical information on the use of this area is limited. Because of diminished immunogenicity, hepatitis B and rabies vaccines should not be given in the buttock at any age. Persons who were given hepatitis B vaccine in the buttock should be tested for immunity and reimmunized if antibody concentrations are inadequate.

When the upper, outer quadrant of the buttocks is used for large-volume passive immunization, such as IM administration of large volumes of immune globulin, care must be taken to avoid injury to the nerve. The site selected should be well into the upper, outer mass of the gluteus maximus, away from the central region of the buttocks, and the needle should be directed anteriorly—that is, if the patient is lying prone, perpendicular to the table's surface, not perpendicular to the skin plane. The ventrogluteal site may be less hazardous for IM injection because it is free of major nerves and vessels. This site is the center of a triangle whose boundaries are the anterior superior iliac spine, the tubercle of the iliac crest, and the upper border of the greater trochanter.

Vaccines containing adjuvants (eg, aluminum-adsorbed DTaP, DT, dT, hepatitis B, and hepatitis A) must be injected deep in the muscle mass. They should not be administered subcutaneously or intracutaneously because they can cause local irritation, inflammation, granuloma formation, and necrosis. Immune Globulin (IG), Rabies Immune Globulin (RIG), and other similar products for passive immunoprophylaxis also are injected intramuscularly except when RIG is infiltrated around the site of a bite wound.

* For a review on intramuscular injections, see Bergeson PS, Singer SA, Kaplan AM. Intramuscular injections in children. *Pediatrics.* 1982;70:944–948

The needles used for IM injections should be long enough to reach the substance of the muscle. For certain very young, small infants, a ⅝-inch long needle may be adequate. Ordinarily, a needle ⅞- to 1-inch long is required to ensure penetration of the thigh muscle in healthy 4-month-old infants and of the thigh or deltoid in toddlers and older children. The deltoid is preferred for immunization of adolescents and young adults. The needle length should be from 1 to 2 inches depending on the vaccine recipient's weight (eg, 1- to 1.5 inches for males ≤120 kg; 1 inch for females <70 kg; 1.5 inches for females 70–100 kg; and 2 inches for males >120 kg and females >100 kg). A 22- to 25-gauge needle is appropriate for most IM vaccines.

Serious complications of IM injections are rare. Reported events include broken needles, muscle contracture, nerve injury, bacterial (staphylococcal, streptococcal, and clostridial) abscesses, sterile abscesses, skin pigmentation, hemorrhage, cellulitis, tissue necrosis, gangrene, local atrophy, periostitis, cyst or scar formation, and inadvertent injection into a joint space.

Subcutaneous injections can be given in the anterolateral aspect of the thigh or the upper arm by inserting the needle in a pinched-up fold of skin and subcutaneous tissue. A 23- or 25-gauge needle, ⅝- to ¾-inch long, is recommended. Immune responses after subcutaneous administration of hepatitis B and recombinant rabies vaccine are reduced compared with those after IM administration, and these vaccines should not be given by the subcutaneous route. In patients with a bleeding diathesis, the risk of bleeding after IM injection can be minimized by vaccine administration immediately after the patient's receipt of replacement factor, use of a 23-gauge (or smaller) needle, and immediate application of direct pressure to the immunization site for at least 2 minutes. Certain vaccines (eg, *Haemophilus influenzae* type b vaccines, except PRP-OMP [PedvaxHIB]) recommended for IM injection may be given subcutaneously to persons at risk for hemorrhage after IM injection, such as persons with hemophilia. For these vaccines, immune responses and clinical reactions after either IM or subcutaneous injection generally have been reported to be similar.

Intradermal (ID) injections usually are given on the volar surface of the forearm. Because of the decreased antigenic mass administered with ID injections, attention to technique is essential to ensure that the material is not injected subcutaneously. A 25- or 27-gauge needle is recommended.

A patient should be restrained adequately if indicated before any injection. When multiple vaccines are administered, separate sites ordinarily should be used if possible, especially if 1 of the vaccines contains DTaP. When necessary, 2 vaccines can be given in the same limb at a single visit. The thigh is the preferred site for 2 simultaneous IM injections because of its greater muscle mass. The distance separating the 2 injections is arbitrary but should be sufficient (eg, 1 to 2 inches apart) so that local reactions are unlikely to overlap. Multiple vaccines should not be mixed in a single syringe unless specifically licensed and labeled for administering in 1 syringe. A different needle and syringe should be used for each injection. Although most experts recommend "aspiration" by gently pulling back on the syringe before the injection is given, there are no data to document the necessity for this procedure. If blood appears after negative pressure, the needle should be withdrawn and a new site selected.

A brief period of bleeding at the injection site is common and usually can be controlled by gentle pressure for several minutes.

Managing Injection Pain

Concerns and resulting anxiety about injections are common at any age. Current immunization schedules sometimes require children to receive 3 or more injections during a single visit. Although most children older than 5 years of age usually accept immunization with minimal opposition, a significant number of older children react vigorously or refuse to receive the injection. Effective practical techniques can be used to ameliorate some of the discomfort of injections.

A planned approach to managing the child before, during, and after immunization is helpful for children of any age. Truthful and empathetic preparation for injections is more beneficial for older than for younger children. Parents should be advised never to threaten their children with injections or use them as a punishment for inappropriate behavior.

If possible, parents should have a role in comforting their child, rather than in restraining them. For younger children, parents may soothe, stroke, and calm the child. For older children, parents should be coached to distract their child (see Nonpharmacologic Techniques, p 20).

INJECTION TECHNIQUE AND POSITION

A rapid plunge of the needle through the skin may reduce discomfort associated with skin penetration. The Z-track method of injection also is reported to decrease associated pain; traction is applied to the skin and subcutaneous tissues before insertion of the needle and released after the needle is withdrawn, so that the injection track superficial to the muscle is displaced from the track within the muscle to seal the medication into the muscle. The limb should be positioned to allow relaxation of the muscle to be injected. For the deltoid, some flexion of the arm may be required. For the anterolateral thigh, some degree of internal rotation may be helpful. Infants may exhibit less pain behavior when held on the lap of a parent or other caregiver. Older children may be more comfortable sitting on a parent's lap or examination table edge, hugging their parent chest to chest while an immunization is administered.

If multiple injections are to be given, administering them simultaneously at multiple sites by different providers, eg, right and left anterolateral thighs, may reduce some of the anticipation of the next injection. Allowing older children some choice in selecting the site to be injected may be helpful by allowing a degree of control.

TOPICAL ANESTHETIC TECHNIQUES

Some physical techniques and topically applied agents reduce the pain of injection. Pressure at the site for 10 seconds before injection reduces the pain of injection. Ice provides only 1 to 2 seconds of analgesia at the injection site and, therefore, is not recommended. Local anesthetic agents may be administered by several routes. Eutectic mixture of local anesthetic (EMLA) cream, which is applied topically under an occlusive dressing, has been evaluated in multiple placebo-controlled, randomized clinical trials and has been demonstrated to provide pain relief during the injection and for the next 24 hours. Because EMLA requires 1 hour to work adequately, planning usually is necessary, such as applying the cream before an office visit or immediately on arrival. Lidocaine also may be delivered by iontophoresis to a depth of 8 to 10 mm in about 10 minutes, but the electric current causes some discomfort. Vapocoolant spray provides rapid transient analgesia at the injection site and is inexpensive. Studies comparing EMLA and vapocoolant spray at the time of administration demonstrate comparable efficacy.

Additional studies need to be performed on the use of local anesthetic agents to better establish their safety and effectiveness when used to manage injection pain and to assure that their use does not interfere with the immune response, particularly to subcutaneous injections.

NONPHARMACOLOGIC TECHNIQUES

Sucrose placed on the tongue or on a pacifier ameliorates discomfort in newborn infants but has little effect beyond the immediate postnatal period. Stroking or rocking a child following an injection decreases crying and other pain behaviors. For older children, breathing and distraction techniques, such as "blowing the pain away," use of "party blowers," pinwheels, or soap bubbles, telling children stories, reading books, or the use of music, are all effective. Techniques that involve the child in a fantasy or reframe the experience with the use of suggestion ("magic love" or "pain switch") also are effective but may require prior training.

The younger the child, the greater the reliance on technique and pharmacologic approaches. As the child becomes older, distraction and other psychological approaches in addition to pharmacologic and technical approaches to pain reduction are increasingly effective.

Scheduling Immunizations

A vaccine is intended to be administered to a person who is capable of an appropriate immunologic response and who likely will benefit from the protection given. However, optimal immunologic response for the person must be balanced against the need to achieve effective protection against disease. For example, pertussis-containing vaccines may be less immunogenic in early infancy than later in infancy, but the benefit of conferring early protection in young infants dictates that immunization should be given despite a lessened serum antibody response. In some developing countries, OPV vaccine is given at birth, in accordance with recommendations of the World Health Organization, for a similar reason.

With parenterally administered live-virus vaccines, the inhibitory effect of residual specific maternal antibody determines the optimal age of administration. For example, live-virus measles vaccine in use in the United States has suboptimal rates of successful immunization during the first year of life mainly because of transplacentally acquired maternal antibody.

An additional factor in selecting an immunization schedule is the need to achieve a uniform and regular response. With some products, a response is achieved after 1 dose; for others, it is achieved only after multiple doses. Live-virus rubella vaccine is an example of a vaccine that evokes a regular predictable response at highly acceptable rates after a single dose. In contrast, some persons respond to only 1 or

2 types of poliovirus(es) after a single dose of poliovirus vaccine. Hence, multiple doses are given to produce antibody against all 3 types, thereby ensuring complete protection for the person and maximum response rates for the population. A single dose of some vaccines (mostly inactivated or killed antigens) confers less than optimal response in the recipient. As a result, several doses are needed to complete the primary immunization, and periodic booster doses (eg, with tetanus and diphtheria toxoids) are administered to maintain immunologic protection.

Most of the widely used vaccines are considered safe and effective when administered simultaneously, although limited data are available for many products. This information is particularly important for scheduling immunizations for children with lapsed or missed immunizations and for persons preparing for foreign travel (see Simultaneous Administration of Multiple Vaccines, p 26). Limited data and theoretical concerns indicate possible impaired immune responses to 2 live-virus vaccines given nonsimultaneously but within 28 days (4 weeks) of each other, but there is no evidence that this occurs with current vaccines. Parenterally administered live-virus vaccines not administered on the same day should be given at least 28 days (4 weeks) apart. Recent receipt of OPV vaccine is not a contraindication to MMR vaccine, which should be given at the first available opportunity, according to age-specific recommendations. In the United States as of the year 2000, only IPV is recommended for use.

The schedule in Fig 1.1 (p 22) represents a consensus of the American Academy of Pediatrics (AAP), the Advisory Committee on Immunization Practices of the CDC, and the American Academy of Family Physicians for routine childhood immunization in the year 2000. This schedule is reviewed regularly, and an updated national schedule is issued annually in January to incorporate new vaccines and revised recommendations. Special attention should be given to the footnotes of the schedule because they summarize major recommendations for routine childhood immunization. Combination vaccine products may be given whenever any component of the combination is indicated and its other components are not contraindicated, provided they are approved by the FDA for the child's age.*

Table 1.5 (p 24) gives the recommended schedule for children who were not immunized appropriately during the first year of life.

For children in whom early or rapid immunization is urgent or for children not immunized on schedule, simultaneous immunization with multiple products allows for more rapid protection. In addition, in some circumstances, immunization can be initiated earlier than at the usually recommended ages and doses given at shorter intervals than is recommended routinely (for guidelines, see the immunization recommendations in the disease-specific chapters in Section 3).

The immunization schedule used in the United States may not be appropriate for developing countries because of different disease risks, age-specific immune responses, and vaccine availability. The schedule recommended by the Expanded Programme on Immunization of the World Health Organization should be

* American Academy of Pediatrics Committee on Infectious Diseases. Combination vaccines for childhood immunization: recommendations of the Advisory Committee on Immunization Practices (ACIP), the American Academy of Pediatrics (AAP), and the American Academy of Family Physicians (AAFP). *Pediatrics*. 1999;103:1064–1077

Figure 1.1. **Childhood Immunization Schedule**

Recommended Childhood Immunization Schedule United States, January – December 2000

Vaccines[1] are listed under routinely recommended ages. [Bars] indicate range of recommended ages for immunization. Any dose not given at the recommended age should be given as a "catch-up" immunization at any subsequent visit when indicated and feasible. (Ovals) indicate vaccines to be given if previously recommended doses were missed or given earlier than the recommended minimum age.

Age ▶ / Vaccine ▼	Birth	1 mo	2 mos	4 mos	6 mos	12 mos	15 mos	18 mos	24 mos	4-6 yrs	11-12 yrs	14-16 yrs
Hepatitis B[2]	[Hep B] (Birth–2 mos)											
			[Hep B] (1–4 mos)		[Hep B] (6–18 mos)						(Hep B)	
Diphtheria, Tetanus, Pertussis[3]			DTaP	DTaP	DTaP		[DTaP[3]] (15–18 mos)			DTaP	[Td] (11–16 yrs)	
H. influenzae type b[4]			Hib	Hib	Hib	[Hib] (12–15 mos)						
Polio[5]			IPV	IPV	[IPV[5]] (6–18 mos)					IPV[5]		
Measles, Mumps, Rubella[6]						[MMR] (12–15 mos)				MMR[6]	(MMR[6])	
Varicella[7]						[Var] (12–18 mos)					(Var[7])	
Hepatitis A[8]									[Hep A[8]-in selected areas] (24 mos–12 yrs)			

Approved by the Advisory Committee on Immunization Practices (ACIP), the American Academy of Pediatrics (AAP), and the American Academy of Family Physicians (AAFP)

(For **necessary footnotes** and important information, see next page.)

Figure 1.1. **Childhood Immunization Schedule, continued**

On October 22, 1999, the Advisory Committee on Immunization Practices (ACIP) recommended that Rotashield (RRV-TV), the only US-licensed rotavirus vaccine, no longer be used in the United States (MMWR Morb Mortal Wkly Rep. Nov 5, 1999;48(43):1007). Parents should be reassured that their children who received rotavirus vaccine before July are not at increased risk for intussusception now.

[1] This schedule indicates the recommended ages for routine administration of currently licensed childhood vaccines as of 11/1/99. Additional vaccines may be licensed and recommended during the year. Licensed combination vaccines may be used whenever any components of the combination are indicated and its other components are not contraindicated. Providers should consult the manufacturers' package inserts for detailed recommendations.

[2] **Infants born to HBsAg-negative mothers** should receive the 1st dose of hepatitis B (Hep B) vaccine by age 2 months. The 2nd dose should be at least 1 month after the 1st dose. The 3rd dose should be administered at least 4 months after the 1st dose and at least 2 months after the 2nd dose, but not before 6 months of age for infants.
Infants born to HBsAg-positive mothers should receive hepatitis B vaccine and 0.5 mL hepatitis B immune globulin (HBIG) within 12 hours of birth at separate sites. The 2nd dose is recommended at 1 to 2 months of age and the 3rd dose at 6 months of age.
Infants born to mothers whose HBsAg status is unknown should receive hepatitis B vaccine within 12 hours of birth. Maternal blood should be drawn at the time of delivery to determine the mother's HBsAg status; if the HBsAg test is positive, the infant should receive HBIG as soon as possible (no later than 1 week of age).
All children and adolescents (through 18 years of age) who have not been immunized against hepatitis B may begin the series during any visit. Special efforts should be made to immunize children who were born in or whose parents were born in areas of the world with moderate or high endemicity of hepatitis B virus infection.

[3] The 4th dose of DTaP (diphtheria and tetanus toxoids and acellular pertussis vaccine) may be administered as early as 12 months of age, provided 6 months have elapsed since the 3rd dose and the child is unlikely to return at age 15 to 18 months. Td (tetanus and diphtheria toxoids) is recommended at 11 to 12 years of age if at least 5 years have elapsed since the last dose of DTP, DTaP, or DT. Subsequent routine Td boosters are recommended every 10 years.

[4] Three *Haemophilus influenzae* type b (Hib) conjugate vaccines are licensed for infant use. If PRP-OMP (PedvaxHIB or ComVax [Merck]) is administered at 2 and 4 months of age, a dose at 6 months is not required. Because clinical studies in infants have demonstrated that using some combination products may induce a lower immune response to the Hib vaccine component, DTaP/Hib combination products should not be used for primary immunization in infants at 2, 4, or 6 months of age unless FDA-approved for these ages.

[5] To eliminate the risk of vaccine-associated paralytic polio (VAPP), an all-IPV schedule is now recommended for routine childhood polio vaccination in the United States. All children should receive four doses of IPV at 2 months, 4 months, 6 to 18 months, and 4 to 6 years. OPV (if available) may be used only for the following special circumstances:

1. Mass vaccination campaigns to control outbreaks of paralytic polio.
2. Unvaccinated children who will be traveling in <4 weeks to areas where polio is endemic or epidemic.
3. Children of parents who do not accept the recommended number of vaccine injections. These children may receive OPV only for the third or fourth dose or both; in this situation, health care professionals should administer OPV only after discussing the risk for VAPP with parents or caregivers.
4. During the transition to an all-IPV schedule, recommendations for the use of remaining OPV supplies in physicians' offices and clinics have been issued by the American Academy of Pediatrics (see *Pediatrics*, December 1999).

[6] The 2nd dose of measles, mumps, and rubella (MMR) vaccine is recommended routinely at 4 to 6 years of age but may be administered during any visit, provided at least 4 weeks have elapsed since receipt of the 1st dose and that both doses are administered beginning at or after 12 months of age. Those who have not previously received the second dose should complete the schedule by the 11- to 12-year-old visit.

[7] Varicella (Var) vaccine is recommended at any visit on or after the first birthday for susceptible children, ie, those who lack a reliable history of chickenpox (as judged by a health care professional) and who have not been immunized. Susceptible persons 13 years of age or older should receive 2 doses, given at least 4 weeks apart.

[8] Hepatitis A (Hep A) is shaded to indicate its recommended use in selected states and/or regions; consult your local public health authority. (Also see *MMWR Morb Mortal Wkly Rep.* Oct 01, 1999;48(RR-12): 1-37).

Table 1.5. **Recommended Immunization Schedules for Children Not Immunized in the First Year of Life***

Recommended Time/Age	Immunization(s)[†]	Comments
Younger Than 7 Years		
First visit	DTaP, Hib,[‡] HBV, MMR	If indicated, tuberculin testing may be done at same visit. If child is 5 y of age or older, Hib is not indicated in most circumstances.
Interval after first visit		
1 mo (4 wk)	DTaP, IPV, HBV, Var[§]	The second dose of IPV may be given if accelerated poliomyelitis immunization is necessary, such as for travelers to areas where polio is endemic.
2 mo	DTaP, Hib,[‡] IPV	Second dose of Hib is indicated only if the first dose was received when younger than 15 mo.
≥8 mo	DTaP, HBV, IPV	IPV and HBV are not given if the third doses were given earlier.
Age 4–6 y (at or before school entry)	DTaP, IPV, MMR[‖]	DTaP is not necessary if the fourth dose was given after the fourth birthday; IPV is not necessary if the third dose was given after the fourth birthday.
Age 11–12 y	See Fig 1.1, p 22	
7–12 Years		
First visit	HBV, MMR, dT, IPV	
Interval after first visit		
2 mo (8 wk)	HBV, MMR,[‖] Var,[§] dT, IPV	IPV also may be given 1 mo after the first visit if accelerated poliomyelitis immunization is necessary.
8–14 mo	HBV,[¶] dT, IPV	IPV is not given if the third dose was given earlier.
Age 11–12 y	See Fig 1.1, p 22	

* Table is not completely consistent with all package inserts. For products used, also consult manufacturer's package insert for instructions on storage, handling, dosage, and administration. Biologics prepared by different manufacturers may vary, and package inserts of the same manufacturer may change. Therefore, the physician should be aware of the contents of the current package insert. Vaccine abbreviations: HBV indicates hepatitis B virus; Var, varicella; DTaP, diphtheria and tetanus toxoids and acellular pertussis; Hib, *Haemophilus influenzae* type b conjugate; IPV, inactivated poliovirus; MMR, live measles-mumps-rubella; dT, adult tetanus toxoid (full dose) and diphtheria toxoid (reduced dose), for children 7 years of age or older and adults.

Table 1.5. **Recommended Immunization Schedules for Children Not Immunized in the First Year of Life,* continued**

† If all needed vaccines cannot be administered simultaneously, priority should be given to protecting the child against the diseases that pose the greatest immediate risk. In the United States, these diseases for children younger than 2 years usually are measles and *Haemophilus influenzae* type b infection; for children older than 7 years, they are measles, mumps, and rubella. Before 13 years of age, immunity against hepatitis B and varicella should be ensured. DTaP, HBV, Hib, MMR, and Var can be given simultaneously at separate sites if failure of the patient to return for future immunizations is a concern. For further information on pertussis and poliomyelitis immunization, see the respective chapters (Pertussis, p 435, and Poliovirus Infections, p 465).

‡ See *Haemophilus influenzae* Infections, p 262, and Table 3.11 (p 268).

§ Varicella vaccine can be administered to susceptible children any time after 12 months of age. Unimmunized children who lack a reliable history of varicella should be immunized before their 13th birthday.

‖ Minimal interval between doses of MMR is 1 month (4 wk).

¶ HBV may be given earlier in a 0-, 2-, and 4-month schedule.

consulted (http://www.who.org/). Modifications may be made by the ministries of health in individual countries, based on local considerations.

Interchangeability of Vaccine Products

Similar vaccines made by different manufacturers may differ in their components and formulation and may elicit different immune responses. Such vaccines have been considered interchangeable when administered according to their licensed indications, although data documenting interchangeability sometimes are limited. Vaccines that can be used interchangeably according to their licensed indication during a vaccine series include diphtheria and tetanus toxoids, live and inactivated polio vaccines, hepatitis A vaccines, hepatitis B vaccines, and rabies vaccines (see Rabies, p 475).

Any of the licensed Hib conjugate vaccines are considered interchangeable for primary as well as for booster immunization (see *Haemophilus influenzae* Infections, p 262).

When feasible, the same DTaP vaccine product should be used for the first 3 doses of the pertussis immunization series (see Pertussis, p 435). No data exist on the safety, immunogenicity, or efficacy of different DTaP vaccines when administered interchangeably in the primary series. However, in the circumstances in which the type of DTaP product(s) received previously is not known or the previously administered product(s) is not readily available, any of the DTaP vaccines licensed for use in the primary series may be used. For the fourth and fifth doses, any licensed product is acceptable, irrespective of prior vaccines received. These recommendations may change as data become available about the response to different DTaP vaccines administered interchangeably in a primary series or as the fourth or fifth doses.

Simultaneous Administration of Multiple Vaccines

Most vaccines can be safely and effectively administered simultaneously. No contraindications to the simultaneous administration of multiple vaccines routinely recommended for infants and children are known. Immune responses to one vaccine generally do not interfere with those to other vaccines; exceptions include interference among the 3 oral poliovirus serotypes in trivalent OPV vaccine and concurrent administration of cholera and yellow fever vaccines. Simultaneous administration of IPV, MMR, varicella, or DTaP vaccines has resulted in rates of seroconversion and of side effects similar to those observed when the vaccines are administered at separate times. Because simultaneous administration of common vaccines is not known to affect the efficacy or safety of any of the routinely recommended childhood vaccines, simultaneous administration of all vaccines (DTaP, IPV, MMR, varicella, hepatitis B, and Hib vaccines) appropriate for the age and previous immunization status of the recipient is recommended. Simultaneous administration of multiple vaccines can raise immunization rates significantly.

For persons preparing for foreign travel, multiple vaccines generally can be given concurrently. An exception is the simultaneous administration of yellow fever and cholera vaccines. Antibody responses to both cholera and yellow fever vaccines are decreased if given simultaneously or within a short time of each other. If possible, these vaccines should be separated by at least 3 weeks; alternatively, cholera vaccine could be omitted since its effectiveness is limited and few indications for its use exist.

If both vaccines are necessary and time constraints exist, these vaccines can be given simultaneously or within a 3-week period with the understanding that antibody responses may not be optimal.

When vaccines commonly associated with substantial local or systemic reactions (eg, cholera, parenteral typhoid vaccines, and plague) are given simultaneously, the reactions can be accentuated. Thus, in most circumstances, if feasible, these vaccines should be given on separate occasions.

Lapsed Immunizations

A lapse in the immunization schedule does not require reinstitution of the entire series. If a dose of DTaP, IPV, Hib, or hepatitis B vaccine is missed, immunizations should be given at the next visit as if the usual interval had elapsed. The medical charts of children in whom immunizations have been missed or postponed should be flagged to remind health care professionals to complete immunization schedules at the next available opportunity.

Unknown or Uncertain Immunization Status

A physician may encounter some children with an uncertain immunization status. Many young adults and some children do not have adequate documentation of immunizations, and recollection by the parent or guardian may be of questionable validity. In general, these persons should be considered disease susceptible, and appropriate immunizations should be administered. No evidence indicates that administration of MMR, varicella, Hib, hepatitis B, or poliovirus vaccine to already immune recipients is harmful; dT, rather than DTaP should be given to those 7 years of age or older.

Immunizations Received Outside the United States

Persons immunized in other countries, including international adoptees, refugees, and exchange students, should be immunized according to recommended schedules in the United States for healthy infants, children, and adolescents (see Fig 1.1 and Table 1.5, p 22 and p 24). Only written documentation should be accepted as evidence of prior immunization. In general, written records may be considered valid if the vaccines, dates of administration, number of doses, intervals between doses, and age of the patient at the time of immunization are comparable to that of the current US schedule. Although some vaccines with inadequate potency have been produced in other countries, most vaccines used worldwide are produced with adequate quality control standards and are reliable. However, immunization records for children, especially children from an orphanage, from some areas (eg, Eastern Europe, Russia and other countries of the former Soviet Union, and China) may not accurately reflect protection because of inaccurate or unreliable records, lack of vaccine potency, or other problems, such as recording MMR but giving a product that did not contain one of the components (eg, rubella). Therefore, it may be reasonable to check antibody titers on these children. For any child who has received immunizations outside of the United States, if any question exists about whether the immunizations were administered or were immunogenic, the best course is to repeat them.

Vaccine Dose

The recommended doses of vaccines are derived from experimental trials and clinical experience. Reduction in the recommended doses can result in an inadequate response and continuing susceptibility of the recipient. Exceeding the recommended dose also may be hazardous. Excessive local concentrations of injectable inactivated vaccines might result in enhanced tissue or systemic reactions, whereas administering an increased dose of a live vaccine constitutes a theoretical but unproven risk.

Reducing or dividing doses of DTP or any other vaccine, including those given to premature or low-birth-weight infants, is not indicated. The efficacy of this practice in reducing the frequency of adverse events has not been demonstrated. Such a practice also might confer less protection against disease than that achieved with the recommended doses. A diminished antibody response in both term and premature infants to reduced doses of DTP has been reported. A previous immunization with a dose that was less than the standard dose or one administered by a nonstandard route should not be counted, and the patient should be reimmunized as appropriate for age.

Active Immunization of Persons Who Recently Received Immune Globulin

Live-virus vaccines given parenterally can have diminished immunogenicity when given shortly before or during a period of several months after receipt of immune globulins. High doses of immune globulin have been demonstrated to inhibit the response to measles vaccine for a prolonged period. The duration of inhibition varies directly with the dose of immune globulin administered. Inhibition of immune response to rubella, while of shorter duration than measles, also has been demonstrated. The appropriate suggested interval between immune globulin administration and measles immunization will vary with the indication for immune globulin (which determines the dose) and specific product (eg, Immune Globulin vs Immune Globulin Intravenous); suggested intervals are given in Table 3.35 (p 390). If immune globulin must be given within 14 days after administration of measles or measles-containing vaccines, these live-virus vaccines should be administered again after the period specified in Table 3.35 (p 390) unless serologic testing at an appropriate interval after immune globulin administration indicates that adequate serum antibodies were produced.

The effect of administration of immune globulin on the antibody response to varicella vaccine is not known. Because of potential inhibition of the response, varicella vaccine should not be administered after receipt of an immune globulin preparation or a blood product (except washed red blood cells), as recommended for measles vaccine (see Table 3.36, p 391). In addition, immune globulin preparations, if possible, should not be administered for 14 days immunization. If an immune globulin preparation is given in this interval, the vaccine recipient should be reimmunized after the period specified in Table 3.35 (p 390) or tested for varicella immunity at that time and reimmunized if seronegative.

In contrast with live-virus vaccines given parenterally, administration of immune globulin preparations has not been demonstrated to cause significant inhibition of the immune responses to inactivated vaccines and toxoids. For example, concurrent administration of recommended doses of Hepatitis B Immune Globulin, Tetanus Immune Globulin, or RIG and the corresponding inactivated vaccine or toxoid in postexposure prophylaxis does not impair the efficacy of vaccine and provides immediate and long-term immunity, ie, active and passive immunoprophylaxis. Standard doses of the corresponding vaccines are recommended. Increases in the vaccine dose volume or number of immunizations are not indicated. Vaccines should be administered at sites different from that of intramuscularly administered immune globulin. For further information, see chapters on specific diseases in Section 3.

Administration of hepatitis A vaccine together with IG has been recommended for situations in which immediate *and* prolonged protection against HAV infection is desired. Although this combined active-passive immunization has been demonstrated to result in significantly lower serum antibody concentrations than those induced by vaccine administration only, these concentrations are still many times higher than those considered protective and seroconversion rates are not affected. The reduced immunogenicity, therefore, is not considered clinically significant.

A possible exception to the lack of inhibition of immune responses to inactivated vaccines may be the effect of Respiratory Syncytial Virus Immune Globulin Intravenous (RSV-IGIV) on antibody responses to some inactivated vaccines. However, the data are inconclusive, and supplemental doses of these vaccines for RSV-IGIV recipients are not indicated. Other than deferral of MMR and varicella vaccines, as previously discussed, these recipients should be immunized according to the recommended schedule for routine childhood immunization (see Fig 1.1, p 22). The RSV monoclonal antibody (palivizumab), which is given by the intramuscular route, does not interfere with response to vaccines.

Administration of immune globulin preparations does not interfere with antibody responses to yellow fever or OPV vaccines. Hence, OPV and yellow fever vaccines can be administered simultaneously with or at any time before or after immune globulin, such as to travelers whose departure is imminent.

Tuberculin Testing

Recommendations for tuberculin testing (see Tuberculosis, p 593) are independent of those for immunization. Tuberculin testing at any age is not required before administration of live-virus vaccines, such as MMR, varicella, or yellow fever. A tuberculin skin test can be applied at the same visit that these vaccines are administered. Because measles vaccine temporarily can suppress tuberculin activity, if tuberculin testing is indicated and cannot be done at the same time as measles immunization, tuberculin testing should be postponed for 4 to 6 weeks. The effect of live-virus varicella and yellow-fever vaccines on tuberculin skin test reactivity is not known.

Record Keeping and Immunization Registries

PATIENTS' PERSONAL IMMUNIZATION RECORDS

Each state health department has developed an official immunization record. This record should be given to the parents of every newborn infant and should be accorded the status of a birth certificate or passport and retained with vital documents for subsequent referral. Physicians should cooperate with this endeavor by recording immunization data in this record and by encouraging patients not only to preserve the record, but also to present it at each visit to a health care professional.

The immunization record is especially important for patients who move frequently. It facilitates an accurate patient medical record, enables the physician to evaluate the child's immunization status, and fulfills the need for documentation of immunizations for child care and school attendance and for admission to other institutions and organizations.

Many states are developing computer-based immunization registries to help remind parents and health care providers when immunizations are due or overdue and determine for health care professionals the immunization needs of their patients at the time of each visit. These registries also will serve to measure immunization coverage. The AAP urges physicians to cooperate with state and local health officials in providing needed immunization information.

Until such registries are functioning reliably, parents and physicians must rely on the personal immunization record to document each child's immunization status.

PHYSICIANS' IMMUNIZATION RECORDS

Every physician should ensure that the immunization history of each patient is maintained in a permanent confidential record that can be reviewed easily and updated when subsequent immunizations are administered. The format of the record should facilitate identification and recall of patients in need of immunization.

Records of children whose immunizations have been delayed or missed should be flagged to indicate the need to complete immunizations. For data that are required by the National Childhood Vaccine Injury Act of 1986, as well as data recommended by the AAP to be recorded in the patient's medical record for each immunization, see Informing Patients and Parents (p 4).

Vaccine Safety and Contraindications

RISKS AND ADVERSE EVENTS

All licensed vaccines in the United States are safe and effective, but no vaccine is absolutely safe and completely effective. Some vaccine recipients will have an untoward reaction, and some will not always be fully protected. The goal of vaccine development is to achieve the highest degree of protection with the lowest rate of untoward effects.

Risks of immunization may vary from trivial and inconvenient to severe and life-threatening. When developing immunization recommendations, vaccine benefits and safety are weighed against the risks of natural disease to the person and to the community. Recommendations attempt to maximize disease prevention and to minimize risk by providing specific advice on dose, route, and timing of the vaccine and by delineating persons who should be immunized and circumstances that warrant precaution or contraindicate immunization.

Common vaccine side effects usually are mild to moderate in severity and without permanent sequelae. Because such reactions are intrinsic to the immunizing antigen or some other component of the vaccine, they occur frequently and are unavoidable. Examples include local inflammation after administration of DTaP vaccine and fever and rash 1 to 2 weeks after administration of measles vaccine.

Sterile abscesses have occurred at the site of injection of several inactivated vaccines. The abscesses presumably result from the irritating nature of the vaccine or its adjuvant; in some instances, they may be caused by inadvertent subcutaneous inoculation of a vaccine intended for intramuscular use.

Rarely, serious adverse effects of immunization occur that can result in permanent sequelae or be life-threatening. These individual events are not predictable. In the United States, vaccine-associated paralytic poliomyelitis after administration of OPV vaccine to an apparently healthy child will no longer occur with the change to an IPV only vaccine schedule (see Childhood Immunization Schedule, Fig 1.1, p 22).

The occurrence of an adverse event after immunization does not prove that the vaccine caused the symptoms or signs. Vaccines are administered to infants and children during a period in their lives when certain clinical conditions most often become manifest (eg, seizure disorders). Association of an adverse clinical event with a specific vaccine is suggested if the event occurs at a significantly higher rate in recipients than in unimmunized groups of similar age and residence, or the same event occurs after sequential doses of the same vaccine. For most live-virus vaccines, definitive causative association between the vaccine and a subsequent illness requires isolating the vaccine strain from the patient.

Although a specific condition occurring in a single person after immunization does not provide sufficient evidence to establish that the condition was caused by the vaccine, reporting of adverse events after immunization is important because, in conjunction with other reports, it may provide clues to an unanticipated adverse reaction.

REPORTING OF ADVERSE EVENTS

Before administering a subsequent dose of any vaccine, parents and patients should be questioned about adverse effects and possible reactions after previous doses. No recommendations can anticipate all possible contingencies, particularly with newly licensed vaccines. Physicians should be alert to possible deviations from the expected outcome. Unexpected events occurring soon after administration of any vaccine, particularly those severe enough to require medical attention, should be described in detail in the patient's medical record and a VAERS (Vaccine Adverse Event Reporting System) report should be made, as subsequently described.

The National Childhood Vaccine Injury Act of 1986 requires physicians and other health care professionals who administer vaccines to maintain permanent immunization records and to report occurrences of certain adverse events stipulated in the act (see Appendix III, p 759) to VAERS.* The vaccines to which these requirements, as of January 2000, apply are measles, mumps, rubella, varicella, polio, hepatitis B, pertussis, diphtheria, tetanus, and *Haemophilus influenzae* B (see Record Keeping and Immunization Registries, p 30).

Clinically significant adverse events other than those listed in Appendix III, (p 759), or those occurring after administration of other vaccines, also should be reported to VAERS. Forms (see Fig 1.2, p 33) can be obtained from VAERS.

All reports of possible adverse events after administration of any vaccine, irrespective of the age of the recipient, are accepted. Submission of a report does not necessarily denote that the vaccine caused the adverse event. All patient-identifying information is kept confidential. Written notification that the report has been received is provided to the person submitting the form. Staff from VAERS will contact the reporter for follow-up of the patient's condition at 60 days and at 1 year after serious adverse events.

VACCINE SAFETY DATALINK PROJECT

To supplement the VAERS program, which is primarily a passive surveillance system, the CDC formed partnerships with 4 large health maintenance organizations to establish the Vaccine Safety Datalink (VSD) project, an active surveillance system designed to continually evaluate vaccine safety. The VSD project includes data on more than 6 million people. Medical records of the study population are monitored for potential adverse events resulting from immunization. The VSD project allows for planned vaccine safety studies, as well as for timely investigations of emerging vaccine safety concerns. The VSD concept to evaluate vaccine safety has been proven to be sound; previously known associations between febrile seizures and DTP immunization (day of immunization) and MMR immunization (days 8–14 after immunization) have been replicated in the study. Notable new findings from completed studies include the following: (1) MMR vaccine does not increase the occurrence of chronic arthropathy in women; (2) risk of aseptic meningitis followed Jeryl Lynn–derived strain of mumps virus vaccine in MMR vaccine is not increased; and (3) a second dose of MMR vaccine may result in a greater frequency of adverse events in the 10- to 12-year-old age group than in the 4- to 6-year-old age group. Additional studies are evaluating the risk of multiple sclerosis after hepatitis B immunization, the association of immunization with diabetes mellitus, MMR immunization and inflammatory bowel disease, and several other vaccine safety issues.

VACCINE INJURY COMPENSATION

The National Vaccine Injury Compensation Program is a no-fault system in which persons thought to have suffered an injury or death as a result of administration of a covered vaccine may seek compensation. Claims arising from covered vaccines must first be adjudicated through the program before civil litigation can be pursued. Developed as an alternative to civil litigation and operational since 1988, the program has reduced lawsuits against health care professionals and manufacturers, and helped to ensure a stable vaccine supply and marketplace.

* See Appendix I, Directory of Resources, p 743.

Figure 1.2. **VAERS form.**

For directions for completing form, see http://www.fda.gov/cber/vaers/new.htm/

VAERS

VACCINE ADVERSE EVENT REPORTING SYSTEM
24 Hour Toll-free information line 1-800-822-7967
P.O. Box 1100, Rockville, MD 20849-1100
PATIENT IDENTITY KEPT CONFIDENTIAL

For CDC/FDA Use Only
VAERS Number ______
Date Received ______

Patient Name:	Vaccine administered by (Name):	Form completed by (Name):
Last First M.I.	Responsible Physician ______	Relation to Patient ☐ Vaccine Provider ☐ Patient/Parent ☐ Manufacturer ☐ Other
Address	Facility Name/Address	Address *(if different from patient or provider)*
City State Zip	City State Zip	City State Zip
Telephone no. (____)______	Telephone no. (____)______	Telephone no. (____)______

1. State
2. County where administered
3. Date of birth __/__/__ (mm dd yy)
4. Patient age
5. Sex ☐M ☐F
6. Date form completed __/__/__ (mm dd yy)

7. Describe adverse event(s) (symptoms, signs, time course) and treatment, if any

8. Check all appropriate:
☐ Patient died (date __/__/__ mm dd yy)
☐ Life threatening illness
☐ Required emergency room/doctor visit
☐ Required hospitalization (_____days)
☐ Resulted in prolongation of hospitalization
☐ Resulted in permanent disability
☐ None of the above

9. Patient recovered ☐ YES ☐ NO ☐ UNKNOWN

10. Date of vaccination __/__/__ (mm dd yy) Time______ AM PM

11. Adverse event onset __/__/__ (mm dd yy) Time______ AM PM

12. Relevant diagnostic tests/laboratory data

13. Enter all vaccines given on date listed in no. 10

	Vaccine (type)	Manufacturer	Lot number	Route/Site	No. Previous doses
a.					
b.					
c.					
d.					

14. Any other vaccinations within 4 weeks prior to the date listed in no. 10

	Vaccine (type)	Manufacturer	Lot number	Route/Site	No. Previous doses	Date given
a.						
b.						

15. Vaccinated at:
☐ Private doctor's office/hospital ☐ Military clinic/hospital
☐ Public health clinic/hospital ☐ Other/unknown

16. Vaccine purchased with:
☐ Private funds ☐ Military funds
☐ Public funds ☐ Other /unknown

17. Other medications

18. Illness at time of vaccination (specify)

19. Pre-existing physician-diagnosed allergies, birth defects, medical conditions (specify)

20. Have you reported this adverse event previously? ☐ No ☐ To health department ☐ To doctor ☐ To manufacturer

Only for children 5 and under

22. Birth weight ____ lb. ____ oz.

23. No. of brothers and sisters

21. Adverse event following prior vaccination (check all applicable, specify)

	Adverse Event	Onset Age	Type Vaccine	Dose no. in series
☐ In patient				
☐ In brother or sister				

Only for reports submitted by manufacturer/immunization project

24. Mfr. / imm. proj. report no.

25. Date received by mfr. / imm. proj.

26. 15 day report? ☐ Yes ☐ No

27. Report type ☐ Initial ☐ Follow-Up

Health care providers and manufacturers are required by law (42 USC 300aa-25) to report reactions to vaccines listed in the Table of Reportable Events Following Immunization. Reports for reactions to other vaccines are voluntary except when required as a condition of immunization grant awards.

Form VAERS-1

The program is based on a Vaccine Injury Table (VIT; see Appendix III, p 759) listing the vaccines covered by the program, as well as injuries, disabilities, illnesses, and conditions (including death) for which compensation may be awarded. The VIT defines the time during which the first symptoms or significant aggravation of an injury must appear after immunization. If an injury listed in the VIT is proven, claimants receive a "legal presumption of causation," thus avoiding the need to prove causation in an individual case. If the claim pertains to conditions not listed in the VIT, claimants may prevail if they prove causation.

Additional information about the Program and the VIT are available from the following:

National Vaccine Injury Compensation Program
Health Resources and Services Administration
Parklawn Bldg, Room 8A-46
5600 Fishers Ln
Rockville, MD 20857
Telephone: 800-338-2382
Web site: http://www.hrsa.dhhs.gov/bhp/vicp/

Persons wishing to file a claim for a vaccine injury should telephone or write to the following:

United States Court of Federal Claims
717 Madison Pl, NW
Washington, DC 20005-1011
Telephone: 202-219-9657

PRECAUTIONS AND CONTRAINDICATIONS

Precautions and contraindications to immunization are described in specific chapters on vaccine-preventable diseases and in the manufacturer's product labeling (ie, package insert). A contraindication indicates that a vaccine should not be administered. In contrast, a precaution specifies a situation in which vaccine may be indicated if, after careful assessment, the benefit of immunization to the individual patient is judged to outweigh the risk. Contraindications and precautions may be generic and apply to all vaccines, or they may be specific to one or more vaccines.

Minor illness with or without fever does not contraindicate immunization. Most vaccines are intended for use in healthy persons or in persons whose diseases or conditions are not affected by immunization. For optimal safety, vaccines should not be used if an undesirable side effect or adverse reaction to the vaccine may seriously affect or be confused with an underlying illness. A common situation is the child needing immunization who has a minor illness with or without fever (temperature, ≥38°C [≥100°F]). No evidence indicates an increased risk of adverse events or a reduction in effectiveness associated with immunization administered during a minor illness. Deferring immunization in such situations constitutes a missed opportunity and frequently results in unimmunized or inadequately immunized children who may develop or transmit vaccine-preventable disease.

Fever per se is not a contraindication to immunization. For the child with an acute febrile illness (temperature, ≥38°C [≥100°F]), guidelines for immunization are based on the physician's assessment of the child's illness and the specific vaccines the child is scheduled to receive. However, if fever or other manifestations suggest a moderate or serious illness, the child should not be immunized until recovered. Specific recommendations are as follows:

- ***Live-virus vaccines.*** Minor respiratory, gastrointestinal, or other illnesses with or without fever do not contraindicate the use of live-virus vaccines, such as MMR or varicella. Children with febrile upper respiratory tract infections have serologic responses similar to those of well children after immunization. The potential benefit of immunization at the recommended age, irrespective of the presence of a minor illness, outweighs the possible increased risk of vaccine failure.
- ***DTaP.*** Mild illnesses (eg, upper respiratory tract illnesses) do not contraindicate administration of DTaP. However, a moderate or severe illness with or without fever is a reason to delay immunization, in part because evolving signs and symptoms associated with the illness may be difficult to distinguish from a vaccine reaction.
- ***Child with frequent febrile illnesses.*** A child who has moderate or severe febrile illnesses at the time of scheduled immunizations should be asked to return as soon as the current febrile illness resolves so that immunization can be completed.
- ***Immunocompromised children.*** Special consideration needs to be given to immunocompromised children, such as those with congenital immunodeficiencies, human immunodeficiency virus infection, malignant neoplasm, or recipients of immunosuppressive therapy (see Immunocompromised Children, p 56).

A concise summary of contraindications to and precautions for immunizations is given in the Standards for Pediatric Immunization Practices (see Appendix II, p 748).

HYPERSENSITIVITY REACTIONS TO VACCINE CONSTITUENTS

Hypersensitivity reactions to constituents of vaccines are rare. In some instances, although symptoms appear soon after a vaccine is administered, differentiation between an allergic reaction to the vaccine and a reaction to an environmental allergen is not possible. Facilities and personnel should be available for treating immediate hypersensitivity reactions in all settings where vaccines are administered. This recommendation does not preclude administration of vaccines in school-based or other nonclinic settings. Whenever possible, patients should be observed for an allergic reaction for 15 to 20 minutes after receiving immunization(s).

The 4 types of hypersensitivity reactions considered related to vaccine constituents are (1) allergic reactions to egg-related antigens; (2) mercury sensitivity in some recipients of mercury-containing immune globulins and some vaccines (see Thimerosal content of some vaccines and immune globulin preparations, p 36); (3) antibiotic-induced allergic reactions; and (4) hypersensitivity to other vaccine components, including the infectious agent.

Allergic Reactions to Egg-Related Antigens. Current measles and mumps vaccines are derived from chick embryo fibroblast tissue cultures but do not contain significant amounts of egg cross-reacting proteins. Recent studies indicate that children with egg allergy, even those with severe hypersensitivity, are at low risk for anaphylactic reactions to these vaccines, singly or in combination (ie, MMR), and that skin testing with dilute vaccine is not predictive of an allergic reaction to immunization. Most immediate hypersensitivity reactions following MMR appear to be reactions to other vaccine components, such as gelatin or neomycin. Therefore, children with egg allergy routinely may be given MMR, measles, or mumps vaccine without prior skin testing.

Current yellow fever and influenza vaccines contain egg proteins and on rare occasions may induce immediate allergic reactions, including anaphylaxis. Skin testing with yellow fever vaccines is recommended before administration to persons with a history of systemic anaphylactic symptoms (generalized urticaria, hypotension, or manifestations of upper or lower airway obstruction) after egg ingestion. Skin testing also has been used for children with severe anaphylactic reactions to eggs who are to receive influenza vaccine, but these children generally should not receive influenza vaccine because of the risk of reaction, the likely need for yearly immunization, and the availability of chemoprophylaxis against influenza infection (see Influenza, p 351). Less severe or local manifestations of allergy to egg or to feathers are not contraindications to yellow fever or influenza vaccine administration and do not warrant vaccine skin testing.

An egg-sensitive person can be tested with vaccine (eg, yellow fever vaccine) before its use as follows:

- ***Scratch, prick, or puncture test.*** A drop of 1:10 dilution of the vaccine in physiologic saline is applied at the site of a superficial scratch, prick, or puncture on the volar surface of the forearm. Positive (histamine) and negative (physiologic saline) control tests also should be used. The test is read after 15 to 20 minutes. A positive test result is a wheal 3 mm larger than that of the saline control, usually with surrounding erythema. The histamine control must be positive for valid interpretation. If the result of this test is negative, an ID test is performed.
- ***Intradermal test.*** A dose of 0.02 mL of a 1:100 dilution of the vaccine in physiologic saline is injected intradermally; positive- and negative-control skin tests are performed concurrently. A wheal 5 mm or larger than the negative control with surrounding erythema is considered a positive reaction.

If these test results are negative, the vaccine may be given. If the child's test result is positive, the vaccine still may be given using a desensitization procedure if immunization is considered warranted because of a person's risk from the disease. A suggested protocol is subcutaneous administration of the following successive doses of vaccine at 15- to 20-minute intervals as follows:

1. 0.05 mL of 1:10 dilution
2. 0.05 mL of full strength
3. 0.10 mL of full strength
4. 0.15 mL of full strength
5. 0.20 mL of full strength

Scratch, prick, or puncture tests with other allergens have resulted in fatalities in highly allergic persons. **Although such untoward effects have not been reported for vaccine testing, all skin tests and desensitization procedures should be performed by trained personnel experienced in the management of anaphylaxis.** Necessary medications and equipment should be readily available (see Treatment of Anaphylactic Reactions, p 51).

Thimerosal content of some vaccines and immune globulin preparations. Thimerosal is a mercury-containing preservative that has been used as an additive to biologics and vaccines since the 1930s because of its effectiveness in preventing bacterial and fungal contamination, particularly in open multidose containers. Because of the acknowledged value of reducing exposures to mercury, vaccine manufacturers, the FDA, other public health service agencies, and the AAP are working together to remove thimerosal from vaccines that contain this compound without causing disruptions in the recommended childhood immunization schedule. Vaccines that contain thimerosal include some DTaP and Hib products, DT, dT, one hepatitis B product, all influenza vaccines, meningococcal vaccine, one pneumococcal vaccine, and one rabies vaccine. None of the live-virus vaccines contain thimerosal. A complete listing of thimerosal content of vaccines has been published.*

Information about the goal of obtaining a vaccine supply free of vaccines that contain thimerosal, changes in thimerosal content of vaccines, and additional recommendations will be updated on the AAP Web site (http://www.aap.org/). The only nonvaccine biologics that contain thimerosal in active production and US distribution are Rh_0 (D) Immune Globulin, Vaccinia Immune Globulin, Bio Port Corporation's Human Immune Globulin, and certain antivenins. Immune Globulin Intravenous does not contain preservatives including thimerosal.

Antibiotic-Induced Allergic Reactions. Antibiotic reactions have been suspected in persons with known allergies who received vaccines containing trace amounts of antibiotics (see package insert for each product for specific listing). Proof of a causal relationship is difficult and often impossible to confirm.

The IPV vaccine contains trace amounts of streptomycin, neomycin, and polymyxin B. Live-virus measles, mumps, rubella (singly or in combination as MMR), and varicella vaccines have trace quantities of neomycin. Some persons allergic to neomycin may experience a delayed-type local reaction 48 to 96 hours after administration of IPV, MMR, or varicella vaccines. The reaction consists of an erythematous pruritic papule. This minor reaction is of little importance compared with the benefit of immunization and should not be considered a contraindication. However, if a person has a history of anaphylactic reaction to neomycin, neomycin-containing vaccines should not be used. No currently recommended vaccine contains penicillin or its derivatives.

Hypersensitivity to Other Vaccine Components, Including the Infectious Agent. Some live-virus vaccines, such as MMR, varicella, and yellow fever, contain gelatin as a stabilizer. Persons with a history of food allergy to gelatin rarely develop anaphylaxis after receipt of gelatin-containing vaccines. Skin testing is a consideration for these persons before administration of a gelatin-containing vaccine, but no protocol or reported experience is available. Because gelatin used in the United States as a vaccine stabilizer usually is porcine, and food gelatins may be derived solely from bovine sources, a negative food history does not exclude the possibility of an immunization reaction.

Plague, cholera, and parenterally administered inactivated whole-cell typhoid vaccines infrequently are associated with local and, occasionally, systemic reactions, usually of a toxic rather than a hypersensitivity nature. Such reactions occur with DTaP vaccines but are much less frequent than with DTP vaccines. On occasion, urticarial or anaphylactic reactions have occurred in recipients of DTP, DTaP,

* American Academy of Pediatrics Committee on Infectious Diseases and Committee on Environmental Health. Thimerosal in vaccines: an interim report to clinicians. *Pediatrics.* 1999;104:570–574

DT, dT, or tetanus toxoid vaccine. Tetanus and diphtheria antigen-specific antibodies of the IgE type have been identified in some of these patients. Although attributing a specific sensitivity to vaccine components is difficult, an immediate, severe, or anaphylactic allergic reaction to one of these vaccines is a contraindication to subsequent immunization of the patient with the specific product. A transient urticarial rash, however, is not a contraindication to further doses (see Pertussis, p 435).

Persons who have high serum concentrations of tetanus IgG antibody, usually as the result of frequent booster immunizations, can have an increased incidence and severity of reactions to subsequent vaccine administration (see Tetanus, p 563).

Reactions resembling serum sickness have been reported in approximately 6% of patients after a booster dose of human diploid rabies vaccine, probably due to sensitization to human albumin that had been altered chemically by the virus-inactivating agent. Measles and rabies vaccines contain albumin, a derivative of human blood. Because of effective donor screening and product manufacturing processes, the FDA believes the risk for transmission of any viral disease from albumin in these vaccines is rare.

Japanese encephalitis virus vaccine has been associated with generalized urticaria and angioedema, sometimes with respiratory distress and hypotension occurring within minutes of immunization to as long as 2 weeks after immunization. The pathogenesis of such reactions is not understood. Persons with a history of urticaria are at increased risk for an adverse reaction. Vaccine recipients should be observed for 30 minutes after immunization and warned about the possibility of delayed urticaria and potentially life-threatening angioedema.

Significant hypersensitivity reactions occurring as a result of pneumococcal, Hib, hepatitis B, hepatitis A, or poliovirus vaccines are rare.

MISCONCEPTIONS ABOUT VACCINE CONTRAINDICATIONS

Some health care professionals inappropriately consider certain conditions or circumstances to be contraindications to immunization. Common conditions or circumstances that are **not** contraindications include the following:

- Mild acute illness with low-grade fever or mild diarrheal illness in an otherwise well child
- The convalescent phase of illness
- Current antimicrobial therapy
- Reaction to a previous DTaP or DTP dose that involved only soreness, redness, or swelling in the immediate vicinity of the immunization site or temperature of less than 40.5°C (105°F)
- Prematurity. The appropriate age for initiating most immunizations in the prematurely born infant is the usually recommended chronologic age. Vaccine doses should not be reduced for preterm infants (see Preterm Infants, p 54, and Hepatitis B, p 289).
- Pregnancy of mother or other household contact. Vaccine viruses in MMR vaccine are not transmitted by vaccine recipients. Although varicella vaccine virus has been transmitted by a healthy vaccine recipient to contacts, the frequency is rare, only mild or symptomatic infection has been reported, and use of this vaccine is not

contraindicated by pregnancy of either the child's mother or other household contacts (see Varicella-Zoster Infections, p 624).

- Recent exposure to an infectious disease
- Breastfeeding. The only vaccine virus that has been isolated from human milk is rubella vaccine virus. No evidence indicates that human milk from women immunized against rubella is harmful to infants.
- A history of nonspecific allergies or relatives with allergies
- Allergies to penicillin or any other antibiotic, except anaphylactic reactions to neomycin or streptomycin (see Hypersensitivity Reactions to Vaccine Constituents, p 35). These reactions occur rarely, if ever. None of the vaccines licensed in the United States contain penicillin.
- Allergies to duck meat or duck feathers. No vaccine available in the United States is produced in substrates containing duck antigens.
- Family history of seizures in a person considered for pertussis or measles immunization (see Children With a Personal or Family History of Seizures, p 68)
- Family history of sudden infant death syndrome in children considered for DTaP immunization
- Family history of an adverse event, unrelated to immunosuppression, after immunization
- Malnutrition

Reporting of Vaccine-Preventable Diseases

Most vaccine-preventable diseases are reportable throughout the United States. Public health officials depend on health care professionals to report promptly to state or local health departments suspected cases of vaccine-preventable disease. These reports are transmitted weekly to the CDC and are used to detect outbreaks, monitor disease-control strategies, and evaluate national immunization practices and policies.

Standards for Pediatric Immunization Practices (see Appendix II, p 748)

In 1992, national *Standards for Pediatric Immunization Practices* were recommended by the National Vaccine Advisory Committee, approved by the US Public Health Service, and endorsed by the AAP. These standards are recommended for use by all health care professionals providing care in public or private health care settings who are involved in the administration of vaccines or management of immunization services for children. Their use is intended to improve preschool immunization rates, prevent vaccine-preventable disease outbreaks, and achieve the national objectives for immunization.

Parental Misconceptions About Immunizations

Misconceptions about the need for and safety of routine childhood immunizations are potential causes of delayed immunization, underimmunization, or both in the United States. Several common misconceptions of parents have been addressed by the CDC (*6 Common Misconceptions About Vaccination and How to Respond to Them,* National Immunization Program, CDC, 1996; available at: http://www.cdc.gov/nip/publications/6mishome.htm). In an effort to inform parents further, the AAP has published a brochure entitled *Immunizations: What You Should Know.* These documents address common questions about routine childhood immunizations, including the following:

- **"Why should children be immunized when most vaccine-preventable diseases have been eliminated in the United States?"** While immunizations have dramatically reduced the incidence of a number of childhood diseases in the United States, many of these diseases remain prevalent in other areas of the world and easily could be introduced into the United States and without immunization could spread quickly. Unimmunized children also will be at risk throughout their lives, including when they travel to countries where vaccine-preventable diseases are endemic.
- **"Do immunizations work? Haven't most people who get a vaccine-preventable disease been immunized?"** A few people do not respond to vaccines, but most childhood vaccines are 85% to 98% effective. Therefore, while some immunized children will develop the disease, the vast majority are protected.
- **"Aren't some vaccine lots more dangerous than others?"** All vaccines are licensed and monitored before and after release by the FDA. No evidence indicates that individual lots of commonly used vaccines differ in safety.
- **"Isn't giving children more than one immunization at a time dangerous?"** Numerous studies have shown that recommended routine childhood immunizations can be given safely at the same time.

Health care professionals should obtain and distribute copies of CDC and AAP immunization documents, as well as the vaccine information statements, to parents to address their questions and concerns. These resource materials can assist parents to make informed decisions about immunizing their children. Other sources of objective vaccine information are available (see the following list of selected authoritative Web sites) that can help health care professionals respond to questions and misconceptions about immunizations and vaccine-preventable diseases.

Alleged adverse events following immunization initially may be published in the mass media. Some parents will want immediate answers to their questions. Health care professionals should refer to the following Web sites to help them address the questions posed by parents. Efforts usually are made to address questions raised by the media within 24 to 48 hours. Alternatively, physicians can call the CDC Hotline at 1-800-232-2522.

In addition, the **National Network for Immunization Information** (NNII), an initiative of the Infectious Diseases Society of America, the Pediatric Infectious Diseases Society, the AAP, and the American Nurses Association, provides education and communication about immunization issues. Immunization information can be found on the NNII Web site at http://www.idsociety.org/vaccine/. The NNII also recommends additional reliable resources for current immunization information.

- **Questions and Answers About Vaccine Safety** (http://www.cdc.gov/nip/vacsafe)
- **Key Health Communication Messages: Vaccine Safety and Injury Compensation** (http://www.cdc.gov/nip/news/keymess.htm)

- **What Would Happen If We Stopped Immunizations?** (http://www.cdc.gov/nip/vacsafe/fs/valuefs.htm)
- **Vaccine Safety Fact Sheets** (with index to topics) (http://www.cdc.gov/nip/vacsafe/fs/vaxsaft.htm)
- **American Academy of Pediatrics** (www.aap.org)

Other Web sites for vaccine and immunization information include the following:

- **Institute for Vaccine Safety** (http://www.vaccinesafety.edu)
- **Immunization Action Coalition** (http://www.immunize.org)
- **National Vaccine Program Office** (http://www.cdc.gov/od/nvpo/)

PASSIVE IMMUNIZATION

Passive immunization entails administration of preformed antibody to a recipient. Passive immunization is indicated in the following general circumstances for prevention or amelioration of infectious diseases:

- When persons are deficient in synthesis of antibody as a result of congenital or acquired B-lymphocyte defects, alone or in combination with other immunodeficiencies
- When a person susceptible to a disease is exposed to or has a high likelihood of exposure to that infection, especially when that person has a high risk of complications from the disease (eg, a child with leukemia exposed to varicella or measles), or when time does not permit adequate protection by active immunization alone (eg, some postexposure situations involving measles, rabies, or hepatitis B)
- Therapeutically, when a disease is already present, antibody may ameliorate or aid in suppressing the effects of a toxin (eg, foodborne or wound botulism, diphtheria, or tetanus) or suppress the inflammatory response (eg, Kawasaki disease)

Passive immunization or serotherapy has been accomplished with several different types of products. The choice is dictated by the types of products available, the type of antibody desired, the route of administration, timing, and other considerations. These products include Immune Globulin (IG) and specific ("hyperimmune") immune globulin preparations given intramuscularly (eg, Hepatitis B Immune Globulin [HBIG]), Immune Globulin Intravenous (IGIV), specific (hyperimmune) immune globulins given by the intravenous (IV) route (eg, Respiratory Syncytial Virus IGIV [RSV-IGIV]), human plasma, and antibodies of animal origin.

Indications for administration of immune globulin preparations other than those relevant to infectious diseases are not reviewed in the *Red Book*. Examples include immune thrombocytopenic purpura and Guillain-Barré syndrome.

Whole blood and blood components for transfusion (including plasma) from registered blood banks in the United States are tested for the presence of bloodborne pathogens, including syphilis, hepatitis B virus, hepatitis C virus (HCV), human immunodeficiency virus (HIV)-1, HIV-2, and human T-lymphotropic viruses (HTLV-I and II), (see Blood Safety, p 88). A similar array of tests is performed by US-licensed establishments that collect plasma used only to manufacture plasma derivatives, such as IGIV, IG, and specific immune globulins. United

States–licensed IG and specific immune globulin preparations have not transmitted any of these diseases. Hepatitis C virus transmission in 1994 was associated with administration of IGIV produced by 1 manufacturer, and, as a result of this outbreak, the US Food and Drug Administration (FDA) now requires that IGIV and other immune globulin preparations for intravenous administration undergo additional manufacturing procedures that inactivate or remove viruses.

Immune Globulin

Immune Globulin is derived from the pooled plasma of adults by an alcohol-fractionation procedure. It consists primarily of the immunoglobulin (Ig) fraction (at least 95% IgG and trace amounts of IgA and IgM), is sterile, and is not known to transmit hepatotropic viruses, HIV, or any other infectious disease agent. Immune Globulin is a concentrated protein solution (approximately 16.5% or 165 mg/mL) containing specific antibodies in proportion to the infectious and immunization experience of the population from whose plasma it was prepared. Large numbers of donors (at least 1000 donors per lot of final product) are used to ensure inclusion of a broad spectrum of antibodies.

Immune Globulin is recommended for intramuscular (IM) administration. Because some recipients experience local pain and most experience local discomfort, IG should be administered deep into a large muscle mass, usually in the gluteal region or anterior thigh of a child (see Site and Route of Immunization, p 16). The amount of discomfort is lessened if the IG is at room temperature when administered. No more than 5 mL ordinarily should be administered in 1 site in an adult or large child; lesser amounts per site (1-3 mL) should be given to small children and infants. Administration of more than 20 mL at any one time is seldom, if ever, warranted.

Peak serum concentrations of antibodies usually are achieved 48 to 72 hours after intramuscular administration. The serum half-life generally is 3 to 4 weeks. Some investigators have used slow subcutaneous administration in special circumstances, such as for immunodeficient patients.

Intravenous use of IG is contraindicated. Intradermal use of IG is not recommended.

INDICATIONS FOR THE USE OF IG

Replacement Therapy in Antibody-Deficiency Disorders. The usual dosage is 100 mg/kg (equivalent to 0.66 mL/kg) per month intramuscularly. Customary practice is to administer twice this dose initially and to adjust the interval (2 to 4 weeks) between administration of the doses, based on the trough IgG concentrations and on the clinical response (absence of or decrease in infections). In most cases, however, IG has been replaced by IGIV. Studies in adolescents and adults with antibody deficiencies indicate that slow subcutaneous administration of IG is safe, less expensive than IGIV, convenient, and suitable for home therapy. Systemic allergic reactions occurred in fewer than 1% of infusions, and local tissue reactions generally were mild.

Hepatitis A Prophylaxis. Immune Globulin can prevent clinical disease resulting from hepatitis A virus in exposed susceptible persons when given within 14 days of exposure. Indications include foreign travel by children younger than 2 years of age and postexposure prophylaxis (see Hepatitis A, p 280).

Measles Prophylaxis. Immune Globulin administered to exposed, measles-susceptible persons will prevent or modify infection if given within 6 days of exposure (see Measles, p 385).

ADVERSE REACTIONS TO IG

- The most common problem encountered with the use of IG is discomfort and pain at the site of administration (which is lessened if the preparation is at room temperature at the time of injection). Less common reactions include flushing, headache, chills, and nausea.
- Serious reactions are uncommon; these may involve chest pain or constriction, dyspnea, or anaphylaxis and systemic collapse. An increased risk of systemic reaction results from inadvertent intravenous administration. Persons requiring repeated doses of IG have been reported to experience systemic reactions, such as fever, chills, sweating, uncomfortable sensations, and shock.
- Because IG contains trace amounts of IgA, persons who are selectively serum IgA-deficient in rare cases can develop anti-IgA antibodies and react to a subsequent dose of IG, whole-blood transfusion, or plasma infusion with systemic symptoms, including chills, fever, and shock-like symptoms. In the rare cases in which reactions related to anti-IgA antibodies have occurred, use of IgA-depleted IGIV preparations may reduce the likelihood of further reactions. Because of the rarity of these reactions, routine screening for IgA deficiency is not recommended.
- Healthy persons given IG may develop antibodies against heterologous IgG allotypes. Usually, this phenomenon has no clinical significance; however, on rare occasions, a systemic reaction can result.
- Immune Globulin Intravenous, most IG, and specific immune globulin preparations do not contain thimerosal (see Thimerosal content of some vaccines and immune globulin preparations, p 36).

PRECAUTIONS FOR THE USE OF IG

- Caution should be used when giving IG to a patient with history of adverse reactions to IG.
- Although systemic reactions to IG are rare (see Adverse Reactions to IG, above), epinephrine and other means of treating acute reactions should be immediately available.
- Immune Globulin is not approved by the FDA for use in patients with severe thrombocytopenia or any coagulation disorder that would preclude intramuscular injection. In such cases, use of IGIV is preferred.
- Screening for IgA deficiency is not recommended routinely for potential recipients of IG (see Adverse Reactions to IG).

Specific Immune Globulins

Specific immune globulins, termed "hyperimmune globulins," differ from other immune globulin preparations in the selection of donors and may differ in the number of donors whose plasma is included in the pool from which the product is prepared. Donors known to have high titers of the desired antibody, either naturally acquired or stimulated by immunization, are selected. These preparations are prepared by the same procedure as other immune globulin preparations. Specific immune globulin preparations for use in infectious diseases include HBIG, Rabies Immune Globulin, Tetanus Immune Globulin, Varicella-Zoster Immune Globulin, Cytomegalovirus (CMV) IGIV, and RSV-IGIV. An intramuscularly administered monoclonal antibody preparation for prevention of RSV is available. Recommendations for use of these globulins are given in the discussion of specific diseases in Section 3. The precautions and adverse reactions for IG and IGIV also are applicable to the specific immune globulins.

Immune Globulin Intravenous

Immune Globulin Intravenous is derived from pooled plasma of adults by an alcohol-fractionation procedure, which is modified by individual manufacturers so as to yield a product suitable for IV use. The donor pool is like that of IG. The FDA specifies that all preparations must have a minimum concentration of measles, diphtheria, polio, and hepatitis B antibodies. Antibody concentrations against common pathogens, such as *Streptococcus pneumoniae,* vary widely between products and even among lots of the same product. Immune Globulin Intravenous consists primarily of the immunoglobulin fraction (more than 95% IgG and trace amounts of IgA and IgM). The protein content varies, depending on the product; both liquid and dried products are available. Immune Globulin Intravenous does not contain thimerosal.

INDICATIONS FOR THE USE OF IGIV

During the 1980s, IGIV was developed as an infusion product that allowed patients with primary immunodeficiencies to receive enough immune globulin at monthly intervals to protect them from infection until their next infusion. Since then, the FDA and the National Institutes of Health have expanded the recommended uses for IGIV (see Table 1.6, p 45).* This product also may be useful for other conditions. Since November 1997, a shortage of IGIV has existed in the United States because of production impediments related to compliance and withdrawals based on the theoretical risk for contamination with the Creutzfeldt-Jakob disease (CJD) agent. Other problems include increased administration for approved and unapproved uses, wastage, and export of IGIV. In August 1998, the US Surgeon General recommended that plasma derivatives including IGIV be withdrawn only if the blood donor developed variant CJD (see Blood Safety, p 88). The FDA is using several methods to improve IGIV distribution to patients. Clinicians should review

* Centers for Disease Control and Prevention. Availability of immune globulin intravenous for treatment of immune deficient patients: United States, 1997–1998. *MMWR Morb Mortal Wkly Rep.* 1999;48:159–162

Table 1.6. **US Food and Drug Administration and National Institutes of Health (NIH) Recommendations for Use of Immune Globulin Intravenous.**

Primary immunodeficiencies
Kawasaki disease
Pediatric human immunodeficiency virus infection
Chronic B-cell lymphocytic leukemia
Recent bone marrow transplantation in adults
Immune-mediated thrombocytopenia
Chronic inflammatory demyelinating polyneuropathy*

* Approved only by the NIH Consensus Development Conference.

their IGIV use to ensure consistency with current recommendations. The use of IGIV for other conditions needs to be supported by adequate scientific evidence of effectiveness.

Approval by the FDA of specific indications for a manufacturer's IGIV product is based on availability of data from one or more clinical trials. Thus, not all licensed products are approved for each of the indications listed in Table 1.6 (see above); in some cases only a single product has the indication in its product label. Therapeutic differences among IGIV products of different manufacturers may exist but have not been demonstrated. Recommended indications in children and adolescents for the prevention or treatment of infectious diseases include the following:

- ***Replacement therapy in antibody-deficiency disorders.*** The usual dosage of IGIV in immunodeficiency syndromes is 300 to 400 mg/kg of body weight administered once a month by IV infusion. Dosage and frequency of infusions, however, should be based on the effectiveness in the individual patient. Effective dosages have ranged from 200 to 800 mg/kg monthly. Maintenance of a trough IgG concentration of at least 500 mg/dL (5 g/L) has been demonstrated to correlate with clinical response.
- ***Kawasaki disease.*** Administration of IGIV within the first 10 days of the illness shortens the duration of fever and decreases the frequency of coronary artery abnormalities (see Kawasaki disease, p 360).
- ***Pediatric HIV infection.*** The value of IGIV in children with HIV infection has been evaluated in several trials. The Working Group on Antiretroviral Therapy and Medical Management of Infants, Children, and Adolescents with HIV Infection* has recommended IGIV therapy for children with any of the following: (1) significant recurrent bacterial infections despite appropriate antimicrobial prophylaxis in infants and children who have humoral immune defects, (2) absence of detectable antibody to measles in children who have received 2 doses of measles vaccine and who live in regions with a high prevalence of measles, (3) HIV-associated thrombocytopenia despite antiretroviral therapy, and

* Antiretroviral therapy and medical management of pediatric HIV infection and 1997 USPHS/IDSA report on the prevention of opportunistic infections in persons infected with human immunodeficiency virus. *Pediatrics.* 1998;102(suppl):999–1085

(4) chronic bronchiectasis that is suboptimally responsive to antimicrobial and pulmonary therapy.

- ***Hypogammaglobulinemia in chronic lymphocytic leukemia.*** Administration of IGIV to adults with this disease has been demonstrated to reduce the incidence of serious bacterial infections, although its cost-effectiveness has been questioned.
- ***Bone marrow transplantation.*** Immune Globulin Intravenous may reduce the incidence of infection and death but not acute graft-vs-host disease (GVHD) in pediatric bone marrow recipients. In adult transplant recipients, IGIV decreases the incidence of interstitial pneumonia (presumably caused by CMV), reduces the risk of sepsis and other bacterial infections, decreases the incidence of acute GVHD (but not overall mortality), and, in conjunction with ganciclovir, is effective in the treatment of some patients with CMV pneumonia.

Immune Globulin Intravenous has been used in many other conditions.

- ***Low-birth-weight infants.*** Results of some clinical trials have indicated that IGIV decreases the incidence of late-onset infections in infants who weigh less than 1500 g at birth, but other studies have not confirmed these results. Trials have varied in IGIV dosage, time of administration, and other aspects of study design. A large multicenter placebo-controlled trial, however, concluded that IGIV was beneficial for very-low-birth-weight infants. At present, IGIV is not recommended for routine use in preterm infants to prevent late-onset infection.
- ***Equal to other therapy.*** Guillain-Barré syndrome.
- ***May be useful.*** Anemia because of parvovirus B19, patients with stable multiple myeloma who are at high risk for recurrent infection, CMV-negative recipients of CMV-positive organs, hypogammaglobulinemic neonates with a risk factor for infection or morbidity, intractable epilepsy, systemic vasculitic syndromes, warm-type autoimmune hemolytic anemia, neonatal alloimmune thrombocytopenia when unresponsive to other treatments, immune-mediated neutropenia, decompensation in myasthenia gravis, dermatomyositis, polymyositis, and severe thrombocytopenia that is unresponsive to other treatments.

ADVERSE REACTIONS TO IGIV

The reported incidence of adverse events associated with the administration of IGIV ranges from 1% to 15% but usually is less than 5%. Most of these reactions are mild and self-limited. Severe reactions occur infrequently and usually do not contraindicate further IGIV therapy. Adverse events include the following:

- Pyrogenic reactions marked by high fever, chills, and systemic symptoms
- Minor systemic reactions with headache, myalgia, anxiety, light-headedness, nausea, or vomiting
- Vasomotor or cardiovascular manifestations, marked by flushing, changes in blood pressure, and tachycardia
- Aseptic meningitis
- Hypersensitivity reactions
- Acute renal failure

Anaphylactic reactions induced by anti-IgA can occur in patients with primary antibody deficiency who have a total absence of circulating IgA and have IgG antibodies to IgA. These reactions are rare in panhypogammaglobulinemic persons and potentially more common in patients with selective IgA deficiency and subclass IgG deficiencies. In the rare instances in which reactions related to anti-IgA antibodies have occurred, use of IgA-depleted IGIV preparations will reduce the likelihood of further reactions. Avoidance of anaphylactic reactions, however, may require the use of globulin preparations that are completely devoid of IgA. Because of the extreme rarity of these reactions, screening for IgA deficiency is not recommended routinely.

An outbreak of hepatitis C occurred in the United States in 1994 among recipients of IGIV lots from a single domestic manufacturer. Procedures and requirements in the preparation of IGIV subsequently have been instituted to prevent transmission of HCV by IGIV.

PRECAUTIONS FOR THE USE OF IGIV

- Caution should be used when giving IGIV to a patient with a history of adverse reactions to immune globulin.
- Because systemic reactions to IGIV may occur (see Adverse Reactions to IGIV), epinephrine and other means for treating acute reactions should be immediately available.
- Adverse reactions often can be alleviated by reducing either the rate or the volume of infusion. For patients with repeated severe reactions unresponsive to these measures, hydrocortisone, 1 to 2 mg/kg, can be given intravenously 30 minutes before infusion. Using a different IGIV preparation or pretreatment with diphenhydramine, acetaminophen, or aspirin also may be helpful.
- Seriously ill patients with compromised cardiac function who are receiving large volumes of IGIV may be at increased risk of vasomotor or cardiac complications manifested by elevated blood pressure, cardiac failure, or both.
- Screening for IgA deficiency is not recommended routinely for potential recipients of IGIV (see Adverse Reactions to IGIV).

Human Plasma

The use of human plasma for control of infectious diseases should be limited. Human plasma has been administered to patients with burns in an attempt to control *Pseudomonas* infections, but data are insufficient to substantiate this use. Plasma infusions have been useful for treating infants who have protein-losing enteropathy. Plasma infusions also have been substituted for IG for some patients with IgG antibody deficiency when they develop adverse reactions to IG or fail to respond to treatment with IG; however, these immunodeficient patients can be managed with IGIV (or by slow subcutaneous administration of IG).

Antibodies of Animal Origin (Animal Antisera)

Products of animal origin are derived from serum of horses. Experimental products prepared in other species also may be available. These products are derived by concentrating the serum globulin fraction with ammonium sulfate. Some, but not all, products also are subjected to an enzyme digestion process in an attempt to decrease reactions to foreign proteins.

Use of the following products is discussed in the disease-specific chapters in Section 3:

- Botulism antitoxin (equine), trivalent (types A, B, E)
- Diphtheria antitoxin (equine)
- Equine tetanus antitoxin (not available in the United States)
- Rabies equine globulin (equine rabies antiserum) (not available in the United States)

INDICATIONS FOR USE OF ANIMAL ANTISERA

Antibody-containing products prepared from animal sera pose a special risk to the recipient, and the use of such products should be limited strictly to certain indications for which specific IG preparations of human origin are not available (eg, diphtheria and botulism).

REACTIONS TO ANIMAL SERA

Before any animal serum is injected, the patient must be questioned about asthma, allergic rhinitis, urticaria, and previous injections of animal sera. Patients with a history of asthma or allergic symptoms, especially from exposure to horses, can be dangerously sensitive to the animal sera and should be given serum only with the utmost caution. Those who previously have received animal sera are at increased risk of developing allergic reactions and serum sickness after administration of sera from the same animal species.

SENSITIVITY TESTS FOR REACTIONS TO ANIMAL SERA

Each patient who is to be given an animal serum should be skin tested before its administration.

Whereas intradermal (ID) skin tests have resulted in fatalities, the scratch test usually is safe. Therefore, scratch tests always should precede the ID tests. Nevertheless, any sensitivity test always should be performed by trained personnel familiar with treatment of acute anaphylaxis; necessary medications and equipment should be readily available (see Treatment of Anaphylactic Reactions, p 51).

Scratch, Prick, or Puncture Test.* Apply 1 drop of a 1:100 dilution of the serum in preservative-free isotonic sodium chloride to the site of a superficial scratch, prick, or puncture on the volar aspect of the forearm. Positive (histamine) and negative (physiologic saline) control tests for the scratch test also should be applied. A positive test result is a wheal with surrounding erythema at least 3-mm larger than the negative control test, read at 15 to 20 minutes. The histamine control must be positive for valid interpretation. If the scratch test result is negative, an ID test is performed.

Intradermal Test.* A dose of 0.02 mL of 1:1000 saline-diluted serum (enough to raise a small wheal) is administered. Positive and negative control tests as described for the scratch test also should be applied. If the test result is negative, it should be repeated using a 1:100 dilution. For persons with negative history for

* Antihistamines may inhibit reactions in the scratch, prick, or puncture tests, and in the intradermal skin test. Hence, testing should not be performed for at least 24 hours or, preferably, 48 hours after receipt of these drugs.

both animal allergy and prior exposure to animal serum, the 1:100 dilution may be used initially if a scratch, prick, or puncture test result with the serum is negative. Interpretation is the same as for the scratch test.

Positive test results not due to an irritant reaction indicate sensitivity, but a negative skin test result is not an absolute guarantee of lack of sensitivity. Therefore, animal sera should be administered with caution even to persons whose test results are negative. Immediate hypersensitivity testing is performed to identify IgE-mediated disease and does not predict other immune reactions, such as serum sickness.

If the intradermal test is positive or if the history for systemic anaphylaxis after previous administration of serum is highly suggestive in a person for whom the need for the serum is unquestioned, desensitization can be undertaken (see Desensitization to Animal Sera, below).

If the history and sensitivity tests are negative, the indicated dose of serum can be given intramuscularly. The patient should be observed afterwards for at least 30 minutes. Intravenous administration may be indicated if a high concentration of serum antibody is imperative, such as for the treatment of diphtheria or botulism. In these instances, the serum should be diluted and slowly administered intravenously according to the manufacturers' instructions. The patient should be monitored carefully for signs or symptoms of anaphylaxis.

DESENSITIZATION TO ANIMAL SERA

Tables 1.7 (p 50) and 1.8 (p 50) serve as guides for the desensitization procedures for administration of animal sera. Either the intravenous (IV) (Table 1.7) or the intradermal (ID), subcutaneous, or intramuscular regimens (Table 1.8) may be chosen. The IV route is considered safest because it offers better control. The desensitization procedure should be performed by trained personnel familiar with treatment of anaphylaxis and with appropriate drugs and equipment available (see Treatment of Anaphylactic Reactions, p 51). Some physicians advocate the concurrent use during the procedure of an oral or parenteral antihistamine (such as diphenhydramine), with or without IV hydrocortisone or methylprednisolone. If signs of anaphylaxis occur, aqueous epinephrine should be administered immediately (see Treatment of Anaphylactic Reactions, p 51). Administration of sera under the protection of a desensitization procedure must be continuous because after administration is interrupted, protection from desensitization is lost.

TYPES OF REACTIONS TO ANIMAL SERA

The following reactions can occur as the result of administration of animal sera. Of these, only anaphylaxis is mediated by IgE antibodies, and, thus, occurrence can be predicted by prior skin testing results.

Acute Febrile Reactions. These reactions usually are mild and can be treated with antipyretics. Severe febrile reactions should be treated with antipyretics, tepid water sponge baths, or other available methods to reduce the temperature.

Serum Sickness. Manifestations, which usually begin 7 to 10 days (occasionally as late as 3 weeks) after the primary exposure to the foreign protein, consist of fever, urticaria, or a maculopapular rash (90% of cases); arthritis or arthralgia; and lymphadenopathy. Local edema can occur at the serum injection site a few days before the systemic signs and symptoms appear. Angioedema, glomerulonephritis, Guillain-

Table 1.7. Desensitization to Serum—Intravenous (IV) Route

Dose Number*	Dilution of Serum in Isotonic Sodium Chloride	Amount of IV Injection, mL
1	1:1000	0.1
2	1:1000	0.3
3	1:1000	0.6
4	1:100	0.1
5	1:100	0.3
6	1:100	0.6
7	1:10	0.1
8	1:10	0.3
9	1:10	0.6
10	Undiluted	0.1
11	Undiluted	0.3
12	Undiluted	0.6
13	Undiluted	1.0

* Administer consistently at 15-minute intervals.

Table 1.8. Desensitization to Serum—Intradermal (ID), Subcutaneous (SC), and Intramuscular (IM) Routes

Dose Number*	Route of Administration	Dilution of Serum in Isotonic Sodium Chloride	Amount of ID, SC, or IM Injection, mL
1	ID	1:1000	0.1
2	ID	1:1000	0.3
3	SC	1:1000	0.6
4	SC	1:100	0.1
5	SC	1:100	0.3
6	SC	1:100	0.6
7	SC	1:10	0.1
8	SC	1:10	0.3
9	SC	1:10	0.6
10	SC	Undiluted	0.1
11	SC	Undiluted	0.3
12	IM	Undiluted	0.6
13	IM	Undiluted	1.0

* Administer consistently at 15-minute intervals.

Barré syndrome, peripheral neuritis, and myocarditis also can occur. However, serum sickness may be mild and resolve spontaneously within a few days to 2 weeks. Persons who previously have received serum injections are at an increased risk after readministration; manifestations in these patients usually occur shortly (from hours to 3 days) after administration of serum. Antihistamines can be helpful for management of serum sickness for the alleviation of pruritus, edema, and urticaria. Fever, malaise, arthralgia, and arthritis can be controlled in most patients by administration of aspirin or other nonsteroidal anti-inflammatory agents. Corticosteroids may be helpful for controlling serious manifestations that are controlled poorly by other agents; prednisone or prednisolone in therapeutic dosages (1.5 to 2 mg/kg per day) for 5 to 7 days is an appropriate regimen.

Anaphylaxis. The rapidity of onset and the overall severity of anaphylaxis may vary considerably. Anaphylaxis usually begins within minutes of exposure to the causative agent, and, in general, the more rapid the onset, the more severe the overall course. Major manifestations are the following: (1) cutaneous: pruritus, flushing, urticaria, and angioedema; (2) respiratory: hoarse voice and stridor, cough, wheeze, dyspnea, and cyanosis; (3) cardiovascular: a rapid, weak pulse, hypotension, and arrhythmias; and (4) gastrointestinal: cramps, vomiting, diarrhea, and dry mouth. Anaphylaxis is a medical emergency.

Treatment of Anaphylactic Reactions

Personnel administering biologic products or serum should be prepared to recognize and treat anaphylaxis. The necessary medications, equipment, and staff competent to maintain the patency of the airway and to manage cardiovascular collapse must be immediately available.

The emergency treatment of anaphylactic reactions is based on the type of reaction. In all instances, epinephrine is the primary drug. Mild symptoms of pruritus, erythema, urticaria, and angioedema should be treated with epinephrine injected intramuscularly or subcutaneously, followed by diphenhydramine, hydroxyzine, or other antihistamine given orally or parenterally (see Tables 1.9 and 1.10, p 52 and p 53). Epinephrine administration may be repeated every 5 to 15 minutes. If the patient's condition improves with this management and remains stable, a long-acting epinephrine injection may be given and an oral antihistamine prescribed for the next 24 hours.

Treatment of more severe or potentially life-threatening systemic anaphylaxis involving severe bronchospasm, laryngeal edema, shock, and cardiovascular collapse necessitates additional therapy. Maintenance of the airway and oxygen administration should be instituted promptly. Intravenous epinephrine may be indicated; for this use, it must be diluted from the 1:1000 aqueous base using physiologic saline (see Table 1.9, p 52). A slow continuous infusion is preferable to repeated bolus administration. Nebulized albuterol or IV aminophylline is indicated for bronchospasm (see Table 1.10, p 53). Rapid IV infusion of physiologic saline, Ringer's lactate, or other isotonic solution adequate to maintain blood pressure must be instituted to compensate for the loss of circulating blood volume that occurs.

In some cases, the use of an inotropic agent, such as dopamine (see Table 1.10, p 53), titrated to maintain blood pressure may be necessary. The combination of histamine H_1- and H_2-receptor-blocking agents (see Table 1.10, p 53) can be synergistic in effect and should be used. Corticosteroids probably should be used in all cases of anaphylaxis except those that are mild and have responded promptly to initial therapy (see Table 1.10, p 53). Corticosteroids do not exert an immediate effect, however, and should not be considered primary drugs.

All patients showing signs and symptoms of anaphylaxis, regardless of severity, should be observed for several hours. Biphasic and protracted anaphylaxis may be

Table 1.9. Epinephrine in the Treatment of Anaphylaxis*

Subcutaneous or intramuscular administration

Epinephrine 1:1000 (aqueous): 0.01 mL/kg per dose repeated every 10–20 min.† Usual dose:

- Infants—0.05–0.1 mL
- Children—0.1–0.3 mL
- Adolescents—0.3–0.5 mL

Intravenous administration‡

Epinephrine 1:1000 (aqueous): 0.1 mL/kg diluted to 1:10 000 with physiologic saline. Dose may be repeated every 10–20 min. A continuous infusion should be started if repeated doses are required. One milligram (1 mL) of 1:1000 dilution of epinephrine added to 250 mL of 5% dextrose in water, resulting in a concentration of 4 µg/mL, is infused initially at a rate of 0.1 µg/kg per minute and increased gradually to 1.5 µg/kg per minute to maintain blood pressure.

* **In addition to epinephrine, maintenance of an airway and administration of oxygen are critical.**

† If agent causing anaphylactic reaction was given by injection, epinephrine can be injected into the same site to slow absorption.

‡ If intravenous access cannot be obtained, IM dose can be injected into posterior one third of sublingual area.

mitigated with early administration of oral corticosteroids but has occurred despite adequate initial management. Therefore, patients should be observed even after remission of immediate symptoms; however, a specific period of observation has not been established. A period of observation of 4 hours would be reasonable for mild episodes and perhaps as long as 24 hours for severe episodes.

Anaphylaxis occurring in persons already taking ß-adrenergic blocking agents presents a unique situation. In such persons, the manifestations are likely to be more profound and significantly less responsive to epinephrine and other ß-adrenergic agonist drugs. More aggressive therapy with epinephrine may be adequate to override the receptor blockade in some patients. The use of IV glucagon for cardiovascular manifestations and inhaled atropine for management of bradycardia or bronchospasm also has been recommended in this situation.

Table 1.10. **Dosages of Commonly Used Secondary Drugs in the Treatment of Anaphylaxis**

Drug	Dose*
H_1-blocking agents (antihistamines)	
Diphenhydramine	Oral, IM, IV: 1–2 mg/kg every 4–6 h (100 mg, maximum single dose)
Hydroxyzine	Oral, IM: 0.5–1 mg/kg every 4–6 h (100 mg, maximum single dose)
H_2-blocking agents (also antihistamines)	
Cimetidine	IV: 5 mg/kg, slowly during 15 min every 6–8 h (300 mg, maximum single dose)
Ranitidine	IV: 1 mg/kg, slowly during 15 min every 6–8 h (50 mg, maximum single dose)
Corticosteroids	
Hydrocortisone	IV: 100–200 mg every 4–6 h
Methylprednisolone	IV: 1.5–2 mg/kg every 4–6 h (60 mg, maximum single dose)
Prednisone	Oral: 1.5–2 mg/kg, single morning dose, (60 mg, maximum single dose), use corticosteroids as long as needed
$ß_2$-agonist	
Albuterol	Nebulizer solution: 0.5% (5 mg/mL), 0.05–0.15 mg/kg per dose in 2–3 mL isotonic sodium chloride, maximum of 5.0 mg per dose every 20 min for 1–2 h or 0.5 mg/kg per hour by continuous nebulization (15 mg/h, maximum dose)
Other	
Dopamine	IV: 5–20 µg/kg per minute. Mixing 150 mg of dopamine with 250 mL of saline or 5% dextrose in water will produce a solution that, if infused at the rate of 1 mL/kg per hour, will deliver 10 µg/kg per minute. The solution must be free of bicarbonate, which may inactivate dopamine.
Aminophylline	IV: 4–6 mg/kg in 20 mL saline by rapid drip every 6 h or 0.9–1.1 mg/kg per hour continuous infusion

* IM indicates intramuscular; IV, intravenous.

Immunization in Special Clinical Circumstances

Preterm Infants

Prematurely born infants, including infants of low birth weight, should be immunized at the usual chronologic age in most cases. Some studies suggest a reduced immune response in very-low-birth-weight infants (≤1500 g) immunized by the usual schedule. Additional data are required to better define the optimal immunization schedule for these infants. Vaccine dosages should not be reduced for preterm infants. If an infant is still in the hospital at 2 months of age, the immunizations routinely scheduled at that age should be given, including diphtheria and tetanus toxoids and acellular pertussis (DTaP), *Haemophilus influenzae* type B (Hib) conjugate, and inactivated poliovirus (IPV) vaccine (see Fig 1.1, p 22).

The optimal time to initiate hepatitis B immunization in preterm infants with birth weights less than 2 kg whose mothers are hepatitis B surface antigen (HBsAg)-negative has not been determined. Seroconversion rates in low-birth-weight infants in whom immunization was initiated shortly after birth have been reported in some studies to be lower than rates in preterm infants immunized at a later age and in term infants immunized shortly after birth. Hence, initiation of immunization in preterm infants with a birth weight of less than 2 kg whose mothers are HBsAg-negative should be delayed until just before hospital discharge if the infant weighs 2 kg or more or until approximately 2 months of age when other immunizations are given (see Fig 1.1, p 22, and Hepatitis B, p 289).

Preterm infants with birth weights less than 2 kg whose mothers are HBsAg-positive should receive Hepatitis B Immune Globulin (HBIG) within 12 hours of birth and concurrent hepatitis B vaccine at different sites (see Hepatitis B, p 289). If the maternal HBsAg status is not known, vaccine also should be given in accordance with recommendations for the infant of an HBsAg-positive mother (see Hepatitis B, p 289). The maternal HBsAg status should be determined, and HBIG should be given to the infant if the mother is HBsAg-positive. If the birth weight is less than 2 kg and the maternal status cannot be determined within the initial 12 hours of life, HBIG should be given. This initial vaccine dose should not be counted in the required 3 doses to complete the immunization series. The maternal HBsAg status will determine the subsequent schedule for completion of hepatitis B immunization (see Hepatitis B, p 289).

Preterm infants in whom chronic respiratory tract disease develops should be given influenza immunization annually in the fall once they reach 6 months of age. To protect premature infants and infants with other chronic conditions before this age, the family and other caregivers, including hospital personnel, should be immunized against influenza (see Influenza, p 351). In addition, infants with a history of premature birth, chronic lung disease, or both may benefit from immunoprophylaxis with palivizumab or Respiratory Syncytial Virus Immune Globulin Intravenous (see Respiratory Syncytial Virus, p 483).

Pregnancy

Immunization during pregnancy poses theoretical risks to the developing fetus. Although no evidence indicates that vaccines in use today have detrimental effects on the fetus, pregnant women should receive a vaccine only when the vaccine is unlikely to cause harm, the risk for disease exposure is high, and the infection would pose a significant risk to the mother or fetus. When a vaccine is to be given during pregnancy, delaying administration until the second or third trimester, when possible, is a reasonable precaution to minimize concern about possible teratogenicity.

The only vaccines routinely recommended for administration during pregnancy in the United States, provided they are otherwise indicated (either for primary or booster immunization), are those for tetanus, diphtheria, and influenza. Pregnant women who have not received a diphtheria and tetanus toxoid (dT) booster during the last 10 years should be given a booster dose, and those who are unimmunized or only partially immunized should complete the primary series. In developing countries with a high incidence of neonatal tetanus, dT routinely is administered during pregnancy without evidence of adverse effects and with striking reductions in the occurrence of neonatal tetanus.

Studies indicate that women in the second and third trimesters of pregnancy and the early puerperium, even in the absence of underlying risk factors, are at increased risk of complications and hospitalization from influenza. Therefore, the Advisory Committee on Immunization Practices (ACIP) of the Centers for Disease Control and Prevention (CDC) recommends that influenza vaccine be administered to all women who will be beyond 14 weeks of pregnancy during the influenza season (see Influenza, p 351).

Pneumococcal immunization can be given to a pregnant woman at high risk for serious or complicated illness from these infections. Hepatitis A or B immunizations, if indicated, should be given to pregnant women. Although data on the safety of these vaccines for the developing fetus are not available, no risk would be expected because the vaccines contain either formalin-inactivated virus (hepatitis A) or noninfectious surface antigen (hepatitis B). In contrast, infection with either agent in a pregnant woman can result in severe disease in the mother and, in the case of hepatitis B, chronic infection in the newborn. Thimerosal-free hepatitis B vaccines are recommended.

Pregnancy is a contraindication to administration of all live-virus vaccines, except when susceptibility and exposure are highly probable and the disease to be prevented poses a greater threat to the woman or fetus than does the vaccine. Although only a theoretical risk to the fetus of a live-virus vaccine exists, the background rate of anomalies in uncomplicated pregnancies may result in a defect that could be attributed inappropriately to a vaccine. Therefore, live vaccines should be avoided during pregnancy. However, yellow fever vaccine may be given to pregnant women who are at substantial risk of imminent exposure to infection, such as in some circumstances of international travel. Pregnant women who previously received complete or partial immunization against poliovirus may be given IPV vaccine. For unimmunized women, IPV vaccine is recommended for all doses (see Poliovirus Infections, p 465).

Because measles, mumps, rubella, and varicella vaccines are contraindicated for pregnant women, efforts should be made to immunize susceptible women against these illnesses before they become pregnant. Although of theoretical concern, no case of embryopathy caused by rubella vaccine has been reported. Accumulated evidence demonstrates that inadvertent administration of rubella vaccine to susceptible pregnant women rarely, if ever, causes congenital defects. The effect of varicella vaccine on the fetus, if any, is unknown. The manufacturer, in collaboration with CDC, has established the VARIVAX Pregnancy Registry to monitor the maternal and fetal outcomes of women who inadvertently are given varicella vaccine 3 months before or at any time during pregnancy. Reporting of cases is encouraged and may be done by telephone (1-800-986-8999). A pregnant mother or other household member is not a contraindication for varicella immunization of a child in that household. Transmission of vaccine virus from an immunocompetent vaccine recipient to a susceptible person has been reported only rarely and only in the presence of a rash (see Varicella-Zoster Infections, p 624).

Immunocompromised Children

PRIMARY AND SECONDARY IMMUNE DEFICIENCIES

The safety and effectiveness of vaccines in persons with immune deficiency are determined by the nature and degree of immunosuppression. Immunocompromised persons vary in their degree of immunosuppression and susceptibility to infection. These children represent a heterogeneous population with regard to immunization. Immunodeficiency conditions can be grouped into primary and secondary (acquired) disorders. Primary disorders of the immune system generally are inherited and include disorders of B-lymphocyte (humoral) immunity, T-lymphocyte (cell)-mediated immunity, complement, and phagocytic function. Secondary disorders of the immune system are acquired and occur in persons with human immunodeficiency virus (HIV) infection or acquired immunodeficiency syndrome, malignant neoplasms, or transplantation and in persons receiving immunosuppressive or radiation therapy (see Table 1.11, p 57). Experience with vaccine administration in immunocompromised children is limited. In most situations, theoretical considerations are the only guide to vaccine administration because experience with specific vaccines in patients with most specific disorders is lacking. However, considerable data in HIV-infected infants provide reassurance about the low risk of adverse events in these patients after immunization.

Live vaccines. In general, persons who are severely immunocompromised or in whom immune status is uncertain should not receive live vaccines, either viral or bacterial, because of the risk of disease from the vaccine strains. Although precautions, contraindications, and suboptimal efficacy of immunizations in immunocompromised patients are emphasized, some immunocompromised children may benefit from special-use as well as routinely administered immunizations.

Inactivated vaccines. Inactivated vaccines and immune globulin preparations should be used when appropriate, since the risk of complications from these preparations is not increased in immunocompromised persons. However, the immune responses of immunocompromised children to inactivated vaccines (eg, DTaP,

Table 1.11. **Immunization of Children and Adolescents With Primary and Secondary Immune Deficiencies***

Category	Specific Immunodeficiency	Vaccine Contraindications	Effectiveness and Comments
Primary			
B-lymphocyte (humoral)	X-linked and common variable agammaglobulinemia	OPV† and live bacterial; consider measles and varicella	Effectiveness of any vaccine dependent on humoral response is doubtful; IGIV interferes with measles and possibly varicella response
	Selective IgA deficiency and selective subclass IgG deficiency	OPV†; other live vaccines seem to be safe, but caution is urged	All vaccines probably effective Vaccine response may be attenuated
T-lymphocyte (cell-mediated and humoral)	Severe combined	All live vaccines‡§	Effectiveness of any vaccine dependent on humoral or cellular response is doubtful
Complement	Deficiency of early components (C1, C4, C2, C3)	None	All routine vaccines probably effective Pneumococcal and meningococcal vaccines recommended
	Deficiency of late components (C5-C9), properdin, factor B	None	All routine vaccines probably effective Meningococcal vaccine recommended
Phagocytic function	Chronic granulomatous disease Leukocyte adhesion defect Myeloperoxidase deficiency	Live bacterial vaccines§	All routine vaccines probably effective Influenza vaccine should be considered to decrease secondary infection

Table 1.11. **Immunization of Children and Adolescents With Primary and Secondary Immune Deficiencies,* continued**

Category	Specific Immunodeficiency	Vaccine Contraindications	Effectiveness and Comments
Secondary			
	HIV/AIDS	OPV,[†] BCG, withhold MMR and varicella in severely immunocompromised children	MMR, varicella, and all inactivated vaccines, including influenza, may be effective[‖]
	Malignant neoplasm, transplantation, immunosuppressive or radiation therapy	Live viral and bacterial, depending on immune status[‡§]	Effectiveness of any vaccine depends on degree of immune suppression

* OPV indicates oral poliovirus; IGIV, Immune Globulin Intravenous; Ig, immunoglobulin; HIV, human immunodeficiency virus; AIDS, acquired immunodeficiency syndrome; BCG, bacille Calmette-Guérin; and MMR, measles, mumps, rubella.

† OPV vaccine is no longer recommended for routine use in the United States.

‡ Live viral vaccines: MMR, OPV, varicella.

§ Live bacterial vaccines: BCG and Ty21a *Salmonella typhi* vaccine.

‖ HIV-infected children should receive Ig after exposure to measles (see Measles, p 385) and may receive varicella vaccine if CD4 count ≥25% (see Varicella-Zoster Infections, p 624).

hepatitis B, inactivated poliovirus, Hib, pneumococcal, and influenza) may vary and may be inadequate. Therefore, the vaccine's immunogenicity in these children may be reduced substantially. In children with secondary immunodeficiency, the ability to develop an adequate immunologic response depends on when immunosuppression occurs. In children in whom immunosuppressive therapy is discontinued, an adequate response usually occurs between 3 months and 1 year after discontinuation of the immunosuppressive therapy. Influenza vaccine should be given to immunosuppressed children before each influenza season. In children with malignant neoplasms, influenza immunization should be given no less than 3 to 4 weeks after chemotherapy is discontinued and when peripheral granulocyte and lymphocyte counts greater than 1000 cells/µL (1.0×10^9/L) are achieved.

Primary immunodeficiencies. Live vaccines are contraindicated for most patients with B-lymphocyte defects except IgA deficiency and for all patients with T-lymphocyte–mediated disorders of immune function (see Table 1.11, p 58). Measles and varicella vaccines should be considered for children with B-lymphocyte disorders; however, antibody response may not occur because of the underlying disease and because the patient is receiving Immune Globulin Intravenous (IGIV) periodically. Fatal poliomyelitis and measles vaccine virus infections have occurred in children with disorders of T-cell function after administration of live-virus vaccines. Oral poliovirus vaccine is no longer recommended for routine use in the United States.* Inactivated vaccine should be administered if available for a given disease. Children with deficiency in antibody-synthesizing capacity are incapable of developing an antibody response to vaccines and should receive regular doses of immune globulin (usually IGIV) to provide passive protection against many infectious diseases. Specific immune globulins (eg, Varicella-Zoster Immune Globulin [VZIG]) are available for postexposure prophylaxis for some infections. Children with milder B-lymphocyte and antibody deficiencies have an intermediate degree of vaccine responsiveness and may require monitoring of postimmunization antibody titers to confirm vaccine immunogenicity.

Children with early or late complement deficiencies can receive all immunizations, including live vaccines. Children with phagocyte function disorders, including chronic granulomatous disease and leukocyte adhesion defect, can receive all immunizations except live bacterial vaccines (bacille Calmette-Guérin [BCG] and Ty21a *Salmonella typhi*). Most experts believe that live viral vaccines are safe to administer to children with complement deficiencies and phagocyte disorders.

Secondary (acquired) immunodeficiencies. Several factors should be considered in immunization of children with secondary immunodeficiencies, including the underlying disease, the specific immunosuppressive regimen (dose and schedule), and the infectious disease and immunization history of the patient. Live vaccines generally are contraindicated because of the increased risk of serious adverse effects. Exceptions are children with HIV infection who are not severely immunocompromised in whom measles, mumps, rubella (MMR) vaccine is recommended (see HIV Infections, p 325) and in whom varicella vaccine should be considered if CD4

* American Academy of Pediatrics Committee on Infectious Diseases. Prevention of poliomyelitis: recommendations for use of only inactivated poliovirus vaccine for routine immunization. *Pediatrics*. 1999;104:1404–1406

values are 25% or more (see Varicella-Zoster Infections, p 624). The use of varicella vaccine in children with acute lymphocytic leukemia in remission should be considered because the risk of natural varicella outweighs the risk from the attenuated vaccine virus (see Varicella-Zoster Infections, p 624).

Live-virus vaccines usually are withheld for an interval of at least 3 months after immunosuppressive cancer chemotherapy has been discontinued. The exception is corticosteroid therapy (see Corticosteroids, p 61). This interval is based on the assumption that immune response will have been restored in 3 months and that the underlying disease for which the immunosuppressive therapy was given is in remission or under control. However, the interval may vary with the intensity and type of immunosuppressive therapy, radiation therapy, underlying disease, and other factors. Therefore, a definitive recommendation often is not possible concerning an interval after cessation of immunosuppressive therapy when live-virus vaccines can be administered safely and effectively. In vitro testing of immune function may provide guidelines for safe timing of immunizations in individual patients.

Other considerations. Because patients with congenital or acquired immunodeficiencies may not have an adequate response to an immunizing agent, they may remain susceptible despite having received an appropriate vaccine. Specific serum antibody titers should be determined after immunization to assess immune response and guide management of future exposures and further immunization.

Persons with certain immune deficiencies may benefit from specific immunizations directed at preventing infection by organisms to which they are particularly susceptible. Examples include administration of pneumococcal and meningococcal vaccines to persons with splenic dysfunction, asplenia (see Asplenic Children, p 66), and complement deficiencies who are at increased risk of infection with encapsulated bacteria. Also, influenza immunization is indicated for children with splenic dysfunction, asplenia, and phagocyte function deficiencies to prevent influenza and reduce the risk of secondary bacterial infections that may occur. Most experts advise administration of routinely recommended inactivated and subunit vaccines.

Household contacts. Immunocompetent siblings and other household contacts of persons with an immunologic deficiency should not receive oral poliovirus vaccine because the vaccine virus may be transmitted to the immunocompromised person. However, siblings and household contacts should receive live MMR and influenza vaccines if indicated because transmission of the vaccine viruses does not occur. Varicella vaccine is recommended for susceptible contacts of immunocompromised children because transmission of varicella vaccine virus from healthy persons is rare, and disease, if it develops, is mild. No precautions need be taken after immunization unless the vaccine recipient develops a rash, particularly a vesicular rash. In such instances, the vaccine recipient should avoid direct contact with immunocompromised susceptible hosts for the duration of the rash. If contact inadvertently occurs, administration of VZIG is not indicated because the risk of transmission is low. Also, when transmission has occurred, the virus has maintained its attenuated characteristics. In most instances, antiviral therapy is not necessary but can be given if disease occurs (see Varicella-Zoster Infections, p 624).

CORTICOSTEROIDS

Children who receive corticosteroid therapy can become immunocompromised. The minimal amount of systemic corticosteroids and duration of administration sufficient to cause immunosuppression in an otherwise healthy child are not well defined. The frequency and route of administration of corticosteroids, the underlying disease, and concurrent other therapy are other factors affecting immunosuppression. Despite these uncertainties, sufficient experience exists to recommend empiric guidelines for administration of live-virus vaccines to previously healthy children receiving corticosteroid therapy for nonimmunocompromising conditions. Many clinicians consider a dosage equivalent to 2 mg/kg per day or greater of prednisone or equivalent to a total of 20 mg/d or greater for children who weigh more than 10 kg, particularly when given for more than 14 days, sufficient to raise concern about the safety of immunization with live-virus vaccines. Accordingly, guidelines for administration of live-virus vaccines to recipients of corticosteroids are as follows:

- ***Topical therapy or local injections of corticosteroids.*** Administration of topical corticosteroids, either on the skin or in the respiratory tract (ie, by aerosol) or eyes, and intra-articular, bursal, or tendon injections of corticosteroids usually do not result in immunosuppression that would contraindicate administration of live-virus vaccines. However, live-virus vaccines should not be administered if clinical or laboratory evidence of systemic immunosuppression results from prolonged application until corticosteroid therapy has been discontinued for at least 1 month.
- ***Physiologic maintenance doses of corticosteroids.*** Children who are receiving only maintenance physiologic doses of corticosteroids can receive live-virus vaccines during corticosteroid treatment.
- ***Low or moderate doses of systemic corticosteroids given daily or on alternate days.*** Children receiving less than 2 mg/kg per day of prednisone or its equivalent, or less than 20 mg/d if they weigh more than 10 kg, can receive live-virus vaccines during corticosteroid treatment.
- ***High doses of systemic corticosteroids given daily or on alternate days for fewer than 14 days.*** Children receiving 2 mg/kg per day or more of prednisone or its equivalent, or 20 mg or more daily if they weigh more than 10 kg, can receive live-virus vaccines immediately after discontinuation of treatment. Some experts, however, would delay immunization until 2 weeks after corticosteroid therapy has been discontinued, if possible (ie, if the patient's condition allows temporary cessation).
- ***High doses of systemic corticosteroids given daily or on alternate days for 14 days or more.*** Children receiving 2 mg/kg per day or more of prednisone or its equivalent, or 20 mg or more daily if they weigh more than 10 kg, should not receive live-virus vaccines until corticosteroid therapy has been discontinued for at least 1 month.
- ***Children with a disease that, in itself, is considered to suppress the immune response and who are receiving systemic or locally administered corticosteroids.*** These children should not be given live-virus vaccines except in special circumstances.

These guidelines are based on concerns about vaccine safety in recipients of high doses of corticosteroids. In addition, when deciding whether to administer live-virus vaccines, the potential benefits and risks of immunization for an individual patient and in specific circumstances should be considered. For example, some experts recommend immunization of a patient at increased risk of a vaccine-preventable infection (and its complications) if, despite corticosteroid therapy, the patient does not have clinical evidence of immunosuppression.

The guidelines also are based on considerations of safety concerning live-virus vaccines and do not necessarily correlate with those for optimal vaccine immunogenicity. For example, some children receiving moderate doses of prednisone, such as 1.5 mg/kg per day, for several weeks or longer may have a less than optimal serum antibody response to some vaccine antigens. Nevertheless, unless immunization can be deferred temporarily until corticosteroids are discontinued without compromising the likelihood of immunization, children should be immunized to enhance the likelihood of protection in the case of exposure to disease. In contrast, some children receiving relatively high doses of corticosteroids (eg, 30 mg/d of prednisone) may respond adequately to immunization.

HODGKIN DISEASE

Patients with Hodgkin disease should be immunized with pneumococcal vaccine according to age-specific recommendations (see Pneumococcal Infections, p 452); they also should receive Hib vaccine according to age-specific recommendations (see *Haemophilus influenzae* Infections, p 262). These patients are at increased risk for invasive pneumococcal infection; most experts believe that they also are at increased risk for invasive Hib infection. The antibody response is likely to be best when patients are immunized at least 10 to 14 days before initiation of therapy for Hodgkin disease. During active chemotherapy and shortly thereafter, the antibody responses to the pneumococcal vaccine are impaired. However, the ability of these patients to respond improves rapidly, and immunization as early as 3 months after cessation of chemotherapy is reasonable. Patients who received vaccine during chemotherapy or radiation therapy should be reimmunized 3 months after discontinuation of the therapy.

TRANSPLANT RECIPIENTS

Many factors can affect the immunity to vaccine-preventable diseases for a child recovering from successful bone marrow transplantation (BMT), including the donor's immunity, type of transplantation (ie, autologous or allogeneic, blood or hematopoietic cell, or solid organ), interval since the transplant, receipt of immu nosuppressive medications, and graft-vs-host disease (GVHD). Although many children who are transplant recipients acquire the immunity of the donor, some will lose serologic evidence of immunity. Retention of donor immune memory can be facilitated if recalled by antigenic stimulation soon after transplantation. Clinical studies of BMT recipients indicate that pretransplant administration of diphtheria and tetanus toxoids to the bone marrow donor and immediate post-transplant administration to the recipient can facilitate response to these antigens. In these studies, serum antibody titers did not increase when immunization of the recipient was delayed until 5 weeks after transplantation. In theory, these results could be expected with other inactivated vaccine antigens, including pertussis, Hib, hepatitis B, IPV, and pneumococcal vaccines.

The risk of acquiring diphtheria or tetanus during the year after bone marrow transplantation is very low. Some experts elect to reimmunize all children without serologic evaluation, while others base the decision to reimmunize against diphtheria and tetanus on adequacy of serologic titers obtained 1 year after transplantation. Adequate immune responses can be obtained with 3 doses of diphtheria and tetanus toxoids (dT) at 12, 14, and 24 months after transplantation in persons 7 years of age or older. In persons younger than 7 years of age, DTaP or DT can be used. No data are available on safety and immunogenicity of pertussis immunization for BMT recipients. Persons with tetanus-prone wounds sustained during the first year after transplantation should be given Tetanus Immune Globulin (TIG), regardless of their tetanus immunization status.

Data on which to base recommendations for reimmunization against Hib or *Streptococcus pneumoniae* are limited. Doses of Hib conjugate vaccine appear to provide some protection if given at 12, 14, and 24 months after BMT for recipients of any age. In 1 study, time after transplantation was the most important factor for determining the immune response to pneumococcal polysaccharide vaccine, with the greatest response observed when the vaccine was administered 2 or more years after transplantation. Some experts recommend a multiple-dose schedule of pneumococcal vaccine at 12 and 24 months after transplantation depending on the age of the patient. The second dose of pneumococcal vaccine is not a booster dose but provides a second opportunity for pneumococcal immunization for persons who fail to respond to the first dose. In patients undergoing autologous BMT, preharvest immunization with an Hib-conjugate vaccine resulted in higher anti-Hib antibody concentrations for 2 years after transplantation compared with patients not immunized before harvest. Similar benefit in transplant recipients was noted when allogenic bone marrow donors were immunized before harvest.

Two years after BMT, MMR often is given if the recipient is presumed immunocompetent; data indicate that healthy survivors at that time can receive these live-virus vaccines without untoward effects. A second dose of MMR should be given 1 month (4 weeks) or more after the first dose unless serologic response to measles is demonstrated after the first dose. The benefit of a second dose in this population has not been evaluated. Patients with chronic GVHD should not receive MMR vaccine because of concern about resulting latent virus infection and its sequelae. Susceptible persons who are exposed to measles should receive passive immunoprophylaxis (see Measles, p 385). Varicella vaccine is contraindicated for BMT recipients fewer than 24 months after BMT. Use of varicella vaccine for BMT recipients is restricted to research protocols in which the vaccine may be considered 24 months or more after BMT for recipients who are presumed immunocompetent. Passive immunization with VZIG is recommended for susceptible persons with known exposure to varicella (see Varicella-Zoster Infections, p 624).

Only IPV vaccine should be given to transplant recipients and their household contacts. Bone marrow transplant recipients should be immunized with IPV vaccine at 12, 14, and 24 months after BMT. The effectiveness of giving additional doses is not known; more data are needed on optional methods and timing of IPV immunization. Recipients can be tested for immunity, but serologic tests for antibody titers against polioviruses are not readily available in commercial or state laboratories.

Influenza vaccine is not effective when given within the initial 6 months after BMT, but immunization may provide protection when given at 1 year after BMT. Because the risk of disease is substantial, influenza vaccine should be administered annually during early autumn (see Influenza, p 351) to persons who underwent BMT more than 6 months before, even if the interval is less than 12 months.

The immunogenicity of hepatitis B vaccine in BMT recipients has not been assessed adequately. Based on the response of these patients to other protein antigens, initiation of a 3-dose series at 12, 14, and 24 months after transplantation followed by postimmunization serologic testing for antibody to hepatitis B surface antigen is reasonable. Additional doses (maximum of 3) are given to vaccine nonresponders. Routine administration of hepatitis A vaccine is not recommended but may be considered 12 months or more after BMT for persons who have chronic liver disease or chronic GVHD, persons from hepatitis A endemic areas, or persons in areas experiencing outbreaks. Hepatitis A immunization requires 2 doses given 6 to 12 months apart.

For children who are scheduled to undergo solid-organ transplantation and who are older than 12 months of age, if previously immunized, serologic antibody titers for measles, mumps, rubella, and varicella should be performed. Children who are susceptible should be given MMR vaccine, varicella vaccine, or both before transplantation. The preferred time to give these vaccines is at least 1 month before transplantation. Serum antibody titers to measles, mumps, rubella, and varicella should be measured in all patients 1 or more years after transplantation. Information about the use of live-virus vaccines in patients after solid-organ transplantation is limited. Annual influenza immunization is indicated, as recommended for BMT recipients. The use of passive immunization (ie, immune globulin administration) should be based on serologic evidence of susceptibility and exposure to disease.

Household and health care worker contacts of BMT and solid organ transplant recipients should have immunity to or be immunized against hepatitis A, influenza, polio, MMR, and varicella.

Because of limited data on immunization of transplant recipients, immunization schedules vary in different centers.

HIV INFECTION (SEE ALSO HIV INFECTION, P 325)

Data on the use of currently available live-virus and bacterial vaccines in HIV-infected children are limited, but complications have been reported after BCG and measles immunizations. One case of vaccine-related measles pneumonitis was reported in a severely immunocompromised child 1 year after measles immunization. Because of reports of severe measles in symptomatic HIV-infected children, including fatalities in as many as 40% of cases, measles immunization (given as MMR) is recommended for HIV-infected children in most circumstances, including children who are symptomatic but are not severely immunocompromised, as well as those who are asymptomatic. Vaccine should be given at 12 months of age to enhance the likelihood of an appropriate immune response. In a measles epidemic, vaccine should be given at an earlier age, such as at 6 to 9 months of age followed by the routinely recommended dose at 12 months of age (or 1 month [28 days] after this initial dose) (see Measles, p 385). The second dose after the 12-month immunization may be administered as soon as 1 month (28 days) later in an attempt to induce seroconversion as early as possible. However, severely immunocompromised patients with HIV infection, as defined by low CD4+ T-lymphocyte counts or low percentage of total circulating lymphocytes, should not receive measles vaccine (see HIV Infection, p 325, and Table 3.24, p 327).

After the potential risks and benefits are weighed, varicella vaccine should be considered for asymptomatic or mildly symptomatic HIV-infected children with age-specific CD4+ T-lymphocyte percentages of 25% or more (see Varicella-Zoster Infections, p 624).* Children with asymptomatic or symptomatic HIV infection also should receive other routinely recommended childhood vaccines, including DTaP, IPV, hepatitis B, and Hib conjugate vaccines, according to the recommended schedule (see Fig 1.1, p 22). Annual influenza immunization of HIV-infected persons is recommended (see Influenza, p 351). Pneumococcal immunization also is indicated based on age- and vaccine-specific recommendations (see Pneumococcal Infections, p 452). Data are limited on the effect of routine immunizations on HIV RNA viral load in children. Some studies in adults have demonstrated transient increases of HIV RNA levels after immunization with influenza or pneumococcal vaccine, while other studies have shown no increase. No evidence indicates that this transient increase enhances progression of disease. In children, 1 study demonstrated no increase of HIV RNA levels after influenza or DTP (diphtheria and tetanus toxoids and pertussis) immunization, while another study found only transient increases in viral load in 5 of 16 children given influenza vaccine. Additional studies are needed in infants and children given all routine immunizations.

In the United States, BCG is contraindicated for HIV-infected patients. In areas of the world with a high incidence of tuberculosis, the World Health Organization (WHO) recommends giving BCG to HIV-infected children who are asymptomatic.

Routine or widespread screening to detect asymptomatic HIV-infected children before routine immunization is not recommended. Children without clinical manifestations of or known risk factors for HIV infection should be immunized in accordance with the recommendations for routine childhood immunization.

Since the ability of HIV-infected children to respond to vaccine antigens likely is related to the degree of immunosuppression at the time of immunization and may be inadequate, these children should be considered potentially susceptible to vaccine-preventable diseases, even after appropriate immunization, unless a recent serologic test demonstrates adequate antibody concentrations. Hence, passive immunoprophylaxis or chemoprophylaxis after exposure to these diseases should be considered even if the child previously has received the recommended vaccines.

Vaccine-type varicella-zoster virus rarely has been transmitted from healthy persons. Therefore, household contacts of HIV-infected persons can be immunized with live-virus varicella vaccine (see Varicella-Zoster Infections, p 624). No precautions are needed after immunization of healthy children who do not develop a rash.

---

* American Academy of Pediatrics Committee on Infectious Diseases. Varicella vaccine update. *Pediatrics*. 2000;105:136–141

Vaccine recipients who develop a rash should avoid direct contact with susceptible immunocompromised hosts for the duration of the rash. If the immunocompromised contact develops varicella, it will be mild, and use of VZIG to prevent transmission is not indicated.

ASPLENIC CHILDREN

The asplenic state results from the following: (1) surgical removal of the spleen, (2) certain diseases, such as sickle cell disease (functional asplenia), or (3) congenital asplenia. All asplenic infants, children, adolescents, and adults, regardless of the reason for the asplenic state, have an increased risk for fulminant bacteremia, which is associated with a high mortality rate. Susceptibility to fulminant bacteremia is determined largely by the underlying disease. In comparison with healthy children who have not undergone splenectomy, the mortality rate from septicemia is increased 50-fold in children who have had splenectomy after trauma and approximately 350-fold in children with sickle cell disease, and the rate may be even higher in children who have had splenectomy for thalassemia. The risk of bacteremia is higher in younger children than in older children, and it may be greater during the years immediately after splenectomy. Fulminant bacteremia, however, has been reported in adults as many as 25 years after splenectomy.

Streptococcus pneumoniae is the most important pathogen in asplenic children. Less common causes of bacteremia include Hib, *Neisseria meningitidis,* other streptococci, *Escherichia coli, Staphylococcus aureus,* and gram-negative bacilli, such as *Salmonella* species, *Klebsiella* species, and *Pseudomonas aeruginosa.* Persons who are functionally or anatomically asplenic also are at increased risk for fatal malaria and severe babesiosis.

Pneumococcal vaccine is indicated for all asplenic children 2 years of age and older; the conjugate vaccine, when licensed, will be recommended beginning at 2 months of age (see Pneumococcal Infections, p 452). Reimmunization of recipients of the polysaccharide vaccine after 3 to 5 years is recommended for children with asplenia who are 10 years of age or younger and for older children and adults who were immunized initially at least 5 years before. Only 1 reimmunization is recommended. Immunization against Hib infections should be initiated at 2 months of age, as recommended for otherwise healthy young children (see Fig 1.1, p 22) and for all previously unimmunized children with asplenia. Quadrivalent meningococcal polysaccharide vaccine also should be administered to asplenic children 2 years of age and older (see Meningococcal Infections, p 396). The efficacy of meningococcal vaccine in asplenic children is not certain, although this vaccine probably is as effective as pneumococcal polysaccharide vaccine. No known contraindication exists to giving these vaccines at the same time in separate syringes at different sites. Since the currently licensed meningococcal vaccine is an unconjugated polysaccharide vaccine, it may not be as effective for preventing disease in children younger than 5 years of age as it is in older persons.

Daily antimicrobial prophylaxis against pneumococcal infections is recommended for many asplenic children, irrespective of immunization status. For infants with sickle cell anemia, oral penicillin prophylaxis against invasive pneumococcal disease should be initiated as soon as the diagnosis is established and preferably by 2 months of age. Although the efficacy of antimicrobial prophylaxis has been proven only in patients with sickle cell anemia, other asplenic children at particularly high risk, such as those with malignant neoplasms or thalassemia, also should receive daily chemoprophylaxis. Less agreement exists about the need for prophylaxis for children who have had splenectomy after trauma. In general, antimicrobial prophylaxis (in addition to immunization) should be strongly considered for all asplenic children younger than 5 years of age and for at least 1 year after splenectomy.

The age at which chemoprophylaxis is discontinued often is an empirical decision. Based on a multicenter study, prophylactic penicillin can be discontinued at approximately 5 years of age in children with sickle cell anemia who are receiving regular medical attention and who have not had a severe pneumococcal infection or a surgical splenectomy. The appropriate duration of prophylaxis for children with asplenia due to other causes is unknown. Some experts continue prophylaxis throughout childhood and into adulthood for particularly high-risk patients with asplenia.

For antimicrobial prophylaxis, oral penicillin V (125 mg twice a day for children younger than 5 years of age and 250 mg twice a day for children 5 years of age and older) usually is recommended. Some experts recommend amoxicillin (20 mg/kg per day). In recent years, the proportion of pneumococcal isolates that have intermediate or high-level resistance to penicillin has increased in most areas of the United States. Ongoing surveillance for resistant pneumococci is needed to determine whether changes to the recommended chemoprophylaxis will be required.

When antimicrobial prophylaxis is used, its limitations must be stressed to parents and patients. They should recognize that some bacteria capable of causing fulminant sepsis are not susceptible to the antimicrobial agents given for prophylaxis. Parents should be aware that all febrile illnesses are potentially serious in asplenic children and that immediate medical attention should be sought because the initial signs and symptoms of fulminant bacteremia can be subtle. When bacteremia is a possibility, the physician should hospitalize the child, obtain specimens for blood and other cultures as indicated, and immediately begin treatment with an antimicrobial regimen effective against *S pneumoniae, H influenzae,* and *N meningitidis.* In some clinical situations, other antibiotics, such as aminoglycosides, may be indicated. If an asplenic child travels or resides in an area where medical care is not accessible, an appropriate antibiotic should be readily available and the child's caregiver instructed in appropriate use.

Whenever possible, alternatives to splenectomy should be considered. Management options include postponement of splenectomy for as long as possible in congenital hemolytic anemias, preservation of accessory spleens, performance of partial splenectomy for benign tumors of the spleen, conservative (nonoperative) management of splenic trauma, or, when feasible, repair rather than removal, and, if possible, avoidance of splenectomy when immunodeficiency is present (eg, Wiskott-Aldrich syndrome).

Children With a Personal or Family History of Seizures

Infants and children with a personal or family history of seizures are at increased risk for having a seizure after receipt of DTP or measles (usually as MMR) vaccines. In most cases, these seizures are brief, self-limited, and generalized and occur in conjunction with fever. These characteristics indicate that such vaccine-associated seizures are usually febrile seizures. No evidence indicates that these seizures cause permanent brain damage or epilepsy, aggravate neurologic disorders, or affect the prognosis for children with underlying disorders.

In the case of pertussis immunization during infancy, however, administration of DTaP could coincide with or hasten the inevitable recognition of a disorder associated with seizures, such as infantile spasms or epilepsy, and cause confusion about the role of pertussis immunization. Hence, pertussis immunization in infants with recent seizures should be deferred until a progressive neurologic disorder is excluded or the cause of the earlier seizure has been determined. In contrast, measles immunization is given at an age when the cause and nature of a child's recent seizure and neurologic status are more likely to have been established. This difference provides the basis for the recommendation that measles immunization should not be deferred for children with recent seizures.

A family history of seizure disorders is not a contraindication to pertussis or measles immunization or a reason to defer immunization. Postimmunization seizures in these children usually are febrile in origin, have a benign outcome, and are not likely to be confused with manifestations of a previously unrecognized neurologic disorder. In addition, many children have a family history of seizures and would remain susceptible to pertussis and measles if family history were a contraindication to immunization.

Specific recommendations for pertussis and measles immunization of children with a personal or family history of seizures are given in the respective disease-specific chapters (see Pertussis, p 435, and Measles, p 385); detailed discussion and recommendations about pertussis immunization of children with neurologic disorders also are given.

Children With Chronic Diseases

Some chronic diseases make children more susceptible to the severe manifestations and complications of common infections. In general, immunizations recommended for healthy children should be given to children with these disorders. However, for children with immunologic disorders, live-virus vaccines usually are contraindicated; the major exception is MMR for HIV-infected children who are not severely immunocompromised (see Immunocompromised Children, p 56). Children with certain chronic diseases (eg, cardiorespiratory, allergic, hematologic, metabolic, and renal disorders and cystic fibrosis) are at increased risk for complications of influenza, pneumococcal infection, or both and should receive influenza and/or pneumococcal vaccine (see Influenza, p 351, and Pneumococcal Infections, p 452). Persons with chronic liver disease are at risk for severe clinical manifestations of acute infection with hepatitis A virus (HAV). Therefore, these children should be immunized with HAV vaccine after 2 years of age (see Hepatitis A, p 280).

The appropriateness of administering a live-virus vaccine to a specific child with a rare disorder (eg, galactosemia or renal tubular acidosis) is problematic, particularly if the disease may impair the immune response to the vaccine. The experience in some of these disorders is minimal or nonexistent, and the physician should seek guidance from a specialist before administering the vaccine(s).

Active Immunization After Exposure to Disease

Since not all susceptible persons receive vaccines before exposure, active immunization may be considered for a person who has been exposed to a specific disease. The following situations are the most commonly encountered (see the disease-specific chapters in Section 3 for detailed recommendations).

- ***Measles.*** Live-virus measles vaccine given within 72 hours of exposure will provide protection against measles in some cases. Determining the time of exposure may be difficult because infected persons can spread measles virus for 3 to 5 days before the appearance of a rash and for 1 to 2 days before the onset of symptoms.

  Immune Globulin (IG) intramuscularly in a dose of 0.25 mL/kg (maximum dose, 15 mL), given within 6 days of exposure, also can prevent or modify measles in a healthy susceptible person. Since measles morbidity is high in children younger than 1 year of age, administration of IG is recommended for infants exposed to measles and for immunocompromised and pregnant persons. Exposed immunocompromised persons should receive 0.5 mL/kg of IG (maximum dose, 15 mL).
- ***Varicella.*** Varicella vaccine is recommended for use in susceptible immunocompetent children and household contacts within 3 days of the appearance of the rash in the index case (see Varicella-Zoster Infections, p 624). Susceptible immunocompromised children should be given passive protection with VZIG as soon as possible after contact with an infected person (see Varicella-Zoster Infections, p 624).
- ***Hepatitis B.*** Postexposure immunization is highly effective if combined with passive antibody. Administration of HBIG does not inhibit active immunization with hepatitis B virus (HBV) vaccine. For postexposure prophylaxis in a newborn infant whose mother is an HBsAg carrier, hepatitis B immunization is essential. For percutaneous or mucosal exposure to HBV, combined active and passive immunization is recommended for susceptible persons (see Hepatitis B, p 289). Persons with continuing household or sexual contact with an HBsAg carrier also should be immunized.
- ***Hepatitis A.*** Available data are insufficient to recommend HAV vaccine alone for postexposure prophylaxis. Immune Globulin should be administered to household, sexual, and other contacts of HAV cases as soon as possible after exposure. If ongoing exposure to HAV is likely, IG and the first dose of HAV vaccine may be administered simultaneously at different sites.
- ***Tetanus.*** In wound management, unimmunized or incompletely immunized persons should be given tetanus toxoid immediately in addition to TIG, depending on the nature of the wound and the immunization history of the person (see Table 3.58, p 566).
- ***Rabies.*** Postexposure active and passive immunization is an essential aspect of the immunoprophylaxis for rabies (see Rabies, p 475).

- ***Mumps and Rubella.*** Exposed susceptible persons are not necessarily protected by postexposure administration of live-virus vaccine. However, a common practice for persons exposed to mumps or rubella is to administer vaccine to presumed susceptible persons so that permanent immunity will be afforded by the immunization if mumps or rubella does not result from the current exposure. Administration of live-virus vaccine is recommended for exposed adults born in the United States after 1956 who have not previously had mumps or rubella or been immunized against mumps or rubella.

Children in Residential Institutions

Children housed in institutions pose special problems for control of certain infectious diseases. Ensuring appropriate immunization is important because of the risk of transmission within the facility and because the conditions that led to institutionalization may increase the risk of complications from the disease. All children entering a residential institution should have received appropriate routine immunizations for their age (see Fig 1.1 and Table 1.5, p 22 and p 24). If they have not been immunized appropriately, arrangements should be made to administer these immunizations as rapidly as possible. Employees should be familiar with standard precautions and procedures for handling contaminated blood and body fluids and for accidental trauma involving these fluids. Employees should be aware of children infected with HBV to ensure prompt and appropriate management in these circumstances. Specific diseases of concern include the following (see the disease-specific chapters in Section 3 for detailed recommendations):

- ***Measles.*** Epidemics can occur among susceptible children in institutional settings. Recommendations for managing children in an institutional setting when a case of measles is recognized are as follows: (1) within 72 hours of exposure, administer live measles virus vaccine (as MMR) to all susceptible children 1 year of age or older for whom immunization is not contraindicated, and (2) administer IG in a dose of 0.25 mL/kg, or 0.5 mL/kg to immunocompromised children (maximum dose, 15 mL) as soon as possible and within 6 days of exposure to all exposed susceptible children younger than 1 year of age. These IG recipients will still require live-virus vaccine (as MMR) at 12 months of age or thereafter, depending on the age and dose of IG administration (see Table 3.35, p 390, for the appropriate interval between IG administration and MMR immunization).
- ***Mumps.*** Epidemics may occur among susceptible unimmunized children in institutions. The major hazards are disruption of activities, the need for acute nursing care in difficult settings, and occasional serious complications (eg, in the susceptible adult attendants).

  If mumps is introduced into a setting where susceptible persons reside, no prophylaxis is available to limit the spread or modify the disease in a susceptible person. Immune Globulin is not effective; Mumps Immune Globulin is not available. Although mumps virus vaccine may not be effective after exposure, the vaccine should be administered to susceptible persons to protect against future exposures.

- ***Influenza.*** Influenza can be devastating in a residential or custodial institutional setting. Rapid spread, intensive exposure, and underlying disease can result in a high risk of severe illness that may affect many residents simultaneously or in close sequence. Current measures for control of influenza in institutions include the following: (1) a program of annual influenza immunization of residents and staff, and (2) appropriate use of chemoprophylaxis during influenza A epidemics. When considering the use of chemoprophylaxis, health care professionals often can obtain information on which strains of influenza are prevalent in the community from local and state health department personnel.
- ***Pertussis.*** Since progressive developmental delay may have resulted in a deferral of pertussis immunization, many children in an institutional setting may not be immunized fully or may be immunized incompletely against pertussis. Because pertussis vaccine does not cause progressive neurologic disease and because pertussis disease poses a greater risk than pertussis immunization to a specific child, children who are not fully immunized and are younger than 7 years of age should be immunized against pertussis. If pertussis is recognized, infected patients and their close contacts should receive chemoprophylaxis.
- ***Hepatitis A.*** Outbreaks of hepatitis A affecting residents and staff can occur in institutions for custodial care by fecal-oral transmission. Infection usually is mild or asymptomatic in young children but can be severe in adults. Although an effective HAV vaccine is available for children 2 years of age and older, the role of this vaccine in helping to control or prevent outbreaks in these settings has not been determined. If an outbreak occurs, susceptible residents and staff members in close personal contact with patients should receive IG (0.02 mL/kg intramuscularly).
- ***Hepatitis B.*** Children living in residential institutions for developmentally disabled children and their caregivers are assumed to be at increased risk for acquiring HBV infection. The high prevalence of HBV markers among children living in these facilities indicates that HBV infections have the propensity for spread in an institutional setting, presumably by exposure to blood and body fluids containing HBV. Factors associated with high prevalence of HBV markers include crowding, high client-staff ratios, and lack of in-service educational programs for the staff. In the presence of such factors, the prevalence of HBV increases with the duration of time spent at the institution. Thus, residents and staff entering or already residing in residential institutions for the developmentally disabled should be immunized against HBV; preimmunization serologic screening for HBV markers probably is not cost-effective.

  After parenteral or sexual exposure to an institutionalized patient recognized to be an HBsAg carrier, unimmunized, susceptible patients or staff should receive active and passive immunoprophylaxis.
- ***Pneumococcal Infections.*** Children with severe physical or mental disabilities, particularly children who are bedridden, who suffer from a compromised respiratory status, or who are capable of only limited physical activity, may benefit from pneumococcal vaccine (see Pneumococcal Infections, p 452).

- ***Varicella.*** Varicella is very contagious and can occur in a high percentage of susceptible children in an institutional setting. All healthy children, 1 year of age or older, who lack a reliable history of varicella should be immunized. Prophylaxis with VZIG (see Table 3.74, p 631) during outbreaks currently is recommended only for immunocompromised susceptible children at risk for serious complications or death from varicella.
- ***Other Infections.*** Other organisms causing diseases that spread in institutions, for which no immunizations are available, include *Shigella, E coli* O157:H7, *Streptococcus pyogenes, Staphylococcus aureus,* respiratory tract viruses except influenza virus, cytomegalovirus, rotavirus, astroviruses, enteric adenoviruses, caliciviruses, *Giardia lamblia, Cryptosporidium,* scabies, and lice.

Children in Military Populations

In general, children of active-duty military personnel require the same immunizations as their civilian counterparts. If delay in pertussis immunization is recommended for any reason, parents should be warned that the risk of contracting the disease in countries where pertussis immunization is not administered routinely is significantly higher than that in countries where effective vaccine is used. For military dependents going overseas, the risk of exposure to HAV and HBV, measles, pertussis, diphtheria, polio, yellow fever, Japanese encephalitis, and other infections may be increased and may necessitate additional immunizations (see Foreign Travel, p 77). In these instances, the choice of immunizations will be dictated by the country of proposed residence, expected travel, and the age and health of the child. For information on the risk of specific diseases in different countries and preventive measures, see Foreign Travel (p 77) or consult the CDC Web site (http://www.cdc.gov).

Adolescent* and College Populations

Adolescents and young adults may not be protected against all vaccine-preventable diseases. This age group may include persons who escaped natural infection and who (1) were not immunized with all recommended vaccines, (2) received appropriate vaccines but at too young an age (eg, measles vaccine before 12 months of age), (3) received incomplete immunization regimens (eg, only 1 or 2 doses of HBV vaccine), or (4) failed to respond to vaccines administered at the appropriate ages.

To assure age-appropriate immunization, all children should have a routine preadolescent appointment at 11 to 12 years of age for the following purposes: (1) immunize persons who previously have not received 2 doses of MMR, (2) give varicella and/or hepatitis B vaccines as indicated, (3) provide a booster dose of diphtheria and tetanus (dT) toxoids, and (4) provide other immunization and preventive services that are indicated. Additional vaccines that may be indicated at this preadolescent visit include influenza, pneumococcal, and hepatitis A vaccines. Specific indications for each of these vaccines are given in the respective disease-specific chapter in Section 3.

---

* Centers for Disease Control and Prevention. Vaccine-preventable diseases: improving vaccination coverage in children, adolescents, and adults. A report on recommendations from the Task Force on Community Preventive Services. *MMWR Morb Mortal Wkly Rep.* 1999;48(RR-8):1–15

Appointments for needed doses of vaccine that are not administered during the aforementioned visit should be scheduled. During all subsequent adolescent visits, the person's immunization status should be reviewed and deficiencies should be corrected, including completion of the 3-dose HBV vaccine series.

School immunization laws encourage "catch-up" programs for older adolescents. Accordingly, school and college health services should establish a system to ensure that all students are protected against vaccine-preventable diseases. Many colleges are implementing the American College Health Association (ACHA) recommendations for prematriculation immunization requirements, mandating protection from measles, mumps, rubella, tetanus, diphtheria, polio, varicella, and HBV. In addition, *Neisseria meningitidis* vaccine is recommended by the ACHA and by some colleges and universities.

- ***Measles.*** Many colleges and universities have experienced measles outbreaks during the past decade, delaying efforts to eliminate this disease from the United States. To prevent measles outbreaks and ensure high levels of immunity among young adults on college and university campuses, the ACHA has recommended that colleges and universities require 2 doses of measles vaccine as a condition for matriculation. The first dose is required on or after the first birthday; the interval between the first and second dose must be at least 1 month. In addition, in post–high school educational settings, the AAP recommends a 2-dose measles immunization schedule, given as MMR vaccine, for persons born after 1956.
- ***Rubella.*** Adolescents and adults should be considered susceptible to rubella if documentation of immunity is lacking. Immunizing adolescents and adults in college reduces the chance of outbreaks and helps to prevent congenital rubella syndrome.
- ***Varicella.*** Varicella immunity is desirable in adolescents and in adults, especially adults in colleges and universities and nonpregnant women of childbearing age.* Adults, adolescents, and children with a reliable history of varicella can be assumed to be immune, and immunization is not necessary. Because approximately 70% to 90% of persons 18 years of age or older without a reliable history of varicella also will be immune, serologic testing of persons 13 years of age or older and immunization of persons who are seronegative may be cost-effective. If serologic testing is performed, a tracking system for seronegative persons should be developed to assure that susceptible persons are immunized. However, serologic testing is not required because varicella vaccine is well tolerated in those immune from prior disease. In some situations, universal immunization may be easier to implement than serologic testing and tracking.
- ***Hepatitis B.*** Hepatitis B virus vaccine is recommended for administration to all adolescents, especially those who have one or more risk factors for HBV infection. Risk factors include multiple sexual partners (defined as more than 1 partner within the previous 6 months), a sexually transmitted disease, sexually active homosexual or bisexual behavior, injection drug use, and occupation or training involving contact with blood or body fluids.

* American Academy of Pediatrics Committee on Infectious Diseases. Varicella vaccine update. *Pediatrics.* 2000;105:136–141

- ***Diphtheria, Tetanus, and Pertussis.*** The adult-type diphtheria and tetanus toxoids, dT, should be given at 11 to 12 years of age and no later than 16 years of age. Thereafter, booster immunization with dT is given every 10 years. Studies are underway to address the need for pertussis immunization in adolescents and adults.
- ***Influenza.*** Epidemic influenza can affect any closed population. Physicians responsible for health care in schools and colleges should consider annual influenza immunization of students, particularly students residing in dormitories or students who are members of athletic teams, to decrease morbidity and minimize disruption of routine activities during epidemics.
- **Neisseria meningitidis.** Immunization of college students is recommended by the ACHA. Pediatricians should inform and educate students and parents about the risk of meningococcal disease and the existence of a safe and effective vaccine and immunize students at their request or if educational institutions require its use for admission.
- ***Other Recommendations.*** Because adolescents and young adults frequently undertake international travel, their immunization status and travel plans should be reviewed 2 or more months before departure to allow time to administer any needed vaccines (see Foreign Travel, p 77).

  Some physicians are unaware of the risks of vaccine-preventable diseases to adolescents and young adults and do not give priority to immunization. Pediatricians should assist in providing information on immunization and vaccine-preventable disease to others who care for adolescents in their communities and should work to heighten awareness of the importance of immunizing adolescents and young adults.

  The possible occurrence of diseases such as measles, mumps, rubella, hepatitis A and B, pertussis, influenza, and *N meningitidis* infections in a school or college should be reported promptly to local health officials.

Health Care Personnel*

Adults whose occupations place them in contact with patients with contagious diseases are at increased risk for contracting vaccine-preventable diseases and, if infected, for transmitting them to their patients. Staff at residential institutions and health care personnel, including physicians, nurses, students, and ancillary personnel, should protect themselves and susceptible patients by receiving appropriate immunizations. Physicians, hospitals, and schools for health care professionals should have a major role in implementing these policies. Vaccine-preventable infections of special concern to those involved in the health care of children are as follows (see the disease-specific chapters in Section 3 for further recommendations):

- ***Rubella.*** Outbreaks of rubella among health care personnel have been reported. Although the disease is mild in adults, the risk to a fetus necessitates documentation of rubella immunity in hospital personnel of both sexes. Persons for whom the risk of rubella infection is increased include hospital personnel in pediatrics,

* Centers for Disease Control and Prevention. Immunization of health-care workers: recommendations of the Advisory Committee on Immunization Practices and the Hospital Infection Control Practices Advisory Committee (HICPAC). *MMWR Morb Mortal Wkly Rep.* 1997;46(RR-18):1–42

physicians and nurses working in pediatric and obstetric ambulatory care (including emergency departments), and all persons working in health care areas in which pregnant women are encountered. Persons should be considered immune only on the basis of serologic tests or documented proof of rubella immunization on or after 12 months of age; a history of rubella is unreliable and should not be used in judging immune status. All susceptible persons should be immunized with MMR (or monocomponent rubella vaccine if immunity to measles and mumps has been documented) before initial or continuing contact with pregnant patients.

Although birth before 1957 generally is considered acceptable evidence of rubella immunity, health care facilities should consider recommending a dose of MMR vaccine to unimmunized workers born before 1957 who lack laboratory evidence of rubella immunity. Rubella immunization or laboratory evidence of rubella immunity is particularly important for female health care personnel born before 1957 who can become pregnant.

- ***Measles.*** Because measles in health care personnel has contributed to spread of this disease during outbreaks, evidence of immunity to measles should be required for health care personnel born after 1956 who will have direct patient contact. Proof is established by a physician-documented illness, a positive serologic test for antibody, or documented receipt of 2 doses of live-virus measles vaccine on or after the first birthday. Workers born before 1957 generally have been considered immune to measles. However, since measles cases have occurred in health care personnel in this age group, health care facilities should consider offering at least 1 dose of measles-containing vaccine to workers who lack proof of immunity to measles, particularly in communities with ongoing measles transmission.
- ***Mumps.*** Transmission of mumps in health care facilities can be disruptive and costly. Adults born before 1957 generally have been considered immune to mumps; those born in 1957 or later are considered immune if they have documentation of a single dose of mumps vaccine received after their first birthday or laboratory evidence of immunity.
- ***Hepatitis B.*** Vaccine is recommended for all health care personnel, including physicians, who are likely to be exposed to blood or blood-containing body fluids. The Occupational Safety and Health Administration of the US Department of Labor has issued a regulation requiring employers of workers at risk for occupational exposure to HBV to offer HBV immunization to these employees at the employer's expense.
- ***Influenza.*** Certain groups of patients, such as those with chronic cardiovascular or pulmonary disease, are at high risk for serious or complicated influenza infection. Because medical personnel can transmit influenza to their patients and because nosocomial outbreaks can occur, influenza immunization programs for hospital personnel and other health care professionals should be organized each autumn. Because immunization is not recommended for infants younger than 6 months of age, personnel working in nurseries and infant wards should be immunized.
- ***Varicella.*** Assurance of varicella immunity is recommended for all susceptible health care personnel. In health care institutions, serologic screening of personnel who have a negative or uncertain history of varicella is likely to be cost-effective.

Varicella immunization is recommended for susceptible persons by the ACIP of the CDC.*

- On occasion, susceptible health care personnel adequately immunized with measles, mumps, rubella, varicella, or HBV vaccines fail to develop serologic evidence of immunity against one or more of these antigens. In those instances, an additional dose (or 1 to 3 additional doses of HBV vaccine) can be given 4 to 6 weeks later, followed by serologic testing. Failure to develop immunity thereafter suggests that further immunization is unlikely to induce seroconversion.
- ***Tuberculosis.*** Comprehensive infection control measures, regular tuberculin skin testing, and, if indicated, antituberculous therapy are the recommended strategies for the prevention and control of tuberculosis among health care personnel. Immunization with BCG is not recommended for personnel in most circumstances. According to current CDC recommendations, BCG immunization should be considered on an individual basis in settings with a high prevalence of multidrug-resistant *Mycobacterium tuberculosis* infection in situations in which transmission of resistant organisms is likely and in facilities where comprehensive infection control precautions against *M tuberculosis* transmission have been implemented and have failed.†

Refugees and Immigrants

Prevention of infectious diseases in refugee and immigrant children presents special problems because of the diseases to which these children have been exposed and the immunization practices unique to their native countries. In 1996, a new subsection was added to the Immigration and Naturalization Act (INA) requiring for the first time that persons seeking an immigrant visa for permanent residency show proof of having received the recommended vaccines, as established by the Advisory Committee on Immunization Practices of the CDC, before immigration. While these regulations now apply to all immigrant children entering the United States, international adoptees have been exempted temporarily from the overseas immunization requirements. Adoptive parents are required to sign a waiver indicating their intention to comply with the CDC immunization requirements after arrival in the United States. Refugees are not required to meet the INA immunization requirements at the time of initial entry into the United States but must show proof of immunization at the time they apply for permanent residency, typically within 3 years of arrival.

Refugee children who resided in processing camps for a few months or more often received medical care, including selected immunizations; however, they often arrive in the United States underimmunized. For refugee children whose immunizations are not up-to-date for age, as documented by a written immunization record (see Immunizations Received Outside the United States, p 27), required vaccines

* Centers for Disease Control and Prevention. Prevention of varicella: recommendations of the Advisory Committee on Immunization Practices (ACIP). *MMWR Morb Mortal Wkly Rep.* 1996;45(RR-11): 1–36 and Prevention of varicella: update recommendations of the Advisory Committee on Immunization Practice (ACIP). *MMWR Morb Mortal Wkly Rep.* 1999;48:(RR-6):1–5

† Centers for Disease Control and Prevention. The role of the BCG vaccine in the prevention and control of tuberculosis in the United States: a joint statement by the Advisory Council for the Elimination of Tuberculosis and the Advisory Committee on Immunization Practices. *MMWR Morb Mortal Wkly Rep.* 1996;45(RR-4):1–18

as indicated for their age should be administered simultaneously (see Fig 1.1 and Table 1.5, p 22 and p 24).

Tuberculosis is an important public health problem of refugees and immigrants. Refugees and immigrants have accounted for a substantial and increasing proportion of new cases of tuberculosis in the United States during the past decade. For recommendations about diagnosis and treatment, see Tuberculosis, p 593.

All refugees and immigrants from hepatitis B–endemic areas, particularly eastern Asia and Africa, should be screened for HBsAg by serology. Most of the HBsAg carriers are asymptomatic, and transmission can be limited by universal infant HBV immunization and administration of HBV vaccine to susceptible household contacts of all ages. Serologic screening of all pregnant refugees and immigrants for HBsAg is necessary to identify women whose infants need active and passive immunoprophylaxis. Person-to-person (horizontal) transmission of this infection has been documented in immigrant populations from endemic areas among preschool and early school-age children without a known carrier in the family.

Foreign Travel

Foreign travel requires consideration of additional vaccines to prevent hepatitis A, cholera, yellow fever, meningococcal disease, typhoid fever, rabies, and Japanese encephalitis, in addition to hepatitis B, measles, polio, tetanus, and diphtheria. These vaccines may be required or recommended depending on the destination and type of foreign travel (see Table 1.12, p 78). In addition, immunizations for all children should be brought up-to-date along with the routinely recommended vaccines before foreign travel. Travelers to tropical and subtropical areas often risk exposure to malaria, dengue fever, and other diseases for which vaccines are not available. For travelers at risk, malaria chemoprophylaxis, insect precautions, and care in hygiene associated with food and liquids are important preventive behaviors (see Malaria, p 381).

An excellent source of information is the publication *Health Information for International Travel* (known as the "Yellow Book," see p 3) published approximately every 2 years by the CDC. Every other week, the CDC also publishes *Summary of Health Information* (known as the "Blue Sheet"), which lists areas infected with yellow fever and cholera and gives changes reported by the CDC and the WHO in the official recommendations for entry into certain countries. Local and state health departments and travel clinics also can be consulted for updated information. Information from the CDC Information Service can be accessed by fax (888-232-3299) or by the Internet (http://www.cdc.gov/travel/index.htm).

ROUTINE IMMUNIZATIONS

Infants and children embarking on international travel should receive routine immunizations appropriate for their ages. These are DTaP, IPV, Hib, MMR, varicella, and HBV vaccines (see Fig 1.1, p 22). To ensure immunity before departure, some vaccines should be given on an accelerated schedule (see Table 1.12, p 78).

For polio immunization of children traveling to polio-endemic areas (the western hemisphere was declared free of wild-type polio in 1994), 3 doses of IPV vaccine should be administered before departure. If necessary, the doses may be given at

Table 1.12. **Recommended Immunizations for Travelers to Developing Countries***

Immunizations	Length of Travel: Brief, <2 wk	Intermediate, 2 wk to 3 mo	Long-term Residential, >3 mo
Review and complete age-appropriate childhood schedule (see text for details) • DTaP, poliovirus vaccine, and *Haemophilus influenzae* type b vaccine may be given at 4-wk intervals if necessary to complete the recommended schedule before departure • Measles: 2 additional doses given if younger than 12 mo of age at first dose • Varicella • Hepatitis B†	+	+	+
Yellow fever‡	+	+	+
Hepatitis A§	+	+	+
Typhoid fever§	±	+	+
Meningococcal disease‖	±	±	±
Rabies¶	±	+	+
Japanese encephalitis‡	±	±	+

* See disease-specific chapters in Section 3 for details. For further sources of information, see text. DTaP indicates diphtheria and tetanus toxoids and acellular pertussis; +, recommended; and ±, consider.

† If insufficient time to complete 6-month primary series, accelerated series can be given (see text for details).

‡ For endemic regions (see *Health Information for International Travel*, p 3). For high-risk activities in areas experiencing outbreaks, vaccine is recommended even for brief travel.

§ Indicated for travelers who will consume food and liquids in areas of poor sanitation.

‖ For endemic regions of Africa, during local epidemics, and travel to Saudi Arabia for the Hajj.

¶ Indicated for person with high risk of animal exposure, and for travelers to endemic countries.

4-week intervals, although 6- to 8-week intervals are preferred. Children should then receive a supplemental dose at 4 to 6 years of age (see Poliovirus Infections, p 465).

Importation of measles remains an important source for measles cases in the United States. Therefore, persons traveling abroad should be immune to measles not only for protection, but also to minimize importation of measles by susceptible hosts. Persons should be considered susceptible to measles unless they have documentation of appropriate immunization, physician-diagnosed measles, or laboratory evidence of immunity to measles or were born in the United States before 1957. For persons born after 1956, 2 doses of measles vaccine at or after 1 year of age are required for evidence of immunity (see Measles, p 385).

Hepatitis B vaccine is now recommended for all children but particularly should be considered for travelers of all ages going to areas where the infection is highly endemic, such as countries in Asia and Africa (see Hepatitis B, p 289). Risk factors for hepatitis B include close contact with the local population for a prolonged period (>6 months), contact with blood or blood-containing body fluids, or sexual contact with residents of these areas. An accelerated dosing schedule is approved for one hepatitis B vaccine (Engerix-B*), during which the first 3 doses are given at 0, 1, and 2 months. This schedule may benefit travelers who have insufficient time (ie, <4 months) before departure to complete the standard 3-dose schedule. If the accelerated schedule is used, a fourth dose should be given at 12 months (see Hepatitis B, p 289).

IMMUNIZATIONS REQUIRED OR RECOMMENDED BECAUSE OF RISK OF DISEASE

Depending on the destination, planned activity, and length of stay, other immunizations may be required or recommended (see Table 1.12, p 78, and disease-specific chapters in Section 3).

Immunoprophylaxis against hepatitis A is indicated for susceptible persons traveling to areas with intermediate or high rates of HAV infection. This includes all areas of the world except Australia, Canada, Japan, New Zealand, and Western Europe. Both of the inactivated vaccines and Immune Globulin (IG) are effective for immunoprophylaxis. For persons 2 years of age and older, vaccine is preferred, but IG is an acceptable alternative. To ensure immediate protection for persons whose departure is imminent, both IG and vaccine may be given concurrently at different sites (see Hepatitis A, p 280). For children younger than 2 years of age, IG is indicated since hepatitis A vaccine is not approved in the United States for use in this age group.

Yellow fever vaccine, an attenuated live-virus vaccine, is required by some countries as a condition of entry. The vaccine is recommended to be given 10 days before travel to areas in the yellow fever endemic zones. Boosters are given every 10 years. Countries actually reporting cases of yellow fever and countries in the endemic zone for yellow fever (areas with the appropriate ecology for transmission, but without reported cases), lie in the Amazon region of South America and between 15° north and 10° south of the equator in Africa. Other countries not in these zones may require immunization of persons arriving from an infected or endemic region. The CDC Health Information for International Travel and the travel section of the CDC Web page (http://www.cdc.gov/travel/index.htm) or another authority should be consulted to help make a decision about immunization. The vaccine is available in the United States only in centers designated by state health departments. Whenever possible, immunization with this live-virus vaccine should be delayed until age 9 months of age or older to minimize the risk of vaccine-associated encephalitis. Infants younger than 4 months of age should never receive yellow fever vaccine. Infants between 4 and 9 months of age should be considered for immunization if travel to an area of ongoing epidemic yellow fever cannot be avoided and a high level of protection against mosquito bites is not possible.

The currently available whole-cell inactivated cholera vaccine has limited efficacy and uncomfortable side effects and is no longer required by any country. Despite WHO recommendations to the contrary, some local authorities may require documentation of immunization. In such cases, a single dose of vaccine is sufficient

* SmithKline Beecham, Philadelphia, Pa.

to satisfy local requirements. If cholera vaccine is given, it should be administered, if possible, at least 3 weeks apart from yellow fever vaccine. If this schedule is not possible, the yellow fever vaccine should be given first (see Simultaneous Administration of Multiple Vaccines, p 26).

Typhoid vaccine is recommended for travelers who may be exposed to contaminated food or water. In particular, those who will reside or visit areas with poor sanitation, those with a longer duration of travel, and those who visit remote areas are at greatest risk. Three typhoid vaccines are available for civilian use in the United States: an oral vaccine containing live-attenuated *S typhi* (Ty21a strain), a parenteral Vi capsular polysaccharide (ViCPS) vaccine, and an older, whole-cell inactivated vaccine (see *Salmonella* Infections, p 501). Because the whole-cell inactivated vaccine causes substantially more adverse reactions and is no more effective than the other two vaccines, the choice usually will be between the oral and the ViCPS vaccines. For specific recommendations see *Salmonella* Infections (p 501). Since antibiotics and the antimalarial drug mefloquine (but not chloroquine) can inhibit the growth of the vaccine strain of *S typhi,* the orally administered vaccine should be given at least 24 hours before or after administration of any of these agents. The oral vaccine capsules need to be refrigerated. Typhoid immunization is not a substitute for careful selection of food and drink.

Meningococcal polysaccharide vaccine (quadrivalent groups A, C, Y, and W-135) should be offered for travelers to areas where epidemics occur frequently, such as sub-Saharan Africa, India, and Nepal, and to countries with current meningococcal A or C epidemics. Saudi Arabia requires a certificate of immunization for pilgrims to Mecca or Medina. The travel section of the CDC Web page (http://www.cdc.gov/travel/index.htm) should be consulted.

Rabies immunization should be offered to children who will be living for more than 1 month in areas where they may encounter rabid animals (particularly dogs in developing countries) or if they engage in activities entailing increased risk of rabies transmission (eg, spelunking). The 3-dose preexposure series may be given as intradermal or intramuscular injections, depending on the vaccine product given (see Rabies, p 475). Administration of chloroquine (and possibly mefloquine) for malaria chemoprophylaxis may decrease the immunogenicity of intradermal rabies immunization. Persons who are taking these agents should receive rabies immunization by the intramuscular route. In the event of a bite by a potentially rabid animal, all travelers should be counseled to thoroughly clean the wound with soap and water and then promptly receive postexposure treatment, including booster doses of rabies vaccine.

Japanese encephalitis (JE) virus, which is spread by the dusk-to-dawn–biting, *Culex* mosquitoes, is a potential risk in Southeast Asia, China, Eastern Russia, and the Indian subcontinent. This vaccine should be offered to persons who will be spending 1 month or longer in endemic areas during the transmission season, especially if travel will include rural farming areas, and to those traveling to areas of epidemic transmission regardless of duration. The geographic and seasonal risks are documented in the CDC Yellow Book. Because potentially severe immediate and delayed allergic reactions to JE vaccine occur in approximately 0.5% of recipients, the potential benefits and risks of vaccine use should be considered carefully. No data are available on vaccine safety and efficacy in infants younger than 1 year of age. Immunization requires 3 doses administered subcutaneously on days 0, 7, and 30 and should be completed at least 10 days before travel to an endemic area to observe for potential allergic reactions. If time constraints necessitate an abbreviated schedule, vaccine can be given at 0, 7, and 14 days (see Arboviruses, p 170).

Influenza immunization may be warranted for foreign travelers, depending on the destination, duration of travel, risk of acquisition (based in part on the season of the year), and the traveler's underlying health status. The influenza season is different in the northern and southern hemispheres. Because epidemic strains may differ, the antigenic composition of influenza vaccines used in North America may be different from those used in the Southern Hemisphere (see Influenza, p 351).

Skin testing for tuberculosis before departure is recommended for intermediate- and long-term travelers who will reside and work in developing countries. Some countries may require BCG vaccine for issuance of work and residency permits for expatriate workers and their families. Follow-up is recommended on return from the endemic area.

Other considerations. In addition to vaccine-preventable diseases, international travelers to the tropics will be exposed to other diseases, including malaria, which is one of the most important threats. For recommendations on appropriate use of chemoprophylaxis, including recommendations for pregnant women, infants, and breastfeeding mothers, see Malaria (p 381).

Prevention of mosquito bites will decrease the risk of malaria, dengue fever, and other arbovirus diseases. Appropriate personal protective measures, particularly during the malaria mosquito–biting period from dusk to dawn, can be highly effective. These preventive measures include wearing long-sleeved cotton shirts and long trousers; application of insect repellent, such as DEET,* to exposed skin; and use of window screens and bed nets. DEET-containing repellents should not exceed a concentration of 20% to 30% and should be used sparingly, applied only to exposed areas of skin, and washed off when the child comes indoors. Insect sprays and soaks containing the residual insecticide permethrin may be applied to clothing and bed nets.

Traveler's diarrhea is a significant problem that may be mitigated by attention to foods and beverages ingested and appropriately treating suspected water sources. Chemoprophylaxis generally is not recommended, but educating families about self-treatment, particularly oral rehydration, is important. During foreign travel, some families may want to carry an antimotility agent and an antimicrobial agent for self-treatment (see *Escherichia coli* Diarrhea, p 243). Enteric bacteria, viruses, and parasites are transmitted in some areas by contaminated water and food supplies.

---

* N, N-diethyl-meta-toluamide.

Recommendations for Care of Children in Special Circumstances

CHEMICAL-BIOLOGICAL TERRORISM*

The threat that chemical and biological weapons will be used on a civilian population in an act of domestic terrorism is increasing. Casualties among adults and children could be significant in such an event. Federal, state, and local authorities have begun extensive planning to meet a chemical-biological incident by developing methods of rapid identification of potential agents and protocols for management of victims without injury to health care personnel. Children would be affected disproportionately by a chemical or biological weapons release for several reasons. Physiologic factors that confer a greater risk of injury to children include their relatively higher minute ventilation, the increased permeability of skin, and a relatively large body surface area that can result in hypothermia if skin decontamination (by showering) is not performed in a controlled environment. The preverbal child may be difficult to assess and triage properly. The protective gear that must be worn by health care personnel to safely manage victims reduces dexterity and the ability to care for small children. Finally, potentially life-saving antimicrobial agents, antidotes, vaccines, and other pharmacologic agents have not been studied adequately in children; for many agents, pediatric doses have not been established. Current management strategies from the Centers for Disease Control and Prevention are available on its Web site (http://www.bt.cdc.gov). Table 2.1 (p 84) lists major early clinical manifestations after exposure to various agents. An algorithm for skin decontamination following exposure to a chemical or biological agent is given in Figure 2.1. (p 87) Table 2.2 (p 86) gives recommended diagnostic procedures, isolation, and treatment of children after exposure to various agents.

* American Academy of Pediatrics Committee on Environmental Health and Committee on Infectious Diseases. Chemical and biological terrorism and its impact on children. *Pediatrics.* 2000;105:662–670

Table 2.1. Prominent Early Clinical Manifestations After Exposure to Chemical-Biological Agents*

Manifestations†	Agents/Diseases
Respiratory	
Influenza-like illness	Q fever, smallpox, tularemia, RMSF
Pharyngitis	Ebola, Lassa fever
Dyspnea and stridor	Anthrax
Pneumonitis	Phosgene, Q fever, Hantavirus, tularemia, plague
Bronchospasm	Nerve agents
Dermatologic	
Vesiculation‡	Smallpox
Petechiae, purpura or bullae‡	Ebola, Lassa fever, Hantavirus, RMSF
Ulcers	Anthrax, tularemia
Corrosive injury or burns	Mustard gas, chlorine, ammonia
Cardiovascular	
Collapse, shock	Ricin, Hantavirus
Bradyarrhythmias	Nerve agents
Hematologic	
Hemorrhage	T-2 toxin
Neurologic	
Peripheral	
Weakness, hypotonia	Nerve agents, botulism
Fasciculations	Nerve agents
Central	
Apathy, disorientation, coma	Ebola
Seizures	Nerve agents
Meningitis	Anthrax
Renal	
Oliguria	Hantavirus
Gastrointestinal	
Rebound tenderness	Anthrax
Hematemesis, melena	Anthrax
Diarrhea	Shiga toxin, staphylococcal enterotoxin

* This table does not include all possible agents. Only the agents believed most likely to be used in a chemical-biological attack are included. RMSF indicates Rocky Mountain spotted fever.

† The spectrum of clinical manifestations for many of these agents can be protean. The symptoms and signs noted in this table are those that likely would make someone initially seek medical attention and are based on the route of exposure during an attack (eg, the manifestations of anthrax differ for an inhalation vs foodborne exposure). Fever, headache, vomiting, and diarrhea are common early manifestations of many illnesses.

‡ Many of the diseases that cause petechiae or vesicular skin lesions initially start as macular or papular rashes.

Table 2.2. **Biological Weapons: Recommended Diagnostic Procedures, Isolation, and Treatment of Children**

Agent	Incubation Period	Diagnostic Sample(s)	Isolation Precautions	Treatment Options	Prophylaxis*	Comments
Anthrax	1–60 d	Blood culture, blood smear; skin lesions or tissue culture or fluorescent antibody (FA) staining	Standard; contact for skin lesions	Ciprofloxacin[†] or doxycycline[‡] or (penicillin G and streptomycin)[§] vaccine, if available	Ciprofloxacin[†] or doxycycline[‡]	Alternative agents: gentamicin, erythromycin, chloramphenicol
Brucellosis	5–60 d	Culture of blood or bone marrow; acute and convalescent serum samples	Standard; contact if lesions are draining	Doxycycline[‡] and rifampin; IF younger than 8 y of age, use trimethoprim-sulfamethoxazole (TMP-SMX)	Doxycycline[‡] and rifampin	TMP-SMX; TMP-SMX may substitute for rifampin with doxycycline
Plague	2–3 d	Culture or FA staining of blood, sputum, lymph node aspirate	Droplet	Streptomycin or gentamicin; doxycycline or chloramphenicol	Doxycycline[‡]; tetracycline	TMP-SMX is alternative; chloramphenicol for meningitis
Q fever	10–40 d	Acute and convalescent serum samples	Standard	Doxycycline[‡] or tetracycline[‡]	Doxycycline[‡]; tetracycline[‡]	
Tularemia	2–10 d	Sputum or tissue culture[‖]; FA available; acute and convalescent serum samples	Standard	Streptomycin or gentamicin	Doxycycline[‡]; tetracycline[‡]	
Smallpox	7–17 d	Culture of pharyngeal swab or lesions	Airborne; contact	Cidofovir[¶]	None available (vaccine effective if available)	

Table 2.2. **Biological Weapons: Recommended Diagnostic Procedures, Isolation, and Treatment of Children, continued**

Agent	Incubation Period	Diagnostic Sample(s)	Isolation Precautions	Treatment Options	Prophylaxis*	Comments
Botulism	1–5 d	Serum for toxin if <3 d since exposure; culture and toxin testing of stool or gastric secretions; nerve conduction testing	Standard	Antitoxin (CDC#)	If ingested, induced vomiting, gastric lavage, purgation, and high enemas may benefit	Aminoglycosides potentiate paralysis; antitoxin after exposure for asymptomatic children not usually given
Staphylococcal enterotoxin B	1–6 h	Culture of nasal swab specimen; examine serum and urine specimens for toxin	Standard	Supportive care	None available	
Ricin			Standard	Supportive care	None available	

* Prophylaxis should be initiated only after consultation with public health officials in situations in which exposure is highly likely. The duration of prophylaxis has not been determined for most agents.

† If susceptibility unknown. Ciprofloxacin is not approved by the US Food and Drug Administration (FDA) for persons younger than 18 years of age but is indicated for potentially serious or life-threatening infections.

‡ Tetracyclines, including doxycycline, are not FDA-approved and usually are contraindicated for children younger than 8 years of age, but treatment is warranted for selected serious infections.

§ Penicillin should be used only if the organism is known to be susceptible.

‖ Special media required for culture. Laboratory hazard; only immunized technicians should ordinarily process cultures.

¶ Pediatric dose not established.

\# Centers for Disease Control and Prevention Drug Service, 404-639-3670 (weekdays, 8-4:30 eastern time) or 404-639-2888 (weekends, nights, holidays).

Figure 2.1. Determination of whether to perform topical decontamination following exposure to a chemical or biological agent.

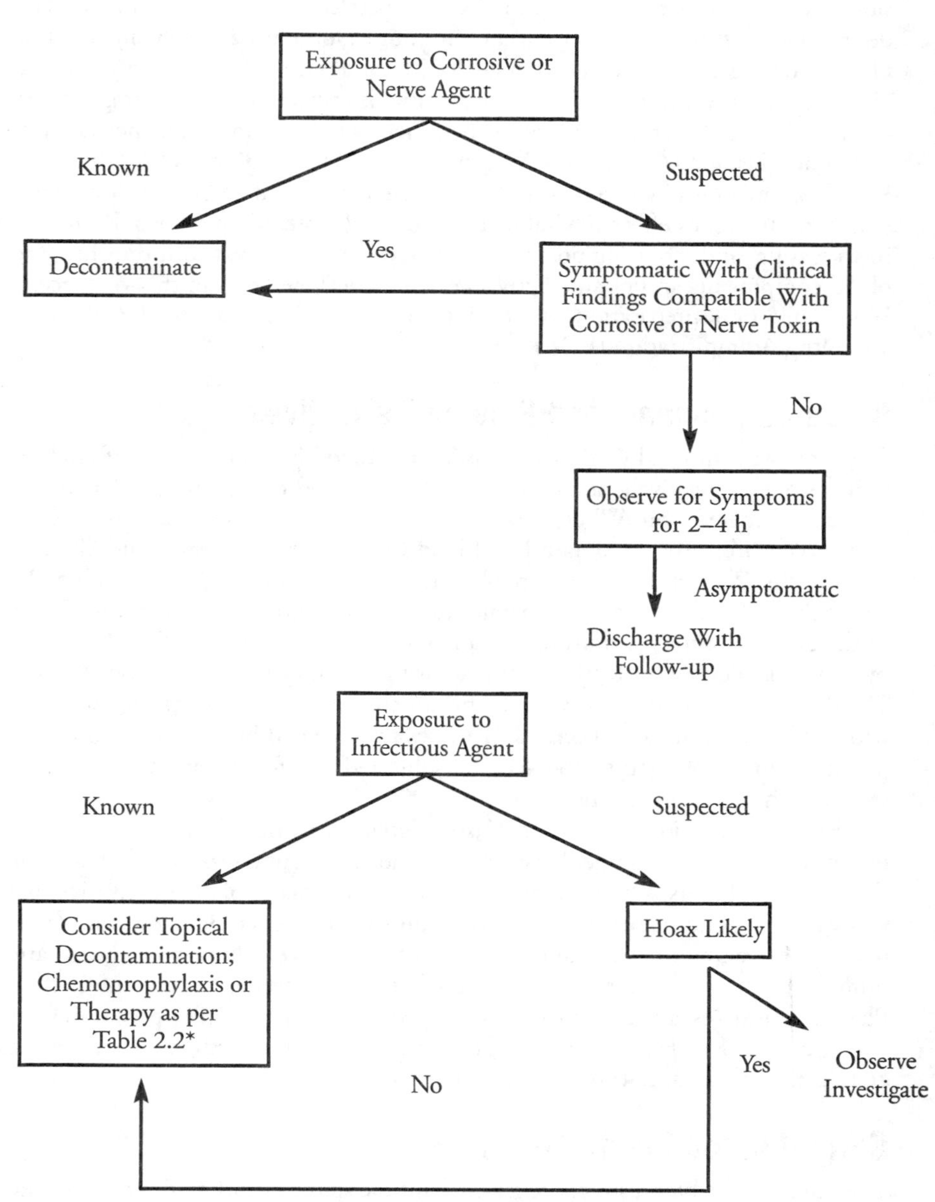

* If exposure to infectious agent likely but agent unknown, public health officials should be contacted to determine whether prophylaxis is warranted.

Blood Safety: Reducing the Risk of Transfusion-Transmitted Infections

In the United States, the risk of transmission of infectious agents through transfusion of blood components (Red Blood Cells, Platelets, and Plasma) and plasma derivatives (clotting factor concentrates, immune globulins, and protein-containing plasma volume expanders) is extremely low. Nevertheless, continued vigilance, including improved surveillance and reporting, is crucial to avert the tragic repercussions that undetected emerging agents, such as human immunodeficiency virus (HIV) and hepatitis C virus (HCV) can effect. The vast majority of HIV and HCV transmissions by blood and blood products occurred before development and introduction of effective viral inactivation and screening methods. Recognizing, investigating, and reporting potential adverse events associated with transfusion of blood components and plasma derivatives are critical elements in this vigilance. Blood collection, preparation, and testing are regulated carefully by the US Food and Drug Administration (FDA).

Blood Components and Plasma Derivatives

The most well-known blood product is Whole Blood, although Whole Blood transfusions are relatively uncommon. The term **blood components** refers to products prepared from Whole Blood using conventional blood-bank methods, such as centrifugation, to obtain Red Blood Cells, Platelets, Plasma, and White Blood Cells. Platelets alone also are obtained through apheresis, in which blood passes through a machine that separates the platelets and returns other components to the donor. Plasma for transfusion can be prepared from Whole Blood or collected by apheresis. Plasma for further manufacturing also may be derived from Whole Blood (recovered plasma) or collected by apheresis (Source Plasma). In contrast with blood components, **plasma derivatives** are prepared by manufacturing; plasma from many donors is pooled and subjected to a fractionation process that separates the desired proteins.

From an infection standpoint, plasma derivatives differ from blood components in several ways. For example, for economic and therapeutic reasons, plasma from thousands of donors is pooled, and, therefore, recipients of plasma derivatives have vastly greater donor exposure than do component recipients. Before introduction of donor screening for HIV and more effective viral inactivation procedures, large numbers of persons who received clotting factor concentrates became infected. Plasma derivatives are able to withstand vigorous viral inactivation processes that would destroy Red Blood Cells and Platelets; component inactivation strategies are at an earlier phase of research and development.

Current Blood Safety Measures

The safety of the blood supply relies on multiple steps, including donor interview and selection, donor screening by serologic tests and other markers of infection, and viral inactivation procedures for plasma-derived products (see Table 2.3, p 89).

Table 2.3. **Blood Donor Screening Measures***

Measure	Targeted Infectious Agents
General interview and screening	
• Previous safety of donor (ie, no deferral in effect)	Bloodborne phase of multiple agents
• General health, current illness, temperature at time of donation	Bloodborne phase of multiple agents
• Donor confidential unit exclusion option	Bloodborne phase of multiple agents
• Reminder to notify blood collector of illness (eg, fever, diarrhea) following donation or of any other pertinent information recalled	Bloodborne phase of multiple agents
Specific risk factor history	
• High-risk sexual behaviors or injection drug use in donor or donor's partner(s)	HIV, HCV, HBV, HTLV
• Geographic risks (travel and residence)	Malaria, new HIV groups
• History of specific infections	HIV, HBV, HCV, other hepatitis agents, parasites (malaria, Chagas disease, babesiosis)
• Previous parenteral exposure to blood via transfusion or occupational exposure; not lifetime deferral	HIV, HCV, HBV
Laboratory screening	HIV-1 and HIV-2 (HIV antibody and HIV-1 p24 antigen), HCV (antibody), HBV (HBsAg and anti-HBc) (ALT generally is performed but not recommended by the FDA), HTLV I/II (antibodies), syphilis

* Screening of Source Plasma (paid) donors is similar, but not identical. For example, because human T-lymphotropic virus (HTLV)-I and HTLV-II are cell-borne agents, Source Plasma donations are not tested for anti-HTLV-I/II. They are not tested for hepatitis B core antibody (anti-HBc). Donors are tested for syphilis at least every 4 months. Additional measures are used for paid Source Plasma donors, including 2 negative screening procedures to become a qualified donor, establishment of residence in community, negative incarceration history, and negative opiate screen. HIV indicates human immunodeficiency virus; HCV, hepatitis C virus; HBV, hepatitis B virus; HBsAg, hepatitis B surface antigen; ALT, alanine aminotransferase; and FDA, US Food and Drug Administration.

Blood screening involves 2 phases: donor screening and blood testing. Blood donors are interviewed to exclude persons with a history of exposures or behaviors that increase their risk for an infectious agent. All blood donations are screened routinely for syphilis, hepatitis B virus (HBV), HCV, human T-lymphotropic viruses (HTLVs) type I and II, and HIV type 1 (HIV-1) and type 2 (HIV-2); selected donations also are screened for cytomegalovirus (CMV). In 1997, approximately 232 000 whole blood units were disqualified in the United States because of positive results on screening tests.

Look-back Programs

If a repeated donor reveals a new or previously undisclosed risk factor on questioning or is found to be infected with certain infectious agents, product retrieval and notification of the party to whom the product was shipped (hospital, transfusion service, or physician) are conducted by blood establishments according to FDA guidance documents and recommendations. Records are reviewed to determine whether any previous donations pose a threat to recipients. For example, an earlier donation may have been made during the "window period" of a viral infection when the donor was viremic but serologic tests were not yet positive. A look-back program is initiated when a repeated donor is determined to have a repeatedly reactive screening test result for HIV or HCV. The first phase is that any remaining components that may contain the infectious agent are located and destroyed. During the second phase, potentially exposed recipients are notified, counseled, and tested.

In 1999 in the United States, a major effort was initiated to notify hundreds of thousands of persons who may have acquired HCV infection from blood transfusions before the introduction of effective screening of blood donations. Two approaches were used to identify these transfusion recipients: (1) a targeted (or directed) approach to identify prior transfusion recipients of donors who tested positive for antibody to HCV after screening tests were implemented (1990 and later) and (2) a general approach to identify all persons who received transfusions before July 1992 (when the more sensitive and specific multiantigen HCV test was implemented). The general notification and education campaign was aimed at providers and the public. Persons who received a transfusion of blood or blood components before July 1992 should seek counseling and testing for HCV infection. Health care professionals should routinely ascertain their patients' transfusion history and probe for risk factors for prior transfusion, such as hematologic disorders, major surgery, trauma, and premature birth.

Transfusion-Transmitted Agents: Known Threats and Potential Pathogens

Any infectious agent that has a blood phase potentially may be transmitted by blood transfusion. Whether an agent is a substantial threat depends on several factors: prevalence in donors, tolerance of the agent to processing and storage, infectivity, pathogenicity, and the recipient's health status. Table 2.4 (p 91) lists major known transfusion-transmitted infections and some of the emerging agents under investigation; these agents are described briefly as follows.

1. **Viruses**

   Although blood donations are screened for several viruses, there is a small residual risk of infection, resulting almost exclusively from donations collected during the window period of infection, which is the period soon after infection during which a blood donor is infectious but screening tests are negative.

   HIV (p 325), HCV (p 302), HBV (p 289). The Retrovirus Epidemiology Donor Study, a National Institutes of Health–funded study of blood donors, provides mathematical estimates of risk for several viruses based on window periods, incidence of infection in the population, and donation intervals in repeated donors (Table 2.4, p 91). The probability of infection in recipients

Table 2.4. Selected Known and Potential Transfusion-Transmitted Agents*

Agents and Products	Transfusion-transmitted	Pathogenic	Estimated per Unit Risk of Contamination (US Studies, Except as Noted)
Viruses for which all blood donors tested			
HIV	Yes	Yes	1 in 676 000
HCV	Yes	Yes	1 in 127 000
HBV	Yes	Yes	1 in 63 000
HTLV types I and II	Yes	Yes	1 in 641 000
Other viruses			
CMV	Yes	Yes	Majority of donors harbor virus
Parvovirus B19	Yes	Yes	1 in 10 000
HAV	Yes	Yes	1 in 1 million
HGV	Yes	Unknown	1–2 in 100
TTV	Yes	Unknown	1 in 10 (Japan), 1 in 50 (Scotland)
HHV-8	Unknown	Yes	Unknown
Bacteria			
Red Blood Cells	Yes	Yes	1 in 500 000 *(Yersinia enterocolitica)*
Platelets			
Random donor	Yes	Yes	1 in 12 500
Apheresis	Yes	Yes	1 in 19 500
Parasites[†]			
Malaria	Yes	Yes	1 in 4 million
Chagas *(Trypanosoma cruzi)*	Yes	Yes	Unknown
Prion			
CJD/vCJD	Unknown	Yes	Unknown
Tick-borne			
Babesia species	Yes	Yes	Unknown
Rocky Mountain spotted fever	Yes	Yes	Unknown
Colorado tick fever virus	Yes	Yes	Unknown
Borrelia burgdorferi	Unknown	Yes	Unknown
Ehrlichia species	Unknown	Yes	Unknown

* HIV indicates human immunodeficiency virus; HCV, hepatitis C virus; HBV, hepatitis B virus; HTLV, human T-lymphotropic virus; CMV, cytomegalovirus; HAV, hepatitis A virus; HGV, hepatitis G virus; TTV, transfusion-transmitted virus; HHV, human herpesvirus; CJD, Creutzfeldt-Jakob disease; and vCJD, variant CJD. For additional information, see Goodnough LT, Brecher ME, Kanter MH, AuBuchon JP. Transfusion medicine: first of two parts: blood transfusion. *N Engl J Med.* 1999;340:438-447; Goodnough LT, Brecher ME, Kanter MH, AuBuchon JP. Transfusion medicine: second of two parts: blood conservation. *N Engl J Med.* 1999;340:525–533; and National Institutes of Health Consensus Development Panel on Infectious Disease Testing for Blood Transfusions. Infectious disease testing for blood transfusions. Bethesda, MD: National Institutes of Health; 1995:1–29.

† Other transfusion-transmitted agents include *Toxoplasma gondii* and leishmanial species.

who are exposed to these viruses is approximately 90% for HIV and HCV and 70% for HBV. The current estimated risks of contamination per unit for HIV, HCV, and HBV are shown in Table 2.4 (p 91). These risks are expected to decrease with the introduction of nucleic acid testing of donors, which will reduce the window period.

Human T-Lymphotropic Viruses I and II (p 101). Infections with HTLV are relatively common in certain geographic areas and in specific populations: HTLV-I in Japan, the Caribbean, and southern United States and HTLV- II in North American aboriginals and injection drug users. Blood is screened routinely for HTLV-I and HTLV-II. Risk of exposure through transfusion is estimated per unit at 1 in 641 000. Human T-lymphotropic virus is less likely to lead to infection than HIV, HBV, or HCV, with an approximate 27% seroconversion rate in persons in the United States who receive blood from infected donors.

Cytomegalovirus (p 227). Immunocompromised persons, including premature infants, bone marrow and solid organ transplant recipients, and others, are at risk of severe, life-threatening illness from transfusion-transmitted CMV. Consequently, only blood from donors who lack CMV antibodies is given to these persons. Leukoreduction also reduces the risk of CMV transmission, since CMV resides in a latent phase within white blood cells.

Parvovirus B19 (p 423). Blood donations are not screened for parvovirus B19 since infection with parvovirus B19 is relatively ubiquitous in humans. Seroprevalence rates in adult blood donors range from 29% to 79%. Estimates of parvovirus B19 viremia in blood donors have ranged from 0.0 to 2.6 per 10 000. Parvovirus, like CMV, usually does not cause severe disease in immunocompetent hosts but may be a threat to certain persons (eg, nonimmune pregnant women, persons with hemoglobinopathies such as sickle-cell disease and thalassemia, and immunocompromised patients). Transmission of parvovirus B19 from single-donor components is thought to occur rarely; however, pooled plasma derivatives frequently are positive for parvovirus B19 DNA since parvovirus B19 lacks a lipid envelope, making it resistant to solvent and detergent treatment. Persons with hemophilia have elevated rates of seropositivity to parvovirus B19 compared with age-matched control subjects; however, the clinical significance of parvovirus B19 among persons with hemophilia is uncertain. To increase safety, some manufacturers of blood products test for parvovirus DNA.

Hepatitis A (p 280). Infection with hepatitis A virus (HAV) leads to a relatively short period of viremia, and a chronic carrier state does not occur. Cases of posttransfusion HAV infection have been reported but are rare. Clusters of HAV infections transmitted from clotting factor concentrates have occurred among persons with hemophilia in Europe during the early 1990s and in South Africa and more recently in the United States. Like parvovirus, HAV lacks a lipid envelope and may survive solvent and detergent treatment.

2. Other Viruses

Two viruses (hepatitis G virus [HGV] and transfusion-transmitted [TT] virus) have been discovered recently, by using new molecular biology techniques, in an attempt to find the cause(s) of posttransfusion hepatitis that cannot be traced to known hepatotropic viruses. One other virus (human herpesvirus [HHV]-8) is being evaluated as a possible bloodborne pathogen.

Hepatitis G Virus (see p 308). Hepatitis G virus and the related GVB-C strain have undergone extensive investigation since their discovery in 1995. In the United States, 1% to 2% of donors are viremic, as defined by the presence of viral nucleic acid in their blood. Although HGV is transfusion transmissible, it is less likely to lead to infection in exposed persons than agents such as HIV or HCV. The HGV has not been established as a true pathogen or even to be hepatotropic, despite its name. The HGV seems to be destroyed by viral inactivation steps used for plasma products, so only component recipients are at risk (see Hepatitis G, p 308). There is no approved test for donor screening, and there is no evidence that implementation of such a test would provide any benefit.

Transfusion-Transmitted Virus. A significant proportion of donors seem to carry TT virus, which was discovered in 1997. Approximately 10% of Japanese and 2% of United Kingdom donors are viremic. Transmission by transfusion has been shown, and fecal-oral transmission also is possible. So far, no clear disease associations with this virus have been established.

Human Herpesvirus 8. Human herpesvirus 8 has been associated with Kaposi sarcoma (KS) in persons with HIV infection, with non-HIV KS, and with certain rare malignant neoplasms. The nucleic acid of HHV-8 and antibodies to HHV-8 have been detected in blood donors (antibody-positive donors likely still harbor HHV-8, as with CMV and other herpes viruses), but transfusion transmission has not been documented. Seroepidemiologic studies suggest that HHV-8 is more likely sexually transmitted than bloodborne (see Human Herpesvirus 8, p 324).

3. Bacteria

Although major advances in blood safety have been made, bacterial contamination of blood products remains an important cause of transfusion reaction, and efforts to detect such contamination should be a routine part of transfusion reaction evaluation. However, suspicion of bacterial contamination often is low, and appropriate testing is not regularly performed for proper detection. For these reasons, bacterial contamination of blood products may be underestimated and unrecognized.

Bacterial contamination of **Platelets** is common in comparison with contamination with viruses. Contamination most often arises from donor skin flora, which enters the bag during blood collection, but may occur during subsequent processing steps as well. Less often, the donor has inapparent bacteremia at the time of donation. The predominant bacteria contaminating platelets is *Staphylococcus epidermidis. Bacillus* species and more virulent organisms, such as *Staphylococcus aureus* and various gram-negative bacteria, also have been reported. Transfusion reactions due to contaminated platelets are likely underrecognized, because episodes of bacteremia with skin organisms are common in patients requiring platelets and the link to the transfusion may not be suspected. Because of the increasing risk of bacterial overgrowth with time, the shelf life of platelets stored at 20°C to 24°C (68°F–75°F) is 5 days.

Red Blood Cell units are much less likely to contain bacteria at the time of transfusion because of the different storage temperatures. Red Blood Cell refrigeration kills or inhibits growth of most bacteria, which are able to grow in platelets, because platelets must be stored at room temperature. Certain bacteria, most notably *Yersinia enterocolitica,* may contaminate Red Blood Cells since this organism survives cold storage. *Yersinia enterocolitica* may cause inapparent donor bacteremia, and cases of septic shock and death due to transfusion-transmitted *Y enterocolitica* are well documented.

The study of *Ba*cterial *Con*tamination of Blood and Blood Products (BaCon study) is an ongoing collaborative effort by the American Association of Blood Banks (AABB), American Red Cross (ARC), Department of Defense (DoD), and Centers for Disease Control and Prevention (CDC) to evaluate transfusion reactions associated with bacterial contamination of blood and blood products.

The BaCon study materials have been developed to assist in educating hospital personnel and encourage proper detection and reporting of episodes of transfusion reaction caused by bacterial contamination of blood and blood products. When a case meets criteria for transfusion reaction, clinical personnel should complete BaCon report forms. Appropriate steps then will be taken by transfusion service personnel, who will contact blood collection facility personnel. Blood collection facility personnel will notify their coordinating organization (AABB, ARC, or DoD). Otherwise, transfusion services should follow their standard operating procedure for investigation and their usual mechanism of reporting to the blood collection facility or blood bank as required by law. When a fatality occurs, reporting to the FDA also is required.

The BaCon study Web site is a resource for blood banks or hospitals that have not received or need additional materials. The BaCon study protocol case criteria, case report forms, and further information can be found at http://www.cdc.gov/ncidod/hip/bacon/. Clinical personnel and transfusion services also may contact CDC directly for guidance about case reporting and evaluation at 404-639-6413.

4. Parasites

Several parasitic agents have been reported to cause transfusion-transmitted infection, including malaria, Chagas disease, babesiosis, toxoplasmosis, and leishmaniasis. Donors are asked about their travel history and disease from or treatment for malaria. Reducing transfusion transmission of parasites is crucial in endemic regions, but increasing travel to and immigration from endemic areas has led to a need for increased vigilance in the United States.

Malaria (see p 381). Approximately 2 to 3 cases of transfusion-associated malaria are reported each year in the United States, despite donor screening for malaria risk factors.

Chagas Disease (see American Trypanosomiasis, p 591). The immigration of millions of persons from *Trypanosoma cruzi*–endemic areas (parts of Central and South American and Mexico) and increased international travel have raised concern about the potential for transfusion-transmitted Chagas disease. Cases of transfusion-transmitted Chagas disease have been reported in North America.

Babesiosis (see p 181). The most commonly reported transfusion-associated tick-borne infection in the United States is babesiosis. Prolonged carriage of *Babesia* organisms has been shown, and some carriers may be well enough to donate blood. Most cases of transfusion-transmitted infection due to *Babesia microti* reported in the United States have occurred in New England, where the parasite is endemic. Transfusion-transmitted babesiosis due to a related organism labeled WA-1 has been reported from Washington State. The parasite survives blood banking conditions and is transmissible by transfusion of Red Blood Cells and Platelet concentrates.

5. **Transmissible Spongiform Encephalopathies: Prion Disease** ***Creutzfeldt-Jakob Disease and Variant Creutzfeldt-Jakob Disease (p 471).*** Creutzfeldt-Jakob disease (CJD) and variant CJD (vCJD) are fatal neurologic illnesses believed to be caused by unique agents known as prions (see Transmissible Spongiform Encephalopathies, p 471).

   CJD. Risk factors for CJD were added to the donor questionnaire in 1995, and blood components and plasma derivatives from donors who developed CJD or had a risk factor for CJD were withdrawn. These policies led in part to shortages of some plasma derivatives, and in 1998 a decision based on a review of current knowledge was made to rescind the policy of withdrawing plasma derivatives. The risk of CJD transmission through blood is considered theoretical. Laboratory experiments using animal models suggest prion infectivity may be present in blood, but epidemiologic evidence is reassuring, since no confirmed cases of CJD resulting from receipt of blood transfusion have been reported. Case-control studies have not found an association with receipt of blood and development of CJD. No cases of CJD in persons with hematologic conditions that require frequent transfusion, such as sickle cell disease and thalassemia, have been reported. Studies of recipients of blood from donors who subsequently developed CJD and surveillance for CJD among persons with hemophilia also have not detected evidence of CJD. Collectively, these epidemiologic data suggest that the risk of CJD, if any, from transfusion, must be rare.

   vCJD. Variant CJD clinically and pathologically is distinct from CJD. Surveillance has been established in the United States for emergence of vCJD, but to date, cases have not been reported. The vCJD has had a major effect on blood safety policies in the United Kingdom: to prevent recipient exposure to plasma from a donor in whom vCJD later develops, plasma from UK residents is no longer used to make plasma derivatives. Also, leukoreduction from all blood components has been initiated in the United Kingdom and other European countries with the goal of reducing possible white blood cell–associated infectivity. In the United States, donors who have been diagnosed with vCJD are deferred permanently. Potential donors who have spent 6 months (cumulatively) or more in the United Kingdom between January 1, 1980, and December 31, 1996, should be deferred indefinitely.

6. **Tick-borne Infections (see Prevention of Tick-borne Infections, p 159)** Agents transmitted via tick bites are receiving attention as emerging infections in the United States. Several types of tick-borne agents are of concern in North America (see Prevention of Tick-borne Infections, p 159). Babesiosis is the most commonly reported transfusion-transmitted tick-borne infection. Rocky Mountain spotted fever and Colorado tick fever associated with transfusion are rare. Lyme disease and ehrlichiosis have not been associated with transfusion.

Improving Blood Safety

A number of strategies have been proposed or recently implemented to further reduce the risk of transmission of infectious agents through blood and blood products. Various safety strategies are as follows.

Improving Laboratory Tests

SHORTENING THE WINDOW PERIOD

The window period for HIV, HCV, and HBV may be shortened by use of tests to detect nucleic acid, because nucleic acid is detectable for days or weeks before currently used antibody or antigen tests become positive. Estimates are that nucleic acid tests will reduce the HIV window period from 16 days to 13 to 14 days. For HCV, nucleic acid tests could reduce the window period from 70 to 80 days to 10 to 30 days and reduce the per-unit risk of HCV from estimates of 1 in 127 000 to 1 in 500 000 to 1 million. Nucleic acid tests have been introduced to detect HIV and HCV in Source Plasma donations and in the majority of Whole Blood donations.

RESPONDING TO GENETIC DIVERSITY: "BIOLOGIC MOVING TARGETS"

Laboratory tests for detecting rapidly changing agents must be revised appropriately in response to genetic diversity. For example, HIV test kits have been modified and will require future modification to include new strains as they are discovered. Not all serologic tests consistently detect HIV-1 group O (outlier) infections, which are common in some West and Central African countries but rare in the United States.

Elimination of Infectious Agents

AGENT INACTIVATION

Virtually all plasma derivatives, including Immune Globulin Intravenous (IGIV) and clotting factors, are treated to eliminate viruses that may be present despite screening measures. Methods used for this include treatment with a solvent and a detergent. Techniques to treat blood components to eliminate pathogens are progressing rapidly. Solvent- and detergent-treated Pooled Plasma for transfusion is available in the United States, and methods of treating single-donor Plasma are under study. Because of their fragility, pathogen inactivation of Red Blood Cells and Platelets is more difficult. However, several methods have been developed, such as addition of psoralens followed by exposure to UV-A to reduce the levels of HIV and hepatotropic viruses. Clinical trials of these treated components are underway.

The spectrum of infectious agents killed by different methods varies. For example, solvent and detergent treatment dissolves the lipid envelope of HIV, HBV, and HCV but is not effective against non–lipid enveloped viruses, such as HAV, parvovirus B19, and TT virus. Thus, a theoretical risk exists that solvent- and detergent-treated products may be unsafe if a new non–lipid enveloped viral pathogen emerges. Some methods, such as psoralens and UV light, destroy both viruses and bacteria and, thus, may help solve the problem of bacterial contamination.

AGENT REMOVAL

Another proposed strategy under FDA review is leukoreduction, whereby filters are used to remove donor white blood cells. Several countries have adopted this practice. The concentration of intracellular or cell-associated agents would be reduced (eg, viruses such as CMV, Epstein-Barr virus, HHV-8, and HTLV).

In addition, some experts believe that the theoretical risk of transmission of vCJD through blood may be reduced by white blood cell removal. Noninfectious benefits of this process include reducing febrile transfusion reactions related to white blood cells and their products and reducing the immune modulation associated with transfusion. White blood cells may have a key role in this immune modulation process, which has been speculated to increase the risks of cancer and wound infections in blood recipients.

Decreasing Exposure to Blood Products

ALTERNATIVES TO HUMAN BLOOD PRODUCTS

Many alternatives to human blood products have been developed. Established alternatives include recombinant clotting factors for patients with hemophilia and factors, such as erythropoietin, used to stimulate Red Blood Cell production. New agents include several Red Blood Cell substitutes currently in clinical trials. These products include human hemoglobin extracted from Red Blood Cells, recombinant human hemoglobin, animal hemoglobin, and various oxygen-carrying chemicals.

AUTOLOGOUS TRANSFUSION

Another means of decreasing recipient exposure is autologous transfusion. Blood may be donated by the patient several weeks before a surgical procedure (preoperative autologous donation) or, alternatively, donated immediately before surgery and replaced with a volume expander (acute normovolemic hemodilution). In either case, the patient's blood can be reinfused if needed. Autologous blood is not completely risk free, since bacterial contamination may occur.

Blood recycling techniques (autotransfusion) are also in this category. During surgery, blood lost by the patient may be collected, processed, and reinfused to the patient.

SHORTAGES OF PLASMA DERIVATIVES

Periodically, shortages of plasma derivatives occur. Factors that contribute to these shortages have included the following: (1) production impediments related to compliance, (2) withdrawals of plasma products because of the theoretical risk of contamination with CJD agent (although, currently, derivatives would be withdrawn only if a plasma donor were diagnosed with vCJD), (3) increase in off-label use of some products (eg, IGIV), (4) waste, and (5) hoarding of product because of concerns about scarcity. For recommendations for use of IGIV, see Indications for the Use of IGIV, p 44.

Strategies to Prevent Harm to Those Exposed to Contaminated Blood

PREEXPOSURE STRATEGIES

Receipt of HBV vaccine is recommended for patients with bleeding disorders who receive clotting factor concentrates (see Hepatitis B, p 289), and HAV vaccine also should be given to this group (see Hepatitis A, p 280).

Strategies to Improve Surveillance

National programs for surveillance include pathogen- and disease-specific systems (eg, HIV, viral hepatitis) and programs that focus on donors and recipients of blood and plasma products. In addition, large-scale repositories of specimens from donors and recipients have been used to study infectious complications of transfusions.

Transfusion-transmitted infection surveillance is crucial and must be coupled with the capacity to rapidly investigate reported cases and to implement measures needed to prevent further infections. A surveillance system was implemented in the United States to specifically address the issue of bacterial contamination (BaCon). Serious adverse reactions and product problems should be reported to the manufacturer (or, alternatively, to the supplier for transmission to the manufacturer). Practitioners also may report such information directly to the FDA through MEDWATCH. This can be done by telephone (1-800-FDA-1088), fax (1-800-FDA-0178), Internet (http://www.fda.gov/medwatch/report/hcp.htm), or mail (see MEDWATCH, p 726). This reporting is voluntary, but it is considered vital for monitoring product safety.

HUMAN MILK

Breastfeeding provides numerous health benefits to young infants, including protection against morbidity and mortality from infectious diseases of bacterial, viral, and parasitic origin. While providing an ideal source of infant nutrition, largely uncontaminated by environmental pathogens, human milk contains protective factors, including cells, specific secretory antibodies, nonimmune factors such as glycoconjugates, and anti-inflammatory components. In their gastrointestinal tracts, breastfed infants have high concentrations of protective bifidobacteria and lactobacillus, which increase resistance to pathogenic organisms. Increasing evidence indicates that human milk may modulate development of the infant's immune system. Protection by human milk is established most clearly for pathogens causing gastrointestinal tract infection. In addition, human milk seems to provide protection against otitis media, invasive *Haemophilus influenzae* type b infection, respiratory syncytial virus infection, and other causes of upper and lower respiratory tract infections.

The American Academy of Pediatrics (AAP) Committee on Nutrition issues statements and publishes a manual on infant feeding that provides further information about the benefits of breastfeeding and recommended feeding practices.* In the *Pediatric Nutrition Handbook,* and in the AAP policy statement on human milk,† questions about immunization of lactating mothers and breastfeeding infants, transmission of infectious agents via human milk, and potential effects on breastfeeding infants of antimicrobial agents administered to lactating mothers also are addressed.

Immunization of Mothers and Infants

EFFECT OF MATERNAL IMMUNIZATION

Women who have not received the recommended immunizations before or during pregnancy may be immunized during the postpartum period regardless of lactation status. No evidence exists for concern about the potential presence in maternal milk of live viruses from vaccines if the mother is immunized during lactation. Lactating women may be immunized, as recommended for other adults, to protect against measles, mumps, rubella, tetanus, diphtheria, influenza, *Streptococcus pneumoniae,* hepatitis A virus, hepatitis B virus, and varicella. If previously unimmunized or if traveling to a highly endemic area, a lactating mother may be given inactivated poliovirus vaccine. Rubella seronegative mothers who could not be immunized during pregnancy should be immunized during the postpartum period.

EFFICACY OF IMMUNIZATION IN BREASTFED INFANTS

The immunogenicity of some currently recommended vaccines is enhanced by breastfeeding, but the importance of these observations in their efficacy is unknown. Although high concentrations of antipoliovirus antibody in milk of some mothers theoretically could interfere with the immunogenicity of oral polio vaccine, no such association has been demonstrated. Infants should be immunized according to the recommended schedule regardless of the infant's mode of feeding.

Transmission of Infectious Agents Via Human Milk

BACTERIA

Mastitis and breast abscesses have been associated with the presence of bacterial pathogens in human milk. In general, infectious mastitis resolves with continued lactation during antibiotic therapy and does not pose a significant risk for the healthy term infant. Breast abscesses occur rarely and have the potential to rupture into the ductal system, releasing large numbers of organisms, such as *Staphylococcus aureus,* into milk. In general, feeding an infant using a breast affected by an abscess is not recommended. However, some experts recommend that infant feeding using the affected breast may resume once the mother is treated adequately with an appropriate antimicrobial agent and the abscess is drained surgically. Even when breastfeeding is interrupted on the affected breast, breastfeeding may continue on the opposite (unaffected) breast.

* American Academy of Pediatrics Committee on Nutrition. *Pediatric Nutrition Handbook.* 4th ed. Elk Grove Village, IL: American Academy of Pediatrics; 1998

† American Academy of Pediatrics Work Group on Breastfeeding. Breastfeeding and the use of human milk. *Pediatrics.* 1997;100:1035–1039

Women with tuberculosis who have been treated appropriately for 2 or more weeks and who are otherwise considered noncontagious may breastfeed. Women with active tuberculosis suspected of being contagious should refrain from breastfeeding or any other close contact with the infant because of potential transmission through respiratory tract droplets (see Tuberculosis, p 593). *Mycobacterium tuberculosis* rarely causes mastitis or a breast abscess, but if a breast abscess caused by *M tuberculosis* is present, breastfeeding should be discontinued until the mother is no longer contagious.

Expressed human milk can become contaminated with a variety of bacterial pathogens, including *Staphylococcus* species and gram-negative enteric bacilli. Outbreaks of gram-negative bacterial infections in neonatal intensive care units occasionally have been attributed to contaminated human milk specimens that have been collected or stored improperly. Human milk fed to infants from women other than the biologic mother should be treated according to the guidelines of the Human Milk Banking Association of North America. Routine culturing or heat treatment of a mother's milk fed to her infant has not been demonstrated to be necessary or cost-effective (see Human Milk Banks, p 102).

VIRUSES

Cytomegalovirus. Cytomegalovirus (CMV) may be shed intermittently in human milk. Although transmission of CMV through human milk has occurred, disease in the neonate is uncommon, presumably because of passively transferred maternal antibody. Preterm infants, however, are at greater potential risk of symptomatic disease and sequelae than are term infants. Infants born to CMV-seronegative women who seroconvert during lactation and premature infants with low concentrations of transplacentally acquired maternal antibodies to CMV can develop symptomatic disease with sequelae from acquiring CMV through breastfeeding. Decisions about breastfeeding of premature infants by mothers known to be CMV-seropositive should consider the potential benefits of human milk and the risk of CMV transmission. Pasteurization of milk seems to inactivate CMV; freezing milk at –20°C (–4°F) will decrease viral titers but does not reliably eliminate CMV.

Hepatitis B. Hepatitis B surface antigen (HBsAg) has been detected in milk from HBsAg-positive women. However, studies from Taiwan and England have indicated that breastfeeding by HBsAg-positive women does not increase significantly the risk of infection among their infants. In the United States, infants born to known HBsAg-positive women should receive Hepatitis B Immune Globulin (HBIG) and hepatitis B virus vaccine, effectively eliminating any theoretical risk of transmission through breastfeeding. There is no need to delay initiation of breastfeeding until after the infant is immunized. Immunoprophylaxis of infants with hepatitis B vaccine alone also provides protection, but optimal therapy of infants born to HBsAg-positive mothers includes hepatitis B virus vaccine and HBIG (see Hepatitis B, p 289).

Hepatitis C. Hepatitis C virus (HCV) RNA and antibody to HCV have been detected in milk of mothers infected with HCV. Transmission of HCV via breastfeeding has not been documented in anti-HCV positive, anti–human immunodeficiency virus (HIV)-negative mothers. Mothers infected with HCV should be counseled that transmission of HCV by breastfeeding theoretically is possible but has not been documented. According to current guidelines of the US Public Health Service, maternal HCV infection is not a contraindication to breastfeeding. The decision to breastfeed should be based on informed discussion between a mother and her health care professional.

Human Immunodeficiency Virus. Human immunodeficiency virus has been isolated from human milk and can be transmitted through breastfeeding. The risk of transmission is higher for women who acquire HIV infection during lactation (ie, postpartum) than in women with preexisting infection. In populations, such as in the United States, in which the risk of mortality from infectious diseases and malnutrition is low and in which safe and effective alternative sources of feeding are available readily, HIV-infected women should be counseled not to breastfeed their infants or donate milk. All pregnant women in the United States should be counseled and encouraged to be tested for HIV infection. In areas where infectious diseases and malnutrition are important causes of mortality early in life, the World Health Organization (WHO) recommends that if a mother is infected with HIV, replacement of human milk to reduce the risk of HIV transmission may be preferable provided that the risk of replacement feeding is less than the potential risk of HIV transmission. The WHO policy stresses the need for continued support for breastfeeding by mothers who are HIV-negative or of unknown HIV status, improved access to HIV counseling and testing, and government efforts to ensure uninterrupted access to nutritionally adequate human milk substitutes (see HIV Infection, p 325).

Human T-Cell Lymphotropic Virus Type I. This retrovirus, which is endemic in Japan, the Caribbean, and parts of South America, is associated with development of malignant neoplasms and neurologic disorders among adults. Epidemiologic and laboratory studies suggest that mother-to-infant transmission of human T-cell lymphotropic virus type I (HTLV-I) occurs primarily through breastfeeding. Women in the United States who are HTLV-I seropositive should be advised not to breastfeed.

Human T-Cell Lymphotropic Virus Type II. Human T-cell lymphotropic virus type II (HTLV-II), also a retrovirus, has been detected among American and European injection drug users and some indigenous Native American groups. Although apparent maternal-infant transmission has been reported, the rate and timing of transmission have not been established. Until additional data about possible transmission through breastfeeding become available, women in the United States who are seropositive should be advised not to breastfeed.

Herpes Simplex Virus Type 1. The virus has been isolated from human milk in the absence of vesicular lesions or drainage from the breast or concurrent positive cultures from the maternal cervix, vagina, or throat. Cases of transmission of herpes simplex virus type 1 (HSV-1) after breastfeeding in the presence of maternal breast lesions have been reported. Since development of extragenital lesions seems to occur more often with primary than with recurrent HSV infection, some experts recommend that women with primary mucocutaneous disease should not breastfeed their infants until all lesions have resolved and viral shedding has ceased. Women with herpetic lesions on their breasts should refrain from breastfeeding; active lesions elsewhere should be covered.

Rubella. Both wild and vaccine strains of rubella virus have been isolated from human milk. However, the presence of rubella virus in human milk has not been associated with significant disease in infants, and transmission is more likely to occur through other routes. Women with rubella or women who have just been immunized with rubella live-attenuated virus vaccine need not refrain from breastfeeding.

Varicella. Whether varicella vaccine virus is secreted in human milk or whether the virus would infect a breastfeeding infant is unknown. Therefore, varicella vaccine may be considered for a susceptible breastfeeding mother if the risk of exposure to natural varicella-zoster virus is high. For recommendations for use of varicella-zoster immune globulin and varicella vaccine for contacts of a breastfeeding mother in whom varicella develops, see Varicella-Zoster Infections (p 624).

HUMAN MILK BANKS

Some conditions, such as premature delivery, may preclude breastfeeding. In these cases, infants may be fed milk collected from their own mothers or from unrelated individual donors. The potential for transmission of infectious agents through human milk requires appropriate selection and screening of donors and careful collection, processing, and storage of milk. Currently, US donor milk banks that belong to the Human Milk Banking Association of North America voluntarily follow guidelines drafted in consultation with the US Food and Drug Administration and the Centers for Disease Control and Prevention. These guidelines include screening of all donors for antibodies to HIV-1, HIV-2, HTLV-I, HTLV-II, HBsAg, hepatitis C, and syphilis. Donor milk is dispensed only on prescription after it is heat-treated at 56°C (133°F) or greater for 30 minutes and bacterial cultures reveal no growth. Milk from the birth mother of a premature infant does not require processing if fed to her infant, but proper storage needs to be assured.

Heat treatment at 56°C (133°F) or greater for 30 minutes reliably eliminates bacteria, inactivates HIV, and decreases the titers of other viruses, but heating to 56°C (133°F) in 1 study did not completely eliminate CMV. Holder pasteurization (62.5°C [144.5°F] for 30 minutes) reliably inactivates HIV and CMV and will eliminate or significantly decrease titers of most other viruses.

Freezing at –20°C (–4°F) will eliminate HTLV-I and will decrease the concentration of CMV but will not destroy most other viruses or bacteria. Although few data are available about appropriate microbiologic quality standards for fresh, unpasteurized, expressed milk, the Human Milk Banking Association of North America recommends use of only specimens with fewer than 104 colony-forming units per milliliter of nonpathogenic bacteria. The presence of gram-negative bacteria, *S aureus,* or α- or ß-hemolytic streptococci precludes use of milk specimens.

Antimicrobial Agents in Maternal Milk

Antimicrobial agents taken by a lactating mother often can appear in her milk. A general guideline is that an antimicrobial agent is safe to administer to a lactating woman if it is safe to administer to an infant. The AAP Committee on Drugs has reviewed the risks to infants of specific antimicrobial agents taken by lactating mothers.* Recommendations are included in Table 2.5 (p 104). Although important exceptions exist, the majority of antimicrobial agents that might be taken by lactating mothers are compatible with breastfeeding. When treatment with metronidazole is indicated for the lactating mother, the infant's exposure can be minimized by alteration of the dosing schedule and temporary interruption of breastfeeding. For example, for treatment of *Trichomonas vaginalis* infection, a single 2-g dose of metronidazole may be taken by the lactating mother, after which she should pump and discard her milk for 24 hours and then resume breastfeeding. The alternative is a 10-day course with a cessation of breastfeeding during that time. Women receiving chloramphenicol should not breastfeed because of the theoretical risk of idiosyncratic and dose-related bone marrow suppression in the breastfeeding infant.

The AAP Committee on Drugs considers maternal use of isoniazid to be compatible with breastfeeding. While potential hepatotoxic effects in breastfeeding infants are a concern, no adverse effects have been demonstrated. The infant should receive pyridoxine (see Tuberculosis, p 593). Although not evaluated by the Committee on Drugs, maternal use of the fluoroquinolones, such as ciprofloxacin, norfloxacin, and ofloxacin, is not recommended during breastfeeding by many experts because these compounds are excreted in human milk in high concentrations and, based on experimental data in immature animals, might affect cartilage development of weight-bearing joints of infants. In addition, a case of pseudomembranous colitis associated with ciprofloxacin self-administered by the mother has been reported in a 2-month-old breastfed infant. In 1 study, norfloxacin was found not to be excreted in detectable concentrations in human milk. Therefore, some experts consider the use of norfloxacin to be compatible with breastfeeding.

Maternal use of tetracycline usually is compatible with breastfeeding, since absorption of the drugs by the breastfeeding infant is negligible. However, some experts recommend that use of tetracycline by a lactating mother should be avoided, if possible, because of the potential for staining of the infant's unerupted teeth.

The amount of drug an infant receives from a lactating mother depends on a number of factors, including maternal dose, frequency and duration of administration, absorption, and distribution characteristics of the drug. When a lactating woman receives appropriate doses of an antimicrobial agent, the concentration of the compound in her milk usually is less than the equivalent of a therapeutic dose for the infant. A breastfed infant who requires antimicrobial therapy should receive recommended doses directly, even if the same agent is administered to the mother.

The characteristics of the recipient infant should be considered when assessing the potential effect of specific antimicrobial agents taken by the mother. The maturity of the infant at birth, the chronologic postpartum age, the infant's clinical prob-

* American Academy of Pediatrics Committee on Drugs. The transfer of drugs and other chemicals into human milk. *Pediatrics*. 1994;93:137–150

Table 2.5. **Antimicrobial Agents Taken by Mothers That May Be a Cause for Concern for Breastfeeding Women***

Maternal Antimicrobial Agent	Reported Sign or Symptom in Infant or Possible Cause for Concern	Committee on Drugs Evaluation
Chloramphenicol	Possible idiosyncratic bone marrow suppression	Unknown effect on breastfeeding infant but may be of concern
Metronidazole	In vitro mutagen; may discontinue breastfeeding for 12–24 h to allow excretion of dose when single-dose therapy is given to mother	Unknown effect on breastfeeding infant but may be of concern
All fluoroquinolones	Theoretically may affect cartilage development of weight-bearing joints	Not evaluated
Isoniazid	None; acetyl metabolite also secreted; may be hepatotoxic	Usually compatible with breastfeeding
Nalidixic acid	Hemolysis in infant with G6PD deficiency	Usually compatible with breastfeeding
Nitrofurantoin	Hemolysis in infant with G6PD deficiency	Usually compatible with breastfeeding
Sulfonamides	Caution in infant with jaundice or G6PD deficiency and in ill, stressed, or premature infant	Usually compatible with breastfeeding

* G6PD indicates glucose-6-phosphate dehydrogenase.

lems, and the pattern of breastfeeding will alter the possible risk. If an infant has glucose-6-phosphate dehydrogenase deficiency, maternal use of nalidixic acid, nitrofurantoin, or sulfonamides should be avoided (see Table 2.5, above). With premature, jaundiced, stressed, or ill infants, maternal use of sulfonamide compounds should be avoided. In addition, pharmacokinetic properties of the antimicrobial agent may be helpful for deciding about the safety of a new agent whose appearance in milk is unknown. If the drug is not orally bioavailable (ie, it must be given parenterally), it will not be absorbed from milk by the infant.

Another consideration is the potential for interaction of drugs the mother is receiving and drugs an infant is receiving. Hence, physicians caring for infants who are breastfeeding should be aware of the medications the mother is taking and their potential for adverse interaction with drugs that might be prescribed for the infant. When making the decision about use of appropriate antimicrobial agents for a lactating woman, the physician should weigh the benefits of breastfeeding against the potential risk to the breastfeeding infant of exposure to a drug. In most cases, the benefits exceed the risks. The circumstance would be rare in which the only effective medication for treatment of maternal infection would be contraindicated because of risks to the infant.

Children in Out-of-Home Child Care*

Infants and young children who are cared for in groups have an increased rate of certain infectious diseases and an increased risk for acquiring antibiotic-resistant organisms. Prevention and control of infection in out-of-home child care settings is influenced by several factors, including the following: (1) caregivers' practice of personal hygiene and immunization status, (2) environmental sanitation, (3) food handling procedures, (4) the ages and immunization status of children, (5) the ratio of children to caregivers, (6) the physical space and quality of the facilities, and (7) frequency of use of antimicrobial agents in children in child care. Adequately addressing problems of infection control in child care settings requires collaborative efforts of public health officials, licensing agencies, child care providers, physicians, nurses, parents, employers, and other members of the community.

Child care programs should require that all children and staff receive age-appropriate immunizations and routine health care. In addition, these programs have the opportunity to provide young, inexperienced parents with day-to-day instruction in child development, hygiene, appropriate nutrition, and management of minor illnesses.

Classification of Care Service

Child care services commonly are classified by the type of setting, the number of children in care, ages of the children, and their health status. **Small-family child care** is defined as out-of-home care provided in a private residence where a provider cares for fewer than 6 unrelated children. **Large-family child care** is defined as out-of-home care provided in a private residence for 7 to 12 children. **Center child care** is provided in a nonresidential facility and usually serves 13 or more children in a part-day or full-day program. **Sick-child care** describes specialized programs designed to provide care for mildly ill children who are excluded from regular child care programs. All 50 states license out-of-home child care; however, licensing is directed toward center-based child care; few states or municipalities license small or family run child care programs.

Grouping of children by age varies in different programs, but in child care centers, grouping often consists of **infants** (birth to 12 months of age), **toddlers** (13–35 months of age), **preschoolers** (36–59 months of age), and **school-age** children (5–12 years of age).

Infants and toddlers require diapering or assistance in using a toilet, explore the environment with their mouths, have poor control over their secretions and excretions, have immature immune systems, and require hands-on contact with care providers. In addition, toddlers have frequent direct contact with other toddlers. Therefore, child care programs that provide infant and toddler care need to give special attention to infection control measures.

---

* This chapter is modified from recommendations formulated and revised by a joint committee of the American Academy of Pediatrics and the American Public Health Association (*Caring for Our Children. National Health and Safety Performance Standards: Guidelines for Out-of-Home Child Care Programs.* Washington, DC: American Public Health Association; 2000).

Management and Prevention of Illness

The modes of transmission of bacteria, viruses, parasites, and fungi within child care settings are listed in Table 2.6 (p 107). In most instances, the risk of introducing an infectious agent into a child care group is related directly to prevalence of the agent in the population and to the number of susceptible children in that group. Transmission of an agent within the group depends on the following: (1) characteristics such as mode of spread, infective dose, and survival in the environment; (2) frequency of asymptomatic infection or carrier state; and (3) immunity to the respective pathogen. Transmission also can be affected by characteristics of the child care providers, particularly hygienic aspects of child handling, by environmental practices, and by ages and immunization status of the children enrolled. Appropriate and thorough hand washing is the most important factor for reducing transmission of disease in child care settings. Children infected in a child care group subsequently can transmit infection not only within the group, but also within their households and the community.

The major options for management of ill or infected children in child care and for controlling spread of infection include the following: (1) antimicrobial treatment, prophylaxis, or immunization when appropriate; (2) exclusion of ill or infected children from the facility; (3) provision of alternative care at a separate site; (4) cohorting to provide care (ie, inclusion of infected children in a group with separate staff and facilities); (5) limiting admission of newly enrolled children; and (6) closing the facility (a rarely exercised option). Recommendations for controlling the spread of specific infectious agents differ according to the epidemiology of the pathogen (see disease-specific chapters in Section 3).

Certain general and disease-specific infection control procedures in child care programs reduce acquisition and transmission of communicable diseases within and outside the programs. Among these procedures are the following: (1) review of child and employee illness records, including current immunization records; (2) hygienic and sanitary procedures for toilet use and toilet training; (3) hand-washing procedures (the single most important measure for preventing infection) and enforcement of hand-washing procedures; (4) environmental sanitation; (5) personal hygiene for children and staff; (6) sanitary handling of food; (7) communicable disease surveillance and reporting; and (8) management of pets. Specific staff policies that include training procedures for full- and part-time employees and staff illness exclusion policies also aid in the control of infectious diseases. Health departments should have plans for responding to reportable and nonreportable communicable diseases in child care programs and should provide training, written information, and technical consultation to child care programs when requested. Evaluation of the health status of each child should be performed by a qualified staff member each day, on entry of the child at the site and during the day. Parents should be encouraged to share information with child care staff about their child's acute and chronic illnesses and medication use. Parents should be required to report their child's immunization status on a regular ongoing basis.

Table 2.6. **Modes of Transmission of Organisms in Child Care Settings**

Mode of Transmission*	Bacteria	Viruses	Other†
Fecal-oral	*Campylobacter* organisms, *Clostridium difficile, Escherichia coli* O157:H7, *Salmonella* organisms, *Shigella* organisms	Astrovirus, calicivirus, enteric adenovirus, enteroviruses, hepatitis A virus, rotaviruses	*Cryptosporidium parvum, Enterobius vermicularis, Giardia lamblia*
Respiratory	*Bordetella pertussis, Haemophilus influenzae* type b, *Mycobacterium tuberculosis, Neisseria meningitidis, Streptococcus pneumoniae,* group A streptococcus	Adenovirus, influenza, measles, mumps, parainfluenza, parvovirus B19, respiratory syncytial virus, rhinovirus, rubella, varicella-zoster virus	...
Person-to-person via skin contact	Group A streptococcus, *Staphylococcus aureus*	Herpes simplex virus, varicella-zoster virus	Agents causing pediculosis, scabies, and ringworm
Contact with blood, urine, and/or saliva	...	Cytomegalovirus, hepatitis B and C viruses, herpes simplex virus	...

* The potential for transmission of microorganisms in the child care setting by food and animals also exists (see Appendix V, Clinical Syndromes Associated With Foodborne Diseases, p 767, and Appendix VII, Diseases Transmitted by Animals, p 773).

† Parasites, fungi, mites, and lice.

Recommendations for Inclusion or Exclusion

Mild illness is common among children, and most children will not need to be excluded from their usual source of care for mild respiratory tract illnesses, because transmission is likely to have occurred before symptoms developed in the child or is a result of contact with children with asymptomatic infection. The risk of illness can be reduced by following common-sense hygienic practices.

Exclusion of sick children (and adults) from out-of-home child care settings has been recommended when such exclusion could reduce the likelihood of secondary cases. In many situations, the expertise of the program's medical consultant and that of the responsible local and state public health authorities are helpful for determining the benefits and risks of excluding children from their usual care program. Most states have laws about isolation of persons with communicable diseases. Local or state health departments should be contacted about these laws, and authorities in these areas should be notified about cases of reportable communicable diseases and unusual outbreaks of other illnesses involving children or adults in the child care environment (see Appendix VIII, Nationally Notifiable Infectious Diseases in the United States, p 777).

Children should be excluded from the child care setting for the following reasons:

- Illness that prevents the child from participating comfortably in program activities.
- Illness that results in a greater need for care than the staff can provide without compromising the health and safety of other children.
- The child has any of the following conditions: fever, lethargy, irritability, persistent crying, difficult breathing, or other manifestations of possible severe illness.
- Diarrhea or stools that contain blood or mucus.
- *Escherichia coli* O157:H7 or *Shigella* infection, until diarrhea resolves and 2 stool cultures are negative for these organisms.
- Vomiting 2 or more times during the previous 24 hours, unless the vomiting is determined to be caused by a noncommunicable condition and the child is not in danger of dehydration.
- Mouth sores associated with drooling, unless the child's physician or local health department authority states that the child is noninfectious.
- Rash with fever or behavioral change, until a physician has determined the illness is not a communicable disease.
- Purulent conjunctivitis (defined as pink or red conjunctiva with white or yellow eye discharge, often with matted eyelids after sleep and eye pain or redness of the eyelids or skin surrounding the eye), until examined by a physician and approved for readmission, with treatment.
- Tuberculosis, until the child's physician or local health department authority states that the child is noninfectious.
- Impetigo, until 24 hours after treatment has been initiated.
- Streptococcal pharyngitis, until 24 hours after treatment has been initiated.
- Head lice (pediculosis), until after the first treatment.
- Scabies, until after treatment has been given.
- Varicella, until all lesions have dried and crusted (usually 6 days) (see Varicella-Zoster Infections, p 624).
- Pertussis, until 5 days of appropriate antibiotic therapy (which is to be given for a total of 14 days) has been completed (see Pertussis, p 435).
- Mumps, until 9 days after onset of parotid gland swelling.
- Measles, until 4 days after onset of rash.
- Hepatitis A virus (HAV) infection, until 1 week after onset of illness or jaundice (if symptoms are mild).

Most minor illnesses do not constitute a reason for excluding a child from child care. Examples of illnesses and conditions that do not necessitate exclusion include nonpurulent conjunctivitis (defined as pink conjunctiva with a clear, watery eye discharge without fever, eye pain, or eyelid redness), rash without fever and without behavioral change, parvovirus B19 infection in an immunocompetent host, cytomegalovirus (CMV) infection, hepatitis B virus (HBV) carrier (see p 113 for possible exceptions), and human immunodeficiency virus (HIV) infection (see p 114 for possible exceptions). Asymptomatic children who excrete an enteropathogen usually do not need to be excluded, except when an infection with enterohemorrhagic *E coli,* including *E coli* O157:H7, or with a *Shigella* species has occurred in the child care program. Because these infections are transmitted easily and can be severe, exclusion is warranted until 2 stool cultures are negative for the organism (see *Escherichia coli* Diarrhea, p 243, and *Shigella* Infections, p 510).

During the course of an identified outbreak of any communicable illness in a child care setting, a child determined to be contributing to the transmission of the illness at the program may be excluded. The child may be readmitted when the risk of transmission is determined to be no longer present.

Infectious Diseases—Epidemiology and Control

(Also see chapters on the specific diseases in Section 3.)

ENTERIC DISEASES

The close personal contact and poor hygiene of young children provide ready opportunities for spread of enteric bacteria, viruses, and parasites in child care groups. Although many enteropathogens can cause diarrhea among children in child care, enteric pathogens transmitted by the person-to-person route, such as rotaviruses, enteric adenoviruses, astroviruses, caliciviruses, *Shigella, E coli* O157:H7, *Giardia lamblia,* and *Cryptosporidium parvum,* have been the principal organisms implicated in outbreaks; infrequently, *Salmonella, Clostridium difficile,* and *Campylobacter* species have been associated with disease in children in child care. Most reptiles carry *Salmonella* organisms, and small reptiles (like turtles) that could be handled by children can transmit *Salmonella* organisms (or other bacteria) to these children.

The most important aspect of enteric disease in child care is the association of increased frequency of diarrhea and HAV infection with young children who are not toilet trained. Fecal contamination of the environment is frequent in child care programs and is highest in infant and toddler areas where enteric disease and HAV infection occur most frequently. Enteropathogens are spread by the fecal-oral route, either directly (by person-to-person transmission) or indirectly (by toys and other objects, environmental surfaces, and food). The risk of food contamination can be increased when staff caring for diapered children also prepare or serve food. Several enteric pathogens, including rotaviruses, HAV, *Giardia lamblia* cysts, and *Cryptosporidium parvum* oocysts, survive on environmental surfaces for periods ranging from hours to weeks.

Child care programs can be a major source of HAV spread within the community. Hepatitis A virus differs from most other diseases in child care centers because symptomatic illness occurs primarily among adult contacts of infected asymptomatic children. To recognize outbreaks and initiate appropriate control measures, health care personnel and staff need to be aware of this epidemiologic characteristic (see Hepatitis A, p 280). Vaccine for HAV should be considered for the staff of child care centers with ongoing or recurrent outbreaks and in communities where cases in a child care center are a major source of HAV infection.

The single most important procedure to minimize fecal-oral transmission is frequent hand washing combined with staff training and monitoring of staff procedures. A child in whom acute diarrhea or jaundice develops while in child care should be moved to a separate area, away from contact with other children, until the child can be removed by a parent or guardian. Exclusion for acute diarrhea should continue until the diarrhea ceases; children with *Shigella* infection also should receive antimicrobial therapy before readmission. The child with symptomatic HAV infection should be excluded until 1 week after the onset of illness. Asymptomatic children without diarrhea who excrete enteropathogens other than *E coli* O157:H7 or *Shigella* do not require treatment or exclusion from child care in the absence of specific public health indications. Asymptomatic excretion illustrates the need for frequent hand washing and environmental cleaning in out-of-home child care facilities.

RESPIRATORY TRACT DISEASES

Organisms spread by the respiratory route include those causing acute upper respiratory tract infections or those associated with invasive diseases, such as *Haemophilus influenzae* type b, *Streptococcus pneumoniae, Neisseria meningitidis, Bordetella pertussis,* and *Mycobacterium tuberculosis.* Possible modes of spread of respiratory tract viruses include aerosols, respiratory droplets, and direct hand contact with contaminated secretions, toys, and other objects. The viral pathogens responsible for respiratory tract disease in child care settings are those that cause disease in the community, including respiratory syncytial virus, parainfluenza virus, influenza virus, adenovirus, and rhinovirus. The incidence of viral infections of the respiratory tract is increased in child care settings.

Hand washing may decrease the incidence of acute respiratory tract disease among children in child care. However, exclusion from child care of children with respiratory tract symptoms associated with the common cold, croup, bronchitis, pneumonia, sinusitis, or otitis media probably will not decrease the spread of infection. Children with such conditions should be separated from other children in the program if their illness is characterized by one or more of the following conditions: (1) a specified cause is identified that requires exclusion, (2) the illness limits the child's comfortable participation in child care activities, or (3) the illness results in a greater need for care than can be provided by the staff without compromising the health and safety of other children.

Transmission of *H influenzae* type b may occur among unimmunized young children in group child care, especially children younger than 24 months of age. Transmission can originate from an asymptomatic carrier or a carrier with a respiratory tract infection. Appropriate immunization of children with an *H influenzae* type b conjugate vaccine prevents the occurrence of disease and decreases the rate of carriage, thereby decreasing the risk of transmission to others. In an outbreak of invasive *H influenzae* type b disease in child care, rifampin prophylaxis may be indicated for contacts (see *Haemophilus influenzae* Infections, p 262).

Infections caused by *N meningitidis* occur in all age groups. The highest attack rates occur in children younger than 1 year of age. Close contact for an extended period for children and staff exposed to an index case of meningococcal disease predisposes to secondary transmission. Because outbreaks may occur in child care settings, chemoprophylaxis is indicated for exposed child care contacts (see Meningococcal Infections, p 396).

The risk of primary invasive disease due to *S pneumoniae* among children in child care settings is increased. Secondary spread of *S pneumoniae* in child care centers has been reported, but the degree of risk of secondary spread in child care facilities is unknown. Prophylaxis of contacts after the occurrence of a single case of invasive *S pneumoniae* disease is not recommended.

Group A streptococcal infection among children in child care has not been a common problem. A child with proven group A streptococcal infection should be excluded from classroom contact until 24 hours after initiation of antibiotic therapy. While outbreaks of streptococcal pharyngitis in these settings have occurred, the risk of secondary transmission after a single case of severe invasive group A streptococcal infection remains low. Chemoprophylaxis of contacts after a single case of severe invasive group A streptococcal infection in child care facilities is not recommended (see Group A Streptococcal Infections, p 526).

Infants and young children with tuberculosis are not as contagious as adults with *M tuberculosis* disease, because children are less likely to have cavitary pulmonary lesions and are unable to forcefully expel large numbers of organisms into the air. If approved by health officials, children may attend a child care group after chemotherapy is begun and when they are considered noninfectious to others. Infants and young children who have both HIV and *M tuberculosis* infections may need to be excluded from group child care. Because an adult with tuberculosis poses a hazard to children in a child care group, tuberculin screening with a Mantoux skin test of all adults who have contact with children in a child care setting is recommended before the contact is initiated. Adults with HIV and tuberculosis may not have a reaction to a tuberculin skin test (see Tuberculosis, p 593). The need for periodic subsequent tuberculin testing of persons without clinically important reactions should be based on their risk of acquiring a new infection and local or state health department recommendations. Care providers found to have active tuberculosis should be excluded from the center and not be allowed to care for children until chemotherapy has rendered them noninfectious to others (see Tuberculosis, p 593).

Parvovirus B19. The spectrum of illness produced by parvovirus B19 includes asymptomatic infection in 20% of infected persons; erythema infectiosum, which is the most common manifestation of illness and usually occurs in children; arthritis in adults; chronic anemia in immunocompromised hosts; aplastic crisis; and fetal hydrops. Isolation or exclusion of immunocompetent persons with parvovirus B19 infection in child care settings is unwarranted because little or no virus is present in respiratory tract secretions at the time of occurrence of the rash of erythema infectiosum. In addition, because fewer than 1% of pregnant teachers during erythema infectiosum outbreaks would be expected to experience an adverse fetal outcome, exclusion of pregnant women from employment in child care or teaching is not recommended (see Parvovirus B19, p 423).

VARICELLA-ZOSTER VIRUS

Children with varicella who have been excluded from child care may return on the sixth day after onset of rash or sooner if all lesions have dried and crusted. All staff members and parents should be notified when a case of varicella occurs; they should be informed about the greater likelihood of serious infection in susceptible adults and adolescents and of the potential for fetal damage if infection occurs during pregnancy. Approximately 5% of adults will be susceptible to varicella-zoster virus. Susceptible adults should be offered varicella vaccine, unless medically contraindicated. Susceptible child care staff who are pregnant and exposed to children with varicella should be referred to a qualified physician or other professional for counseling and management within 24 hours of the exposure. The Centers for Disease Control and Prevention (CDC) recommends the use of varicella vaccine in susceptible persons within 72 hours after exposure to varicella.

Exclusion of staff members or children with herpes zoster (shingles) whose lesions cannot be covered should be based on criteria similar to those for varicella. Herpes zoster lesions that can be covered pose little risk to susceptible persons, since transmission usually occurs from direct contact with fluid from lesions. Lesions should be covered by clothing or a dressing until they have crusted. Thorough hand washing is warranted whenever contact with fluid from a lesion has occurred.

HERPES SIMPLEX VIRUS

Children with herpes simplex virus (HSV) gingivostomatitis who do not have control of oral secretions (drooling) should be excluded from child care when active lesions are present. Although HSV can be transmitted from a mother to her fetus or newborn infant, maternal HSV infections that are a threat to offspring usually are acquired by the infant during birth from genital infections of the mother; therefore, maternal exposure to HSV in a child care setting carries little risk for her fetus. Care providers should be instructed on the importance of hand washing and other measures for limiting transfer of infected material from children with varicella-zoster virus or HSV infection (eg, saliva, tissue fluid, or fluid from a skin lesion).

CMV INFECTION

Spread of CMV from asymptomatic infected children in child care to their mothers or to child care providers is the most important consequence of child care–related CMV infection (see Cytomegalovirus Infection, p 227). Children enrolled in child care programs are more likely to acquire CMV than children cared for primarily at home. The highest rates (eg, 70%) of viral excretion occur in children between 1 and 3 years of age, and excretion often continues for years. Studies of CMV seroconversion among child care providers have found annualized seroconversion rates of 8% to 20%. Exposure to CMV with the increased rate of acquisition that occurs in child care staff most likely leads to an increased rate of gestational CMV infection in seronegative staff and an increased risk of congenital CMV infection in their offspring. Women who are seropositive before pregnancy are not at risk from exposure to children, but seropositive women whose CMV infection reactivates during pregnancy have a small (approximately 1 in 500) risk of having an infant with congenital CMV infection; only about 5% of these infected infants have sequelae, which are mild and consist mostly of moderate hearing loss.

Transmission of CMV requires direct contact with virus-containing secretions. Therefore, careful attention to hygiene, specifically hand washing, is critical. Avoiding contact with secretions is recommended to prevent infection in child care providers. However, the effectiveness of these measures in an environment in which CMV is ubiquitous has not been determined. Because CMV excretion is so prevalent, attempts at isolation or segregation of children who excrete CMV are impractical and inappropriate. Similarly, testing of children to detect CMV excretion is inappropriate because excretion often is intermittent, and results of testing can be misleading.

In view of the risk of CMV infection in child care staff and the potential consequences of gestational CMV infection, child care staff should be counseled about the risks. This counseling may include testing for serum antibody to CMV to determine the child care provider's immunity against CMV, but routine serologic testing currently is not recommended.

BLOODBORNE VIRUS INFECTIONS

Hepatitis B virus, HIV, and hepatitis C virus (HCV) are bloodborne pathogens. Although the risk of contact with blood containing one of these viruses is low in the child care setting, appropriate infection control practices will prevent transmission of bloodborne pathogens if exposure occurs.

Hepatitis B Virus. Transmission of HBV in the child care setting has been described but occurs rarely. Because of a low risk for transmission, children known to be HBV carriers (hepatitis B surface antigen [HBsAg]-positive) may attend child care in most circumstances.

Transmission of HBV in a child care setting is most likely to occur through direct exposure to blood after an injury or from bites or scratches that break the skin and introduce blood or body secretions from an HBV carrier into another person. Indirect transmission through environmental contamination with blood or saliva is possible but has not been documented in the child care setting in the United States. Because saliva contains much less virus than does blood, the potential infectivity of saliva is low. Infectivity of saliva has been demonstrated only when inoculated through the skin of gibbons and chimpanzees.

On the basis of limited data, the risk of disease transmission from a child or staff member who is an HBV carrier but who behaves normally and is without injury, generalized dermatitis, or bleeding problems is minimal. This slight risk usually does not justify exclusion of a child who is an HBV carrier from child care or the necessity of HBV immunization of the child's contacts at the care program, most of whom already should be protected by prior HBV immunization as part of their routine immunization schedule.

Routine screening of children for HBV carrier status before admission to child care is not justified. The admission of a child previously identified to be an HBV carrier with one or more risk factors for transmission of bloodborne pathogens (eg, biting, frequent scratching, generalized dermatitis, or bleeding problems) should be assessed by the child's physician, child care provider, or program director. The responsible public health authority should be consulted when appropriate. Regular assessment of behavioral risk factors and medical conditions of enrolled HBV carriers is necessary and requires that the child care director and primary child care providers are informed about enrollment of a known HBV carrier.

Children who bite pose an additional concern. Existing data in humans suggest a small risk of HBV transmission from the bite of an HBV carrier. For victims of bites by HBV carriers, prophylaxis with Hepatitis B Immune Globulin (HBIG) and hepatitis B immunization is recommended for susceptible persons (see Hepatitis B, p 289).

The risk of HBV acquisition when a susceptible child bites an HBV carrier is unknown. A theoretical risk exists if HBsAg-positive blood enters the oral cavity of the biter, but transmission by this route has not been reported. Although data on risks of transmission are limited, most experts would not give HBIG to a susceptible biting child who does not have oral mucosal disease when the amount of blood transferred is small.

In the common circumstance in which the HBsAg status of both the biting child and the victim is unknown, the risk of HBV transmission is extremely low because of the expected low seroprevalence of HBsAg in most groups of preschool-age children, the low efficiency of disease transmission from bites, and routine HBV immunization of preschool children. Because all preschool children attending child care settings should be immunized, concern about bites and HBV transmission associated with breaks in the skin is minimal. Serologic testing generally is not warranted for the biting child or the recipient of the bite, but each situation should be evaluated individually.

Efforts to reduce the risk of disease transmission in child care through hygienic and environmental standards in general should focus primarily on precautions for blood exposures and limiting potential saliva contamination of the environment. Toothbrushes should not be shared among children. Accidents that lead to bleeding or contamination with blood-containing body fluids by any child should be handled as follows: (1) disposable gloves should be used when cleaning or removing any blood or blood-containing body fluid spills; (2) the area should be disinfected with a freshly prepared solution of 1:10 household bleach applied for at least 30 seconds and wiped after the minimum contact time; (3) persons involved in cleaning contaminated surfaces should avoid exposure of open skin lesions or mucous membranes to blood or blood-containing body fluids and to wound or tissue exudates; (4) hands should be washed thoroughly following exposure to blood or blood-containing body fluids after gloves are removed; (5) disposable towels or tissues should be used and properly discarded, and mops should be rinsed in the disinfectant; (6) blood-contaminated paper towels, diapers, and other materials should be placed in a plastic bag with a secure tie for disposal; and (7) personnel should be educated about standard precautions for handling blood or blood-containing material.

HIV Infection (see also HIV Infection, p 325). The risk of transmission of HIV infection to children in the child care setting seems negligible. Children who enter child care should not be required to be HIV tested or to disclose their HIV status. No need exists to restrict placement of HIV-infected children without risk factors for transmission of bloodborne pathogens in child care facilities to protect other children or personnel in these settings. Because HIV-infected children whose status is unknown may attend child care, standard precautions should be adopted for handling spills of blood and blood-containing body fluids and wound exudates of all children, as described in the preceding HBV section.

The decision to admit HIV-infected children to child care is best made on an individual basis by qualified persons, including the child's physician, who are able to evaluate whether the child will receive optimal care in the program and whether an HIV-infected child poses a significant risk to others. Specifically, admission of each HIV-infected child with one or more potential risk factors for transmission of bloodborne pathogens (eg, biting, frequent scratching, generalized dermatitis, or bleeding problems) should be assessed by the child's physician and the program director. A responsible public health authority should be consulted as appropriate. Although biting, theoretically, is a possible mode of transmission of bloodborne illness, such as HIV infection, the risk of such transmission is believed to be rare. If a bite results in blood exposure to either person involved, the US Public Health Service recommends postexposure follow-up, including consideration of postexposure prophylaxis. Information about a child who has immunodeficiency, irrespective of cause, should be available to caregivers who need to know how to help protect the child against other infections. For example, immunodeficient children exposed to measles or varicella should immediately receive postexposure immunoprophylaxis (see Measles, p 385, and Varicella-Zoster Infections, p 624).

Available data provide no reason to support that HIV-infected adults will transmit HIV to children during the course of their normal duties. Therefore, HIV-infected adults who do not have open and uncoverable skin lesions, other conditions that would allow contact with their body fluids, or a transmissible infectious disease may care for children in child care programs. However, immunosuppressed adults with HIV infection may be at increased risk for acquiring infectious agents from children and should consult their physicians about the safety of their continuing child care work.

Hepatitis C Virus. The transmission risks of HCV infection in child care settings are unknown. The general risk of HCV infection from percutaneous exposure to infected blood is estimated to be 10 times greater than that of HIV but lower than that of HBV. Transmission of HCV via contamination of mucous membranes or broken skin probably has a risk intermediate between that for blood infected with HIV and HBV. Standard precautions outlined under the HBV section should be followed to prevent infection with HCV.

IMMUNIZATIONS

Routine immunization at the appropriate age is important for children in child care because preschool-age children can have high age-specific incidence rates of measles, rubella, *H influenzae* type b disease, varicella, and pertussis. Outbreaks of mumps in child care settings have not been reported, but any cluster of susceptible persons can sustain transmission.

Written documentation of immunizations appropriate for age should be provided by parents or guardians of all children enrolling in child care. Unless contraindications exist, immunization records should demonstrate the following as shown in the Recommended Childhood Immunization Schedule (see p 22).

- One dose of DTaP (diphtheria and tetanus toxoids and acellular pertussis or DTP) vaccine by 3 months of age, 2 doses by 5 months of age, 3 doses by 7 months of age, and 4 doses by 19 months of age
- One dose of inactivated poliomyelitis vaccine (IPV) or OPV by 3 months of age, 2 doses by 5 months of age, and 3 doses by 19 months of age (see Poliovirus Infections, p 465). Beginning in the year 2000, an all-IPV vaccine schedule is recommended for routine childhood immunization in the United States.

- One dose of MMR (measles-mumps-rubella) vaccine by 16 months of age
- One or more doses of *H influenzae* type b conjugate vaccine (see *Haemophilus influenzae* Infections, p 262, for the age-appropriate recommendations)
- Two doses of HBV vaccine by 7 months of age and 3 doses by 19 months of age
- One dose of varicella vaccine by 19 months of age

Children who have not received recommended age-appropriate immunizations before enrollment should have their immunization series initiated as soon as possible—no later than within 1 month of enrollment—and completed according to Fig 1.1 (p 22) and Table 1.5 (p 24). In the interim, unimmunized or inadequately immunized children should be allowed to attend child care unless a vaccine-preventable disease to which they are susceptible occurs in the child care program. In such a situation, all underimmunized children should be excluded for the duration of possible exposure or until they have completed their immunizations.

Child care providers should have received all immunizations routinely recommended for adults. All staff should have completed a primary series for tetanus and diphtheria, should receive a booster every 10 years, and should have been immunized against measles, mumps, rubella, and poliomyelitis according to guidelines for adult immunization of the Advisory Committee on Immunization Practices of the CDC and the American College of Physicians. Consideration should be given to annual immunization of child care providers against influenza. Hepatitis B virus immunization also should be considered, especially for providers who may manage blood spills.

Child care providers should be asked about a history of varicella. Child care providers with a negative or uncertain history of varicella should be immunized or undergo serologic testing for susceptibility; those who are not immune should be offered varicella vaccine, unless it is contraindicated medically.

Because HAV can cause symptomatic illness in adult contacts and because child care programs have been a source of infection in the community, HAV vaccine in some current circumstances may be justified (see Hepatitis A, p 280). However, since the prevalence of HAV infection does not seem significantly increased in staff members of child care centers in comparison with the prevalence in the general population, routine immunization of staff members is not recommended. During HAV outbreaks, immunization should be considered (see p 283).

Child care providers who have not been immunized against poliomyelitis and who will be caring for infants and children who may have received OPV may become infected and have a small risk of vaccine-associated paralytic poliomyelitis. Transmission can be prevented by appropriate hand washing, especially after diaper changing, and by appropriate immunization of child care providers. Because of the expanded use of IPV, this concern is limited.

General Practices

The following practices are recommended to reduce transmission of infectious agents in a child care setting without losing the developmentally desirable features of child care:

- Each child care facility should have **written policies** for managing child and employee illness in child care.

- **Toilet areas and toilet training equipment** should be maintained in sanitary condition.
- **Diaper changing surfaces** should be nonporous and sanitized between uses. Alternatively, the diaper changing surface should be covered with a paper pad, which is discarded after each use. If the surface becomes wet or soiled, it should be cleaned and sanitized.
- **Diaper changing procedures** should be posted at the changing area. Soiled disposable diapers and soiled disposable wiping cloths should be discarded in a secure, foot-activated, plastic-lined container. Diapers should contain all urine and stool and minimize fecal contamination of children, providers, environmental surfaces, and objects in the child care program. The 2 types of diapers that should be used are modern disposable paper diapers with absorbent gelling material or carboxymethyl cellulose and single-unit reusable systems with an inner cotton lining attached to an outer waterproof covering that are changed as a unit. Clothes should be worn over diapers while the child is in the child care facility. Soiled reusable diapers should be bagged and sent home for laundering.
- **Diaper changing areas** should never be located in food preparation areas and should never be used for temporary placement of food.
- The use of **child-sized toilets** or access to steps and modified toilet seats that provide for easier maintenance should be encouraged in child care programs; the use of potty chairs should be discouraged. If potty chairs are used, they should be emptied into a toilet, cleaned in a utility sink, and disinfected after each use. Staff should sanitize potty chairs, flush toilets, and diaper changing areas with a freshly prepared solution of 1:64 household bleach (¼ cup diluted in 1 gallon of water) applied for 2 minutes, rinsed, and dried.
- **Written procedures for hand washing,** which is the single most important measure for preventing infection, should be established and enforced. Hand-washing sinks should be adjacent to all diaper changing and toilet areas. These sinks should be washed and disinfected at least daily and, when soiled, should not be used for food preparation. These sinks should not be used for rinsing soiled clothing or for cleaning potty chairs. Children should have access to height-appropriate sinks, soap dispensers, and disposable paper towels.
- Written **personal hygiene policies** for staff and children are necessary.
- Written **environmental sanitation policies and procedures** should include cleaning and disinfecting floors, covering sandboxes, cleaning and sanitizing play tables, and cleaning and disinfecting spills of blood or body fluids and wound or tissue exudates. In general, routine housekeeping procedures using a freshly prepared solution of commercially available cleaner (eg, detergents, disinfectant-detergents, or chemical germicides) compatible with most surfaces are satisfactory for cleaning spills of vomitus, urine, and feces. For spills of blood or blood-containing body fluids and of wound and tissue exudates, the material should be removed using gloves to avoid contamination of hands, and the area then should be disinfected using a freshly prepared solution of 1:10 household bleach applied for 30 seconds and wiped with a disposable cloth after the minimum contact time.

- Each item of **sleep equipment** should be used only by a single child and should be cleaned and sanitized before being assigned to another child. Crib mattresses should be cleaned and sanitized when soiled or wet. Sleeping mats should be stored so contact with the sleeping surface of another mat does not occur. Bedding (sheets and blankets) should be assigned to each child and cleaned when soiled or wet.
- Optimally, **toys** that are placed in children's mouths or otherwise contaminated by body secretions should be cleaned with water and detergent, disinfected, and rinsed before handling by another child. All frequently touched toys in rooms that house infants and toddlers should be cleaned and disinfected daily. Toys in rooms for older children (nondiapered) should be cleaned at least weekly and when soiled. The use of soft, nonwashable toys in infant and toddler areas of child care programs should be discouraged.
- **Food** should be handled safely and appropriately to prevent growth of bacteria and to prevent contamination by other enteropathogens, insects, or rodents. Tables and countertops used for food preparation and food service should be cleaned and sanitized between uses and before and after eating. No one who has signs or symptoms of illness, including vomiting, diarrhea, or infectious skin lesions that cannot be covered, or who is infected with potential foodborne pathogens should be responsible for food handling. Hands should be washed using soap and water before handling food. Because of their frequent exposure to feces and children with enteric diseases, staff who work with diapered children should not prepare food for others. Caregivers who prepare food for infants should be especially aware of the importance of careful hand washing. No unpasteurized milk or milk products should be served (see Appendix VI, Potentially Contaminated Food Products, p 770).
- The living quarters of **pets** should be enclosed and kept clean of waste to reduce the risk of human contact with the waste. Hands should be washed after handling all animals or animal wastes. Dogs and cats should be kept away from child play areas, handled only with staff supervision, and be in good health and immunized appropriately for age. Such animals should be given flea, tick, and worm control programs. Reptiles should not be handled by children.
- Written policies, which comply with local and state regulations, for filing and regularly updating each child's **immunization record** should be maintained.
- Each child care program should use the services of a **health consultant** to assist in development and implementation of written policies for the prevention and control of communicable diseases and the provision of related health education to children, staff, and parents.
- The child care provider should, on registering each child, **inform parents of the need to share information about illness** that could be communicable, in the child or in any member of the immediate household, to facilitate prompt reporting of disease and institution of any measures necessary to prevent transmission to others. The child care provider or program director, after consulting with the program's health consultant or the responsible public health official, should follow recommendations of the consultant or public health official for **notification of parents** of children who attend the program about exposure of their child to a communicable disease.

- Local and/or state **public health authorities should be notified** about cases of communicable diseases involving children or care providers in the child care setting.

SCHOOL HEALTH

While clustering of children together in the school setting provides opportunities for spread of infectious diseases, school attendance is important for children and adolescents, and unnecessary barriers and impediments to attending school should be minimized. Determining the likelihood that infection in one or more children will pose a risk for schoolmates depends on an understanding of several factors, including the following: (1) the mechanism by which the organism causing the infection is spread, (2) the ease with which the organism is spread (contagion), and (3) the likelihood that classmates are immune either because of immunization or prior infection. Decisions to intervene to prevent spread of infection within a school should be made through collaboration among school officials, local public health officials, and health care professionals, considering the availability and effectiveness of specific methods of prevention and the risk of serious complications from infection.

Infectious agents are spread through one or more of the following 4 routes of transmission: fecal-oral; respiratory; contact with infected skin; and contact with blood, urine, or body secretions. In the school setting, respiratory secretions and skin contact provide the most frequent means of transmission of microorganisms. In the care of preschool children in out-of-home child care (see Children in Out-of-Home Child Care, p 105) and older children with health problems or developmental disabilities, transmission via the fecal-oral route and through contact with urine also is an important consideration. Specific circumstances, such as care of bleeding injuries or intimate contact between classmates, provide an opportunity for spread via blood and other body fluids.

Generic methods for control and prevention of spread of infection in the school setting include the following:

- For vaccine-preventable diseases, documentation of the immunization status of enrolled children should be reviewed. Schools have a legal responsibility to ensure that students have been immunized against vaccine-preventable disease at the time of enrollment, in accordance with state requirements (see Appendix IV, State Immunization Requirements for School Attendance, p 766). Although the specific diseases vary by state, most require proof of protection against poliomyelitis, pertussis, diphtheria, measles, mumps, and rubella. Hepatitis B immunization is now mandatory in many states. Immunization against varicella, available since 1995, is mandatory in some states. Hepatitis A virus (HAV) immunization is required for school entry in some states. The Centers for Disease Control and Prevention recommends that all states require that children entering elementary school have received varicella vaccine or have other evidence of immunity to varicella. Policies established by a state health department about exclusions of unimmunized children and exemptions for children with certain underlying medical conditions and families with religious objection to immunization should be followed.

- Infected children should be excluded from school until they are no longer considered contagious (for recommendations on specific diseases, see relevant disease-specific chapters in Section 3).
- In many instances, administration of appropriate antimicrobial therapy will limit further spread of infection (eg, streptococcal pharyngitis and pertussis).
- Antimicrobial prophylaxis given to close contacts of children with infections caused by specific pathogens may be warranted in some circumstances (eg, meningococcal infection).
- Temporary school closing can be used in several circumstances: (1) to prevent spread of infection, (2) when an infection is expected to affect a large number of susceptible students, and available control measures are considered inadequate (eg, outbreak of influenza), or (3) when an infection is expected to have a high rate of morbidity or mortality.

Physicians involved with school health should be aware of current public health guidelines to prevent and control infectious diseases. In all circumstances requiring intervention to prevent spread of infection within the school setting, the privacy of children who are infected should be protected.

Diseases Preventable by Routine Childhood Immunization

Students who have received 1 dose of varicella vaccine (2 doses for children immunized after 13 years of age) and 2 doses of measles, mumps, and rubella (MMR) vaccine should be considered immune to these diseases. Students with a history of physician-documented infection or serologic evidence of immunity also are considered immune.

Measles and varicella vaccines have been demonstrated to provide protection in some susceptible persons if administered within 72 hours after exposure. Measles or varicella immunization should be recommended immediately for all nonimmune persons during a measles or varicella outbreak, respectively, except for persons with a contraindication to immunization. Students immunized for measles for the first time under these circumstances should be allowed to return to school immediately.

Mumps vaccine given after exposure has not been demonstrated to prevent infection among susceptible contacts, but immunization should be administered to unimmunized students to protect them from infection from subsequent exposure.

Although rubella infection usually does not pose a major risk to preadolescent school-age children, the immunization status of contacts should be reviewed, and documentation of rubella immunization should be required for previously unimmunized students. Pregnant contacts who have serologically confirmed immunity against rubella early in pregnancy should be reassured. Physician consultation should be recommended for susceptible pregnant women who are exposed to rubella (see Rubella, p 495).

Other Infections Spread by the Respiratory Route

Some pathogens that cause severe, lower respiratory tract disease in infants and toddlers, such as respiratory syncytial virus, are of less concern in healthy school-age children. Respiratory tract viruses, however, are associated with exacerbations of reactive airway disease and an increase in the incidence of otitis media and can cause significant complications for children with chronic respiratory tract disease, such as cystic fibrosis, or for children who are immunocompromised.

Although influenza virus infection is a frequent cause of febrile respiratory tract disease and school absenteeism, mandatory exclusion of children with suspected influenza infection from school is not warranted. Annual influenza immunizations should be given to targeted high-risk groups (see Influenza Vaccine, p 351). Influenza immunization also may be indicated for students to prevent disruption of academic or athletic activities, especially children residing in dormitories or in other circumstances in which close contact occurs.

Mycoplasma pneumoniae causes upper and lower respiratory tract infection in school-age children, and outbreaks of *M pneumoniae* infection occur in communities and schools. The nonspecific symptoms and signs of this infection and the lack of a rapid diagnostic test make distinguishing *M pneumoniae* infection from other causes of respiratory tract illness difficult. Antibiotic therapy does not eradicate the organism or necessarily prevent spread. Thus, intervention to prevent secondary infection in the school setting is difficult.

Symptomatic contacts of students with pharyngitis due to group A streptococcus should be evaluated and treated if streptococcal infection is demonstrated. Infected students may return to school 24 hours after initiation of antimicrobial therapy. Students awaiting results of culture or antigen detection tests who are not receiving antimicrobial therapy may attend school during the culture incubation period unless there is an associated fever or the infection involves a young child with poor hygiene and poor control of secretions. Asymptomatic contacts usually require neither evaluation nor therapy.

Bacterial meningitis in school-age children usually is caused by *Neisseria meningitidis*. Infected persons are not considered contagious after 24 hours of appropriate antibiotic therapy. After hospitalization, they pose no risk to classmates and may return to school. Prophylactic antibiotic therapy is not recommended for school contacts in most circumstances. Close observation of these students is recommended, and they should be evaluated promptly if a febrile illness develops. Students who have been exposed to oral secretions of an infected student, such as occurs during kissing or sharing of food and drink, should receive chemoprophylaxis (see Meningococcal Infections, p 396). Immunization of school contacts with meningococcal vaccine, which contains polysaccharide antigens for serogroups A, C, Y, and W-135, should be considered, in consultation with local public health authorities, if evidence suggests an outbreak within a school due to one of the meningococcal serogroups contained in the vaccine.

Students and staff with documented pertussis should be excluded until they have received 5 days of erythromycin therapy. In some circumstances, chemoprophylaxis is recommended for their school contacts (see Pertussis, p 435).

Children with tuberculosis generally are not contagious, but students who are in close contact with an infected child, teacher, or other adult should be evaluated for infection, including skin testing (see Tuberculosis, p 593). An infected adolescent or adult is almost always the source of infection for young children. If an adult source outside the school is identified (eg, parent or grandparent of a student), efforts should be made to determine whether other students have been exposed to the same source and whether they warrant evaluation for infection.

Children with erythema infectiosum should be allowed to attend school, since the period of contagion occurs before a rash is evident. Parvovirus B19 infection poses no risk of significant illness for healthy classmates, although aplastic crisis can develop in infected children with sickle cell disease and other hemoglobinopathies. The relatively low risk of fetal damage should be explained to pregnant students and teachers exposed to children in the early stages of parvovirus B19 infection, 5 to 10 days before appearance of the rash. These exposed women should be referred to their physician for counseling and possible serologic testing.

Infections Spread by Direct Contact

Infection and infestation of skin, eyes, and hair can spread through direct contact with the infected area or through contact with contaminated hands or fomites, such as hair brushes, hats, and clothing. *Staphylococcus aureus* and group A streptococcus may colonize the skin or the oropharynx of asymptomatic persons. Lesions may develop when these organisms are passed from a person with infected skin to another person. Organisms also can be transmitted to open skin lesions in the same child or to other children. Although most skin infections due to *S aureus* and group A streptococcus are minor and require only topical or oral antibiotic therapy, person-to-person spread should be interrupted by appropriate treatment whenever lesions are recognized. Exclusion of affected children before initiation of therapy is necessary unless the risk for skin contact is low based on location of the lesion and age of the child. Severe and disseminated disease from these pathogens, including toxic shock syndrome and necrotizing fasciitis, occurs rarely.

Herpes simplex virus (HSV) infection of the mouth and skin is common among school-age children. It usually is spread through direct contact with virus from infected lesions. In addition, asymptomatic shedding of virus from oral secretions is common. Infection of the fingers (herpetic whitlow) can occur after direct contact with oral or genital secretions. Cutaneous infection can occur after direct contact with infected lesions or after contact of abraded skin with a contaminated surface, as occurs among wrestlers (herpes gladiatorum) and rugby players (scrum pox). Although asymptomatic shedding of virus from pharyngeal and oral secretions is common, spread of infection requires direct contact with these secretions and, thus, is unlikely to occur during normal school activities. "Cold sore" lesions of herpes labialis identify persons with active and probably recurrent infection, but no evidence suggests that these students pose any greater risk to their classmates than the unidentified asymptomatic shedders. Herpes simplex virus, type 1, the usual cause of oropharyngeal and cutaneous lesions, will infect the majority of persons by adulthood. Most of these infections are asymptomatic and, although sometimes painful, even symptomatic infection poses virtually no risk of serious disease to a healthy school-age child. All children should be advised to avoid direct or indirect (eg, sharing cups and bottles) oral contact with other children and to wash their hands, but excluding symptomatic children with HSV from normal school activities is not justified. Exclusion of students with obvious skin or oral lesions from wrestling or rugby and careful cleaning of wrestling mats after use with a freshly prepared solution of household bleach (¼ cup of bleach diluted in 1 gallon of water) for a minimum of 15 seconds is reasonable. The bleach solution may be wiped off after the minimum contact time or allowed to air dry.

For immunocompromised children and for children with open skin lesions (eg, severe eczema), HSV infection may pose significant risk. Because of the frequency of symptomatic and asymptomatic shedding of HSV among classmates and teachers and staff, careful hygienic practices are the best means of preventing infection.

Infectious conjunctivitis can be caused by bacterial (eg, nontypable *Haemophilus influenzae* and *Streptococcus pneumoniae*) or viral (eg, adenoviruses, enteroviruses, HSV) pathogens. Bacterial conjunctivitis is uncommon in children older than 5 years of age. Infection occurs through direct contact or through contamination of hands followed by autoinoculation. Respiratory tract spread from large droplets also may occur. Topical antibiotic therapy is indicated for bacterial conjunctivitis, which usually is distinguished by a purulent exudate. Herpes simplex virus conjunctivitis usually is unilateral and may be accompanied by vesicles on adjacent skin. Evaluation of HSV conjunctivitis by an ophthalmologist and administration of specific antiviral therapy are indicated. Conjunctivitis due to adenoviruses or enteroviruses is self-limited and requires no specific antiviral therapy. Spread of infection is minimized by careful hand washing, and infected persons should be presumed to be contagious until symptoms have resolved. Except when viral or bacterial conjunctivitis is accompanied by systemic signs of illness, infected children should be allowed to remain in school once any indicated therapy is implemented, unless their behavior is such that close contact with other students cannot be controlled.

Fungal infections of the skin and hair are spread by direct person-to-person contact and through contact with contaminated surfaces or objects. *Trichophyton tonsurans*, the predominant cause of tinea capitis, remains viable for long periods on combs, hair brushes, furniture, and fabric. The fungi that cause tinea corporis (ringworm) are transmissible by direct contact. Tinea cruris (jock itch) and tinea pedis (athlete's foot) occur in adolescents and young adults. The fungi that cause these infections have a predilection for moist areas and are spread through direct contact and through contact with contaminated surfaces. Students with fungal infections of the skin or scalp should be treated, both for their benefit and to prevent spread of infection. Spread of infection by students with tinea capitis may be decreased by use of selenium sulfide shampoos, but treatment requires systemic antifungal therapy (see Tinea Capitis, p 569). Students with tinea capitis who receive treatment may attend school and participate in their usual activities. Children who fail to obtain treatment do not need to be excluded unless the nature of their contact with other students could potentiate spread. Students with tinea cruris, tinea corporis, or tinea pedis should not be excluded from school even before initiation of therapy. Students with tinea capitis should be instructed not to share combs, hair brushes, hats, or hair ornaments with classmates until they have been treated. Students with tinea pedis should be excluded from swimming pools and from walking barefoot on locker room and shower floors until treatment has been initiated.

Sarcoptes scabiei (scabies) and *Pediculus capitis* (head lice) are transmitted primarily through person-to-person contact. Combs, hair brushes, hats, and hair ornaments can transmit head lice, but away from the scalp, lice do not remain viable. Shampooing with an appropriate pediculocide and manually removing nits with combing usually are effective in eradicating viable lice (see Pediculosis, p 427).

Scabies can be transmitted via clothing and bedding to household contacts, but direct skin contact is the predominant means of transmission in the school setting. The parasite survives on clothing for only 3 to 4 days without skin contact. Caregivers who have prolonged skin-to-skin contact with infested students during the school day, because of physical or mental disabilities, may benefit from prophylactic treatment (see Scabies p 506).

Children identified as having scabies or head lice should be excluded from school only until treatment has been started. School contacts generally should not be treated prophylactically.

Infections Spread by the Fecal-Oral Route

For developmentally normal school-age children, pathogens spread through the fecal-oral route constitute a risk only if the infected person fails to maintain good hygiene, including hand washing after toilet use, or if contaminated food is shared between or among schoolmates.

Outbreaks due to HAV can occur in schools, but these outbreaks usually are associated with community outbreaks. Schoolroom exposure generally does not pose an appreciable risk of infection, and Immune Globulin (IG) administration is not indicated. However, if transmission within a school is documented, IG could be used to limit further spread (see Hepatitis A, p 280). Alternatively, HAV vaccine should be considered as a means of prophylaxis and prolonged protection. If an outbreak occurs, consultation with local public health authorities is indicated before initiating interventions.

Enteroviral infections probably are spread by the oral-oral route, as well as by the fecal-oral route. The attack rate is so high during summer and fall epidemics that control measures specifically aimed at the school classroom likely would be futile. Person-to-person spread of bacterial, viral, and parasitic enteropathogens within school settings is infrequent, but foodborne outbreaks due to enteric pathogens can occur. Symptomatic persons with gastroenteritis due to an enteric pathogen should be excluded until symptoms resolve.

Children in diapers at any age and in any setting constitute a far greater risk for spread of gastrointestinal tract infection due to enteric pathogens. Guidelines for control of these infections in child care settings should be applied for developmentally disabled school-age students in diapers (see Children in Out-of-Home Child Care, p 105).

Infections Spread by Blood and Body Fluids*

Contact with the blood and other body fluids of another person requires more intimate exposure than usually occurs in the school setting. The care required for developmentally disabled children, however, may result in exposure of caregivers to urine, saliva, and, in some cases, blood. The application of Standard Precautions for prevention of transmission of bloodborne pathogens, as recommended in out-of-home child care, prevents spread of infection from these exposures (see Children in Out-of-Home Child Care, p 105). School staff who routinely provide acute care

* American Academy of Pediatrics Committee on Pediatric AIDS and Committee on Infectious Diseases. Issues related to human immunodeficiency virus transmission in schools, child care, medical settings, the home and community. *Pediatrics*. 1999;104:318–324

for children with epistaxis or bleeding from injury should wear gloves and use good hand-washing technique immediately after glove removal to protect themselves from bloodborne pathogens. Staff at the scene of an injury or bleeding incident who do not have access to gloves need to use some type of barrier to avoid exposure to blood or blood-containing materials, use good hand-washing technique, and adhere to proper protocols for handling contaminated material. Routine use of these precautions avoids the necessity of identifying children known to be infected with human immunodeficiency virus (HIV), hepatitis B virus (HBV), or hepatitis C virus (HCV) and acknowledges that unrecognized infection poses at least as much risk as the identified child.

During adolescence, the likelihood of infection due to HBV, HIV, and other sexually transmitted diseases (STDs) increases in proportion to sexual activity. All children should be immunized against HBV before age 13 years of age, and adolescents should be instructed in appropriate methods of prevention of STDs.

Students infected with HIV, HBV, or HCV do not need to be identified to school personnel. Since HIV-, HBV-, and HCV-infected children and adolescents will not be identified, policies and procedures to manage potential exposures to blood or blood-containing materials should be established and implemented. Parents and students should be educated about the types of exposure that present a risk for school contacts. Although the student's right to privacy should be maintained, decisions about activities at school should be made by parents or guardians together with a physician on a case-by-case basis, keeping the health needs of the infected student and the student's classmates in mind.

Prospective studies to aid in determining the risk of transmission of HIV, HBV, or HCV during contact sports among high school students have not been performed, but the available evidence indicates that the risk is extremely low. Guidelines for management of bleeding injuries have been developed for college and professional athletes in recognition of the possibility of unidentified HIV, HBV, or HCV infection in any competitor. Recommendations developed by the American Academy of Pediatrics (AAP) for prevention of transmission of HIV and other bloodborne pathogens in the athletic setting were issued in 1999.*

- Athletes infected with HIV, HBV, or HCV should be allowed to participate in all competitive sports.
- The physician should respect the right of infected athletes to confidentiality. This includes not disclosing the patient's infection status to other participants or the staff of athletic programs.
- Athletes should not be tested for bloodborne pathogens because they are sports participants.
- Pediatricians are encouraged to counsel athletes who are infected with HIV, HBV, or HCV that they have a very small risk of infecting other competitors. Infected athletes can consider choosing a sport in which this risk is relatively low. This may be protective for other participants and for infected athletes themselves, reducing their possible exposure to bloodborne pathogens other

* American Academy of Pediatrics Committee on Sports Medicine and Fitness. Human immunodeficiency virus and other blood-borne viral pathogens in the athletic setting. *Pediatrics.* 1999;104:1400–1403

than the one(s) with which they are infected. Wrestling and boxing probably have the greatest potential for contamination of injured skin by blood. The AAP opposes boxing as a sport for youth.

- Athletic programs should inform athletes and their parents that the program is operating under the policies of the 4 recommendations above and that the athletes have a very small risk of becoming infected with a bloodborne pathogen.
- Clinicians and staff of the athletic programs should aggressively promote HBV immunization among athletes and among coaches, athletic trainers, equipment handlers, laundry personnel, and any other persons at risk of exposure to athletes' blood as an occupational hazard. All athletes should, if possible, receive HBV immunization.
- Each coach and athletic trainer must receive training in first aid and emergency care and in the prevention of transmission of bloodborne pathogens in the athletic setting. These staff members can then help to implement these recommendations.
- Coaches and members of the health care team should educate athletes about the precautions described in these recommendations and about the greater risks of transmission of HIV and other bloodborne pathogens through sexual activity and needle sharing during the use of illicit drugs, including anabolic steroids. Athletes should be told not to share personal items, such as razors, toothbrushes, and nail clippers, that might be contaminated with blood.
- The following precautions should be adopted in sports with direct body contact and other sports in which an athlete's blood or other bodily fluids visibly tinged with blood may contaminate the skin or mucous membranes of other participants or staff members of the athletic program. Even if these precautions are adopted, the risk that a participant or staff member may become infected with a blood-borne pathogen in the athletic setting will not be entirely eliminated.
- In some states, depending on state law, schools may need to comply with Occupational Safety and Health Administration (OSHA) regulations* for prevention of bloodborne pathogens. The athletic program must determine what rules apply. Compliance with OSHA regulations is a reasonable and recommended precaution even if this is not specifically required by the state.
  - Athletes must cover existing cuts, abrasions, wounds, or other areas of broken skin with an occlusive dressing before and during participation. Caregivers should cover their own damaged skin to prevent transmission of infection to or from an injured athlete.
  - Disposable, water-impervious vinyl or latex gloves should be worn to avoid contact with blood or other bodily fluids visibly tinged with blood and any object, such as equipment, bandages, or uniforms, contaminated with these fluids. Hands should be cleaned with soap and water or an alcohol-based antiseptic handwash as soon as possible after gloves are removed.
  - Athletes with active bleeding should be removed from competition as soon as possible and the bleeding stopped. Wounds should be cleaned with soap and water. Skin antiseptics may be used if soap and water are not available.

---

* American Academy of Pediatrics. *OSHA: Materials to Assist the Pediatric Office in Implementing the Bloodborne Pathogen, Hazard Communication, and Other OSHA Standards.* Elk Grove Village, IL: American Academy of Pediatrics; 1994

Wounds must be covered with an occlusive dressing that will remain intact during further play before athletes return to competition.

- Athletes should be advised to report injuries and wounds in a timely fashion before or during competition.
- Minor cuts or abrasions that are not bleeding do not require interruption of play but can be cleaned and covered during scheduled breaks. During these breaks, if an athlete's equipment or uniform fabric is wet with blood, the equipment should be cleaned and disinfected (see below), or the uniform should be replaced.
- Equipment and playing areas contaminated with blood must be cleaned until all visible blood is gone and then disinfected with an appropriate germicide, such as a freshly made bleach solution containing 1 part bleach in 10 parts of water. The decontaminated equipment or area should be in contact with the bleach solution for at least 30 seconds. The area may be wiped with a disposable cloth after the minimum contact time or be allowed to air dry.
- Emergency care must not be delayed because gloves or other protective equipment is not available. If the caregiver does not have the appropriate protective equipment, a towel may be used to cover the wound until an off-the-field location is reached where gloves can be used during more definitive treatment.
- Breathing (Ambu) bags and oral airways should be available for giving resuscitation. Mouth-to-mouth resuscitation is recommended only if this equipment is not available.
- Equipment handlers, laundry personnel, and janitorial staff must be educated in proper procedures for handling washable or disposable materials contaminated with blood.

INFECTION CONTROL FOR HOSPITALIZED CHILDREN

Isolation Precautions

Nosocomial infections are a major cause of morbidity and mortality in hospitalized children, particularly children in intensive care units. Hand washing before and after each patient contact remains the single most important practice in the control of nosocomial infections. However, additional policies and procedures are required to prevent infection in critically ill pediatric patients. The Hospital Infection Control Practices Advisory Committee (HICPAC) of the Centers for Disease Control and Prevention (CDC) has posted an updated comprehensive set of guidelines for preventing and controlling nosocomial infections, including isolation precautions, employee health recommendations, and guidelines for the prevention of postoperative and device-related infections on its Web site (www.cdc.gov/ncidod/hip/Guide/guide.htm). Additional guidelines are available from the principal infection control societies in the United States, the Society for Healthcare Epidemiology of America, and the Association for Professionals in Infection Control and Epidemiology, as well as specialty societies and regulatory agencies, such as the Occupational Safety and Health Administration. The Joint Commission on Accreditation of Healthcare Organizations has established standards related to infection control. Infection control professionals should be familiar with this increasingly complex array of guidelines, regulations, and standards.

In 1996, HICPAC issued isolation guidelines for the care of hospitalized patients.* These guidelines rely on consistent strategies to prevent the spread of pathogens among hospitalized patients. These recommendations state that "no guideline can address all of the needs of the more than 6000 US hospitals, which range in size from 5 beds to more than 1500 beds and serve different patient populations. Hospitals are encouraged to review the recommendations and to modify them according to what is possible, practical, and prudent." Therefore, with these recommendations as a guide, each institution must create its own specific isolation policies. These isolation policies, supplemented by hospital policies and procedures for other aspects of infection and environmental control and occupational health, should result in policies that are "possible, practical, and prudent" for each hospital.

These guidelines rely on the routine and optimal performance of an expanded set of universal practices, designated **Standard Precautions,** designed for the care of all patients regardless of their diagnosis or presumed infection status, and pathogen- and syndrome-based precautions, designated **Transmission-based Precautions,** to be used when caring for patients who are infected or colonized with pathogens spread by the airborne, droplet, or contact routes. To determine which diseases are reportable, see Appendix VIII (Nationally Notifiable Infectious Diseases in the United States, p 777).

STANDARD PRECAUTIONS

This category of precautions, which extends the CDC's previous **Universal Precautions,** applies to blood, all body fluids, secretions, and excretions except sweat (regardless of whether these fluids, secretions, or excretions contain visible blood), nonintact skin, and mucous membranes. These general barrier techniques are designed to reduce exposure of health care personnel to body fluids containing the human immunodeficiency virus or other bloodborne pathogens, since medical history and examination cannot reliably identify all patients infected with these agents. In addition, **Standard Precautions** may reduce transmission of microorganisms from patients who are not recognized as harboring potential pathogens, such as antibiotic-resistant bacteria. **Standard Precautions** include the following techniques:

- **Hand washing** is necessary after touching blood, body fluids, secretions, excretions, and contaminated items, whether or not gloves are worn. Hands should be washed immediately after removing gloves, between patient contacts, and when otherwise indicated to avoid transfer of microorganisms to other patients or environments.
- **Gloves** (clean, nonsterile) should be worn when touching blood, body fluids, secretions, excretions, and items contaminated with these fluids. Clean gloves should be used before touching mucous membranes and nonintact skin. Gloves

* Garner JS. Hospital Infection Control Practices Advisory Committee. Guideline for isolation precautions in hospitals. *Infect Control Hosp Epidemiol.* 1996;17:53–80

should be changed between tasks and procedures on the same patient after contact with material that may contain a high concentration of microorganisms. Gloves should be promptly removed after use and hand washing performed before touching noncontaminated items and environmental surfaces and before contact with another patient.

- **Masks, eye protection, and face shields** should be worn to protect mucous membranes of the eyes, nose, and mouth during procedures and patient care activities likely to generate splashes or sprays of blood, body fluids, secretions, or excretions.
- **Nonsterile gowns** that are fluid-resistant will protect skin and prevent the soiling of clothing during procedures and patient care activities likely to generate splashes or sprays of blood, body fluids, secretions, or excretions. Soiled gowns should be removed promptly.
- **Patient care equipment** that has been used should be handled in a manner that prevents skin and mucous membrane exposures and contamination of clothing.
- **All used linen** is considered to be contaminated and should be handled, transported, and processed in a manner that prevents skin and mucous membrane exposure and contamination of clothing.
- **Bloodborne pathogen** exposure should be avoided by taking all precautions to prevent injuries when using, cleaning, and disposing of needles, scalpels, and other sharp instruments and devices.
- **Mouthpieces, resuscitation bags, and other ventilation devices** should be readily available in all patient care areas and used instead of mouth-to-mouth resuscitation.

TRANSMISSION-BASED PRECAUTIONS

Transmission-based Precautions are designed for patients documented or suspected to be colonized or infected with pathogens for which additional precautions beyond **Standard Precautions** are necessary to interrupt transmission. The 3 types of transmission on which these precautions are based are airborne, droplet, and contact.

- **Airborne transmission** occurs by dissemination of airborne droplet nuclei (small-particle residue [≤5 μm in size] of evaporated droplets containing microorganisms that remain suspended in the air for long periods), dust particles containing the infectious agent, or fungal spores. Microorganisms spread by the airborne route can be dispersed widely by air currents and may become inhaled by or deposited on a susceptible host within the same room or a long distance from the source patient, depending on environmental factors. Therefore, special air handling and ventilation are required to prevent airborne transmission. Spores of filamentous fungi, such as *Aspergillus*, represent a considerable environmental hazard to severely immunosuppressed patients but are not spread from person to person. Strict environmental controls are important for prevention of such fungal infections, but isolation precautions are not required. High-efficiency particulate air (HEPA) filters also can be used if risk is particularly high (ie, bone marrow transplant recipients). Examples of microorganisms transmitted by airborne droplet nuclei are *Mycobacterium tuberculosis,* measles virus, varicella virus, and disseminated zoster. Specific recommendations in **Airborne Precautions** are as follows:

- Private room (If unavailable, consider cohorting patients with the same disease and consult with an infection control professional.)
- Negative air-pressure ventilation (6–12 air changes per hour) with externally exhausted or HEPA filtered air, if recirculated
- If infectious pulmonary tuberculosis is suspected or proven, respiratory protective devices (ie, National Institute for Occupational Safety and Health–certified personally "fitted" and "sealing" respirator masks, such as the N95 respirator) should be worn at all times.
- Susceptible health care personnel should not enter rooms of patients with measles or disseminated infection with varicella-zoster virus if immune health care personnel are available. If susceptible persons must enter the room of a patient with measles or varicella, a mask should be worn. Persons immune to these viruses need not wear a mask.

- **Droplet transmission** occurs when droplets containing microorganisms generated from the infected person, primarily during coughing, sneezing, and talking and during the performance of certain procedures, such as suctioning and bronchoscopy, are propelled a short distance and deposited on the host's conjunctivae, nasal mucosa, and/or mouth. Because these relatively large droplets do not remain suspended in the air, special air handling and ventilation are not required to prevent droplet transmission; droplet transmission should not be confused with airborne transmission via droplet nuclei, which are much smaller. Specific recommendations in droplet precautions are as follows:
  - Private room (When a private room is not available, the patient should be placed in a room with other patients currently infected with the same organism but with no other communicable infection [cohorting]. If cohorting of patients is not achievable, spatial separation of at least 3 feet between other patients and visitors should be maintained.)
  - Use of a mask if within 3 feet of patient

  Specific illnesses and infections requiring **Droplet Precautions** include the following:
  - Adenovirus
  - Diphtheria (pharyngeal)
  - *Haemophilus influenzae* type b (invasive)
  - Influenza
  - Mumps
  - *Mycoplasma pneumoniae*
  - *Neisseria meningitidis* (invasive)
  - Parvovirus B19 (during the phase of illness before onset of rash in immunocompetent patients; see Parvovirus B19, p 423)
  - Pertussis
  - Plague (pneumonic)
  - Rubella
  - Streptococcal pharyngitis, pneumonia, or scarlet fever in infants and young children

- **Contact Transmission,** the most important and frequent route of transmission of nosocomial infections, is divided into 2 modes: direct and indirect. *Direct-contact* transmission involves a direct body surface–to-body contact and physical transfer of microorganisms between a susceptible host and an infected or colonized person, such as occurs when a person turns a patient, gives a patient a bath, or performs other patient care activities that require direct personal contact. Direct-contact transmission also can occur between 2 patients in which one serves as the source of the infectious microorganisms and the other as a susceptible host. *Indirect-contact* transmission involves contact of a susceptible host with a contaminated intermediate object, usually inanimate, such as contaminated instruments, needles, or dressings, or contaminated hands that are not washed or gloves that are not changed between patients. Specific recommendations in **Contact Precautions** are as follows:

- Private room (cohorting patients is permissible if private room unavailable)
- Gloves (clean, nonsterile) at all times
- Hand washing after glove removal
- Gowns at all times, unless the patient is continent and substantial contact of clothing with patient or environmental surfaces is not anticipated. Gowns should be removed before leaving the patient's environment.

Specific illnesses and infections with organisms requiring **Contact Precautions** include the following:

- Multidrug-resistant bacteria (eg, vancomycin-resistant enterococci, methicillin-resistant *Staphylococcus aureus,* multidrug-resistant gram-negative bacilli) judged by the infection control program, based on current state, regional, or national recommendations, to be of special clinical and epidemiologic significance
- *Clostridium difficile*
- Conjunctivitis, viral and hemorrhagic
- Diphtheria (cutaneous)
- Enteroviruses
- *Escherichia coli* O157:H7
- Hepatitis A virus
- Herpes simplex virus (neonatal, mucocutaneous or cutaneous infection)
- Herpes zoster
- Impetigo
- Major (noncontained) abscesses, cellulitis, or decubitus
- Parainfluenza virus
- Pediculosis (lice)
- Respiratory syncytial virus
- Rotavirus
- Scabies
- *Shigella*
- *Staphylococcus aureus* cutaneous infection
- Viral hemorrhagic fevers (Ebola, Lassa, or Marburg)

Airborne, Droplet, and **Contact Precautions** may be combined for diseases that have multiple routes of transmission. When used alone or in combination, these transmission-based precautions are always to be used in addition to **Standard Precautions,** which are recommended for all patients. The specifications for these categories of isolation precautions are summarized in Table 2.7 (p 132). Table 2.8 (p 133) lists syndromes and conditions that are highly suggestive of contagious infec-

Table 2.7. **Transmission-based Precautions for Hospitalized Patients**

These recommendations are in addition to those for **Standard Precautions** for all patients.

Category of Precautions	Single Room	Masks	Gowns	Gloves
Airborne	Yes, with negative air-pressure ventilation	Yes	No	No
Droplet	Yes*	Yes, masks† for persons close to patient	No	No
Contact	Yes*	No	Yes	Yes

* Preferred but not required. Cohorting of children infected with the same pathogen is acceptable.
† See text.

tion and require empiric isolation precautions pending identification of a specific pathogen. When the specific pathogen is known, isolation recommendations and duration of isolation are given in the pathogen- or disease-specific chapters in Section 3.

PEDIATRIC CONSIDERATIONS

These guidelines generally are easy to understand and apply to the care of hospitalized adults, as well as to children. However, unique differences in pediatric care from that for adults necessitate possible modifications of these guidelines including the following: (1) diaper changing, (2) the use of single-room isolation, and (3) the use of common areas, such as hospital waiting rooms, play rooms, and school rooms.

Since diapering is performed routinely without gloves in infants and preschool-age children in the community, it is not mandatory to wear gloves when diapering hospitalized children. Nevertheless, the use of gloves for diapering could minimize transfer of antibiotic-resistant bacteria and other nosocomial pathogens in the stool of one patient to another. For this reason, the wearing of gloves when diapering is suggested by some experts.

Private rooms are recommended for all patients in **Transmission-based Precautions** (ie, **Airborne, Droplet,** and **Contact**). For patients with an infection requiring **Airborne Precautions,** a single room with negative air pressure is indicated. When a private room is mandated by the possibility of airborne transmission, such as for infants with varicella, a forced-air incubator is not a substitute for a private room because such an incubator does not filter the air discharged into the environment. The guidelines for **Standard Precautions** also state that patients who cannot control body excretions should be in single rooms. Since most young children are incontinent, this recommendation is inappropriate for routine care of uninfected children. For infected patients in settings such as nurseries, intensive care units, and infant wards, single-room isolation for **Droplet** and **Contact Precautions** is recommended. For droplet and contact precautions, if single-room isolation is not possible, an isolation area can be defined within an intensive care unit by curtains, partitions, or other barriers. For newborn infants, separate isolation rooms are not necessary if the following conditions are met:

Table 2.8. **Clinical Syndromes or Conditions Warranting Empiric Precautions in Addition to Standard Precautions to Prevent Transmission of Epidemiologically Important Pathogens Pending Confirmation of Diagnosis***

Clinical Syndrome or Condition†	Potential Pathogens‡	Empiric Precautions§
Diarrhea		
Acute diarrhea with a likely infectious cause in an incontinent or diapered patient	Enteric pathogens‖	Contact
Diarrhea in an adult with a history of recent antibiotic use	*Clostridium difficile*	Contact
Meningitis	*Neisseria meningitidis*	Droplet
Rash or exanthems, generalized, cause unknown		
Petechial or ecchymotic with fever	*N meningitidis*	Droplet
Vesicular	Varicella	Airborne and contact
Maculopapular with coryza and fever	Measles	Airborne
Respiratory tract infections		
Cough, fever, or upper lobe pulmonary infiltrate in a human immunodeficiency virus (HIV)-negative patient or a patient at low risk for HIV infection	*Mycobacterium tuberculosis*	Airborne
Cough, fever, or pulmonary infiltrate in any lung location in an HIV-infected patient or a patient at high risk for HIV infection	*M tuberculosis*	Airborne
Paroxysmal or severe persistent cough during periods of pertussis activity in the community	*Bordetella pertussis*	Droplet
Viral infections, particularly bronchiolitis and croup, in infants and young children	Respiratory syncytial or parainfluenza virus	Contact
Risk of multidrug-resistant microorganisms¶		
History of infection or colonization with multidrug-resistant organisms	Resistant bacteria	Contact
Skin, wound, or urinary tract infection in a patient with a recent hospital or nursing home stay in a facility in which multidrug-resistant organisms are prevalent	Resistant bacteria	Contact
Skin or wound infection		
Abscess or draining wound that cannot be covered	*Staphylococcus aureus,* group A streptococcus	Contact

Table 2.8. **Clinical Syndromes or Conditions Warranting Empiric Precautions in Addition to Standard Precautions to Prevent Transmission of Epidemiologically Important Pathogens Pending Confirmation of Diagnosis,* continued**

* Infection control professionals are encouraged to modify or adapt this table according to local conditions. To ensure that appropriate empiric precautions are implemented, hospitals must have systems in place to evaluate patients routinely according to these criteria as part of their preadmission and admission care.

† Patients with the syndromes or conditions listed may present with atypical signs or symptoms (eg, pertussis in neonates, and adults may not have paroxysmal or severe cough). The clinician's index of suspicion should be guided by the prevalence of specific conditions in the community, as well as clinical judgment.

‡ The organisms listed in this column are not intended to represent the complete, or even most likely, diagnoses, but rather possible causative agents that require additional precautions beyond **Standard Precautions** until they can be excluded.

§ Duration of isolation varies by agent (see Garner JS. Hospital Infection Control Practices Advisory Committee. Guidelines for isolation precautions in hospitals. *Infect Control Hosp Epidemiol.* 1996;17:53-80).

|| These pathogens include enterohemorrhagic *Escherichia coli* O157:H7, *Shigella* organisms, *Campylobacter* organisms, hepatitis A virus, enteric viruses including rotavirus, and *Cryptosporidium* organisms.

¶ Resistant bacteria judged by the infection control program, based on current state, regional, or national recommendations, to be of special clinical or epidemiologic significance.

- Transmission of the infection is not by the airborne route.
- Sufficient space is available for a 4- to 6-ft aisle or area between newborn infant beds.
- An adequate number of sinks for hand washing are available in each nursery room and area.
- Continuing instruction is given to personnel about the mode of transmission of infections.

In contrast, a single room is recommended for children who are not crib-confined and who require **Droplet** or **Contact Precautions** since these young children are unable to limit the spread of their secretions. The exception to the need for a single room is for children infected with the same documented pathogen (eg, respiratory syncytial virus), who can be cohorted.

The CDC isolation guidelines specifically are recommended for the care of hospitalized children. These recommendations should not be extrapolated to schools, out-of-home child care centers, and other settings in which healthy children congregate in shared space.

Occupational Health

Prevention of the transmission of infectious agents between patients and health care personnel is particularly important in pediatric care. Some infections pose increased risk for pregnant health care personnel, principally because of possible adverse effects on the fetus (eg, parvovirus B19, cytomegalovirus, rubella, and varicella), or for personnel who are immunocompromised and at increased risk of severe infection (eg, *M tuberculosis,* measles, herpes simplex virus, and varicella).

The consequences to pediatric patients of acquiring infections from infected adults also are significant. Since children often lack immunity to many common viruses and bacteria, they are a highly susceptible population. Mild illness in adults, such as viral gastroenteritis, upper respiratory tract viral infection (eg, respiratory syncytial virus), varicella-zoster virus infection, pertussis, herpes simplex infection, and tuberculosis, can cause life-threatening disease in infants and children. Those at greatest risk are premature infants, children who have heart disease or chronic pulmonary disease, and immunocompromised patients.

The transmission of infectious agents within hospitals is facilitated by the inevitable close contact between patients and health care personnel. In addition, children do not routinely practice good hygienic practices.

To limit the risks of infection to and from children and health care personnel, hospitals should have established employee health policies and services. It is particularly important to ensure that employees are protected against measles, rubella, mumps, hepatitis B, varicella, influenza, polio, pertussis, tetanus, and diphtheria by establishing appropriate screening and immunization policies.

For non–vaccine-preventable infections, employees should be counseled about exposures and the possible need for leave if they are exposed to, ill with, or a carrier of a specific infectious agent, whether the exposure occurs in the home, community, or health care setting.

Employees should be screened by Mantoux skin testing for tuberculosis. Persons with common infections, such as gastroenteritis, dermatitis, herpes simplex lesions on exposed skin, or upper respiratory tract infections, should be evaluated to determine the resulting risk of transmission to their patients or to other health care personnel.

Employees, including pregnant personnel, should be educated about pathogens for which they are and are not at increased risk if they follow **Standard Precautions.**

Employee education is of paramount importance in infection control. Pediatric health care professionals should be knowledgeable about the modes of transmission of infectious agents, proper hand-washing technique, and the potential serious risks to children of certain mild infections in adults.

Sibling Visits

Sibling visits to birthing centers, postpartum rooms, pediatric wards, and intensive care units are encouraged. Newborn intensive care, with its increasing sophistication, often results in long hospital stays for the sick newborn, making family visits important. Sibling visits in newborn intensive care units are received favorably by parents, and subsequent infection is not increased in the sick or well newborn who has been visited by siblings if guidelines are followed.

Guidelines for sibling visits should be established to maximize opportunities for visiting and to minimize the risks of nosocomial spread of pathogens brought into the hospital by these young visitors. Guidelines may need to be modified by local nursing, pediatric, obstetric, and infectious disease staffs to address specific issues in their hospital settings. Basic guidelines for sibling visits to pediatric patients are as follows:

- Sibling visits should be encouraged in the healthy infant nursery and the newborn intensive care nursery, for chronically and critically ill children, and for other hospitalized children.
- Before the visit, a trained health care professional should interview the parents at a site outside the unit to assess the health of each sibling visitor. No child with fever or symptoms of an acute illness, including an upper respiratory tract infection, gastroenteritis, or dermatitis, should be allowed to visit. Siblings who recently have been exposed to a known communicable disease and are susceptible should not be allowed to visit. These interviews should be documented in the patient's record, and approval for each sibling visit should be noted.
- Asymptomatic siblings who have been exposed recently to varicella but have been immunized previously should be assumed to be immune.
- Adequate observation and monitoring of all visitors by the medical and nursing staff should occur.
- The visiting sibling should visit only his or her sibling.
- Children should carefully wash their hands before patient contact, especially when siblings are newborn infants or are immunocompromised.

Throughout the visit, sibling activity should be supervised by parents or a responsible adult and limited to the mother's or patient's private room or other designated areas.

Similar guidelines should be applied to visits by other relatives and close friends since such visits often are appropriate for children in non–intensive care settings. Medical and nursing staff also should be vigilant about potential communicable diseases in parents and other adult visitors (eg, a relative with a chronic cough who may have tuberculosis; a parent with a cold visiting a highly immunosuppressed child).

Pet Visitation

Pet visitation in the hospital setting can be placed into 2 categories, that of visits by a child's personal pet and pet visitation as a part of child life therapeutic programs. The former is likely to be an issue only for children requiring long-term hospitalization. The latter provides children requiring lengthy hospitalization the opportunity to interact with pets. Guidelines for pet visitation should be established to minimize risks for transmission of infection from pets to humans. The hospital setting and the level of concern for zoonotic disease will influence the establishment of pet visitation policies. The hospital policy should be developed in consultation with pediatricians, infection control practitioners, nursing staff, the hospital epidemiologist, and veterinarians. Basic principles for hospital pet visitation policies are as follows:

- Pets other than cats and dogs should be excluded from the hospital. No reptiles (iguanas, turtles, snakes), amphibians, birds, primates, ferrets, or rodents should be allowed to visit.
- Visiting pets should have a certificate of immunization from a licensed veterinarian and verification that the pet is free from infections or contagious diseases and that immunizations are up to date.
- The pet should be bathed and groomed for the visit.
- Pet visitation is inappropriate in the intensive care unit.

- The visit of the pet should be approved by appropriate hospital personnel (for example, the director of the child life therapeutic program) who should observe the pet for temperament and general health at the time of visit. The pet should be free from obvious bacterial skin infections, from infections caused by superficial dermatophytes, and from ectoparasitic infections (fleas and ticks).
- Pet visitation should be confined to designated areas. Contact should be confined to the petting and holding of animals, as appropriate. All contact should be supervised throughout the visit by appropriate hospital personnel. Supervisors should be familiar with hospital policies for managing animal bites and cleaning spills of pet urine and feces.
- Patients having contact with pets must have approval from a physician or physician representative before animal contact. Documented allergy to dogs or cats should be considered before approving contact. For patients who are immunodeficient or for persons receiving immunosuppressive therapy, the risks from exposure to the microflora of pets may outweigh the benefits of contact. Contact of children with pets should be approved on a case-by-case basis. Care should be taken to protect indwelling catheter sites. These sites should have dressings that provide an effective barrier to pet contact, including licking.
- Children should wash their hands after contact with pets. Concern for contamination of other body sites should be considered on a case-by-case basis.
- The pet policy should not apply to professionally trained guide animals, such as "seeing eye" dogs. These animals are not pets, and separate policies should govern their uses and presence in the hospital.

INFECTION CONTROL IN PHYSICIANS' OFFICES*

Infection control is an integral part of pediatric practice in outpatient settings, as well as in hospitals. All employees should be aware of the routes of transmission and techniques used to prevent transmission of infectious agents. Policies for infection control and prevention should be written, readily available, and enforced. Standard precautions, as outlined for the hospitalized child (see Infection Control for Hospitalized Children, p 127), with modifications by the American Academy of Pediatrics, are appropriate for most patient encounters. Key principles of infection control in an outpatient setting are as follows:

- All health care personnel should wash their hands before and after patient contact. Parents and children should be taught the importance of hand washing.
- Standard precautions should be used when caring for all patients.
- Contact between infected contagious children and uninfected children should be minimized. Policies to deal with children who present with infections, such as varicella or measles, should be implemented. Prompt triage of immunocompromised children should be performed routinely.

* American Academy of Pediatrics Committee on Infectious Diseases. Infection control in physicians' offices. *Pediatrics*. In press

- Alcohol is preferred for skin preparation before immunization and routine venipuncture. Skin preparation for incision, suture, and collection of blood for culture requires iodine; solutions of choice are 1% or 2% tincture of iodine or povidone iodine.
- Needles and sharps should be handled with great care. Needle disposal units that are impermeable and puncture proof should be available next to the spaces used for injection or venipuncture. The containers should not be overfilled and should be kept out of the reach of young children. Policies should be established for removal and incineration or sterilization of contents.
- Policies for management of needle-stick injuries should be in place.
- Standard guidelines for decontamination, disinfection, and sterilization should be followed.
- Judicious use of antimicrobial agents is essential to limit the emergence and spread of drug-resistant bacteria (see Judicious Use of Antimicrobial Agents, p 647).
- Outpatient offices and clinics should develop policies and procedures for communication with local and state health authorities about reportable diseases and suspected outbreaks.
- Ongoing educational programs that encompass appropriate aspects of infection control should be implemented, reinforced, and evaluated on a regular basis.

Sexually Transmitted Diseases in Adolescents and Children

Physicians and other health care professionals perform a critical role in preventing and treating sexually transmitted diseases (STDs) in the pediatric population. Sexually transmitted diseases are a major problem for adolescents; an estimated 25% of adolescents will develop an STD before graduating from high school. For infants and children, detection of an STD is an important warning signal of possible sexual abuse. Sexual abuse of children has been endemic for generations, but its prevalence and potentially devastating psychological effects have been recognized only recently. In addition to the medical evaluation, appropriate social service and law enforcement agencies must be involved whenever sexual abuse is suspected to ensure the child's protection, and counseling must be provided to the child and family.

STDs in Adolescents

EPIDEMIOLOGY

Although the incidence of all reported STDs in the United States has decreased during the past decade, adolescents and young adults continue to have higher age-specific STD rates than any other age group. In the United States in 1998, case report rates for gonorrhea were 31 per 100 000 for adults between 40 and 64 years of age, 176 per 100 000 for adults between 25 and 39 years of age, and 572 per 100 000 for youth between 15 and 24 years of age. The highest age-specific incidence rate for acquired immunodeficiency syndrome (AIDS) in 1997 was 51 per

100 000. This rate occurred among young adults 25 to 39 years of age who presumably acquired their human immunodeficiency virus (HIV) infections about a decade earlier—frequently, during adolescence. In 1998, reports based on AIDS surveillance data indicate substantial declines in perinatally acquired AIDS, reflecting declining perinatal HIV transmission. In the United States in 1998, the rates of chlamydial infection were 1212 per 100 000 for youth between 15 and 24 years of age and 201 per 100 000 for persons 25 to 39 years of age. These data underestimate STDs among sexually experienced adolescents since *all* adolescents, including the one third of US 10th, 11th, and 12th grade students who have never had sexual intercourse, are included in the denominators used to calculate age-specific STD rates.

MANAGEMENT

Pediatricians should screen for STD risk by asking all adolescent patients whether they have ever had sexual intercourse or ever been sexually active. Adolescents at increased risk of STD are listed in Table 2.9, p 140. Physicians can prepare parents and patients for this sensitive question by informing parents of their policies about confidentiality and by ensuring that the annual checkup of every adolescent includes a private interview. More detailed recommendations for preventive health care for adolescents are contained in the American Academy of Pediatrics *Guidelines for Health Supervision III** and the American Medical Association's *Guidelines for Adolescent Preventive Services.*† All 50 states in the United States allow minors to give their own consent for confidential STD diagnosis and treatment.

Most experts recommend that all adolescent women who have had sexual intercourse receive a Papanicolaou smear annually to screen for cervical dysplasia resulting from papillomavirus infection and that all adolescents who have had sexual intercourse be screened for gonorrhea and chlamydia semiannually and receive HIV counseling and syphilis screening annually. All adolescents should receive hepatitis B virus immunization if they were not immunized earlier in childhood (see Recommended Childhood Immunization Schedule, p 22).

For treatment recommendations for specific STDs, see the condition in Section 3 and Table 4.3, Guidelines for Treatment of Sexually Transmitted Diseases in Children and Adolescents According to Syndrome, p 663. Patients with gonorrhea, *Chlamydia trachomatis* infection, and trichomoniasis should be advised to refrain from sexual intercourse until their sexual partners have received presumptive treatment for these infections. "Tests of cure" for patients who receive standard treatment for *Neisseria gonorrhoeae* or *C trachomatis* infection are no longer recommended since the standard regimens are highly effective. If a multiple-dose regimen is used, noncompliance is possible, but results of retesting for chlamydia infection less than 3 weeks after treatment may be falsely positive as a result of residual nonviable organisms. Some experts recommend repeated testing of adolescents 4 to 6 weeks after STD treatment because of the more substantial likelihood of reinfection, either from a current sexual partner who did not obtain treatment or from a new sexual partner.

---

* American Academy of Pediatrics Committee on Psychosocial Aspects of Child and Family Health. *Guidelines for Health Supervision III.* Elk Grove Village, IL: American Academy of Pediatrics; 1997

† Elster AB, Kuznets NJ, eds. *AMA Guidelines for Adolescent Preventive Services (GAPS) Recommendations and Rationale.* Baltimore, MD: Williams & Wilkins; 1994

Table 2.9. **Adolescents Whose History Includes 1 or More of the Following Categories Are Considered at Increased Risk for Contracting a Sexually Transmitted Disease (STD)***

- Sexual contact with person(s) with a known STD or history of STD
- Symptoms or signs of an STD
- Multiple sexual partners
- Street involvement (eg, homelessness)
- Intercourse with new partner during last 2 months
- More than 2 sexual partners during previous 12 months
- No contraception or use of nonbarrier methods
- Injection drug use
- Men who have sex with men
- "Survival sex" (eg, exchanging sex for money, drugs, shelter, or food)

* Modified from Canadian STD Guidelines, 1998 Edition. Health Canada. Available at: http://www.hc-sc.gc.ca/hpb/lcdc/bah

PREVENTION

Pediatricians can contribute to primary prevention of STDs by encouraging adolescent patients to remain abstinent and to postpone their first sexual intercourse for as long as possible. Pediatricians should encourage adolescents who have ever had sexual intercourse to practice "secondary" abstinence (to be celibate), to minimize their lifetime number of sexual partners, to consistently use barrier methods of contraception, and to be aware of the strong association between alcohol or drug use and failure to use barrier contraception. The correct use of male and female condoms and some strategies for encouraging condom use are reviewed in Tables 2.10 and 2.11 (p 141 and p 142).

Diagnosis and Treatment of STDs in Children

Because of the social and legal implications of the diagnosis, STDs in children must be diagnosed using tests with high specificity since the low prevalence of STDs in children increases the probability that rapid detection tests for STDs will give false-positive results. Therefore, tests that allow for isolation of the organism and that have the highest specificities should be used.

Because of the serious implications of the diagnosis of an STD in a child, antimicrobial therapy for children with suspected STDs may need to be withheld until the final outcome of the diagnostic test is known. Cultures for *N gonorrhoeae* and *C trachomatis* should be taken from the vaginal or cervical area and from the rectal area and for *N gonorrhoeae,* also from the pharyngeal areas. Culture and wet mount of vaginal specimens for *Trichomonas vaginalis* and bacterial vaginosis and serum specimens for syphilis, HIV, and hepatitis B virus should be obtained. For more detailed diagnosis and treatment recommendations for specific STDs, see

Table 2.10. **Recommendations for Proper Use of Condoms to Reduce the Risk of Transmission of Sexually Transmitted Diseases***

Male Condoms

- Use a new condom with each act of sexual intercourse.
- Carefully handle the condom to avoid damaging it with fingernails, teeth, or other sharp objects.
- Put condom on after the penis is erect and before genital contact with partner.
- Ensure that no air is trapped in the tip of the condom.
- Ensure that adequate lubrication exists during intercourse, possibly requiring the use of external lubricants.
- Use only water-based lubricants (eg, K-Y Jelly, Astroglide, Aqua-Lube, and glycerin) with latex condoms. Oil-based lubricants (eg, petroleum jelly, shortening, mineral oil, massage oils, body lotions, and cooking oil) can weaken latex.
- Hold the condom firmly against the base of the penis during withdrawal, and withdraw while penis is still erect to prevent slippage.

Female Condoms

- Lubricated polyurethane sheath with a ring on each end, one of which is inserted into the vagina and rests over the cervix like a diaphragm and the other remains outside the vagina and covers the external genitalia (trade name, Reality).
- When a male condom cannot be used appropriately, consider use of a female condom. Instructions about insertion may be needed.

* From Centers for Disease Control and Prevention. 1998 guidelines for treatment of sexually transmitted diseases. *MMWR Morb Mortal Wkly Rep.* 1998;47(RR-1):1–111.

Section 3 and Table 4.3, Guidelines for Treatment of Sexually Transmitted Diseases in Children and Adolescents According to Syndrome, p 663.

Social Implications of STDs in Children

Children can acquire STDs through vertical transmission, by autoinoculation, or by sexual contact. Each of these mechanisms should be given appropriate consideration in the evaluation of a preadolescent child with an STD. Evaluation based solely on suspicion of an STD should not proceed until the STD diagnosis has been confirmed. Factors to be considered in assessing the likelihood of sexual abuse in a child with an STD include whether the child reports a history of sexual victimization, biological characteristics of the STD in question, and the age of the child (see Table 2.12,* p 143).

Anogenital gonorrhea in a prepubertal child indicates sexual abuse in virtually every case. All cases of gonorrhea in children after the neonatal period should be reported to the local child protective service agency for investigation.

Herpes simplex has a short incubation period but can be transmitted by sexual or nonsexual contact with another person or by autoinoculation. In an infant or

* American Academy of Pediatrics Committee on Child Abuse and Neglect. Guidelines for evaluation of sexual abuse of children: subject review [published correction appears in *Pediatrics.* 1999;103: 1049]. *Pediatrics.* 1999;103:186–191

Table 2.11. **Barriers to Condom Use and Ways to Overcome Them***

Perceived Barrier	Intervention Strategy
Decreases sexual pleasure (sensation). Note: Often perceived by those who have never used a condom.	Encourage patient to try Put a drop of water-based lubricant or saliva inside the tip of the condom or on the glans of the penis before putting on the condom Try a thinner latex condom or different brand or more lubrication
Decreases spontaneity of sexual activity	Encourage incorporation of condom use during foreplay Remind patient that peace of mind may enhance pleasure for self and partner
Embarrassing, juvenile, "unmanly"	Remind patient that it is "manly" to protect self and others
Poor fit (too small or too big, slips off, uncomfortable)	Smaller and larger condoms are available
Requires prompt withdrawal after ejaculation	Reinforce the protective nature of prompt withdrawal and suggest substitution of other postcoital sexual activities
Fear of breakage may lead to less vigorous sexual activity	With prolonged intercourse, lubricant wears off and the condom begins to rub. Have a water-soluble lubricant available to reapply.
Nonpenetrative sexual activity	Condoms have been advocated for use during fellatio; unlubricated condoms may prove best for this purpose because of the taste of the lubricant Other barriers, such as dental dams or an unlubricated condom cut down the middle to form a barrier, have been advocated for use during certain forms of non-penetrative sexual activity (eg, cunnilingus and anolingual sex)
Allergy to latex	Polyurethane condoms for women are available commercially A natural skin condom can be used together with a latex condom to protect the male or female from contact with latex

* From Canadian STD Guidelines. 1998 Edition. Health Canada. Available at: http://www.hc-sc.gc.ca/hpb/cdc/bah

toddler still in diapers, genital herpes may arise from any of these mechanisms. In a child whose toilet use activities are independent, the new occurrence of genital herpes should prompt a careful investigation, including a child protective service investigation, for suspected sexual abuse.

Trichomoniasis is transmitted perinatally or by sexual contact. In a perinatally infected infant, the vaginal discharge can persist for several weeks; accordingly, intense social investigation may not be warranted. However, a new diagnosis of trichomoniasis in an older infant or child should prompt a careful investigation, including a child protective service investigation, for suspected sexual abuse.

Table 2.12. **Implications of Commonly Encountered Sexually Transmitted Diseases (STDs) for Diagnosis and Reporting of Sexual Abuse of Infants and Prepubertal Children***

STD Confirmed	Sexual Abuse	Suggested Action†
Gonorrhea‡	Diagnostic§	Report
Syphilis‡	Diagnostic	Report
Human immunodeficiency virus‖	Diagnostic	Report
Chlamydia trachomatis‡	Diagnostic§	Report
Trichomonas vaginalis	Highly suspicious	Report
Condylomata acuminata‡ (anogenital warts)	Suspicious	Report
Herpes (genital location)	Suspicious	Report¶
Bacterial vaginosis	Inconclusive	Medical follow-up

* Adapted from American Academy of Pediatrics Committee on Child Abuse and Neglect. Guidelines for the evaluation of sexual abuse of children: subject review. *Pediatrics* [published correction appears in *Pediatrics*. 1999;103:1049]. 1999;103:186–191

† Reports should be made to the agency mandated in the community to receive reports of suspected sexual abuse.

‡ If not perinatally acquired.

§ Only culture using standard confirmation methods should be used. DNA probes should not be used as a diagnostic method.

‖ If not perinatally or transfusion acquired.

¶ Unless there is a clear history of autoinoculation. Herpes 1 and 2 are difficult to differentiate by current techniques.

Infections that have long incubation periods (eg, papillomavirus infection) and that can be asymptomatic for long periods after vertical transmission (eg, syphilis, HIV infection, *C trachomatis* infection) are more problematic. The possibility of vertical transmission should be considered in these cases, but an evaluation of the patient's circumstances by the local child protective services agency is warranted in most.

While hepatitis B virus, *Gardnerella vaginalis* infection, bacterial vaginosis, scabies, and pediculosis pubis can be transmitted sexually, other modes of transmission may occur. The discovery of any of these conditions in a prepubertal child does not warrant child protective services involvement unless the clinician finds other information that suggests abuse.

Sexual Victimization and STDs

GENERAL CONSIDERATIONS

Child sexual abuse has been defined as the exploitation of a child, either by physical contact or by other interactions, for the sexual stimulation of an adult or of a minor who is in a position of power over the child. Sexual victimization of a child younger than 18 years of age by a caregiver is termed *abuse*; physicians are required by law to report abuse to their state child protective service agency. Sexual victimization of a child or adolescent by a person who is not a caregiver is termed *assault*; if the assault did not involve a gun or knife injury, the patient or parent makes the decision whether to report sexual assault to the local law enforcement authority. In some instances, sexual victimization involves physical contact permitting the transfer of sexually transmitted microorganisms. About 5% of sexually abused children acquire an STD as a result of the victimization.

SCREENING ASYMPTOMATIC SEXUALLY VICTIMIZED CHILDREN FOR STDS

Factors that influence the likelihood that a sexually victimized child will acquire an STD include the regional prevalence of STDs in the adult population, the number of assailants, the type and frequency of physical contact between the perpetrator(s) and the child, the infectivity of the various microorganisms, the child's susceptibility to infection, and whether the child has received intercurrent antibiotic treatment. The time interval between a child's physical contact with an assailant and the medical evaluation influences the likelihood that an exposed child will demonstrate signs or symptoms of an STD.

Because universal screening of sexually abused children in North America has yielded only about 5% with any STD, many experts recommend that screening be reserved for the following situations:

- Perpetrator with known STD or high STD risk (eg, has had multiple sex partners or a history of STD)
- Multiple perpetrators
- Patient or family preference
- All postpubertal patients
- Patient has signs or symptoms of an STD or an infection that can be transmitted sexually
- Prevalence of STDs in the community is high
- STDs in siblings, other children, or adults in the household

See Table 2.13, p 145, if STD testing of a child is to be done.

Most experts recommend universal screening of postpubertal patients because the prevalence of preexisting asymptomatic infection in this group is high. When STD screening is done, it should focus on the likely anatomic sites of infection (as determined by the patient's history or by epidemiologic considerations) and should include assessment for HIV infection if the patient, family, or both consent to serologic screening, assessment for bacterial vaginosis, trichomoniasis, and a Papanicolaou smear in postpubertal patients, and testing for *N gonorrhoeae* infection, *C trachomatis* infection, and syphilis. To preserve the "chain of custody" for information that may later constitute legal evidence, specimens for laboratory analysis obtained from sexually victimized patients should be labeled carefully, and standard hospital procedures for transferring specimens from site to site should be followed carefully.

Table 2.13. **STD Testing in a Child* When Sexual Abuse Is Suspected**

Organism/Syndrome	Specimens
Neisseria gonorrhoeae	Rectal, throat, urethral, and/or vaginal culture(s)
Chlamydia trachomatis	Rectal and urethral cultures
Syphilis	Darkfield examination of chancre fluid, if present; blood for serologic tests at time of abuse and 6, 12, and 24 wk later
Human immunodeficiency virus	Serologic testing of abuser (if possible); serologic testing of child at time of abuse and 6, 12, and 24 wk later
Hepatitis B virus	Serum hepatitis B surface antigen testing of abuser
Herpes simplex virus	Culture of lesion
Bacterial vaginosis	Wet mount and culture of vaginal discharge
Papillomavirus	Biopsy of lesion
Trichomonas vaginalis	Wet mount and culture of vaginal discharge
Pediculosis capitis	Identification of eggs, nymphs, and lice with naked eye or using hand lens

* See text for indications for testing for sexually transmitted diseases (STDs), Screening Asymptomatic Sexually Victimized Children for STDs, p 144).

PROPHYLAXIS AFTER SEXUAL VICTIMIZATION

Most experts do not recommend antimicrobial prophylaxis for abused prepubertal children because their incidence of STDs is low and the risk of spread to the upper genital tract in a prepubertal girl is low. As well, follow-up usually can be ensured. If a test for an STD is positive, treatment can then be given. Factors that may increase the likelihood of infection or that constitute an indication for prophylaxis are the same as those listed under "Screening Asymptomatic Sexually Victimized Children for STDs" (p 144).

Many experts believe that prophylaxis is warranted for postpubertal patients who seek care within 72 hours after an episode of sexual victimization because of the high prevalence of preexisting asymptomatic infection and the substantial risk of pelvic inflammatory disease in this group. All patients who receive prophylaxis should be screened for the relevant STDs (see Table 2.13, above) before treatment is given. Postmenarcheal patients should be tested for pregnancy before antibiotic treatment or emergency contraception is given. Regimens for prophylaxis are presented in Tables 2.14 (children) and 2.15 (adolescents).

Because of the demonstrated effectiveness of prophylaxis to prevent HIV infection after perinatal and occupational exposures, the question arises about HIV prophylaxis for children and adolescents after sexual assault. (See also HIV Infection, Control Measures, p 341 and Table 3.29, p 342.) There are no data on effectiveness or safety of HIV prophylaxis for this indication. The risk of HIV transmission from a single sexual assault that involves transfer of secretions and/or blood is low, but not zero. Prophylaxis with zidovudine plus lamivudine may be considered for patients

Table 2.14. Prophylaxis After Sexual Victimization of Preadolescent Children*

Weight <100 lb (45 kg)	Weight ≥ 100 lb (45 kg)
For coverage of gonorrhea	
1A. Cefixime 8 mg/kg (maximum 400 mg) orally in a single dose	1A. Cefixime 400 mg orally in a single dose
OR	**OR**
1B. Ceftriaxone 125 mg IM in a single dose	1B. Ceftriaxone 125 mg IM in a single dose
PLUS — **For coverage of *Chlamydia trachomatis***	**PLUS**
2A. Azithromycin 20 mg/kg (maximum 1 g) orally in a single dose	2A. Azithromycin 1 g orally in a single dose
OR	**OR**
2B. Erythromycin 50 mg/kg per day divided into 4 doses for 10–14 d	2B. Doxycycline 100 mg twice daily for 7 d
PLUS — **For prevention of hepatitis B virus infection**	**PLUS**
3. Begin or complete hepatitis B virus immunization if not fully immunized	3. Begin or complete hepatitis B virus immunization if not fully immunized
PLUS — **Trichomoniasis and bacterial vaginosis**	**PLUS**
4. Consideration should be given to adding prophylaxis for trichomoniasis and bacterial vaginosis (metronidazole 15 mg/kg per day orally in 3 divided doses for 7 d)	4. Consideration should be given to adding prophylaxis against trichomoniasis and bacterial vaginosis (metronidazole 2 g orally in a single dose)

* IM indicates intramuscularly. See text for discussion of prophylaxis for human immunodeficiency virus infection in children following sexual assault.

who seek care within 24 to 48 hours after an assault if the assault involved the transfer of secretions and particularly if the alleged perpetrator is known or suspected to have HIV infection or to have used intravenous drugs. Consideration may be given to adding a protease inhibitor to the regimen if the assault involved exposure to blood or if other circumstances of the assault seem to confer a high risk. Patients should be tested for HIV infection before postexposure prophylaxis is begun.

Table 2.15. Prophylaxis After Sexual Victimization of Adolescents*

Antibiotic prophylaxis† is recommended to include an empiric regimen to cover *Chlamydia trachomatis*, gonorrhea, trichomoniasis, and bacterial vaginosis

For gonorrhea	Cefixime 400 mg orally in a single dose
	OR
	Ceftriaxone 125 mg intramuscularly in a single dose
	OR
	Ciprofloxacin 500 mg orally in a single dose
	OR
	Ofloxacin 400 mg orally in a single dose
	PLUS
For *C trachomatis*	Azithromycin 1 g orally in a single dose
	OR
	Doxycycline 100 mg orally twice a day for 7 d
	PLUS
For trichomoniasis and bacterial vaginosis	Metronidazole 2 g orally in a single dose
	PLUS
For hepatitis B virus	Hepatitis B virus immunization at time of initial examination, if not fully immunized. Follow-up doses of vaccine should be administered 1 to 2 and 4 to 6 mo after the first dose.
	PLUS
For HIV	Consider offering prophylaxis for HIV depending on circumstances (see Table 3.29, p 342)

Emergency Contraception‡

Oral contraceptive pills containing 50 μg of ethinyl estradiol: 2 pills orally at once, then 2 pills orally 12 h later

OR

Oral contraceptive pills containing 30 μg of ethinyl estradiol: 4 pills orally at once, then 4 pills orally 12 h later

PLUS

An antiemetic

* Adapted from Hampton HL. Care of the woman who has been raped [published correction appears in *N Engl J Med.* 1997;337:56]. *N Engl J Med.* 1995;332:234–237 and Centers for Disease Control and Prevention. 1998 guidelines for treatment of sexually transmitted diseases. *MMWR Morb Mortal Wkly Rep.* 1998;47(RR-1):1–111

† See text for discussion of prophylaxis for human immunodeficiency virus (HIV) infection following sexual assault.

‡ The patient should have a negative pregnancy test before emergency contraception is given.

Medical Evaluation of Internationally Adopted Children for Infectious Diseases*

Approximately 15 000 children from abroad are adopted each year by families in the United States. Asian nations (eg, China, Korea, India, Cambodia, the Philippines, and Vietnam), Central and South American countries (eg, Guatemala and Colombia), and Eastern Europe (eg, Russia, Romania, and Ukraine) account for more than 90% of international adoptees. Africa and the Middle East remain uncommon sources for international adoption. The diverse origins of these children, their unknown backgrounds before adoption (including their parents' background and their living circumstances), and the inadequacy of health care in many developing countries make appropriate medical evaluation of internationally adopted children a difficult and important task.

Internationally adopted children differ from refugee children in terms of their medical evaluation before arrival in the United States and in the frequency of certain infectious diseases. While refugee children who resided in processing camps for some months may have received extensive medical care and treatment, the medical evaluation of international adoptees is extremely variable and often unreliable. All internationally adopted children are required to have a medical examination performed by a physician designated by the United States Department of State in the country of origin before an immigrant visa is issued. However, this examination is limited to screening for certain communicable diseases and for serious physical or mental defects that would prevent the issue of a permanent residency visa and is not a comprehensive assessment of the child's health. Accompanying health documents often are out-of-date, inaccurate, or unreliable. There is no simple method of determining which records may be useful. Reliance on these records may lead to inadequate screening for infectious diseases and delay in initiation or omission of preventive health care, such as immunizations.

In prospective studies of internationally adopted children, infectious diseases are among the most common medical diagnoses (see Table 2.16, p 149) and have been found in as many as 60% of children, depending on their country of origin. Because many of these infections are asymptomatic, the diagnosis must be made by screening tests in addition to history and physical examination. Use of screening tests for certain infections is cost-effective preventive health care for these children and their adoptive families. Other important medical diagnoses include hearing loss and visual abnormalities, growth and developmental retardation, nutritional deficiencies, and congenital anomalies. Suggested screening tests for infectious diseases are indicated in Table 2.17, p 150.

Usually a child should be examined within 2 weeks of arrival in the United States. If the child is suffering from an acute illness or has a chronic condition that needs immediate attention, the child should be examined as soon as possible. Some parents may desire to meet with a physician before adoption to review

* For additional information, see www.cdc.gov and www.who.int and Canadian Paediatric Society. *Children and Youth New to Canada: Health Care Guide.* Ottawa: Canadian Paediatric Society; 1998

Table 2.16. **Infectious Diseases of Importance in International Adoptees**

Bacteria or Disease	Viruses	Protozoa	Helminths	Arthropoda
Campylobacter organisms	Cytomegalovirus	Amebiasis	Ascariasis	Lice
Melioidosis	Hepatitis A	Giardiasis	Filariasis	Scabies
Salmonella organisms	Hepatitis B	Malaria	Hookworm	
Shigella organisms	Hepatitis C	Toxoplasmosis	Liver flukes	
Syphilis	Hepatitis D		Lung flukes	
Tuberculosis	HIV*		Schistosomiasis	
Typhoid fever			Strongyloidiasis	
Leprosy			Tapeworm, including cysticercosis	
			Trichuriasis	

* HIV indicates human immunodeficiency virus.

medical records, if available, or to discuss common medical issues in adoptive children. Parents who have not met with a physician before adoption should notify their physician when their child arrives so they can review basic medical issues.

Some infectious diseases occur with sufficient frequency to be reviewed for all international adoptees. Other less common infectious diseases may be encountered depending on the country of origin of the child. The epidemiology of infectious diseases found in different regions depends partly on the local climate and arthropod vectors.

Viral Hepatitis

The prevalence of markers of hepatitis B virus (HBV) infection ranges from 5% to 50% in internationally adopted children, and the prevalence of hepatitis B surface antigen (HBsAg) ranges from 1% to 15%. Adoptees from Asia, Africa, and certain countries in central and eastern Europe (eg, Romania) and the newly independent states of the former Soviet Union (Russia and Ukraine) have the highest rates of infection. However, rates are not negligible in children coming from institutional care in other countries. Therefore, all children should undergo serologic testing for HBsAg, hepatitis B surface antibody, and hepatitis B core antibody to identify current active infection, past resolved infection, or chronic carrier infection to facilitate appropriate medical care. The HBV test results from the country of origin should not be considered reliable. Because HBV may have a prolonged incubation period, consideration should be given to a repeated evaluation 6 months after adoption, based on the findings of the initial evaluation.

Chronic HBV infection is defined by the serologic persistence of HBsAg for more than 6 months. Children with HBsAg-positive test results should be evaluated to verify the presence of chronic HBV infection, assess for biochemical evidence of chronic liver disease, and assess for severity of disease and possible treatment according to current practice guidelines in consultation with, or by referral to, a specialist knowledgeable in this area.

Table 2.17. Screening Tests for Infectious Diseases in International Adoptees

Hepatitis B virus testing: hepatitis B surface antigen, hepatitis B surface antibody, and hepatitis B core antibody
Human immunodeficiency virus 1 serology
Mantoux intradermal skin test
Stool examination for ova and parasites
Syphilis serology
Complete blood cell count with red blood cell indices
Hepatitis C virus testing (see text)

Whenever possible, susceptible household contacts of children who test positive for HBsAg should be immunized before arrival of the child, but adoption need not be delayed until immunization is completed (see Hepatitis B, p 289). The institution of universal childhood HBV immunization in the United States should help to decrease the risk for school and household contacts of the adopted child.

Children who test negative for HBsAg should receive routine immunization for HBV as soon as possible. All household contacts of a child found to be HBsAg-positive should be immunized appropriately against HBV.

Hepatitis D, which occurs only in conjunction with active HBV replication, may be found in adoptees from Eastern Europe, Africa, South America, and the Middle East. Serologic tests for diagnosis of hepatitis D virus infection are available (see Hepatitis D, p 306), but routine testing is not recommended.

Routine serologic screening for hepatitis A virus (HAV) antibodies is not indicated. Many internationally adopted children acquire HAV infection early in life, and, therefore, acute infections after adoption are rare. Chronic HAV infection does not occur.

Serologic screening for hepatitis C virus infection is not indicated routinely because of the low prevalence of infection in most areas. However, children from China, Russia, Eastern Europe, and Southeast Asia should be screened. Screening of children from other areas should depend on history (eg, receipt of blood products, maternal drug use).

Cytomegalovirus

Cytomegalovirus (CMV) is excreted by approximately half of internationally adopted children, who typically acquired the virus perinatally and suffer no sequelae. Congenital CMV disease is unusual. Because CMV is transmitted readily to susceptible household members from infected children, instructions on the value of appropriate hand washing after contact with urine, diapers, and respiratory tract secretions should be given to adoptive parents. Routine screening for CMV is not recommended because of the high prevalence of CMV infection in children in the United States, particularly those attending child care centers. However, adoptive parents should be counseled about CMV, especially if an adoptive mother is not immune and is contemplating pregnancy.

Intestinal Pathogens

Fecal examinations for ova and parasites by an experienced laboratory identify a pathogen in 15% to 35% of internationally adopted children. Children adopted from Korean foster care, however, consistently have a low prevalence of intestinal parasites. The most common pathogens are *Giardia lamblia*, *Ascaris lumbricoides*, and *Trichuris trichiura*. *Strongyloides stercoralis*, *Entamoeba histolytica*, and hookworm are less frequent. One stool sample generally is sufficient for initial screening unless gastrointestinal tract symptoms are present. In addition, children with diarrhea should have stools cultured for *Salmonella*, *Shigella*, *Yersinia*, *Campylobacter*, and *Escherichia coli* O157:H7 organisms with treatment and follow-up cultures as indicated. Therapy decreases intestinal infection with parasites, but complete eradication may not always occur. Thus, children with enteric symptoms occurring months or even years after arrival in the United States should be evaluated for intestinal parasites.

Tuberculosis

Tuberculosis frequently is encountered in international adoptees with rates of disease 8 to 13 times those in American-born children. Because most tuberculosis occurs within the first several years of arrival, screening with the Mantoux test is particularly important (see Tuberculosis, p 593). Routine chest roentgenograms are not warranted in asymptomatic children in whom the Mantoux test is negative. However, a substantial number of international adoptees may be anergic, and, if this is suspected, the Mantoux test should be repeated. Receipt of bacille Calmette-Guérin (BCG) is not a contraindication for Mantoux testing, and a positive Mantoux test should not be attributed to BCG without further investigation (see Tuberculosis, p 593). When active tuberculosis is found in international adoptees, efforts to isolate and test the responsible organism for drug susceptibilities are imperative because of the high prevalence of drug resistance in many foreign countries.

Syphilis

Congenital syphilis, especially with involvement of the central nervous system, is sometimes undiagnosed and often inadequately treated in many developing nations. Each international adoptee should be screened for syphilis by a reliable serologic test regardless of history or report of treatment given abroad (see Syphilis, p 547). Those found to be reactive should have appropriate supplemental testing to document true positivity and the extent of infection. Those infected should be treated (see Syphilis, p 547).

Human Immunodeficiency Virus Infection

The risk of human immunodeficiency virus (HIV) infection in internationally adopted children depends on the country of origin and on individual risk factors. Because of the rapidly changing epidemiology of HIV infection and because adoptees may come from subgroups at high risk for infection, screening should be considered for all internationally adopted children. Test results for HIV from the adoptee's country of origin should not be considered reliable. Transplacentally acquired maternal antibody in the absence of infection can be present in a child younger than 18 months of age. Hence, positive HIV antibody test results in asymptomatic children of this age require follow-up testing (including HIV, DNA, and polymerase chain reaction) and clinical evaluation (see HIV Infection, p 325).

Other Infectious Diseases

Because scabies and pediculosis are common, families should be instructed to examine adoptees immediately after arrival so family members do not become infested. Diseases such as typhoid fever, malaria, leprosy, or melioidosis are encountered infrequently in internationally adopted children compared with refugee children. While routine screening for these diseases is not recommended, the findings of fever, splenomegaly, respiratory tract symptoms, anemia, or eosinophilia should prompt an appropriate evaluation. Malaria can be diagnosed by obtaining Giemsa-stained thick and thin smears of peripheral blood (see Malaria, p 381).

Clinicians should be aware of the potential diseases and their clinical manifestations in internationally adopted children (see Table 2.17, p 150). Some diseases, such as central nervous system cysticercosis, may have long incubation periods and, thus, may not be detected on initial screening. Therefore, based on the findings of the initial evaluation, consideration should be given to a repeated evaluation 6 months after adoption. The longer the interval from adoption to development of a clinical syndrome, the less likely it can be attributed to a pathogen acquired in the country of origin.

Immunizations

International adoptees frequently are not immunized or are underimmunized. The children should receive necessary immunizations according to recommended schedules in the United States for healthy infants and children (see Fig 1.1 and Table 1.5, p 22 and p 24). Only written documentation should be accepted as evidence of prior immunization. In general, written records may be considered valid if the vaccines, dates of administration, number of doses, intervals between doses, and age of the patient at the time of immunization are comparable to the current US schedule (see Immunizations Received Outside the United States, p 27). Although some vaccines with inadequate potency have been produced in other countries, most vaccines used worldwide are produced with adequate quality control standards and are reliable. However, immunization records for international adoptees from some areas (eg, Eastern Europe, Russia, and China), especially children from an orphanage, may not accurately reflect protection because of inaccurate or unreliable records, lack of vaccine potency, or other problems. Therefore, evaluation of antibody titers may be reasonable for these children. For any international adoptee, if there is any question as to whether the immunizations were administered or were immunogenic, the best course is to repeat them.

Injuries From Discarded Needles in the Community

Injuries from hypodermic needles and syringes discarded in public places by injection drug users are perceived by victims as posing a significant risk for transmission of bloodborne pathogens, especially human immunodeficiency virus (HIV). While these injuries may pose less of a risk than needle-stick injuries that occur in health care settings, the injured person often needs evaluation and counseling. While an estimate of the possibility that the discarded syringe might contain a bloodborne pathogen can be made from the prevalence rates of these infections in the local community, the need to test the injured person usually is not influenced significantly by this assessment.

Management of persons with needle-stick injuries includes acute wound care, consideration of the need for prophylactic management, and prevention. Standard wound cleansing and care is indicated; such wounds rarely require closure. Tetanus toxoid and Tetanus Immune Globulin should be administered according to the immunization status of the victim (see Tetanus, p 563).

Consideration of the need for prophylaxis of infection by bloodborne pathogens, which include hepatitis B virus (HBV), HIV, and hepatitis C virus (HCV), is the next step. Extrapolation from similar injuries in health care settings is inappropriate. Risk of acquisition of various pathogens depends on the ability of the pathogens to survive on fomites, their prevalence rates among local injection drug users, and the probability that the syringe and needle came from a local drug user.

Hepatitis B virus is the hardiest of the major bloodborne pathogens and can survive on fomites for at least several days. While immunity may be present even in the absence of serum antibody to hepatitis B surface antigen in a previously immunized person (see Hepatitis B, p 289), children who have not completed the HBV immunization series should receive an additional dose of vaccine and, if indicated, be scheduled to receive the remaining doses to complete the schedule. Administration of Hepatitis B Immune Globulin (HBIG) usually is not indicated if the child has received the 3-dose regimen of HBV vaccine (see Hepatitis B, p 289). However, experts differ about the need for HBIG at the time of an injury of an incompletely immunized child. If the child has received 2 doses of HBV vaccine 4 or more months previously, the immediate administration of the third dose of vaccine alone should be sufficient in most cases.

Infection with HIV usually is the greatest concern of the family and victim. The need for initial baseline serologic tests for preexisting HIV infection is controversial. Negative results from these initial tests support the conclusion that any subsequent positive test results reflect infection acquired from the needle stick. Since positive baseline tests are rare in this circumstance, a decision needs to be made about whether the expense and discomfort of initial testing is justified. Positive test results require further investigation of their causes, such as perinatal transmission, sexual abuse, or drug use. An alternative option is to obtain and save a baseline serum specimen for later testing for HIV antibody in the unlikely event that a subsequent test result is positive. Counseling is necessary before and after testing (see HIV Infection, p 325).

The risk of HIV transmission from a discarded needle in public places seems to be low, and data are not available on the efficacy of postexposure prophylaxis with antiretroviral drugs in these circumstances for either adults or children. Because of the lack of data, the US Public Health Service is unable to recommend for or against prophylaxis in this setting.* Furthermore, antiretroviral therapy is not without risk and often is associated with significant adverse effects (see HIV Infection, p 325). However, some experts recommend that antiretroviral chemoprophylaxis should be considered when the syringe is available and is believed to contain fresh blood from an HIV-infected person, others if visible blood was present on the syringe or needle, and others if a needle stick occurred. Testing the syringe for HIV is not practical or reliable and can pose a risk of injury. Consultation with a specialist in HIV infection should be obtained before the decision is made of whether to give postexposure chemoprophylaxis. If prophylaxis is to be undertaken, any delay before starting the medications should be minimized (see HIV Infection, p 325). The suggested medication options are similar to those for HIV occupational exposure (see HIV Infection, p 325).

While testing a child for serum HIV antibody immediately after exposure is controversial, follow-up should include testing at 6 months and, perhaps, also at 6 and 12 weeks after injury. Testing also is indicated in the event of an illness consistent with an acute HIV-related syndrome (see HIV Infection, p 325).

The third bloodborne pathogen of concern is HCV. Although transmission by sharing syringes among injection drug users is efficient, the risk of transmission from a discarded syringe is low. In addition, the viability of this virus on fomites is poor. Immune globulin preparations and antiviral drugs have not been demonstrated to protect against HCV infection. The need for testing for HCV is uncertain. If done, testing should be performed at the time of injury and 6 months later. Positive tests should be confirmed by supplemental confirmatory tests (see Hepatitis C, p 325).

Needle-stick injuries of children can be minimized by public health programs on safe needle disposal and by programs for exchange of injection drug users' used syringes and needles for sterile ones. Needle and syringe exchanges reduce improper disposal and the spread of bloodborne pathogens without increasing injection drug use. The American Academy of Pediatrics supports needle-exchange programs in conjunction with drug treatment and within the context of continuing research to document their effectiveness and clarify factors contributing to desired outcomes.

* Centers for Disease Control and Prevention. Management of possible sexual, injecting-drug-use, or other nonoccupational exposure to HIV, including considerations related to antiretroviral therapy: Public Health Service statement. *MMWR Morb Mortal Wkly Rep.* 1998;47(RR-17):1–14

Bite Wounds

As many as 1% of all visits to pediatric emergency centers during the summer months are for treatment of human or animal bite wounds. An estimated 4.7 million dog bites, 400 000 cat bites, and 250 000 human bites occur annually in the United States. The incidence of infection after cat bites can be more than 50%, and infection after dog or human bite wounds can be 15% to 20%. Wild animal bites also are a potential source of serious infection. Parents should be informed about the importance of children avoiding contact with wild animals and of securing garbage containers so that raccoons and other animals will not be attracted to the home and places where children may play. Concern for transmission of rabies should be heightened when a bite is not provoked. Dead animals should be avoided because they may harbor rabies virus in their nervous system tissues and saliva and may be infested with arthropods (fleas or ticks) infected with a variety of bacterial, rickettsial, protozoan, or viral agents.

Generic recommendations for bite wound management are given in Table 2.18 (p 156). Sufficient, prospective, controlled studies on which to base recommendations about the closure of bite wounds are lacking, and, thus, these recommendations should be considered guidelines. In general, recent, noninfected, low-risk lesions may be sutured after thorough wound cleansing, irrigation, and débridement. Use of local anesthesia can facilitate these procedures. Because suturing can enhance the risk of wound infection, some clinicians prefer that small wounds be managed by approximation of the wound edges with adhesive strips or tissue adhesive. Bite wounds on the face, which have important cosmetic considerations, seldom become infected and should be sutured whenever possible. Hand and foot wounds, however, have a high risk of infection and should be managed in consultation with an appropriate surgical specialist. Elevation of injured areas to minimize swelling is important.

Limited data exist about the initiation of antimicrobial therapy for patients with wounds that are not infected overtly. The use of an antimicrobial agent within 8 hours of injury, using a suggested guideline for a 2- to 3-day course of therapy, may decrease the rate of infection. Children at high risk for infection (eg, who are immunocompromised or when joint penetration occurs) should receive empiric therapy. Patients with mild injuries in which the skin only is abraded do not need to be treated with antimicrobial agents.

Guidelines for choice of antimicrobial therapy of human and animal bites are given in Table 2.18 (p 156) and reflect the organisms likely to cause infection for each biting species. Empiric therapy may be modified based upon culture results.

Prophylaxis or treatment for the penicillin-allergic child with a human or animal bite wound is problematic. Activity of erythromycin and tetracycline against *Staphylococcus aureus* and anaerobes is unpredictable, and the use of tetracycline, which has activity against *Pasteurella multocida,* in children younger than 8 years of age must be weighed against the risk of dental staining. Oral or parenteral treatment with trimethoprim-sulfamethoxazole, which is effective against *S aureus, P multocida,* and *Eikenella corrodens,* in conjunction with clindamycin, which is active in vitro against anaerobic bacteria, streptococci, and *S aureus,* may be effective for preventing bite wound infections. Cefotaxime or ceftriaxone can be used as alternative parenteral therapy for penicillin-allergic patients who can tolerate

Table 2.18. **Prophylactic Management of Human or Animal Bite Wounds to Prevent Infection**

Category of Management	Time From Injury: <8 h	Time From Injury: ≥8 h
Method of cleansing	Sponge away visible dirt. Irrigate with a copious volume of sterile saline by high-pressure syringe irrigation.* Do not irrigate puncture wounds.	Same as that for wounds of <8 h duration
Wound culture	No, unless signs of infection exist	Yes, except in wounds more than 24 h after injury and without signs of infection
Débridement	Remove devitalized tissue	Same as that for wounds of <8 h duration
Operative débridement and exploration	Yes, if one of the following: • Extensive wounds (devitalized tissue) • Involvement of the metacarpophalangeal joint (closed fist injury) • Cranial bites by large animal†	Same as that for wounds of <8 h duration
Wound closure	Yes, for nonpuncture bite wounds	No
Assess tetanus immunization status‡	Yes	Yes
Assess risk of rabies from animal bites§	Yes	Yes
Assess risk of hepatitis B from human bites‖	Yes	Yes
Assess risk of human immunodeficiency virus from human bites¶	Yes	Yes

Table 2.18. **Prophylactic Management of Human or Animal Bite Wounds to Prevent Infection, continued**

Category of Management	Time From Injury <8 h	Time From Injury ≥8 h
Initiate antimicrobial therapy#	Yes, for: • Moderate or severe bite wounds, especially if edema or crush injury is present • Puncture wounds, especially if bone, tendon sheath, or joint penetration may have occurred • Facial bites • Hand and foot bites • Genital area bites • Wounds in immunocompromised and in asplenic persons	Same as that for wounds of <8 h duration and for bite wounds with signs of infection
Follow-up	Inspect wound for signs of infection within 48 h	Same as that for wounds of <8 h duration

* Use of an 18-gauge needle with a large-volume syringe is effective. Antibiotic or anti-infective solutions offer no advantage and may increase tissue irritation.
† Radiographic studies in facial injuries are indicated if penetrating central nervous system injury is suspected.
‡ See Tetanus, p 563.
§ See Rabies, p 475.
|| See Hepatitis B, p 289.
¶ See HIV Infection, p 325.
# See Table 2.19 (p 158) for suggested drug choices.

Table 2.19. **Antimicrobial Agents for Human or Animal Bite Wounds**

Source of Bite	Organism(s) Likely to Cause Infection	Antimicrobial Agent			
		Oral Route	Oral Alternatives for Penicillin-Allergic Patients*	Intravenous Route	Intravenous Alternatives for Penicillin-Allergic Patients*
Dog/cat	*Pasteurella* species, *Staphylococcus aureus,* streptococci, anaerobes, *Capnocytophaga, Moraxella, Corynebacterium, Neisseria*	Amoxicillin-clavulanate	Extended-spectrum cephalosporin or trimethoprim-sulfamethoxazole PLUS clindamycin	Ampicillin-sulbactam†	Extended-spectrum cephalosporin or trimethoprim-sulfamethoxazole PLUS clindamycin
Reptile	Enteric gram-negative bacteria, anaerobes	Amoxicillin-clavulanate	Extended-spectrum cephalosporin or trimethoprim-sulfamethoxazole PLUS clindamycin	Ampicillin-sulbactam† PLUS gentamicin	Clindamycin PLUS gentamicin
Human	Streptococci, *S aureus, Eikenella corrodens,* anaerobes	Amoxicillin-clavulanate	Trimethoprim-sulfamethoxazole PLUS clindamycin	Ampicillin-sulbactam†	Extended-spectrum cephalosporin or trimethoprim-sulfamethoxazole PLUS clindamycin

* For patients with history of allergy to penicillin or one of its many congeners, alternative drugs are recommended. In some circumstances, a cephalosporin or other ß-lactam class drug may be acceptable. However, these drugs should not be used for patients with an immediate hypersensitivity (anaphylaxis) to penicillin because approximately 5% to 15% of penicillin-allergic patients also will be allergic to the cephalosporins.

† Ticarcillin-clavulanate may be used as an alternative.

cephalosporins; clindamycin is the alternative for patients who also are cephalosporin-allergic. Metronidazole has an excellent anaerobic spectrum of antibacterial activity and has been used instead of clindamycin for that purpose. Azithromycin displays good in vitro activity against the organisms commonly causing bite wound infections, except for some strains of *S aureus*. Azithromycin may prove to be a useful alternative therapy for children with allergy to ß-lactam antibiotics. To date, clinical trials documenting efficacy of azithromycin for bite wound infections are not available.

Prevention of Tick-borne Infections

Tick-borne infectious diseases in the United States include those caused by bacteria (eg, Lyme disease, tularemia, relapsing fever), rickettsia (eg, Rocky Mountain spotted fever, ehrlichiosis), viruses (eg, Colorado tick fever), and protozoa (eg, babesiosis). Physicians should be aware of the epidemiology of tick-borne infections in their local areas. Prevention of tick-borne diseases is based on avoidance of tick-infested habitats, personal protection against tick bites, reduction of tick populations in the environment, and limiting the length of time ticks remain attached to the human host. Control of tick populations in the field often is not practical. Specific measures for prevention are as follows:

- Physicians, parents, and children should be aware that ticks transmit diseases.
- Tick-infested areas should be avoided whenever possible.
- If a tick-infested area is entered, clothing that covers the arms, legs, and other exposed areas should be worn, pants tucked into boots or socks, and long-sleeved shirts buttoned at the cuff. In addition, permethrin (a synthetic pyrethroid) can be sprayed onto clothes to decrease tick attachment. Permethrin should not be sprayed onto skin.
- Tick and insect repellents that contain DEET* applied to the skin provide additional protection but require reapplication every 1 to 2 hours for maximum effectiveness. While there have been rare reports of serious neurologic complications in children resulting from the frequent and excessive application of DEET-containing insect repellents, the risk is low when they are used properly. DEET should be applied sparingly according to product label instructions and not applied to a child's face, hands, or skin that is irritated or abraded. After the child returns indoors, treated skin should be washed with soap and water.
- Persons should inspect themselves and their children's bodies and clothing daily after possible tick exposure. Special attention should be given to the exposed hairy regions of the body where ticks often attach, including the head and neck in children. Ticks should be removed promptly. For removal, a tick should be grasped with a fine tweezers close to the skin and gently pulled straight out without twisting motions. If fingers are used to remove ticks, they should be protected with tissue and washed after removal of the tick. Care should be taken to avoid squeezing the body of the tick.
- Maintaining tick-free pets also may reduce tick exposure. Daily inspection of pets and removal of ticks are indicated.

* N, N-diethyl-meta-toluamide.

Summaries of Infectious Diseases

Actinomycosis

CLINICAL MANIFESTATIONS: The 3 major types of disease are cervicofacial, thoracic, and abdominal. Cervicofacial lesions are the most common and frequently occur after tooth extraction, oral surgery, or facial trauma or are associated with carious teeth. Localized pain and induration progress to "woody hard" nodular lesions that can be complicated by draining sinus tracts. The infection usually spreads by direct invasion of adjacent tissues. Infection also may contribute to chronic obstructive tonsillitis. Thoracic disease most commonly is secondary to aspiration of oropharyngeal secretions and rarely occurs after esophageal disruption secondary to surgery or nonpenetrating trauma. Disease manifests as pneumonia, which can be complicated by development of abscesses, empyema, and, rarely, pleurodermal sinuses. In abdominal infection, the appendix and cecum are the most frequent sites, and symptoms are similar to those of appendicitis. Slowly developing masses may simulate abdominal or retroperitoneal neoplasms. Intra-abdominal abscesses and peritoneal-dermal draining sinuses eventually occur. Chronic localized disease often forms sinus tracts that drain a purulent discharge.

ETIOLOGY: *Actinomyces israelii* is the usual cause. *Actinomyces israelii*, other *Actinomyces* species, and *Propionibacterium* (a related genus) species are slow-growing gram-positive, anaerobic bacilli that can be part of the normal oral flora.

EPIDEMIOLOGY: *Actinomyces* species are worldwide in distribution. Infection is rare in infants and children. The organisms are components of the endogenous gastrointestinal tract flora. *Actinomyces* are opportunistic pathogens, and disease results from penetrating trauma (including human bite wounds) and from nonpenetrating trauma. Actinomycosis is not contagious.

The **incubation period** varies from several days to several years.

DIAGNOSTIC TESTS: A microscopic demonstration of beaded, branched, gram-positive bacilli in pus or tissue suggests the diagnosis. Acid-fast staining can be used to distinguish *Actinomyces* species, which are acid-fast negative, from *Nocardia* species, which are variably acid-fast. Sulfur granules in drainage or loculations of pus, which usually are yellow and may be visualized microscopically or macroscopically, indicate the diagnosis, when present. A Gram stain of sulfur granules discloses a dense reticulum of filaments; the ends of individual filaments may project around the periphery of the granule, with or without radially arranged hyaline clubs. Immunofluorescent stains for *Actinomyces* species are available. For recovery of the organism, specimens must be collected, transported, and cultured anaerobically on semiselective media.

TREATMENT: Initial therapy should include high-dose intravenous penicillin G or ampicillin for 4 to 6 weeks followed by high doses of oral penicillin, amoxicillin, erythromycin, clindamycin, minocycline, or tetracycline for a total of 6 to 12 months. Minocycline and tetracycline are not recommended for children younger than 8 years of age. Surgical drainage may be necessary.

ISOLATION OF THE HOSPITALIZED PATIENT: Standard precautions are recommended.

CONTROL MEASURES: Good oral hygiene, adequate regular dental care, and careful cleansing of wounds (including human bite wounds) can prevent infection.

Adenovirus Infections

CLINICAL MANIFESTATIONS: The most common site of adenovirus infection is the upper respiratory tract. Manifestations include symptoms of the common cold, pharyngitis, pharyngoconjunctival fever, tonsillitis, otitis media, and keratoconjunctivitis, often associated with fever. Life-threatening disseminated infection, severe pneumonia, meningitis, and encephalitis occasionally occur, especially among young infants and immunocompromised hosts. Adenoviruses are infrequent causes of acute hemorrhagic conjunctivitis, a pertussis-like syndrome, croup, bronchiolitis, hemorrhagic cystitis, and genitourinary tract disease. A few adenovirus serotypes can cause gastroenteritis.

ETIOLOGY: Adenoviruses are DNA viruses; at least 51 distinct serotypes divided into 6 subgenera (A to F) cause human infections. Types 40 and 41 and, to a lesser extent, type 31, have been associated with gastroenteritis.

EPIDEMIOLOGY: Infection in infants and children may occur at any age. Adenoviruses causing respiratory tract infection usually are transmitted by respiratory tract secretions through person-to-person contact, fomites, and aerosols. Because adenoviruses are stable in the environment, fomites may be important in their transmission. Other routes of transmission have not been defined clearly and may vary with age, type of infection, and environmental or other factors. The conjunctiva can provide a portal of entry. Community outbreaks of adenovirus-associated pharyngoconjunctival fever have been attributed to exposure to water from contaminated swimming pools and fomites, such as shared towels. Epidemic keratoconjunctivitis often has been associated with nosocomial transmission in ophthalmologists' offices. Enteric strains of adenoviruses are transmitted by the fecal-oral route. Nosocomial transmission of adenoviral respiratory and gastrointestinal tract infections also occurs. Nosocomial spread often has resulted from exposure to contaminated hands of health care workers and infected equipment, including pneumotonometers and ophthalmologic solutions. The incidence of adenovirus-induced respiratory tract disease is increased slightly in late winter, spring, and early summer. Enteric disease occurs during most of the year and primarily affects children younger than 4 years of age. Adenovirus infections are most communicable during the first few days of an acute illness, but persistent and intermittent shedding for longer periods, even months, is frequent. Asymptomatic infections are common. Reinfection can occur.

The **incubation period** for respiratory tract infection varies from 2 to 14 days; for gastroenteritis, it is 3 to 10 days.

DIAGNOSTIC TESTS: Detection of adenovirus infection by culture or antigen is the preferred diagnostic method. Adenoviruses associated with respiratory tract disease can be isolated from pharyngeal secretions, eye swabs, and feces by inoculation of specimens into a variety of cell cultures. A pharyngeal isolate is more suggestive of recent infection than is a fecal isolate, which may indicate either prolonged carriage or recent infection. Adenovirus antigens can be detected in body fluids of infected persons by immunoassay techniques, which are especially useful for diagnosis of diarrheal disease, because enteric adenovirus types 40 and 41 usually cannot be isolated in standard cell cultures. Enteric adenoviruses also can be identified by electron microscopy of stool specimens. Multiple methods to detect group-reactive hexon antigens in body secretions and tissue have been developed. Also, detection of viral DNA can be accomplished with genomic probes, synthetic oligonucleotide probes, or gene amplification by polymerase chain reaction. Serodiagnosis is based on detecting a 4-fold or greater rise in antibodies to a common adenovirus antigen (eg, hexon). Serodiagnosis is used primarily for epidemiologic studies.

TREATMENT: Supportive.

ISOLATION OF THE HOSPITALIZED PATIENT: In addition to standard precautions, for young children with respiratory tract infection, contact and droplet precautions are indicated for the duration of hospitalization. For patients with conjunctivitis, contact precautions in addition to standard precautions are recommended. For diapered and incontinent children with adenoviral gastroenteritis, contact precautions in addition to standard precautions are indicated for the duration of the illness.

CONTROL MEASURES: Children who participate in group child care, particularly children from 6 months through 2 years of age, are at increased risk of adenoviral respiratory tract infections and gastroenteritis. Measures for preventing spread of adenovirus infection in this setting have not been determined, but frequent hand washing is recommended.

Adequate chlorination of swimming pools is recommended to prevent pharyngoconjunctival fever. Epidemic keratoconjunctivitis associated with ophthalmologic practice can be difficult to control and requires use of single-dose medication dispensing and strict attention to hand washing and instrument sterilization procedures. Effective disinfection can be accomplished by immersion of contaminated equipment in a 1% solution of sodium hypochlorite for 10 minutes or by steam autoclaving.

Health care personnel with known or suspected adenoviral conjunctivitis should avoid direct patient contact for 14 days after the onset of disease in their second eye. Because adenoviruses are particularly difficult to eliminate from skin, fomites, and environmental surfaces, assiduous adherence to hand washing and use of disposable gloves when caring for infected patients are recommended. Production of adenovirus vaccines for use in military personnel has been discontinued.

Amebiasis

CLINICAL MANIFESTATIONS: Clinical syndromes associated with *Entamoeba histolytica* infection include noninvasive intestinal infection, which may be asymptomatic (and most likely due to *Entamoeba dispar*), intestinal amebiasis, acute fulminant or necrotizing colitis, ameboma, and liver abscess. Disease is more severe in the very young, the elderly, and pregnant women. Patients with noninvasive intestinal infection may have ill-defined intestinal tract complaints but generally tolerate the infection. Persons with intestinal amebiasis (amebic colitis) generally have 1 to 3 weeks of increasing diarrhea progressing to grossly bloody dysenteric stools with lower abdominal pain and tenesmus. Weight loss is common, and fever occurs in one third of patients. Symptoms may be chronic and may mimic symptoms of inflammatory bowel disease. Progressive involvement of the colon may produce toxic megacolon, fulminant colitis, ulceration of the colon and perianal area, and, rarely, perforation. Progression may occur in patients inappropriately treated with corticosteroids or antimotility drugs. An ameboma is an annular lesion of the cecum or ascending colon that may be mistaken for colonic carcinoma or as a tender extrahepatic mass mimicking a pyogenic abscess. Amebomas usually resolve with antiamebic therapy and do not require surgery.

In a small percentage of patients, extraintestinal disease may occur with involvement of the lungs, pericardium, brain, skin, and genitourinary tract, but the liver is the most common site. Presentation of liver abscess may be acute with fever and abdominal pain, tachypnea, and liver tenderness and hepatomegaly, or chronic with weight loss, vague abdominal symptoms, and irritability. Rupture of abscesses into the abdomen or chest may lead to death. Pericardial abscesses with tamponade may occur. Evidence of recent intestinal infection frequently is absent.

ETIOLOGY: *Entamoeba histolytica* is an enteric protozoan that has been reclassified into 2 species that morphologically are identical but genetically distinct. *Entamoeba histolytica* and *E dispar* organisms are excreted as cysts or trophozoites in stools of infected persons.

EPIDEMIOLOGY: *Entamoeba histolytica* causes invasive disease, while *E dispar* is a noninvasive parasite that does not cause disease. *Entamoeba histolytica* can be found worldwide but is more prevalent in persons of lower socioeconomic status who live in developing countries where the prevalence of amebic infection may be as high as 50%. Groups at increased risk of amebiasis in developed nations include immigrants from endemic areas, long-term visitors to endemic areas, institutionalized persons, and men who have sex with men. More severe disease is associated with immunosuppression, malnutrition, young age, and residence in tropical countries. Infection with *E histolytica* is transmitted via amebic cysts by the fecal-oral route. Ingested cysts, which are unaffected by gastric acid, undergo excystation in the alkaline small intestine and produce trophozoites that infect the colon. Cysts that subsequently develop are the source of transmission, especially from asymptomatic cyst excreters. Infected patients excrete cysts intermittently, sometimes for years if untreated. Transmission occasionally has been associated with contaminated food, water, and enema equipment.

The **incubation period** is variable, ranging from a few days to months or years, but commonly is 1 to 4 weeks.

DIAGNOSTIC TESTS: Intestinal infection depends on identifying trophozoites or cysts in stool specimens. Examination of serial samples may be necessary. Specimens of stool, endoscopy scrapings (not swabs), and biopsies, should be examined by wet mount within 30 minutes of collection and fixed in formalin and polyvinyl alcohol (available in kits) for concentration and permanent staining. *Entamoeba histolytica* is relatively indistinguishable from the noninvasive more prevalent *E dispar*; trophozoites containing ingested red blood cells are more likely to be *E histolytica*. Polymerase chain reaction, isoenzyme analysis, and antigen detection assays can differentiate *E histolytica* and *E dispar*.

Serum antibody tests may be helpful, primarily for the diagnosis of amebic dysentery (85% positive) and extraintestinal amebiasis with liver involvement (99% positive). Patients who are asymptomatic cyst excreters generally have negative serologic assays for *E histolytica*. In developed nations, 5% of the general population will be seropositive. Results of the standard serologic tests are negative in persons infected with *E dispar*.

Ultrasonography and computed tomography can effectively identify liver abscesses and other extraintestinal sites of infection. Aspirates from a liver abscess usually show neither trophozoites nor leukocytes.

TREATMENT*: Treatment involves elimination of the tissue-invading trophozoites as well as organisms in the intestinal lumen. *Entamoeba dispar* infection does not require treatment. Corticosteroids and antimotility drugs administered to persons with amebiasis can worsen symptoms and the disease process. The following regimens are recommended:

- **Asymptomatic cyst excreters (intraluminal infections):** iodoquinol; alternatively, paromomycin or diloxanide furoate, which are luminal amebicides
- **Patients with mild to moderate intestinal symptoms with no dysentery:** metronidazole (or tinidazole) followed by a therapeutic course of a luminal amebicide
- **Patients with dysentery or extraintestinal disease (including liver abscess):** metronidazole (or tinidazole) followed by a therapeutic course of a luminal amebicide

Dehydroemetine followed by a therapeutic course of a luminal amebicide should be considered for patients for whom treatment of invasive disease has failed. Liver abscess alternatively may be treated with chloroquine phosphate concomitantly with dehydroemetine, followed by metronidazole (or tinidazole).

To prevent spontaneous rupture of an abscess, patients with large liver abscesses may benefit from percutaneous or surgical aspiration.

ISOLATION OF THE HOSPITALIZED PATIENT: Standard precautions are recommended for symptomatic and asymptomatic patients.

* For further information, see also Drugs for Parasitic Infections, p 693.

CONTROL MEASURES: Careful hand washing after defecation, sanitary disposal of fecal material, and treatment of drinking water will control the spread of infection. Sexual transmission may be controlled by the use of condoms.

Amebic Meningoencephalitis and Keratitis
(*Naegleria fowleri, Acanthamoeba* and *Balamuthia* Species)

CLINICAL MANIFESTATIONS: *Naegleria fowleri* can cause a rapidly progressive, almost always fatal, primary amebic meningoencephalitis. Early symptoms include fever, headache, and, sometimes, disturbances of smell and taste. The illness rapidly progresses to signs of meningoencephalitis, including nuchal rigidity, lethargy, confusion, and altered level of consciousness. Seizures are common. Death may occur soon after the onset of symptoms. No distinct clinical features differentiate this disease from fulminant bacterial meningitis.

Granulomatous amebic encephalitis caused by *Acanthamoeba* species and *Balamuthia* (leptomyxid) species has a more insidious onset and progression of manifestations occurring weeks to months after exposure. Signs and symptoms may include personality changes, seizures, headaches, nuchal rigidity, ataxia, cranial nerve palsies, hemiparesis, and other focal deficits. Fever is often low-grade and intermittent. The course may resemble that of a bacterial brain abscess or a brain tumor. Skin lesions (pustules, nodules, ulcers) may be present without central nervous system involvement, particularly in patients with acquired immunodeficiency syndrome.

Amebic keratitis usually due to *Acanthamoeba* species and rarely to other species occurs primarily in persons who wear contact lenses and resembles keratitis caused by herpes simplex, bacteria, or fungi, except for a usually more indolent course. Corneal inflammation, photophobia, and secondary uveitis are the predominant features.

ETIOLOGY: *Naegleria fowleri, Acanthamoeba* species, and *Balamuthia mandrillaris* are small, free-living amoebae.

EPIDEMIOLOGY: *Naegleria fowleri* is found in warm fresh water and moist soil. Most infections with *N fowleri* have been associated with swimming in warm, natural bodies of water, but other sources have included tap water, contaminated and poorly chlorinated swimming pools, and baths. Small outbreaks associated with swimming in a warm lake or swimming pool have been reported. A few cases with no history of contact with water have occurred. Disease has been reported worldwide but is uncommon. In the United States, infection occurs primarily in the summer and usually affects children and young adults. The trophozoites of the parasite directly invade the brain from the nose along the olfactory nerves via the cribriform plate.

The **incubation period** for *N fowleri* infection is several days to 1 week.

The causative organisms, especially *Acanthamoeba* species, of granulomatous amebic encephalitis are distributed worldwide and are found in soil, fresh and brackish water, dust, hot tubs, and sewage. *Balamuthia* species, however, have not been isolated from the environment. Infection occurs primarily in debilitated and immunocompromised persons. However, some patients have had no demonstrable underlying disease or defect. Acquisition probably occurs by inhalation or direct contact with contaminated soil or water. The primary focus of infection is most likely the skin or respiratory tract, and spread to the brain is hematogenous.

Acanthamoeba organisms also cause dendritic keratitis, mimicking herpes keratitis in persons who wear contact lenses and use contaminated saline solutions or tap water rinses for lens care.

The **incubation period** for these infections is unknown.

DIAGNOSTIC TESTS: *Naegleria fowleri* infection can be documented by microscopic demonstration of the motile trophozoites on a wet mount of centrifuged cerebrospinal fluid (CSF). The organism also can be cultured on 1.5% nonnutrient agar layered with enteric bacteria held in Page saline. Immunofluorescent tests to determine the species of the organism are available through the Centers for Disease Control and Prevention. The CSF shows polymorphonuclear pleocytosis, an elevated protein level, a slightly reduced glucose level, and no bacteria.

In infection with *Acanthamoeba* species, cysts can be visualized in sections of brain or corneal tissue and may be present in brain biopsy specimens. The CSF typically shows a mononuclear pleocytosis and an elevated protein but no organisms. *Acanthamoeba* species, but not *Balamuthia* species, also can be cultured by the same method as used for *N fowleri.*

TREATMENT: If meningoencephalitis caused by *N fowleri* is suspected because of the presence of organisms in the CSF, therapy should not be withheld while waiting for the results of confirmatory diagnostic tests. Amphotericin B is the drug of choice, although treatment often is unsuccessful, with only a few cases of complete recovery being documented. Recovery has occurred with therapy with amphotericin B only or combined with other agents, such as miconazole and rifampin. Early diagnosis and institution of high-dose drug therapy is probably important for achieving a satisfactory outcome.

Effective treatment for central nervous system infections caused by *Acanthamoeba* and *Balamuthia* species has not been established. Experimental infections can be prevented or cured by sulfadiazine. While *Acanthamoeba* species usually are susceptible in vitro to a variety of antimicrobial agents (eg, pentamidine, flucytosine, ketoconazole, clotrimazole, and, to a lesser degree, amphotericin B), recovery is rare.

Some patients with keratitis due to *Acanthamoeba* organisms have been treated successfully with combinations of topical propamidine isethionate, neomycin, polyhexamethylene biguanide, and various azoles (eg, miconazole, clotrimazole, fluconazole, or itraconazole), as well as topical corticosteroids. Some patients with skin lesions due to *Acanthamoeba* species have been treated successfully by first washing lesions 3 to 4 times a day with chlorhexidine gluconate and then applying topical ketoconazole cream. Patients also were given intravenous pentamidine and oral itraconazole.

ISOLATION OF THE HOSPITALIZED PATIENT: Standard precautions are recommended.

CONTROL MEASURES: People should avoid swimming in warm, stagnant, polluted fresh water. *Acanthamoeba* organisms are resistant to freezing, drying, and the usual concentrations of chlorine found in drinking water and swimming pools.

Only sterile saline solutions should be used to clean contact lenses.

Anthrax

CLINICAL MANIFESTATIONS: The spectrum of illness in humans includes 3 types of infection: cutaneous (malignant pustule), inhalational (woolsorter's disease), and gastrointestinal anthrax. Cutaneous anthrax, which accounts for 95% of cases, is characterized by a painless lesion, often at the site of a cut or abrasion, that progresses from a papule to a vesicle to necrosis and, eventually, to eschar formation. Case fatality in untreated disease approaches 20%. In inhalational anthrax, 2 stages of disease occur. Mild upper respiratory tract symptoms occur initially; severe dyspnea, cyanosis, tachycardia, tachypnea, diaphoresis, fever, rales, and death may follow approximately 2 to 5 days later. Gastrointestinal tract disease is characterized by 2 distinct syndromes, abdominal and oral pharyngeal. The abdominal form includes abdominal pain and distention, vomiting, bloody diarrhea, and, frequently, toxemia and shock. This form of gastrointestinal tract disease has a case-fatality rate of approximately 50%. Oral-pharyngeal anthrax with profound submental swelling, cervical adenopathy, and fever also has been reported. Septicemia and hemorrhagic meningitis result from hematogenous spread of the organism from the primary site. Disease manifestations are similar in adults and children.

ETIOLOGY: *Bacillus anthracis* is an aerobic, gram-positive, encapsulated, spore-forming, nonmotile rod, which produces several toxins responsible for the clinical manifestations of hemorrhage, edema, and necrosis. Spore size is approximately 1 µm.

EPIDEMIOLOGY: Anthrax is a zoonotic disease endemic in many rural regions of the world. The disease is well controlled in the United States because of appropriate animal immunization programs. Human disease occurs after contact with infected animals or their contaminated products. Spores of *B anthracis* are found on hides, carcasses, hair, wool, bone meal, and other by-products of domesticated and wild animals, such as goats, sheep, cattle, swine, horses, buffalo, and deer. Imported dolls and toys decorated with infected hair or hides have been a source of infection. The spore form of the organism has been found in soil samples from throughout the world, including soil in rural farming regions in several areas of the United States. Spores can remain viable for 40 years or more. Although the last case of inhalational anthrax in a human in the United States was in 1978, the potential for use of *B anthracis* in biological warfare has received attention (see Chemical-Biological Terrorism, p 83).

Cutaneous anthrax, which occurs principally in agricultural and industrial workers, results from contact with infected animals or animal products. Inhalation anthrax is rare and has resulted from inhalation of spores aerosolized during industrial processing of animal by-products or aerosolization of *B anthracis* spores in the laboratory setting. In gastrointestinal tract anthrax, ingestion of contaminated undercooked meat is the mode of acquisition, with deposition of spores in the upper (oral pharyngeal) or lower (usually ileum or cecum) gastrointestinal tract. Discharges from cutaneous lesions are potentially infectious, but person-to-person transmission has not been documented. Accidental infections have occurred in laboratory workers.

The **incubation period** is 1 to 7 days; most cases occur within 2 to 5 days of exposure.

DIAGNOSTIC TESTS: Most diagnoses of cutaneous anthrax are made on clinical grounds. The following procedures can be used for diagnosis: (1) microscopic visualization of *B anthracis* on direct Gram-stained smears and cultures on blood agar of lesions or discharges; for inhalation and gastrointestinal tract anthrax, standard blood cultures should show growth in 6 to 24 hours; (2) fluorescent antibody identification of the organisms in vesicle fluid, cultures, or tissue sections; and (3) detection of antibody to *B anthracis* toxin by enzyme immunoassay or immunoblot. Rapid diagnostic tests for diagnosing anthrax, such as enzyme immunoassay and polymerase chain reaction, are available only at national reference laboratories.

TREATMENT: High-dose intravenous penicillin and doxycycline are the antimicrobial agents of choice and are given for 7 to 10 days. Ciprofloxacin also is recommended for therapy of adults with inhalation anthrax. There are isolated reports of *B anthracis* resistant to penicillin. High-dose penicillin combined with streptomycin, or possibly parenteral ciprofloxacin, should be used for treating patients with meningitis or inhalational anthrax. Ciprofloxacin should not be used for patients younger than 18 years of age unless the possible benefits are considered to be greater than the potential risks, and tetracyclines usually should not be given to children younger than 8 years of age (see Antimicrobial Agents and Related Therapy, p 646). Natural *B anthracis* strains are resistant to extended-spectrum cephalosporins. Erythromycin, chloramphenicol, clindamycin, first-generation cephalosporins, aminoglycosides, and vancomycin are effective in vitro. In the event of biological terrorism, recommendations for treatment and prophylaxis should be consulted (see Chemical-Biological Terrorism, p 83).

ISOLATION OF THE HOSPITALIZED PATIENT: Standard precautions are recommended. Contaminated dressings and bedclothes should be incinerated or steam sterilized to destroy spores.

CONTROL MEASURES: A cell-free inactivated vaccine given as 6 injections is available for persons at significant continuing risk of acquiring anthrax.* The vaccine is mandated for all US military active- and reserve-duty personnel. The vaccine is effective for preventing or significantly reducing the occurrence of cutaneous anthrax in adults, and it causes minimal adverse effects. While protection against aerosol challenge has not been evaluated in humans, multiple studies in animals have shown the vaccine to be effective. No data on vaccine effectiveness or safety in children are available, and the vaccine is not licensed for use in children or pregnant women.

* Available from Bio Port Corporation, Lansing, Mich.

For persons believed to be exposed to an aerosol of *B anthracis,* preventive measures should include chemoprophylaxis with ciprofloxacin for at least 4 weeks; tetracycline or penicillin should be used for those in whom fluoroquinolones are contraindicated, unless resistance is suspected.

Surveillance and control of industrial and agricultural sources of *B anthracis* by public health authorities are important. A suspected or documented case of an anthrax illness should be reported immediately to the local or state health department.

Arboviruses

(Including Western and Eastern Equine Encephalitis, St Louis Encephalitis, Powassan, California Encephalitis (primarily La Crosse virus), Colorado Tick Fever, Dengue, Japanese Encephalitis, Venezuelan Equine Encephalitis, Yellow Fever, and West Nile Encephalitis)

CLINICAL MANIFESTATIONS: Arboviruses (arthropod-borne viruses) are spread by mosquitoes, ticks, or sandflies and produce 4 principal clinical syndromes: (1) central nervous system (CNS) infection (including encephalitis, aseptic meningitis, or myelitis); (2) an undifferentiated febrile illness, often with rash; (3) acute polyarthropathy; and (4) acute hemorrhagic fever, usually accompanied by hepatitis. Infection with some arboviruses produces congenital malformations and spontaneous abortion or, in the prenatal period, congenital perinatal illness.

Selected arboviruses transmitted in the United States and of importance to travelers are shown in Tables 3.1 and 3.2 (p 171 and p 172). With the exception of eastern equine encephalitis (EEE) virus, the other principal arboviruses transmitted in North America, La Crosse (LAC), St Louis encephalitis (SLE), and western equine encephalitis (WEE) viruses, mainly produce asymptomatic infections; clinical illness ranges in severity from a self-limited febrile illness with headache and vomiting (especially in children) to a syndrome of aseptic meningitis or acute encephalitis. Characteristics of SLE include confusion, fever, headache, slow disease progression, lack of focal findings, and generalized weakness and tremor; 7% of cases are fatal. The LAC virus produces acute seizures and focal findings in more than 25% of cases, stupor or coma in 50%, but death in fewer than 1%. Eastern equine encephalitis typically is a fulminant illness leading to coma and death in one third of cases and serious neurologic sequelae in another one third. The clinical severity of WEE is intermediate, with a case-fatality ratio of 4%; neurologic impairment is common in infants. In 1999, West Nile virus was described for the first time in the United States in New York. This virus presents with a nondescript febrile illness associated with rash, arthritis, lymphadenopathy, and meningoencephalitis.

Colorado tick fever (CTF) is an acute, self-limited illness consisting of fever, chills, myalgia, arthralgia, severe headache, and ocular pain. Illness is biphasic in 50% of cases and may be complicated by encephalitis, myocarditis, and, rarely, fatal systemic illness with hemorrhage. Transient but significant leukopenia, thrombocytopenia, and anemia due to infection of bone marrow elements are hallmarks of disease. Infected red blood cells potentially circulate for up to 120 days.

Table 3.1. **Important Arboviral Infections of the Central Nervous System Occurring in the Western Hemisphere***

Disease (Causal Agent)†	Geographic Distribution of Virus	Incubation Period, d
California encephalitis (primarily La Crosse and several other California serogroup viruses)	Widespread in the US and Canada, including the Yukon and Northwest Territories; most prevalent in upper Midwest	5–15
Eastern equine encephalitis (EEE virus)	Eastern seaboard and Gulf states of the US (isolated inland foci); Canada; South and Central America	3–10
Powassan encephalitis (Powassan virus)	Canada; northeastern, north central, and western US	4–18
St Louis encephalitis (SLE virus)	Widespread: central, southern, northeastern, and western US; Manitoba and southern Ontario; Caribbean area; South America	4–14
Venezuelan equine encephalitis (VEE virus)	Florida; Mexico; Central and South America	1–4
Western equine encephalitis (WEE virus)	Central and western US; Canada; Argentina, Uruguay, Brazil	2–10
West Nile encephalitis (West Nile virus)	Asia; Africa; Europe; eastern US	5–15

* Although referred to as encephalitis agents, these arboviral infections may cause encephalitis, aseptic meningitis, paralysis, or other neurologic findings or systemic illness. US indicates United States.

† All are mosquito-borne except Powassan encephalitis virus, which is tick-borne.

Infection with any of the 4 serotypes of dengue virus produces dengue fever, an acute febrile illness with headache, retro-orbital pain, myalgia, arthralgia, rash, nausea, or vomiting. Criteria for dengue hemorrhagic fever (DHF) include fever, any hemorrhage including epistaxis and gum bleeding, thrombocytopenia ($\leq 100 \times 10^3/\mu L$ [$\leq 100 \times 10^9/L$]), and increased capillary fragility and permeability. Fluid leakage into the interstitial, pleural, and peritoneal spaces leads to hemoconcentration, with hematocrit increased by 20% (0.20) or more, pleural effusion, and acute shock. Dengue shock syndrome in addition to findings of DHF includes hypotension and narrow pulse pressure (<20 mm Hg). Untreated DHF is fatal in one third of cases but is fatal in fewer than 3% of cases with fluid resuscitation. Encephalopathy, hepatitis, and myocardiopathy are complications. Maternal infection in the third trimester can be followed by acute perinatal illness with hemorrhage.

Japanese encephalitis (JE) is a severe encephalitis characterized by coma, seizures, paralysis, abnormal movements, and death in one third of cases and serious sequelae in 40% of survivors.

Yellow fever (YF) evolves through 3 periods from a nonspecific febrile illness with headache, malaise, weakness, nausea, and vomiting through a brief period of remission to a hemorrhagic fever with gastrointestinal tract bleeding and hemate-

Table 3.2. **Acute, Febrile Diseases and Hemorrhagic Fevers Caused By Arboviruses in the Western Hemisphere That Are Not Characterized by Encephalitis**

Disease*	Geographic Distribution of Virus	Clinical Syndrome	Incubation Period, d
Yellow fever	Tropical areas of South America and Africa†	Febrile illness, hepatitis, hemorrhagic fever	3–6
Dengue fever and dengue hemorrhagic fever	Tropical areas worldwide: Caribbean, Central and South America, Asia, Australia, Oceania, Africa†	Febrile illness—may be biphasic with rash; hemorrhagic fever and shock	2–7
Mayaro fever	Central and South America	Febrile illness and polyarthritis	1–12
Colorado tick fever	South Dakota, Rocky Mountain and Pacific states; western Canada; Asia	Febrile illness—may be biphasic	1–14
Oropouche fever	Central and South America	Febrile illness	2–6

* All are mosquito-borne except Colorado tick fever, which is tick-borne, and Oropouche fever, which is midge-borne.

† Mosquito vectors *Aedes aegypti* (yellow fever, dengue) and *Aedes albopictus* (dengue) are now found in the United States and could transmit introduced virus.

mesis, jaundice, hemorrhage, cardiovascular instability, albuminuria, oliguria and myocarditis; 50% of cases are fatal.

ETIOLOGY: More than 550 arboviruses are classified in a variety of taxonomic groups, principally in the families Bunyaviridae, Togaviridae, and Flaviviridae (Table 3.3, p 173), with more than 150 associated with human disease.

EPIDEMIOLOGY: Most arboviruses are maintained in nature through cycles of transmission among birds or small mammals by arthropod vectors, such as mosquitoes, ticks, and phlebotomine flies. Humans and domestic animals are infected incidentally as "dead-end" hosts. Important exceptions include dengue, YF, Oropouche, and chikungunya viruses that infected vectors spread from person to person (anthroponotic transmission). Direct person-to-person spread does not occur. Colorado tick fever has been transmitted through transfusion (see Blood Safety, p 88).

In the United States, mosquito-borne arboviral infections usually occur during late summer and early autumn, but in the deep south, EEE cases occur throughout the year. A median of 3 to 5 WEE and EEE cases are reported nationally each year. During SLE and WEE epidemics, persons of all ages may be infected, but cases with clinical illness occur more often at the extremes of age, especially in elderly persons. Urban SLE outbreaks have led to hundreds of cases, occurring disproportionately in lower socioeconomic status neighborhoods and among the homeless. Encephalitis due to LAC virus is transmitted in an endemic pattern in relatively stable wooded foci in the eastern United States. Almost all of the approximately 100 cases that are

Table 3.3. **Taxonomy of Major Arboviruses**

Family	Genus	Representative Agents
Bunyaviridae	Bunyavirus	California serogroup viruses (North and South America, Europe, Asia)
		Oropouche virus (South America)
	Phlebovirus	Sandfly fever virus (Europe, Africa, Asia)
		Toscana virus (Europe)
	Nairovirus	Crimean-Congo hemorrhagic fever virus (Africa, Europe, Asia)
	Hantavirus	Hantaan virus of hemorrhagic fever
Togaviraidae	Alphavirus	Western equine encephalitis virus (North and South America)
		Eastern equine encephalitis virus (North and South America)
		Venezuelan equine encephalitis virus (North and South America)
		Mayaro virus (Central and South America)
		Chikungunya virus (Africa, Asia)
		Ross River virus (Australia, Oceania)
		O'nyong-nyong virus (Africa)
		Sindbis virus (Africa, Scandinavia, northern Europe, Asia, Australia)
Flaviviridae	Flavivirus	St Louis encephalitis virus (North and South America)
		Japanese encephalitis virus (Asia)
		Dengue viruses (types 1–4) (tropics, worldwide)
		Yellow fever virus (South America, Africa)
		Murray Valley encephalitis virus (Australia)
		West Nile virus (Europe, Africa, Asia, North America)
		Tick-borne encephalitis complex viruses (Europe and Asia)
		Powassan virus (North America, Asia)
Reoviridae	Coltivirus	Colorado tick fever virus (United States, Canada, Asia)
Rhabdoviridae	Vesiculovirus	Vesicular stomatitis virus (Western hemisphere)

reported each year are in children younger than 15 years of age. The LAC virus is the most common arboviral cause of encephalitis in children in the United States. Eastern equine encephalitis is the most severe arthropod-borne encephalitis in the United States. The **incubation periods** and geographic distributions of selected medically important arboviral infections are given in Tables 3.1 and 3.2 (p 171 and p 172).

DIAGNOSTIC TESTS: A definitive diagnosis is made by serologic testing of cerebrospinal fluid (CSF) or of adequately timed serum pairs, or by viral isolation. Detection of virus-specific immunoglobulin M antibody in CSF is confirmatory, and its presence in a serum sample is presumptive evidence of recent infection in a patient with acute CNS infection. A greater than 4-fold change in serum antibody titer confirms a case, and elevated antibody titer(s) defines a case as presumptive. Polymerase chain reaction assays to detect several arboviruses have been developed, but they have not been introduced into routine laboratory diagnosis. Serologic testing for dengue and arboviruses transmitted in the United States is available through several commercial, state, research, and reference laboratories. During the acute phase of dengue, YF, CTF, Venezuelan equine encephalitis (VEE), and certain other arboviral infections, virus can be isolated from blood and in VEE, from the throat. In patients with encephalitis, viral isolation should be attempted from CSF or from biopsied or postmortem brain tissue. Serologic results should be interpreted in the context of any previous immunizations with YF and JE vaccines and locations of previous residence and travel.

TREATMENT: Active clinical monitoring and supportive interventions may be lifesaving in DHF, YF, and acute encephalitis.

ISOLATION OF THE HOSPITALIZED PATIENT: In addition to standard precautions, respiratory precautions are recommended for patients with acute VEE and when vector mosquitoes are present (such as in most of the eastern United States during the summer); patients with acute dengue and YF should be sequestered from mosquitoes.

CONTROL MEASURES:

Protection Against Vectors. Public health department–administered mosquito control programs are important for controlling vectors. Personal precautions to avoid mosquito bites include repellents, protective clothing, aerosol insecticides, and staying in screened or air-conditioned locations. Although many vector species are most active during twilight hours, certain vectors of EEE and LAC encephalitis are daytime feeders. *Aedes aegypti,* the vector of dengue and urban YF, is found around houses and indoors, even in well-constructed hotels. Travelers to tropical countries should consider bringing mosquito bed nets and aerosol insecticide sprays.

Active Immunization.

Yellow Fever Vaccine. Live attenuated (17D strain) vaccine is available at state-approved immunization centers. A single dose is accepted by international authorities as providing protection for 10 years and may well confer lifelong immunity.

Immunization is recommended for all persons 9 months of age or older living in or traveling to endemic areas and is required by international regulations for travel to and from certain countries. Infants younger than 4 months of age should not be immunized, because they have increased susceptibility for vaccine-associated encephalitis. The decision to immunize infants between 4 and 9 months of age must balance the infant's risk of exposure (eg, infants older than 4 months who must travel to an area of ongoing endemic or epidemic activity may receive the vaccine if a high degree of protection against mosquito exposure is not feasible) with the theoretical risks of vaccine-associated encephalitis. The YF vaccine can be given concurrently with oral and parenteral typhoid, hepatitis A and B viruses, measles, polio, and meningococcal vaccines; chloroquine; and Immune Serum Globulin. If possible, cholera vaccine, when indicated, should not be given concurrently with YF vaccine; ideally, administration of these immunizations should be separated by at least 3 weeks.

Yellow fever vaccine is prepared in embryonated eggs and contains egg protein, which may cause allergic reactions. Persons who have experienced signs or symptoms of anaphylactic reaction after eating eggs should be excused from immunization and issued a medical waiver letter to fulfill health regulations, or they should undergo skin testing according to the package insert before immunization (also see Hypersensitivity Reactions to Vaccine Constituents, p 35). Pregnant women should not be immunized except in high-risk areas. The YF vaccine should not be given to immunocompromised persons. The decision to immunize patients who have immunocompromising conditions must balance the traveler's risk of exposure and clinical status.

Japanese Encephalitis Vaccine. *The inactivated JE vaccine, derived from infected mouse brain, is not recommended for persons who travel routinely to Asia. Because of a risk of vaccine-associated hypersensitivity reactions (angioedema, generalized urticaria) occurring in 0.3% of vaccine recipients, immunization is recommended only for expatriates living in Asia and for travelers who will be residing in areas where JE virus is endemic or epidemic or who are planning prolonged stays (>30 days) in endemic areas during the transmission season, especially if travel includes rural areas or their activities or itinerary place them at increased risk of exposure (eg, travel into an epidemic focus, bicycling, camping, or other unprotected outdoor activity in a rural area). Current information on locations of JE virus transmission and detailed information on vaccine recommendations can be obtained from the Centers for Disease Control and Prevention (see Appendix I, Directory of Resources, p 743) and from recommendations of the Advisory Committee on Immunization Practices.†

The recommended primary immunization series is 3 doses of 1.0 mL each, administered subcutaneously on days 0, 7, and 30. An abbreviated schedule of 0, 7, and 14 days can be used when the longer schedule is precluded by time constraints. The regimen for children 1 to 3 years of age is identical except that each dose is 0.5 mL. No data are available on vaccine safety and efficacy in infants (younger than 12 months of age).

Other Arboviral Vaccines. An inactivated vaccine for tick-borne encephalitis is licensed in some countries in Europe where the disease is endemic, but it is not available in the United States.

Arcanobacterium haemolyticum Infections

CLINICAL MANIFESTATIONS: Acute pharyngitis due to *Arcanobacterium haemolyticum* often is indistinguishable from that caused by group A streptococci. Fever, pharyngeal exudate, lymphadenopathy, rash, and pruritus are common, but palatal petechiae and strawberry tongue are absent. In almost half of all reported cases, a maculopapular or scarlatiniform exanthem is present, beginning on the

* Produced in Japan and distributed in the United States by Connaught Laboratories, Swiftwater, Pa.

† Centers for Disease Control and Prevention. Inactivated Japanese encephalitis virus vaccine: recommendations of the Advisory Committee on Immunization Practices (ACIP). *MMWR Morb Mortal Wkly Rep.* 1993;42(RR-1):1–15

extensor surfaces of the distal extremities, spreading centripetally to the chest and back and sparing the face, palms, and soles.

Skin and soft tissue infections, including chronic ulceration, cellulitis, paronychia, and wound infection, have been attributed to *A haemolyticum.* Invasive infections, including septicemia, peritonsillar abscess, brain abscess, meningitis, endocarditis, osteomyelitis, and pneumonia, also have been reported.

ETIOLOGY: *Arcanobacterium haemolyticum* is a gram-positive bacillus, formerly classified as *Corynebacterium haemolyticum.*

EPIDEMIOLOGY: Humans are the primary reservoir of *A haemolyticum,* and spread is person-to-person, presumably via droplet respiratory secretions. Pharyngitis occurs primarily in adolescents and young adults. Although long-term pharyngeal carriage with *A haemolyticum* has been described after an episode of acute pharyngitis, isolation of the bacterium from the nasopharynx of asymptomatic persons is rare.

The **incubation period** is unknown.

DIAGNOSTIC TESTS: *Arcanobacterium haemolyticum* can be recovered on blood-enriched agar cultures, but growth may be slow, and hemolytic colonies may not be visible for 48 to 72 hours after inoculation. Detection is enhanced by culture on human or rabbit blood agar because both demonstrate larger colony growth and wider zones of hemolysis than growth on sheep blood agar. Growth also is enhanced by the addition of 5% carbon dioxide. Serologic tests for antibodies to *A haemolyticum* have been used in epidemiologic investigations, but they have not been standardized and are not available commercially.

TREATMENT: Erythromycin is the drug of choice, but to date no prospective therapeutic trials have been performed. *Arcanobacterium haemolyticum* is susceptible in vitro to erythromycin, clindamycin, chloramphenicol, and tetracycline; susceptibility to penicillin is variable. Resistance to trimethoprim-sulfamethoxazole is common.

ISOLATION OF THE HOSPITALIZED PATIENT: Standard precautions are recommended.

CONTROL MEASURES: None.

Ascaris lumbricoides Infections

CLINICAL MANIFESTATIONS: Most infections are asymptomatic, although nonspecific gastrointestinal tract symptoms may occur in some patients. During the larval migratory phase, an acute transient pneumonitis (Löffler syndrome) associated with fever and marked eosinophilia may occur. Acute intestinal obstruction may develop in patients with heavy infections. Children are more prone to this complication because of the smaller diameters of the intestinal lumen and heavy worm burden. Worm migration can cause peritonitis, secondary to intestinal wall penetration, and common bile duct obstruction resulting in acute obstructive jaundice. The adult worms can be stimulated to migrate by stressful conditions (eg, fever, illness, or anesthesia) and by some antihelmintic drugs. *Ascaris lumbricoides* has been found in the appendiceal lumen in patients with acute appendicitis, but a causal relationship is uncertain.

ETIOLOGY: *Ascaris lumbricoides* is the largest and, globally, the most widespread of all human intestinal roundworms.

EPIDEMIOLOGY: The adult worms live in the small intestine. Females produce 200 000 eggs per day, which are excreted in the stool and must incubate in soil for 2 to 3 weeks for the embryo to form and to become infectious. Ingestion of infective eggs from contaminated soil results in infection. Larvae hatch in the small intestine, penetrate the mucosa, and are transported passively by portal blood to the liver and subsequently to the lungs. They then ascend through the tracheobronchial tree to the pharynx, are swallowed, and mature into adults in the small intestine. Infection with *A lumbricoides* is ubiquitous but is most common in the tropics, in areas of poor sanitation, and wherever human feces are used as fertilizer. If the infection is untreated, adult worms can live for 12 to 18 months, resulting in daily excretion of large numbers of ova.

The **incubation period** is prolonged. The interval between ingestion of the egg and the development of egg-laying adults is approximately 8 weeks.

DIAGNOSTIC TESTS: Ova can be detected by microscopic examination of stool. Occasionally, patients pass adult worms from the rectum, from the nose following migration through the nares in febrile patients, and from the mouth in vomitus.

TREATMENT: Pyrantel pamoate in a single dose, albendazole in a single dose, or mebendazole for 3 days is recommended for treatment of asymptomatic and symptomatic infections. In children younger than 2 years of age, in whom experience with these drugs is limited, the risks and benefits of therapy should be considered before drug administration. Reexamination of stool specimens 3 weeks after therapy to determine whether the worms have been eliminated is helpful for assessing therapy but is not essential.

In cases of partial or complete intestinal obstruction due to a heavy worm load, piperazine citrate solution (75 mg/kg per day, not to exceed 3.5 g) may be given through a gastrointestinal tube. Piperazine paralyzes the worms, allowing them to be excreted with intestinal peristalsis. Piperazine should not be used with pyrantel pamoate because the two drugs are antagonistic. Surgical intervention occasionally is necessary to relieve intestinal or biliary obstruction, or for volvulus or peritonitis secondary to perforation. If surgery is performed for intestinal obstruction, massaging the bowel to eliminate the obstruction is preferable to incision of the intestine.

ISOLATION OF THE HOSPITALIZED PATIENT: Standard precautions are recommended.

CONTROL MEASURES: Sanitary disposal of human feces stops transmission. Children's play areas should be given special attention. Vegetables cultivated in areas where human feces are used as fertilizer must be thoroughly cooked or soaked in a dilute iodine solution before eating. Household bleach is ineffective.

Aspergillosis

Clinical Manifestations: Aspergillosis is manifested by noninvasive and invasive disease of the following types:

- Allergic bronchopulmonary aspergillosis manifests as episodic wheezing, expectoration of brown mucus plugs, low-grade fever, eosinophilia, and transient pulmonary infiltrates. This form of aspergillosis occurs most frequently in immunocompetent children with chronic asthma or cystic fibrosis.
- Allergic sinusitis is a far less common allergic response to colonization by *Aspergillus* species than allergic bronchopulmonary syndrome. It occurs in children with nasal polyps or previous episodes of sinusitis or who have undergone sinus surgery and is characterized by symptoms of chronic sinusitis with dark plugs of nasal discharge.
- Aspergillomas and otomycosis are 2 syndromes of nonallergic colonization by *Aspergillus* species in immunocompetent children. Aspergillomas grow in preexisting cavities or bronchogenic cysts without invading pulmonary tissue; almost all patients have underlying lung disease, typically cystic fibrosis. Patients with otomycosis have underlying chronic otitis media with colonization of the external auditory canal by a fungal mat that produces a dark discharge.
- Invasive aspergillosis occurs almost exclusively in immunocompromised patients with neutropenia or an underlying disease (eg, chronic granulomatous disease) or medication use (eg, corticosteroids) that causes neutrophil dysfunction or after cytotoxic chemotherapy or immunosuppressive therapy (eg, organ transplantation). Invasive infection usually involves pulmonary, sinus, cerebral, or cutaneous sites, and the hallmark is angioinvasion with resulting thrombosis, dissemination to other organs, and, occasionally, erosion of the blood vessel wall and catastrophic hemorrhage. Rarely, endocarditis, osteomyelitis, meningitis, infection of the eye or orbit, and esophagitis occur.

Etiology: *Aspergillus* species are ubiquitous and grow on decaying vegetation and in soil. Most infected patients, other than those in whom aspergillomas or otomycosis and allergic bronchopulmonary or sinus disease develop, have impairment in phagocyte function. The risk of aspergillosis is related directly to the duration of neutropenia. The principal route of transmission is inhalation of conidiospores. Nosocomial outbreaks of invasive pulmonary aspergillosis have occurred in which the probable source of the fungus was a nearby construction site or faulty ventilation system. Transmission by direct inoculation of skin abrasions or wounds is less likely. Person-to-person spread does not occur.

The **incubation period** is unknown.

Diagnostic Tests: Dichotomously branched and septate hyphae, identified by microscopic examination of 10% potassium hydroxide wet preparations or of Gomori methenamine–silver nitrate stain of tissue specimens or bronchoalveolar lavage, are suggestive of the diagnosis. Isolation of an *Aspergillus* species in culture is required for definitive diagnosis. The organism usually is not recoverable from blood but is isolated readily from lung, sinus, and skin biopsy specimens cultured on Sabouraud dextrose or brain-heart infusion media (without cycloheximide). *Aspergillus* species may be a laboratory contaminant, but when evaluating results from immunocompromised patients, recovery of this organism suggests etiologic significance. Biopsy of a lesion usually is required to confirm the diagnosis. Serologic tests (antigen or antibody) have no established value in the diagnosis of invasive aspergillosis. In allergic aspergillosis, diagnosis is suggested by a typical clinical syndrome and elevated concentrations of total and *Aspergillus*-specific serum immunoglobulin E, eosinophilia, and a positive skin test to *Aspergillus* antigens. In persons with cystic fibrosis, the diagnosis is more difficult because wheezing, eosinophilia, and a positive skin test unassociated with allergic bronchopulmonary aspergillosis often are present.

TREATMENT: Amphotericin B in high doses (1.0 to 1.5 mg/kg per day) is the treatment of choice for invasive infection (see Drugs for Invasive and Other Serious Fungal Infections, p 672); therapy is continued for 4 to 12 weeks or longer. Some experts also recommend concomitant itraconazole or rifampin, but other experts do not believe the additional drugs offer any benefit. Lipid formulations of amphotericin B also should be considered for children who are intolerant of or in whom the infection is refractory to conventional amphotericin B therapy. Safety and efficacy for children younger than 1 month of age have not been established. Itraconazole alone is an alternative for nonmeningeal cases and for patients who are intolerant of or in whom the infection is refractory to amphotericin B therapy. Also, itraconazole can be substituted for amphotericin B when oral drug can be tolerated in a patient with an itraconazole-susceptible *Aspergillus* isolate causing mild to moderate disease. The safety and efficacy of itraconazole for use in children, however, has not been established. Surgical excision of a localized lesion (eg, sinus debris) often is warranted. Allergic bronchopulmonary or sinus aspergillosis usually is treated with corticosteroids. Systemic antifungal therapy is not indicated for patients with allergic aspergillosis or in nonallergic colonization.

ISOLATION OF THE HOSPITALIZED PATIENT: Standard precautions are recommended.

CONTROL MEASURES: Outbreaks of invasive aspergillosis have occurred among hospitalized immunosuppressed patients during construction in hospitals or at nearby sites. Environmental measures reported to be effective include erecting suitable barriers between patient care areas and construction sites, the cleaning of air handling systems, repair of faulty air flow, and replacement of contaminated air filters. High-efficiency particulate air filters and laminar flow rooms markedly reduce the risk of conidiospores in patient care areas. These latter measures, however, may be expensive and difficult for patients to tolerate. Prophylactic use of nasal instillation or inhalation of amphotericin B has been evaluated in immunocompromised patients with variable results. These trials assumed that colonization preceded invasive disease, an assumption proven incorrect for most patients. Low-dose amphotericin B or itraconazole prophylaxis has been reported in bone marrow transplantation, but controlled trials have not been performed.

Astrovirus Infections

CLINICAL MANIFESTATIONS: Illness is characterized by abdominal pain, diarrhea, vomiting, nausea, fever, and malaise. Illness in the immunocompetent host is self-limited, lasting a median of 5 to 6 days.

ETIOLOGY: Astroviruses are nonenveloped single-stranded RNA viruses with a characteristic starlike appearance when visualized by electron microscopy. Eight antigenic types are known.

EPIDEMIOLOGY: Human astroviruses have a worldwide distribution. Multiple antigenic types cocirculate in the same region. Astroviruses have been detected in as many as 10% of sporadic cases of nonbacterial gastroenteritis. Most astrovirus infections have been detected in children younger than 4 years of age, and these episodes seem to have a winter seasonal peak. Transmission is usually person to person via the fecal-oral route, although outbreaks associated with contaminated food have been documented. Outbreaks tend to occur in closed populations of the young and the elderly, and attack rates are high among hospitalized children and children in child care centers. Excretion lasts a median of 5 days after the onset of symptoms, but asymptomatic excretion after illness can last for several weeks in healthy children. Persistent excretion may occur in immunocompromised hosts. Asymptomatic infections are common.

The **incubation period** is 3 to 4 days.

DIAGNOSTIC TESTS: Commercial tests for diagnosis are not available. The following tests are available in some research and reference laboratories: electron microscopy for detection of viral particles in stool, enzyme immunoassay for detection of viral antigen in stool or antibody in serum, and reverse transcriptase–polymerase chain reaction (RT-PCR) for detection of viral RNA in stool. Of these tests, RT-PCR is the most sensitive.

TREATMENT: Rehydration with oral or intravenous fluid and electrolyte solutions.

ISOLATION OF THE HOSPITALIZED PATIENT: In addition to standard precautions, contact precautions are recommended for diapered or incontinent children with possible or proven astrovirus infection for the duration of the illness.

CONTROL MEASURES: No specific control measures are available. The spread of infection can be reduced by using general measures for control of diarrhea, such as training care providers about infection control procedures, maintaining cleanliness of surfaces and food preparation areas, exclusion of ill child care providers or food handlers, adequate hand washing, and exclusion of ill children or placing ill children in cohorts. A vaccine to prevent astrovirus infection is not available.

Babesiosis

CLINICAL MANIFESTATIONS: Gradual onset of malaise, anorexia, and fatigue typically occur, followed by intermittent fever with temperatures as high as 40°C (104°F) and one or more of the following symptoms: chills, sweats, myalgias, arthralgias, nausea, and vomiting. Less common findings are emotional lability and depression, hyperesthesia, headache, sore throat, abdominal pain, conjunctival injection, photophobia, weight loss, and nonproductive cough. Signs on physical examination generally are minimal, often consisting only of fever, although mild splenomegaly, hepatomegaly, or both are noted occasionally. Many clinical features are similar to those of malaria. The illness can last for a few weeks to several months with a prolonged recovery of as long as 18 months. Severe illness is most likely to occur in persons older than 40 years of age, persons who are asplenic, and persons who are immunocompromised (eg, persons with human immunodeficiency virus infection). Some persons, especially those who have had a splenectomy, can suffer fulminant illness resulting in death or prolonged convalescence.

ETIOLOGY: *Babesia* species that cause babesiosis are intraerythrocytic protozoa. *Babesia microti* and one or more related but genetically and antigenetically distinct organisms are responsible for disease in the United States.

EPIDEMIOLOGY: In the United States, the primary reservoir for *B microti* is the white-footed mouse (*Peromyscus leucopus*), and the primary vector is the tick, *Ixodes scapularis*. This tick also can transmit *Borrelia burgdorferi,* the causative agent of Lyme disease, as well as the causative agent of human granulocytic ehrlichiosis. Humans acquire the infection from bites of infected ticks. The white-tailed deer (*Odocoileus virginianus*) is an important host for the tick but is not a reservoir for *B microti*. An increase in the deer population during the past few decades is thought to be a major factor in the spread of *I scapularis* and in the consequent increase in human cases of babesiosis. Rarely, babesiosis is acquired through blood transfusions. Transplacental or perinatal transmission of babesiosis also has been described. Human cases of babesiosis have been reported in the northeast, midwest, and West Coast of the United States (California, Connecticut, Georgia, Massachusetts, Minnesota, Missouri, New Jersey, New York, Rhode Island, Washington, and Wisconsin). Most human cases of babesiosis occur in the summer or autumn. In endemic areas, asymptomatic infections are common.

The **incubation period** ranges from 1 to 9 weeks.

DIAGNOSTIC TESTS: Babesiosis is diagnosed by microscopic identification of the organism on Giemsa- or Wright-stained thick or thin blood smears. Multiple thick and thin blood smears should be examined in suspected cases or when the initial examination result is negative. Serologic tests for detection of *Babesia* antibodies are available at the Centers for Disease Control and Prevention and at several state reference and research laboratories.

TREATMENT: Since many patients have a mild clinical course and recover without specific antibabesial chemotherapy, therapy is reserved for patients who are moderately or seriously ill. The combination of clindamycin and oral quinine for 7 days or atovaquone and azithromycin for 7 to 10 days is the current therapy of choice. Exchange blood transfusions have been used successfully in asplenic patients with life-threatening babesiosis and should be considered for all severely ill persons with a high level of parasitemia.

ISOLATION OF THE HOSPITALIZED PATIENT: Standard precautions are recommended.

CONTROL MEASURES: Specific recommendations concern prevention of tick bites and are similar to those for Lyme disease and other tick-borne infections (see Prevention of Tick-borne Infections, p 159).

Bacillus cereus Infections

CLINICAL MANIFESTATIONS: Two clinical syndromes are associated with *Bacillus cereus* food poisoning. The first is the emetic syndrome, which is a disease with a short incubation period, similar to that of staphylococcal food poisoning, characterized by nausea, vomiting, and abdominal cramps, with diarrhea in approximately one third of patients. The second is the diarrhea syndrome, which has a longer incubation period similar to that of *Clostridium perfringens* food poisoning and is characterized predominantly by moderate to severe abdominal cramps and watery diarrhea, with vomiting in approximately one fourth of patients. In both syndromes, illness is mild, usually is not associated with fever, and abates within 24 hours.

Bacillus cereus also can cause local skin and wound infections, ocular infections, fulminant liver failure, and invasive disease, including bacteremia, endocarditis, osteomyelitis, pneumonia, brain abscess, and meningitis. Ocular involvement includes panophthalmitis, endophthalmitis, and keratitis.

ETIOLOGY: *Bacillus cereus* is an aerobic and facultatively anaerobic, spore-forming, gram-positive bacillus. The emetic syndrome is caused by a preformed heat-stable toxin. The diarrhea syndrome is caused by in vivo production of a heat-labile enterotoxin. This necrotizing enterotoxin also has tissue necrosis and cytotoxic properties.

EPIDEMIOLOGY: *Bacillus cereus* is ubiquitous in the environment. It frequently is present in small numbers in raw, dried, and processed foods, but it is an uncommon cause of food poisoning in the United States. Spores of *B cereus* are heat-resistant and can survive brief cooking or boiling. Vegetative forms can grow and produce enterotoxins over a wide range of temperatures from 25°C to 42°C (77°–108°F). The disease is acquired by eating food containing preformed toxin, most commonly fried rice, which causes the emetic, short incubation syndrome. Disease also can result from eating food contaminated with *B cereus* spores, which produce toxin in the gastrointestinal tract. Spore-associated disease most commonly is caused by contaminated meat or vegetables and results in the longer incubation period syndrome. Foodborne illness caused by *B cereus* is not transmissible from person to person.

Risk factors for invasive disease due to *B cereus* include history of injection drug use, presence of indwelling intravascular catheters or implanted devices, and immunosuppression. Fulminant *B cereus* endophthalmitis has occurred after penetrating ocular trauma and injection drug use.

The **incubation period** of the emetic syndrome is 1 to 6 hours; for the diarrhea syndrome it is 6 to 24 hours.

DIAGNOSTIC TESTS: For foodborne illness, isolation of *B cereus* in a concentration of 10^5 or more per gram of epidemiologically incriminated food establishes the diagnosis. Since the organism can be recovered from stool samples from some well persons, the presence of *B cereus* in feces or vomitus of ill persons is not definitive evidence for infection unless isolates from several ill patients are demonstrated to be the same serotype or stool cultures from a matched control group are negative. Phage typing, DNA hybridization, plasmid analysis, and enzyme electrophoresis have been used as epidemiologic tools in outbreaks of food poisoning.

In patients with risk factors for serious illness, isolation of *B cereus* from wounds, blood, or normally sterile body fluids can be significant and should not be dismissed as a contaminant. Repeated cultures may help to confirm the diagnosis.

TREATMENT: Persons with *B cereus* food poisoning require only supportive treatment. Oral rehydration or, occasionally, intravenous fluid and electrolyte replacement for patients with severe dehydration is indicated. Antibiotics are not indicated.

In contrast, patients with invasive disease require antibiotic therapy and prompt removal of any potentially infected foreign bodies, such as catheters or implants. *Bacillus cereus* usually is susceptible in vitro to vancomycin, clindamycin, ciprofloxacin, imipenem, and meropenem.

ISOLATION OF THE HOSPITALIZED PATIENT: Standard precautions are recommended.

CONTROL MEASURES: Proper cooking and storage of foods, particularly rice cooked for later use, will help to prevent foodborne outbreaks. Food should be kept at temperatures higher than 60°C (140°F) or rapidly cooled to less than 10°C (50°F) after cooking.

Hand washing and strict aseptic technique in caring for immunocompromised patients or patients with indwelling intravascular catheters are important to minimize invasive disease.

Bacterial Vaginosis

CLINICAL MANIFESTATIONS: Bacterial vaginosis (BV), a syndrome primarily occurring in sexually active adolescent and adult women, is characterized by a vaginal discharge that adheres to the vaginal wall and that usually is malodorous with a fishy odor, nonviscous, homogenous, and white. Bacterial vaginosis may be asymptomatic and is not associated with abdominal pain, significant pruritus, or dysuria.

Vaginitis and vulvitis in prepubertal girls usually have a nonspecific cause and are rarely manifestations of BV. In prepubertal girls, other predisposing causes for vaginal discharge include foreign bodies or other infections due to group A streptococci, *Trichomonas vaginalis,* herpes simplex virus, *Neisseria gonorrhoeae, Chlamydia trachomatis,* or *Shigella* species.

ETIOLOGY: The microbiologic cause of BV has not been delineated clearly. The microbial flora of the vagina are changed, with an overgrowth of *Gardnerella vaginalis, Mycoplasma hominis,* and anaerobic bacteria and a marked decrease in the concentration of hydrogen peroxide–producing lactobacilli. Despite these changes, little or no inflammation of the vaginal epithelium occurs.

EPIDEMIOLOGY: Bacterial vaginosis is the most prevalent vaginal infection in sexually active adolescents and adults. It may occur with other conditions associated with vaginal discharge, such as trichomoniasis or cervicitis. While the evidence for sexual transmissibility of BV is controversial, the condition is uncommon in sexually inexperienced females. Bacterial vaginosis may be a risk factor for pelvic inflammatory disease (PID). Pregnant women with BV are at increased risk for chorioamnionitis, premature rupture of the membranes, premature delivery, and postpartum endometritis. High-risk factors for adverse pregnancy outcomes include prior preterm birth or maternal weight less than 50 kg before pregnancy. Bacterial vaginosis also may be a risk factor for postabortion PID in women with symptomatic or asymptomatic BV before the operation. Bacterial vaginosis and chorioamnionitis may increase the risk of perinatal infection with the human immunodeficiency virus (HIV).

Sexually active women with BV should be evaluated for the presence of sexually transmitted diseases, including syphilis, gonorrhea, *Chlamydia trachomatis* infection, hepatitis B virus infection, and HIV infection, since coinfection may occur. Diagnosing BV in a prepubertal girl raises concern about, but does not prove, sexual abuse.

The **incubation period** for BV is unknown.

DIAGNOSTIC TESTS: The clinical diagnosis of bacterial vaginosis requires the presence of 3 of the following symptoms or signs:

- Homogenous, white, noninflammatory, adherent vaginal discharge that smoothly coats the vaginal walls
- Vaginal fluid pH more than 4.5
- A fishy amine-like odor from vaginal fluid before or after mixing with 10% potassium hydroxide
- Presence of "clue cells" (squamous vaginal epithelial cells covered with bacteria, which cause a stippled or granular appearance and ragged "moth-eaten" borders). In BV, clue cells usually constitute at least 20% of vaginal epithelial cells.

A Gram stain of vaginal secretions is an alternative means of establishing a diagnosis. Numerous mixed bacteria, including small curved rods and cocci, and few of the large gram-positive rods consistent with lactobacilli, are characteristic. Culture for *G vaginalis* is not recommended because the organism may be found in females without BV, including those who are not sexually active.

TREATMENT: The principal goal of treatment is to relieve symptoms and signs of infection. All patients who are symptomatic should be offered treatment regardless of pregnancy status. Nonpregnant patients with symptoms should be treated with metronidazole (1.0 g/d orally in 2 divided doses) for 7 days. Alternative regimens are metronidazole, 2 g orally in a single dose; metronidazole gel, 0.75%, 5 g (1 applicator) intravaginally twice a day for 5 days; clindamycin cream, 2%, 1 applicator (5 g) intravaginally at bedtime for 7 days; and clindamycin, 600 mg/d orally in 2 divided doses for 7 days. Clindamycin cream is oil-based, and for up to 72 hours after completing therapy, it may weaken latex condoms.

For high-risk pregnant women, eg, previous preterm birth or maternal weight less than 50 kg with or without symptoms, metronidazole, 750 mg divided in 3 doses daily for 7 days, is the preferred treatment. Alternative regimens include metronidazole 2 g in a single dose or clindamycin 600 mg/d orally divided in 2 doses for 7 days. Treatment should be provided at the earliest part of the second trimester of the pregnancy. Low-risk symptomatic pregnant women should receive treatment to relieve symptoms. Since treatment of BV in high-risk pregnant women who are asymptomatic might prevent adverse pregnancy outcomes, a follow-up evaluation at 1 month after completion of treatment should be considered to evaluate whether therapy was successful.

For nonpregnant and low-risk pregnant women, routine follow-up visits on completion of therapy for BV are unnecessary if symptoms resolve. Recurrences are common and can be treated with the same regimen given initially. The presence of a vaginal foreign body should be excluded. Routine treatment of male sexual partners is not recommended because it does not influence relapse or recurrence rates.

Treatment of BV in females infected with HIV is the same as for HIV-negative patients and is especially important in women who are pregnant, since BV and chorioamnionitis may increase the risk of perinatal transmission of HIV.

ISOLATION OF THE HOSPITALIZED PATIENT: Standard precautions are recommended.

CONTROL MEASURES: None.

Bacteroides and *Prevotella* Infections

CLINICAL MANIFESTATIONS: *Bacteroides* and *Prevotella* species from the oral cavity can cause chronic sinusitis, chronic otitis media, dental infection, peritonsillar abscess, cervical adenitis, retropharyngeal space infection, aspiration pneumonia, lung abscess, empyema, and necrotizing pneumonia. Species from the gastrointestinal tract flora are recovered in patients with peritonitis, intra-abdominal abscess, pelvic inflammatory disease, postoperative wound infection, and vulvovaginal and perianal infections. Soft tissue infections include synergistic bacterial gangrene and necrotizing fasciitis. Invasion of the bloodstream from the oral cavity or intestinal tract can lead to brain abscess, meningitis, endocarditis, arthritis, or osteomyelitis. Skin involvement includes omphalitis in newborn infants, cellulitis at the site of fetal monitors, human bite wounds, infection of burns adjacent to the mouth or rectum, and decubitus ulcers. Neonatal infections, such as conjunctivitis, pneumonia, bacteremia, or meningitis, occur rarely. Most *Bacteroides* infections are polymicrobial.

ETIOLOGY: Most *Bacteroides* and *Prevotella* organisms associated with human disease are pleomorphic, non–spore-forming, facultatively anaerobic, gram-negative bacilli.

EPIDEMIOLOGY: *Bacteroides* and *Prevotella* infections are caused by endogenous organisms that are part of normal flora of the mouth, gastrointestinal tract, or female genital tract. Members of the *Bacteroides fragilis* group predominate in the gastrointestinal tract flora; members of the *Prevotella melaninogenica* (formerly *Bacteroides melaninogenicus*) and *Prevotella oralis* (formerly *Bacteroides oralis*) groups are more common in the oral cavity. These species cause infection as opportunists, usually after an alteration of the body's physical barrier and in conjunction with other endogenous species. Encapsulation of organisms can enhance abscess formation. Endogenous transmission results from aspiration, spillage from the bowel, or damage to mucosal surfaces from trauma, surgery, or chemotherapy. Mucosal injury and granulocytopenia predispose to infection. Except in infections resulting from human bites, no evidence for person-to-person transmission exists.

The **incubation period** is variable and depends on the concentration of organisms and the site of involvement but generally is 1 to 5 days.

DIAGNOSTIC TESTS: Anaerobic cultures are necessary for recovery of *Bacteroides* and *Prevotella* species. Since infections usually are polymicrobial, aerobic cultures also should be obtained. A putrid odor of pus or other discharges is suggestive evidence of anaerobic infection. Use of anaerobic transport tubes or a sealed syringe is recommended for collection of clinical specimens. Collection of clinical material, especially from the respiratory tract, must avoid contamination of the specimen with anaerobes normally present on mucosal surfaces. Rapid identification techniques are not available.

TREATMENT: Abscesses should be drained when feasible; those involving brain or liver sometimes resolve without drainage if effective antimicrobial agents are administered. Necrotizing lesions should be surgically débrided; the value of hyperbaric oxygenation is controversial.

The choice of antimicrobial agent(s) is based on anticipated or known in vitro susceptibility. *Bacteroides* species infections of the mouth and respiratory tract generally are susceptible to penicillin G, ampicillin, and broad-spectrum penicillins, such as ticarcillin and piperacillin. Clindamycin is active against virtually all mouth and respiratory tract *Bacteroides* and *Prevotella* isolates and is recommended by some experts as the drug of choice for anaerobic infections of the oral cavity and lungs. Some species, including members of the *P melaninogenica* and *P oralis* groups, may produce ß-lactamase and are resistant to ß-lactam drugs. A ß-lactam penicillin active against *Bacteroides* combined with a ß-lactamase inhibitor can be useful to treat these infections (ampicillin-sulbactam, amoxicillin-clavulanate, ticarcillin-clavulanate, or piperacillin-tazobactam). *Bacteroides* species of the gastrointestinal tract usually are resistant to penicillin G but are predictably susceptible to metronidazole, chloramphenicol, and, usually, clindamycin. More than 80% of isolates are susceptible to cefoxitin, ceftizoxime, and imipenem. Cefuroxime, cefotaxime, and ceftriaxone are not reliably effective against *Bacteroides* species of the intestinal tract.

ISOLATION OF THE HOSPITALIZED PATIENT: Standard precautions are recommended.

CONTROL MEASURES: None.

Balantidium coli Infections (Balantidiasis)

CLINICAL MANIFESTATIONS: Most human infections are asymptomatic. Acute infection is characterized by the rapid onset of nausea, vomiting, abdominal discomfort or pain, and bloody or watery mucoid diarrhea. Infected patients can develop chronic intermittent episodes of diarrhea. Rarely, organisms spread to mesenteric nodes, pleura, or liver. Inflammation of the gastrointestinal tract and local lymphatics can result in bowel dilation, ulceration, and secondary bacterial invasion. Colitis produced by *Balantidium coli* often is indistinguishable from that produced by *Entamoeba histolytica.* Fulminant disease can occur in malnourished or otherwise debilitated patients.

ETIOLOGY: *Balantidium coli,* a ciliated protozoan, is the largest pathogenic protozoan known to infect humans.

EPIDEMIOLOGY: Pigs are believed to be the primary reservoir of *B coli.* Cysts excreted in feces can be transmitted directly from hand to mouth or indirectly through fecally contaminated water or food. The excysted trophozoites infect the colon. A person is infectious as long as cysts are excreted. The cysts may remain viable in the environment for months.

The **incubation period** is unknown but may be several days.

DIAGNOSTIC TESTS: Diagnosis of infection is established by scraping lesions during sigmoidoscopy, histologic examination of intestinal biopsy specimens, or by ova and parasite examination of stool. Stool examination is less sensitive, and repeated stool examination may be necessary to diagnose infection, because shedding of organisms can be intermittent. The diagnosis can be established only by demonstrating trophozoites in stool or tissue specimens. Microscopic examination of fresh diarrheal stools must be performed promptly because trophozoites quickly degenerate.

TREATMENT: The drug of choice is tetracycline, which is administered for 10 days in a dose of 40 mg/kg per day up to 2 g, divided into 4 doses. Tetracycline should not be given to children younger than 8 years of age unless the benefits of therapy are greater than the risks of dental staining (see Antimicrobial Agents and Related Therapy, p 646). Alternative drugs are iodoquinol and metronidazole.

ISOLATION OF THE HOSPITALIZED PATIENT: In addition to standard precautions, contact precautions are recommended.

CONTROL MEASURES: Control measures include sanitary disposal of human feces and avoidance of contamination of food and water with porcine feces. Despite chlorination of water, waterborne outbreaks of disease have occurred.

Blastocystis hominis Infections

CLINICAL MANIFESTATIONS: The importance of *Blastocystis hominis* as a cause of gastrointestinal tract disease is controversial. The asymptomatic carrier state is well documented. *Blastocystis hominis* has been associated with symptoms of bloating, flatulence, mild to moderate diarrhea without fecal leukocytes or blood, abdominal pain, and nausea. When *B hominis* is identified in stool from symptomatic patients, other causes of this symptom complex, particularly *Giardia lamblia* and *Cryptosporidium parvum,* should be investigated before assuming that *B hominis* is the cause of the signs and symptoms.

ETIOLOGY: *Blastocystis hominis* is a protozoan grouped with the amebae.

EPIDEMIOLOGY: *Blastocystis hominis* is recovered from 1% to 20% of stool samples examined for ova and parasites. Because transmission is believed to be via the fecal-oral route, the presence of the organism may be a marker for fecal contamination with other pathogens. Transmission from animals also may occur.

The **incubation period** is unknown.

DIAGNOSTIC TESTS: Stool specimens should be preserved in polyvinyl alcohol and stained with hematoxylin or trichrome before microscopic examination. The parasite occurs in varying numbers, and infections may be reported as light to heavy. The presence of 5 or more organisms per high-power (×400 magnification) field suggests heavy infection.

TREATMENT: Indications for treatment are not established. Some experts recommend that treatment should be reserved for patients who have persistent symptoms and in whom no other pathogen or process is found to explain the patient's gastrointestinal tract symptoms. Other experts believe that *B hominis* does not cause symptomatic disease and recommend only a careful search for other causes of the symptoms. In anecdotal reports, metronidazole (20 to 35 mg/kg per day divided into 3 doses for children and 2.25 g/d divided into 3 doses for adults) for 10 days also has been associated with improvement in symptoms. Iodoquinol (40 mg/kg per day divided into 3 doses, maximum 2 g/d) for 20 days has eliminated the organism and ameliorated symptoms in some patients. Controlled treatment trials are not available.

ISOLATION OF THE HOSPITALIZED PATIENT: Standard precautions are indicated.

CONTROL MEASURES: None.

Blastomycosis

CLINICAL MANIFESTATIONS: Infection may be asymptomatic or associated with acute, chronic, or fulminant disease. The major clinical manifestations of blastomycosis are pulmonary, cutaneous, and disseminated disease. Children commonly have pulmonary disease that can be associated with a variety of symptoms and radiographic appearances that may be misdiagnosed as bacterial pneumonia, tuberculosis, sarcoidosis, or malignant neoplasm. Skin lesions can be nodular, verrucous, or ulcerative, often with minimal inflammation. Abscesses generally are subcutaneous but may involve any organ. Disseminated blastomycosis usually begins with pulmonary infection and can involve the skin, bones, central nervous system, abdominal viscera, and kidneys. Intrauterine or congenital infections occur rarely.

ETIOLOGY: The disease is caused by *Blastomyces dermatitidis,* a dimorphic fungus existing in the yeast form at 37°C (98°F) and in infected tissues and in a mycelial form at room temperature and in the soil. Conidia, produced from hyphae of the mycelial form, are infectious for humans.

EPIDEMIOLOGY: Infection is acquired through inhalation of conidia from soil. Person-to-person transmission does not occur. Infection may be epidemic or sporadic and has been reported in the United States, Canada, Africa, and India. Endemic areas in the United States are the southeastern and central states and the midwestern states bordering the Great Lakes. The incidence of infection among persons residing in endemic regions is unknown. Although blastomycosis can occur in immunocompromised hosts, the disease has been reported infrequently in human immunodeficiency virus–infected persons.

The **incubation period** is approximately 30 to 45 days.

DIAGNOSTIC TESTS: Thick-walled, figure-of-eight, broad-based, single-budding yeast forms may be seen in sputum, tracheal aspirates, cerebrospinal fluid, urine, or material from lesions processed with 10% potassium hydroxide or a fungal stain. Children with pneumonia who are unable to produce sputum may require an invasive procedure (eg, open biopsy or bronchoalveolar lavage) to establish the diagnosis. Organisms can be cultured on brain-heart infusion and Sabouraud dextrose agar at room temperature. Chemiluminescent DNA probes are available for identification of *B dermatitidis.* Because there is no skin test available for blastomycosis and available serologic tests lack adequate sensitivity, every effort should be made to obtain appropriate specimens for culture.

TREATMENT: Amphotericin B is the treatment of choice for severe or life-threatening infection (see Drugs for Invasive and Other Serious Fungal Infections, p 672). Oral itraconazole, fluconazole, and ketoconazole have been used for mild or moderately severe infections, either alone or sequentially after a short course of amphotericin B. Safety and efficacy data for these drugs in children are limited. Itraconazole is highly effective for the treatment of nonmeningeal, non–life-threatening infections in adults, but it does not achieve effective concentration in the cerebrospinal fluid. In a multicenter trial in adults, itraconazole was more effective and associated with fewer toxic effects than was ketoconazole. Similarly, compared with itraconazole, ketoconazole has been associated with a higher rate of relapse and disease progression in children.

Oral therapy usually is continued for at least 6 months for pulmonary and extrapulmonary disease. Some experts suggest a longer duration of therapy for patients with osteomyelitis.

Isolation of the Hospitalized Patient: Standard precautions are recommended.

Control Measures: None.

Borrelia
(Relapsing Fever)

Clinical Manifestations: Relapsing fever is characterized by the sudden onset of high fever, shaking chills, sweats, headache, muscle and joint pains, and progressive weakness. A fleeting macular rash of the trunk and petechiae of the skin and mucous membranes sometimes occur. Complications include hepatosplenomegaly, jaundice, epistaxis, cough with pleuritic pain, pneumonitis, meningitis, and myocarditis. Untreated, an initial febrile period of 3 to 7 days terminates spontaneously by crisis. The initial febrile episode is followed by an afebrile period of several days to weeks, then by one or more relapses. Relapses typically become progressively shorter and milder as the afebrile periods lengthen. Infection during pregnancy often is severe and can result in abortion, stillbirth, or neonatal infection.

Etiology: Relapsing fever is caused by certain spirochetes of the genus *Borrelia. Borrelia recurrentis* is the only species that causes louse-borne (epidemic) relapsing fever. Worldwide, at least 15 *Borrelia* species cause tick-borne (endemic) relapsing fever, including *Borrelia hermsii* and *Borrelia turicatae* in North America.

Epidemiology: Transmission is vector-borne, either by body lice *(Pediculus humanus)* or by soft-bodied ticks *(Ornithodoros)*. Louse-borne relapsing fever has been reported recently only in Ethiopia, Eritrea, Somalia, and the Sudan where it sometimes occurs in epidemics, especially among the homeless and in refugee populations. Tick-borne relapsing fever is distributed widely throughout the world and usually occurs sporadically and in small clusters, often within families. Most tick-borne relapsing fever in the United States is caused by *B hermsii*. Infection typically results from tick exposures in rodent-infested cabins in western mountainous areas, including state and national parks. *Borrelia turicatae* infections occur less frequently; most cases have been reported from Texas and often are associated with tick exposures in rodent-infested caves. Soft-bodied ticks have painless bites, feed briefly (10 to 30 minutes), usually at night, so that patients often are unaware of bites. Ticks become infected by feeding on rodents and transmit infection via saliva and other tick fluid when they take subsequent blood meals. Ticks may serve as reservoirs of infection as a result of transovarial and transstadial transmission. In contrast, body lice become infected only by feeding on spirochetemic humans; the infection is transmitted when infected lice are crushed and their body fluids contaminate a bite wound or skin abraded by scratching. Infected body lice and ticks remain contagious throughout their lives. Direct human-to-human transmission does not occur.

The **incubation period** is 4 to 18 days with a mean of 7 days.

DIAGNOSTIC TESTS: Spirochetes can be observed by darkfield microscopy, and in Wright-, Giemsa-, or acridine orange–stained preparations of thin or dehemoglobinized thick smears of peripheral blood or in stained buffy-coat preparations. Organisms are found in blood most frequently during the febrile stage of the illness. Spirochetes are cultured from blood by inoculating Barbour-Stoenner-Kelly medium or by intraperitoneal inoculation of immature laboratory mice. Serum antibodies to *Borrelia* species can be detected by enzyme immunoassay and Western immunoblotting, but the tests are not standardized and are affected by antigenic variations between and within *Borrelia* species and strains. Serologic cross-reactions occur with other spirochetes, including *Borrelia burgdorferi*, the agent causing Lyme disease. Biologic specimens for laboratory testing can be sent to the Division of Vector-borne Infectious Diseases, Centers for Disease Control and Prevention, Fort Collins, CO 80522.

TREATMENT: Treatment with penicillin, tetracyclines, erythromycin, or chloramphenicol effectively produces prompt clearance of spirochetes and remission of symptoms. For children younger than 8 years of age and for pregnant women, penicillin and erythromycin are the preferred drugs. A Jarisch-Herxheimer reaction is seen commonly during the first few hours after initiating antimicrobial therapy. Because this reaction sometimes is associated with transient hypotension due to decreased effective circulating blood volume (especially in louse-borne relapsing fever), patients should be monitored closely during the first 12 hours of treatment. However, the Jarisch-Herxheimer reaction in children typically is mild and usually can be managed with antipyretics alone.

Procaine penicillin or intravenous penicillin G is recommended as initial therapy for persons unable to take oral therapy. For oral therapy, patients can be given standard doses of penicillin V, erythromycin, or tetracycline (if 8 years of age or older). Although single-dose treatment is highly effective for curing louse-borne relapsing fever, less is known about single-dose treatment of tick-borne relapsing fever. Continuing treatment for 5 days will ensure prevention of relapses.

ISOLATION OF THE HOSPITALIZED PATIENT: Standard precautions are recommended. If louse infestation is present, contact precautions also are indicated (see Pediculosis, p 427).

CONTROL MEASURES: Contact with ticks can be limited through use of protective clothing, acaricides, and tick repellents (see Prevention of Tick-borne Infections, p 159). Prevention of rodent access to foundations and attics of homes or cabins also reduces the potential for tick exposure. Dwellings infested with soft ticks should be treated professionally with chemical agents and rodent-proofed. When in a louse-infested environment, body lice can be controlled by bathing and by washing clothing at frequent intervals and by use of pediculicides (see Pediculosis, p 427). Reporting of suspected cases of relapsing fever to health authorities is important for initiating prompt investigation and institution of control measures.

Brucellosis

CLINICAL MANIFESTATIONS: Brucellosis in children frequently is a mild self-limited disease compared with the more chronic disease observed among adults. However, in areas where *Brucella melitensis* is the endemic species, disease can be severe. Onset of illness can be acute or insidious. Manifestations are nonspecific and include fever, night sweats, weakness, malaise, anorexia, weight loss, arthralgia, myalgia, abdominal pain, and headache. Physical findings include lymphadenopathy, hepatosplenomegaly, and, occasionally, arthritis. Serious complications include meningitis, endocarditis, and osteomyelitis.

ETIOLOGY: *Brucella* species are small, nonmotile, gram-negative coccobacilli. The species that infect humans are *Brucella abortus, B melitensis, Brucella suis,* and, rarely, *Brucella canis.*

EPIDEMIOLOGY: Brucellosis is a zoonotic disease of wild and domestic animals. Humans are accidental hosts, contracting the disease by direct contact with infected animals and their carcasses or secretions or by ingesting unpasteurized milk or milk products. Persons in occupations such as farming, ranching, and veterinary medicine, as well as abattoir workers, meat inspectors, and laboratory personnel, are at increased risk. Infection is transmitted by inoculation through cuts and abrasions in the skin, by inhalation of contaminated aerosols, by contact with the conjunctival mucosa, or by oral ingestion. Approximately 100 cases of brucellosis occur annually in the United States, with fewer than 10% of reported cases occurring in persons younger than 19 years of age. Most cases result from travel outside the United States or from ingestion of unpasteurized milk products. Human-to-human transmission rarely has been documented.

The **incubation period** varies from less than 1 week to several months, but most patients become ill within 3 to 4 weeks of exposure.

DIAGNOSTIC TESTS: A definitive diagnosis is established by recovery of *Brucella* organisms from blood, bone marrow, or other tissues. A variety of media will support the growth of *Brucella* species. Laboratory personnel should be alerted to incubate cultures for a minimum of 4 weeks and to use proper precautions for protection against laboratory-acquired infection. Lysis-centrifugation techniques may shorten the time necessary to isolate *Brucella* organisms. A presumptive diagnosis can be made by serologic testing. The serum agglutination test (SAT), which is the most commonly used test, will detect antibodies against *B abortus, B suis,* and *B melitensis,* but not *B canis.* Detection of antibodies against *B canis* requires use of *B canis*–specific antigen. Although a single titer is not diagnostic, most patients with active infection have titers of 1:160 or greater. Lower titers may be found early in the course of infection. Elevated concentrations of immunoglobulin (Ig) G agglutinins are found in acute infection, chronic infection, and relapse. When interpreting

SAT titers, the possibility of cross-reactions of *Brucella* antibodies with those against other gram-negative bacteria, such as *Yersinia enterocolitica* serotype 09, *Francisella tularensis,* and *Vibrio cholerae,* should be considered. To avoid the prozone phenomenon, serum should be diluted to 1:320 or higher before testing. Enzyme immunoassay (EIA) is a sensitive method for determining IgG, IgA, and IgM anti-*Brucella* antibodies, but until better standardization is established, EIA should be used for suspected cases with negative SAT titers or for evaluation of patients with suspected relapse or reinfection. The polymerase chain reaction test has been developed but is not available in most clinical laboratories.

TREATMENT: Prolonged therapy is imperative for achieving a cure. Relapses generally are not caused by development of resistance but rather by premature discontinuation of antimicrobial therapy.

Oral doxycycline (2 to 4 mg/kg per day; maximum, 200 mg/d in 2 divided doses) or, alternatively, tetracycline (30 to 40 mg/kg per day; maximum, 2 g/d in 4 divided doses) given orally should be administered for 4 to 6 weeks. However, tetracyclines should be avoided, if possible, for children younger than 8 years of age. Oral trimethoprim-sulfamethoxazole (trimethoprim, 10 mg/kg per day; maximum, 480 mg/d; and sulfamethoxazole, 50 mg/kg per day; maximum, 2.4 g/d) for 4 to 6 weeks is appropriate therapy for younger patients.

To decrease the incidence of relapse, many experts recommend combination therapy with a tetracycline (or trimethoprim-sulfamethoxazole if tetracyclines are contraindicated) and rifampin (15 to 20 mg/kg per day in 1 or 2 divided doses; maximum, 600 to 900 mg/d). Because of the potential emergence of rifampin resistance, rifampin monotherapy is not recommended.

For treatment of serious infection or of complications, including endocarditis, meningitis, and osteomyelitis, streptomycin (20 mg/kg per day in 2 divided doses; maximum, 1 g/d intramuscularly) or gentamicin (5 mg/kg per day in 3 divided doses) for the first 7 to 14 days of therapy in addition to a tetracycline (or trimethoprim-sulfamethoxazole if tetracyclines are contraindicated) is recommended. In addition, rifampin (20 mg/kg per day) can be used with this regimen to reduce the rate of relapse. For life-threatening complications of brucellosis, such as meningitis or endocarditis, the duration of therapy often is extended for several months.

The benefit of corticosteroids for persons with neurobrucellosis is unproven. Occasionally, a Jarisch-Herxheimer–like reaction occurs shortly after initiation of antimicrobial therapy, but this reaction is rarely severe enough to require corticosteroids.

ISOLATION OF THE HOSPITALIZED PATIENT: In addition to standard precautions, contact precautions are indicated for patients with draining wounds.

CONTROL MEASURES: The control of human brucellosis depends on eradication of *Brucella* species from cattle, goats, swine, and other animals. Pasteurization of milk and milk products for human consumption is especially important to prevent disease in children. The certification of raw milk does not eliminate the risk of transmission of *Brucella* organisms. In endemic areas, enforcement of and education about control measures are crucial.

Burkholderia Infections

CLINICAL MANIFESTATIONS: *Burkholderia cepacia* complex has been associated with severe pulmonary infections in patients with cystic fibrosis and with fatal bacteremia in patients with chronic granulomatous disease, newborn infants, and persons with cancer. *Burkholderia cepacia* also is a nosocomial pathogen that may cause significant bacteremia in children with hemoglobinopathies or malignant neoplasms. Nosocomial infections include wound infections, urinary tract infections, and pneumonia. Pulmonary infections in persons with cystic fibrosis occur late in the course of disease, usually after colonization with *Pseudomonas aeruginosa* has been established. Colonized patients may experience no change in the rate of pulmonary decompensation, become chronically colonized and experience a more rapid decline in pulmonary function, or experience an unexpectedly rapid deterioration in clinical status that results in death. The clinical significance of *Burkholderia gladioli* in persons with cystic fibrosis is unknown. In chronic granulomatous disease, pneumonia is the most common infection caused by *B cepacia* complex; lymphadenitis also has been reported. Disease onset is insidious, with low-grade fever early in the course of disease and signs of systemic toxic effects occurring 3 to 4 weeks later. Pleural effusion is common, and lung abscess has been described.

Burkholderia pseudomallei is the cause of melioidosis in the rural population of Southeast Asia. Melioidosis can manifest as a localized infection or as fulminant septicemia. Localized infection most commonly manifests as pneumonia, but skin, soft tissue, and skeletal infections also occur. In disseminated infection, hepatic and splenic abscesses may occur, and relapses are frequent in severe disease.

ETIOLOGY: The genus *Burkholderia* was proposed in 1992 for 7 species that were previously in *Pseudomonas* homology group II. *Burkholderia* are nutritionally diverse, catalase-producing, non–lactose fermenting, gram-negative bacilli. Species are distinguished primarily on the basis of phenotype and biochemical characteristics. All *Burkholderia* species are animal or plant pathogens but are not significant pathogens in healthy human hosts.

EPIDEMIOLOGY: *Burkholderia* species are water- and soil-borne organisms that can survive for prolonged periods when kept moist. In patients with and without cystic fibrosis, person-to-person spread of *B cepacia* has been documented. Epidemiologic studies of camps and other social events attended by patients from different geographic areas have demonstrated person-to-person transmission. The source for acquisition of *B cepacia* by patients with chronic granulomatous disease has not been identified. Nosocomial spread of *B cepacia* most frequently occurs because of the contamination of disinfectant solutions used to clean reusable patient equipment, such as bronchoscopes and pressure transducers, or to disinfect skin. *Burkholderia gladioli* also has been isolated from sputum from persons with cystic fibrosis and may be mistaken for *B cepacia*. *Burkholderia pseudomallei* is acquired early in life, with the highest seroconversion rates between 6 and 42 months of age. Symptomatic infection can occur as early as 1 year of age. Risk factors for disease include diabetes mellitus and renal insufficiency.

DIAGNOSTIC TESTS: Culture is the appropriate test for diagnosis of *B cepacia* infection. In cystic fibrosis lung infection, culture of sputum on selective agar is recommended to decrease the potential for overgrowth by mucoid *P aeruginosa. Burkholderia cepacia* and *B gladioli* can be identified by polymerase chain reaction, but this assay is not available in most commercial laboratories. Diagnosis of melioidosis can be made by isolation of *B pseudomallei* from blood or an infected site. The indirect hemagglutination assay is used most frequently for serologic diagnosis in young children, and a positive test result is more predictive of infection in this age group than in older children and adults because of the lower seroprevalence in young children. Other rapid assays being developed for diagnosis of melioidosis include direct fluorescent antibody for identification of the organism in sputum, an immunoglobulin M enzyme immunoassay, and DNA probes.

TREATMENT: Meropenem seems to be the most active agent against *B cepacia,* which has variable susceptibility to other agents. *Burkholderia cepacia* also is intrinsically resistant to aminoglycosides and polymyxin B. Agents active against *B pseudomallei* include ceftazidime, piperacillin, chloramphenicol, doxycycline, and trimethoprim-sulfamethoxazole.

ISOLATION OF THE HOSPITALIZED PATIENT: Standard precautions are recommended. Unless recent sputum culture results are available at the time of hospital admission, patients with cystic fibrosis should not be grouped together in the hospital setting.

CONTROL MEASURES: Because some strains of *B cepacia* are highly transmissible and virulence is not well understood, many cystic fibrosis centers have attempted to limit contact of *B cepacia*–colonized and noncolonized patients. For example, specialized cystic fibrosis camps no longer are recommended. Education of patients and families about hand washing and appropriate personal hygiene is recommended.

Caliciviruses

CLINICAL MANIFESTATIONS: Diarrhea and vomiting, frequently accompanied by fever, headache, malaise, myalgia, and abdominal cramps, are characteristic. Symptoms last from 1 day to 2 weeks.

ETIOLOGY: Caliciviruses are nonenveloped RNA viruses. The 3 recognized genera that cause disease in humans are Norwalk-like and Sapporo-like caliciviruses and vesiviruses. Vesiviruses cause vesicular exanthema in humans.

EPIDEMIOLOGY: Human caliciviruses have a worldwide distribution. Outbreaks of gastroenteritis have been detected in all age groups. Multiple antigenic types circulate simultaneously in the same region. Caliciviruses may be a major cause of sporadic cases of gastroenteritis requiring hospitalization, but sensitive diagnostic tools have been applied only recently to study this problem. Most sporadic calicivirus infections have been detected in children younger than 4 years of age. Transmission is via the fecal-oral route, by person-to-person spread, or through contaminated food or water, but often, a route of transmission cannot be determined. Outbreaks tend to occur in closed populations and have a high attack rate. Infections in child care centers have been reported. Common-source outbreaks occur in association with ingestion of contaminated ice, shellfish, salads, and cookies. Airborne transmission and exposure to contaminated surfaces and vomitus have been implicated in outbreaks. Excretion lasts 5 to 7 days after the onset of symptoms in half of the infected persons and can be as long as 13 days. Virus excretion may continue as long as 4 days after symptoms cease. Prolonged excretion can occur in immunocompromised hosts. Asymptomatic, persistent virus excretion has been detected for months after primary calicivirus infections in animals.

The **incubation period** is 12 hours to 4 days.

DIAGNOSTIC TESTS: Commercial tests for diagnosis are not available. The following tests are available in some research and reference laboratories: electron microscopy for detection of viral particles in stool, enzyme immunoassay for detection of viral antigen in stool or antibody in serum, and reverse transcriptase–polymerase chain reaction (RT-PCR) for detection of viral RNA in stool. The most sensitive assays are RT-PCR and serologic testing; electron microscopy is relatively insensitive.

TREATMENT: Supportive, including oral rehydration solution to replace fluids and electrolytes. Antibiotics are contraindicated.

ISOLATION OF THE HOSPITALIZED PATIENT: In addition to standard precautions, contact precautions are recommended for diapered and incontinent children for the duration of illness.

CONTROL MEASURES: No specific control measures are available. The spread of infection can be reduced by generic measures for control of diarrhea, such as training care providers about infection control, maintaining cleanliness of surfaces and food preparation areas, exclusion of care providers or food handlers who are ill, adequate hand washing, and exclusion or grouping of ill children for care. If a mode of transmission can be identified (eg, contaminated food or water) during an outbreak, then specific interventions to interrupt transmission can be effective. Immunization to prevent calicivirus infection is not available.

Campylobacter Infections

CLINICAL MANIFESTATIONS: Predominant symptoms are diarrhea, abdominal pain, malaise, and fever. Stools may contain visible or occult blood. In neonates, bloody diarrhea may be the only manifestation of infection. Abdominal pain can mimic that produced by appendicitis. Mild infection lasts 1 or 2 days and resembles viral gastroenteritis. Most patients recover in less than 1 week, but 20% have a relapse or a prolonged or severe illness. Severe or persistent infection may mimic acute inflammatory bowel disease. Bacteremia is uncommon, but neonatal septicemia occurs occasionally. Immunocompromised hosts may have prolonged, relapsing, or extraintestinal infections. Immunoreactive complications, such as acute idiopathic polyneuritis (Guillain-Barré syndrome), Fisher syndrome, reactive arthritis, Reiter syndrome, and erythema nodosum, may occur during convalescence.

ETIOLOGY: *Campylobacter jejuni* are motile, comma-shaped, gram-negative bacilli that cause gastroenteritis. *Campylobacter fetus* is an infrequent cause of systemic illness in neonates and debilitated hosts. Other *Campylobacter* and *Arcobacter* species may cause similar diarrheal or systemic illnesses.

EPIDEMIOLOGY: The gastrointestinal tract of domestic and wild birds and animals is the reservoir of infection. *Campylobacter jejuni* has been isolated from feces of 30% to 100% of chickens, turkeys, and water fowl. Poultry carcasses usually are contaminated with the organism. Many farm animals and meat sources can harbor the organism, and pets, such as dogs, cats, and hamsters (especially young animals), and birds are potential sources. Transmission of *C jejuni* occurs by ingestion of contaminated food, including unpasteurized milk and untreated water, or by direct contact with fecal material from infected animals or persons. Improperly cooked poultry, untreated water, and unpasteurized milk have been the main vehicles of transmission. Outbreaks among school children have occurred after field trips to dairy farms during which children drank unpasteurized milk. Person-to-person spread occurs occasionally, particularly from young children with fecal incontinence. Outbreaks of diarrhea due to *C jejuni* and *Campylobacter upsaliensis* in child care centers have been reported but seem to be uncommon. Person-to-person transmission also has occurred in neonates of infected mothers and has resulted in nosocomial outbreaks in nurseries. In perinatal infection, *C jejuni* usually causes neonatal gastroenteritis, whereas *C fetus* often results in neonatal septicemia or meningitis. Enteritis occurs in persons of all ages. Communicability is uncommon but is greatest during the acute phase of illness. Convalescent excretion usually is brief, typically 2 to 3 weeks, and is shortened by treatment to 2 to 3 days. *Campylobacter* species are the major organisms detected by the Foodborne Diseases Active Surveillance Network (FoodNet) (see http://www.cdc.gov/ncidod/dbmd/foodnet/) Asymptomatic carriage is uncommon.

The **incubation period** is usually 1 to 7 days but can be longer.

DIAGNOSTIC TESTS: Rapid presumptive diagnosis is possible in laboratories experienced in examining stool smears by darkfield microscopic or Gram-stain techniques, although the sensitivity of these tests is low. *Campylobacter jejuni* can be cultured from feces, and *Campylobacter* species, including *C fetus* can be cultured from blood. Laboratory identification of *C jejuni* in stool specimens requires special isolation techniques, which may not be a routine procedure in some microbiology laboratories. Unless the laboratory uses a filtration method in addition to a selective enrichment medium containing antibiotics to suppress colonic flora, many *Campylobacter* species other than *C jejuni* will not be detected.

TREATMENT:

- When given early during the infection, erythromycin and azithromycin shorten the duration of illness and prevent relapse. Treatment with erythromycin or azithromycin usually eradicates the organism from stool within 2 or 3 days. Tetracycline for children 8 years or older is an alternative agent. A fluoroquinolone, such as ciprofloxacin, is effective, but fluoroquinolones are not approved by the US Food and Drug Administration for persons younger than 18 years of age (see Antimicrobial Agents and Related Therapy, p 645).
- If antimicrobial therapy is given for treatment of gastroenteritis, the recommended duration is 5 to 7 days.
- Antimicrobial agents for resistant or bacteremic strains should be selected on the basis of laboratory susceptibility tests. Bacteremic strains almost always are susceptible to aminoglycosides, meropenem, and imipenem.

ISOLATION OF THE HOSPITALIZED PATIENT: In addition to standard precautions, contact precautions are recommended for diapered and incontinent children for the duration of illness.

CONTROL MEASURES:

- Hand washing after handling raw poultry, washing cutting boards and utensils with soap and water after contact with raw poultry, avoiding contact of fruits and vegetables with the juices of raw poultry, and thorough cooking of poultry are critical.
- Pasteurization of milk and chlorination of water supplies are important.
- Exclude symptomatic persons from food handling, care of patients in hospitals, and care of persons in custodial care and child care centers.
- Infected food handlers and hospital employees who are asymptomatic need not be excluded from work if proper personal hygiene measures, including hand washing, are maintained.
- Outbreaks are uncommon in child care centers, and specific strategies for controlling infection in these settings have not been evaluated. General measures for interrupting enteric transmission in child care centers are recommended (see Children in Out-of-Home Child Care, p 105). Infants and children in diapers with symptomatic *C jejuni* infection should be excluded from child care or cared for in a separate protected area until diarrhea has subsided. Erythromycin treatment may further limit the potential for transmission.
- Stool cultures of asymptomatic exposed children generally are not recommended.

Candidiasis

(Moniliasis, Thrush)

CLINICAL MANIFESTATIONS: Mucocutaneous infection results in oral (thrush) or vaginal candidiasis; intertriginous lesions of the gluteal folds, neck, groin, and axilla; paronychia; and onychia. Chronic mucocutaneous candidiasis can be associated with endocrinologic diseases or progressive immunodeficiency, particularly T-cell lymphocyte deficiency, and may be the presenting sign of human immunodeficiency virus (HIV) infection. Esophagitis and laryngitis may occur in immunocompromised patients. Disseminated or invasive candidiasis occurs in very-low-birth-weight newborns and in immunocompromised or debilitated hosts, can involve virtually any organ or anatomic site, and may be rapidly fatal. The presence of typical retinal lesions may be useful in diagnosis. Candidemia can occur with or without systemic disease in patients with indwelling catheters or in patients receiving prolonged intravenous infusions, especially parenteral alimentation and lipids. Candiduria can occur in patients with indwelling catheters or disseminated disease.

ETIOLOGY: *Candida albicans* causes most infections (60%–80%). Other species, such as *Candida tropicalis, Candida parapsilosis, Candida glabrata, Candida krusei, Candida guilliermondii, Candida lusitaniae, Candida lipolytica,* and *Candida stellatoidea,* also can cause serious infections in compromised hosts. Approximately 200 species of *Candida* have been identified.

EPIDEMIOLOGY: *Candida albicans* is ubiquitous. Like other *Candida* species, it is present on skin and in the mouth, intestinal tract, and vagina of healthy persons. Vulvovaginal candidiasis is associated with pregnancy, and newborn infants can acquire the organism in utero, during passage through the vagina, or postnatally. Mild mucocutaneous infection is common in healthy infants. Person-to-person transmission occurs infrequently. Invasive disease occurs almost exclusively in persons with impaired immunity, and infection arises from endogenous colonized sites. Persons with HIV infection or who are immunodeficient for other reasons, such as neutropenia, diabetes mellitus, or treatment with corticosteroids or cytotoxic chemotherapy, are unusually susceptible. Patients undergoing intravenous hyperalimentation or receiving broad-spectrum antimicrobial agents also have increased susceptibility.

The **incubation period** is unknown.

DIAGNOSTIC TESTS: The presumptive diagnosis of mucocutaneous candidiasis or thrush usually can be made clinically, but thrush-like lesions also can be caused by other organisms or trauma. Both yeast and pseudohyphae can be found in *C albicans*–infected tissue and are identified by microscopic examination of scrapings stained by Gram stain or suspended in 10% to 20% potassium hydroxide. Endoscopy is most useful for the diagnosis of esophagitis. Ophthalmologic examination is required to determine retinal lesions, and lesions in the brain, kidney, liver, or spleen may be detected by ultrasonography or computed tomography.

A definitive diagnosis of invasive candidiasis requires isolation of the organism from an otherwise sterile body fluid or tissue (eg, blood, cerebrospinal fluid, bone marrow, or biopsy specimen) or demonstration of organisms in a tissue biopsy specimen. Cultures that are negative for *Candida* species, however, do not exclude invasive infection in immunocompromised hosts. Recovery of the organism is facilitated and more rapid by blood culture using biphasic or lysis-centrifugation systems. A presumptive species identification of *C albicans* can be made by demonstrating germ tube formation.

TREATMENT:

Mucous Membrane and Skin Infections. Oral candidiasis in immunocompetent hosts is treated with oral nystatin suspension or clotrimazole troches.

Fluconazole or itraconazole may be beneficial for immunocompromised patients with oropharyngeal candidiasis. Although cure rates with fluconazole are greater than with nystatin, relapse rates are comparable. The safety and efficacy of fluconazole for use in infants younger than 6 months of age and of itraconazole for use in children have not been established, although both drugs have been used safely in a limited number of patients of these ages.

Mild esophagitis caused by *Candida* species can be treated with high-dose oral nystatin; more severe disease is treated with fluconazole or itraconazole for a minimum of 14 days or with low-dose intravenous amphotericin B (0.3 mg/kg per day) for at least 5 to 7 days depending on patient factors, such as age, severity of the illness, and degree of immunocompromise.

Skin infections are treated with topical nystatin, miconazole, clotrimazole, amphotericin B, ketoconazole, econazole, or ciclopirox (see Topical Drugs for Superficial Fungal Infections, p 673). Nystatin usually is effective and is the least expensive of these drugs.

Vulvovaginal candidiasis is effectively treated with many topical formulations, including clotrimazole, miconazole, butaconazole, terconazole, and tioconazole. Such topically applied azole drugs are more effective than nystatin. Oral azole agents also are effective and should be considered for recurrent or refractory cases. The recommended oral dose for fluconazole for vaginal candidiasis in adolescents and adults is 150 mg given once.

For chronic mucocutaneous candidiasis, fluconazole and itraconazole are effective drugs. Amphotericin B, given intravenously, also is effective in severe cases. Relapses are common with any of these agents once therapy is terminated; invasive infection is rare.

Keratomycosis is treated with corneal baths of amphotericin B, 1 mg/mL. Patients with cystitis due to *Candida* organisms can be treated successfully with short courses (3 to 5 days) of low-dose amphotericin B intravenously (0.3 mg/kg per day), fluconazole, or bladder irrigation with 50 µg/mL of amphotericin B in sterile water.

Systemic Infections. Amphotericin B is the drug of choice for treating persons with invasive candidiasis (see Drugs for Invasive and Other Serious Fungal Infections, p 672). Duration of therapy will vary with the clinical response and presence or absence of neutropenia. Patients at high risk for morbidity and mortality should be treated for a prolonged period and until all signs and symptoms of infection have resolved. Low-risk patients usually can be treated adequately with a 7- to 10-day course of therapy. Short-course therapy also may be successful for catheter-associated infections, provided the catheter is removed. Liposomal preparations of amphotericin B may be used if significant nephrotoxic effects or suboptimal response is observed with conventional amphotericin B therapy.

Flucytosine (150 mg/kg per day in 4 divided doses, given orally) can be given with amphotericin B if infection is associated with central nervous system involvement by *C albicans.* In vitro and clinical studies suggest synergism of flucytosine and amphotericin B against *C albicans.* The dose of flucytosine must be decreased for patients with renal insufficiency. Peak plasma concentrations should be maintained between 40 and 60 µg/mL; higher concentrations predispose to toxic effects. Adverse effects of flucytosine, especially in azotemic patients, include rash, hepatic dysfunction, gastrointestinal tract bleeding, enterocolitis, and dose-related bone marrow suppression.

Fluconazole has been used successfully to treat disseminated candidiasis, but amphotericin B remains the drug of choice. Patients with disseminated candidiasis in whom treatment with amphotericin B failed have responded to fluconazole. Nonneutropenic adults with candidemia respond equally to fluconazole or amphotericin B.

Chemoprophylaxis of candidal infections in immunocompromised patients with drugs such as oral nystatin, ketoconazole, and fluconazole has been evaluated with variable success. Data from a prospective controlled trial indicate that fluconazole can reduce the risk of mucosal (eg, oropharyngeal and esophageal) candidiasis in patients with advanced HIV disease. An increased incidence of fluconazole-resistant *C krusei* infections has been reported in non–HIV-infected patients receiving prophylactic fluconazole. Adults undergoing bone marrow transplantation had significantly fewer candidal infections when given fluconazole. This finding has not been observed in children. Prophylaxis is not recommended routinely for immunocompromised children, including children with HIV infection.

Isolation of the Hospitalized Patient: Standard precautions are recommended.

Control Measures: Prolonged, broad-spectrum, antimicrobial therapy and use of corticosteroids for susceptible patients promotes overgrowth of and predisposes to infection with *Candida* organisms. Meticulous care of intravascular catheter sites is recommended for any patient requiring long-term intravenous alimentation.

Cat-scratch Disease

(Bartonella henselae)

Clinical Manifestations: The predominant sign of cat-scratch disease (CSD) is regional lymphadenopathy in an immunocompetent person. Fever and mild systemic symptoms occur in 30% of patients. A skin papule often is found at the presumed site of bacterial inoculation and usually precedes development of lymphadenopathy by 1 to 2 weeks. Lymphadenopathy usually involves nodes that drain the site of inoculation and may include cervical, axillary, epitrochlear, or inguinal nodes. The area around affected lymph nodes typically is tender, warm, erythematous, and indurated. In as many as 30% of the cases of CSD, the affected nodes suppurate spontaneously. Occasionally, infection can produce Parinaud oculoglandular syndrome involving the conjunctiva and an ipsilateral preauricular lymph node. Rare clinical manifestations include encephalitis, aseptic meningitis, fever of unknown origin, neuroretinitis, osteolytic lesions, hepatitis, microabscesses in the liver and spleen, pneumonia, thrombocytopenic purpura, and erythema nodosum.

ETIOLOGY: *Bartonella henselae* is the causative organism for most cases of CSD. This conclusion is based primarily on serologic, epidemiologic, and molecular probe rather than culture data, although *B henselae* has been isolated from patients with classic signs of CSD, as well as from domestic cats. *Bartonella henselae* are fastidious, slow-growing, gram-negative bacilli that also have been identified as the causative agent of bacillary angiomatosis and peliosis hepatitis, two infections that have been reported primarily in patients infected with the human immunodeficiency virus. *Bartonella henselae* is closely related to *Bartonella quintana*, the agent of trench fever and also a cause of bacillary angiomatosis.

EPIDEMIOLOGY: Cat-scratch disease is believed to be a relatively common infection, although the true incidence is unknown. Most cases occur in patients younger than 20 years of age. Cats are the common reservoir for human disease, and bacteremia in cats associated with patients with CSD is common. More than 90% of patients have a history of recent contact with cats, often kittens, which usually are healthy. Anecdotal reports of possible transmission by other animals, such as dogs and monkeys, and inanimate objects exist. No evidence of person-to-person transmission exists. However, multiple cases have been observed in families, presumably resulting from contact with the same animal. Infection occurs more frequently in the autumn and winter. Cat fleas may be involved in transmission of *B henselae* between cats.

The **incubation period**, from the time of the scratch to the appearance of the primary cutaneous lesion, is 7 to 12 days and 5 to 50 days (median, 12 days) from appearance of the primary lesion to appearance of lymphadenopathy.

DIAGNOSTIC TESTS: The indirect fluorescent antibody (IFA) test for detection of serum antibody to antigens of *Bartonella* species is useful for the diagnosis of CSD. The IFA test is available through the Centers for Disease Control and Prevention, and the reagents are available to state health departments. Results of IFAs performed in some commercial laboratories have not been reliable. Enzyme immunoassays for detection of antibody to *B henselae* have been developed; however, they have not been demonstrated to be more sensitive or specific than the IFA test. Polymerase chain reaction assays are available in some commercial laboratories. If involved tissue is available, the putative agent of the disease may be visualized by the Warthin-Starry silver impregnation stain; however, this test is not specific for *B henselae.* Pathologic and microbiologic examinations also are useful to exclude other diseases. Histologic findings in lymph node sections are characteristic but not pathognomonic for CSD. Early histologic changes consist of lymphocytic infiltrates with epithelioid granuloma formation, similar to changes in lymphomas and sarcoidosis. Later changes consist of polymorphonuclear leukocyte infiltrates with granulomas that become necrotic and resemble those of tularemia, brucellosis, and mycobacterial infections. A cat-scratch antigen skin test, which was used formerly to confirm the clinical diagnosis, was prepared from aspirated pus from suppurative lymph nodes of patients with apparent CSD. This test is unlicensed and should not be used.

TREATMENT: Management is primarily symptomatic since the disease usually is self-limited, resolving spontaneously in 2 to 4 months. Painful suppurative nodes can be treated with needle aspiration for relief of symptoms; surgical excision generally is unnecessary.

Antibiotic therapy may be considered for acutely or severely ill patients with systemic symptoms, particularly persons with hepatosplenomegaly or persons with large painful adenopathy and immunocompromised hosts. No well-controlled randomized clinical trials have been performed that clearly demonstrate a clinically significant benefit of antimicrobial therapy for CSD. Reports suggest that several oral antibiotics (rifampin, trimethoprim-sulfamethoxazole, azithromycin, and ciprofloxacin) and parenteral gentamicin may be effective in CSD. Doxycycline, erythromycin, and azithromycin are effective for treatment of signs and symptoms associated with bacillary angiomatosis if administered for prolonged periods to immunocompromised persons.

ISOLATION OF THE HOSPITALIZED PATIENT: Standard precautions are recommended.

CONTROL MEASURES: Persons should avoid playing roughly with cats and kittens to minimize cat-induced scratches and bites. Persons with immune deficiencies should avoid contact with cats that scratch or bite, and when obtaining a new pet, they should avoid cats younger than 1 year of age. Immunocompromised persons should wash immediately sites of cat scratches or bites and should not allow cats to lick their open cuts or wounds. Care of cats should include flea control. Testing of cats for *Bartonella* infection is not recommended.

Chancroid

CLINICAL MANIFESTATIONS: Chancroid is an acute ulcerative disease that involves the genitalia. In approximately 30% of cases, chancroid is associated with a painful unilateral inguinal adenitis (bubo). An ulcer begins as a tender erythematous papule, becomes pustular, and erodes over several days, forming a sharply demarcated, somewhat superficial lesion with a serpiginous undermined border. Its base is friable and may be covered with a gray or yellow, necrotic, and purulent exudate. Men typically have single ulcers, while women usually have multiple lesions. Unlike a syphilitic chancre, which is painless, the chancroidal ulcer is painful, tender, and nonindurated. Buboes frequently suppurate and become fluctuant.

Males present with a complaint directly referable to the genital ulcer or to inguinal tenderness. Many females are asymptomatic but can, depending on the site of the ulcer, present with less obvious symptoms, including dysuria, dyspareunia, vaginal discharge, pain on defecation, or rectal bleeding. Constitutional symptoms are unusual.

ETIOLOGY: Chancroid is caused by *Haemophilus ducreyi,* which is a gram-negative coccobacillus.

EPIDEMIOLOGY: Chancroid is a sexually transmitted disease that is associated with poverty, urban prostitution, and illicit drug use (in the United States). It is recently endemic in many areas of the United States and also occurs in discrete outbreaks.

Coinfection with syphilis or herpes simplex virus (HSV) occurs in as many as 10% of patients. Chancroid is a well-established cofactor for transmission of human immunodeficiency virus (HIV). Because sexual contact is the only known route of transmission, the diagnosis of chancroid in infants and young children is strong evidence of sexual abuse.

The **incubation period** is 3 to 10 days.

DIAGNOSTIC TESTS: The diagnosis of chancroid usually is made on the basis of clinical findings and the exclusion of other infections associated with genital ulcer disease, such as syphilis or HSV, or adenopathies, such as lymphogranuloma venereum. Direct examination of clinical material by Gram stain may strongly suggest the diagnosis if large numbers of gram-negative coccobacilli, sometimes in "school of fish" patterns, are seen. Confirmation by recovery of *H ducreyi* from a genital ulcer or lymph node aspirate is the more available alternative diagnostic test. Special culture media and conditions are required for isolation; if chancroid is suspected, the laboratory should be informed. Purulent material recovered from intact buboes is almost always sterile. Fluorescent monoclonal antibody stains and polymerase chain reaction tests can provide more specific diagnosis but are not available in most laboratories.

TREATMENT: Azithromycin, 12 to 15 mg/kg (maximum, 1 g), orally in a single dose or ceftriaxone (250 mg intramuscularly in a single dose) is the preferred therapy. Alternative regimens are erythromycin base, 50 mg/kg per day in divided doses for 7 days (maximum, 500 mg 4 times a day), and ciprofloxacin (500 mg orally twice a day for 3 days). Ciprofloxacin should not be administered to pregnant or lactating women or usually to persons younger than 18 years of age (see Antimicrobial Agents and Related Therapy, p 645). Relapses occur in about 5% of patients; retreatment with the original regimen usually is effective. Patients with HIV infection may need more prolonged therapy. Trimethoprim-sulfamethoxazole is not recommended since resistance is variably present.

Clinical improvement occurs within 7 days of onset of successful therapy, and healing is complete in about 2 weeks. Adenitis often is slow to resolve and may require needle aspiration or surgical incision. Patients should be reexamined 3 to 7 days after starting therapy to verify that healing is occurring. If not, the diagnosis, which has often only been made clinically, may be incorrect and further testing is required.

Patients should be evaluated for other sexually transmitted diseases, including syphilis, hepatitis B virus, *Chlamydia trachomatis*, gonorrhea, and HIV at the time of diagnosis. In particular, since chancroid is a risk factor for HIV infection and an enhancer of its transmission, if initial HIV test results are negative, they should be repeated 3 months later. All persons having sexual contact with patients with chancroid within 10 days before onset of the patient's symptoms need to be examined and treated, even if they are asymptomatic.

ISOLATION OF THE HOSPITALIZED PATIENT: Standard precautions are recommended.

CONTROL MEASURES: Examination and treatment of sexual partners of patients with chancroid are important control measures. "Partner notification" is increasingly used to identify a reservoir of cases of chancroid during outbreaks, usually occurring among prostitutes. This process can lead to epidemic control. Regular condom use may decrease transmission.

CHLAMYDIAL INFECTIONS

Chlamydia pneumoniae

CLINICAL MANIFESTATIONS: Patients may be asymptomatic or mildly to moderately ill with a variety of respiratory tract diseases, including pharyngitis, sinusitis, bronchitis, and pneumonia. In some patients, a sore throat precedes the onset of cough by a week or more. Physical examination may reveal nonexudative pharyngitis and frequently bronchospasm, and chest roentgenogram may reveal an infiltrate. Illness is prolonged and can have a biphasic course.

ETIOLOGY: *Chlamydia pneumoniae* (formerly termed the TWAR strain) is a species of *Chlamydia* that is antigenically, genetically, and morphologically distinct from other *Chlamydia* species. In addition to acute respiratory tract disease, some investigators have associated *C pneumoniae* with atherosclerotic cardiovascular disease. This association is based on the increased frequency of serum antibodies in patients compared with controls, the detection of antigen or DNA in atheromatous plaques, the production of arterial lesions in experimentally infected animals, and small human trials demonstrating that treatment of high-risk patients with macrolides decreases the risk of subsequent cardiovascular events. Large, prospective, randomized trials are underway to further explore this association and to determine whether treatment is beneficial. Other investigators have associated *C pneumoniae* with asthma, Alzheimer disease, multiple sclerosis, and Kawasaki disease, but the evidence supporting any of these associations is limited.

EPIDEMIOLOGY: *Chlamydia pneumoniae* infection is assumed to be transmitted from person to person via infected respiratory tract secretions. An animal reservoir is unknown. The disease occurs worldwide, but in tropical and less developed areas, disease occurs earlier in life than in developed countries in temperate climates. In the United States, *C pneumoniae*–specific serum antibody is present in most adults. Initial infection peaks between 5 and 15 years of age. Recurrent infection is common, especially in adults. Clusters of infection have been reported in groups of children and young adults.

The mean **incubation period** is 21 days.

DIAGNOSTIC TESTS: No reliable diagnostic test is available commercially. The organism can be isolated from nasopharyngeal swabs placed into appropriate transport media and held at 4°C (39°F) until inoculated into cell culture; prolonged nasopharyngeal shedding can occur for months after acute disease. Methods for detecting *C pneumoniae* in clinical specimens are available in research facilities and include a fluorescent antibody test using monoclonal antibody specific for *C pneumoniae* and a polymerase chain reaction (PCR) test. Complement-fixing *Chlamydia* antibodies usually are present in children and adolescents with illness but often are absent in adults, but the test does not distinguish among antibodies to *C pneumoniae, Chlamydia trachomatis,* or *Chlamydia psittaci.* The microimmunofluorescent antibody test is the most sensitive and specific serologic test for infection. A 4-fold serum antibody titer increase, an immunoglobulin (Ig) M–specific titer of 1:16 or greater, or an IgG-specific titer of 1:512 or greater is evidence of current infection. An increase in antibody titer may be delayed for several weeks after onset of illness. Early antimicrobial therapy may suppress the antibody response.

TREATMENT: Erythromycin or tetracycline is recommended. Tetracycline should not be given routinely to children younger than 8 years of age (see Antimicrobial Agents and Related Therapy, p 646). Adolescents and older patients have been treated successfully with erythromycin for 5 to 10 days, but a 14- to 21-day course of therapy may be needed, as prolonged or recurrent symptoms are common. For adolescents and adults, tetracycline or doxycycline for 14 days also is appropriate. In vitro data suggest that *C pneumoniae* is not susceptible to the sulfonamides. The macrolide drugs, azithromycin and clarithromycin, and some of the fluoroquinolones also are effective. The fluoroquinolones are approved for persons 18 years of age and older.

ISOLATION OF THE HOSPITALIZED PATIENT: Standard precautions are recommended.

CONTROL MEASURES: None.

Chlamydia psittaci

(Psittacosis, Ornithosis)

CLINICAL MANIFESTATIONS: Psittacosis (ornithosis) is an acute febrile respiratory tract infection with systemic symptoms and signs that often include fever, a nonproductive cough, headache, and malaise. Extensive interstitial pneumonia can occur with radiographic changes characteristically more severe than what would be expected from physical examination findings. Pericarditis, myocarditis, endocarditis, superficial thrombophlebitis, hepatitis, and encephalopathy are rare complications.

ETIOLOGY: *Chlamydia psittaci* is antigenically and genetically distinct from other *Chlamydia* species. Illness may be caused by *Chlamydia pecorum,* a newly designated species formerly not distinguished from *C psittaci.*

EPIDEMIOLOGY: Birds are the major reservoir of *C psittaci.* Several mammalian species, such as cattle, goats, sheep, and cats, and avian species may become infected and develop systemic and debilitating disease. In the United States, psittacine birds (such as parakeets, parrots, and macaws), especially those smuggled into the country, pigeons, and turkeys are important sources of human disease. Both healthy and sick birds may harbor and transmit the organism, usually via the airborne route in fecal dust or secretions. Excretion of *C psittaci* can be intermittent or continuous for weeks or months. Persons in the environment of infected birds, such as workers at poultry slaughter plants, poultry farms, and pet shops, as well as pet owners, are at high risk of infection. Laboratory personnel working with *C psittaci* also are at high risk. Psittacosis is worldwide in distribution and tends to occur sporadically in any season. Infections are rare in children. Person-to-person transmission from acutely ill patients, presumably via the respiratory route, is rare. Severe illness and abortion have been reported in pregnant women after exposure to infected sheep.

The **incubation period** usually is 7 to 14 days but may be longer.

DIAGNOSTIC TESTS: The usual method of diagnosis is serologic, based on a 4-fold increase in complement fixation (CF) antibody titer between acute and convalescent specimens collected 2 to 3 weeks apart. In the presence of a compatible clinical illness, a single CF titer of 1:32 or greater is considered presumptive evidence of infection. Treatment may suppress the antibody response. The CF test does not distinguish among infections caused by *C psittaci, C pneumoniae, C trachomatis,* or *C pecorum.* A microimmunofluorescence assay that is more specific for *C psittaci* has been developed but is not available widely. Isolation of the agent from the respiratory tract should be attempted only by experienced personnel in laboratories in which strict measures to prevent spread of the organism are used during collection and handling of all specimens for culture.

TREATMENT: A tetracycline is the preferred therapy, except for children younger than 8 years of age. Erythromycin is an alternative drug and is recommended for younger children. The macrolide drugs, azithromycin and clarithromycin as well as chloramphenicol, also are effective. Therapy should be administered for at least 10 to 14 days after defervescence.

ISOLATION OF THE HOSPITALIZED PATIENT: Standard precautions are recommended.

CONTROL MEASURES: Reporting cases of human psittacosis to health authorities is mandated in most states. All birds suspected to be the source of human infection should be seen by a veterinarian for evaluation and management. Birds with *C psittaci* infection should be isolated and treated with chlortetracycline for at least 45 days. Birds with suspected infection that have died or have been killed humanely should be sealed in an impermeable container and transported on dry ice to a veterinary laboratory for testing. All potentially contaminated caging and housing areas should be disinfected thoroughly and aired before reuse because these areas may contain infectious organisms. *Chlamydia psittaci* is susceptible to most household disinfectants and detergents, including 70% alcohol, 1% Lysol, and a 1:100 dilution of household bleach. Persons cleaning cages and other bird housing areas should avoid scattering the contents. Persons exposed to common sources of infection should be observed for development of fever or respiratory tract symptoms; early diagnostic tests should be performed and therapy given if symptoms appear.

Chlamydia trachomatis

CLINICAL MANIFESTATIONS: *Chlamydia trachomatis* is associated with a range of clinical manifestations including the following: (1) neonatal conjunctivitis, (2) trachoma, (3) pneumonia in young infants, (4) genital tract infection, and (5) lymphogranuloma venereum (LGV). Neonatal chlamydial conjunctivitis is characterized by ocular congestion, edema, and discharge developing a few days to several weeks after birth and lasting for 1 to 2 weeks, occasionally much longer. In contrast to trachoma, scars and pannus formation are rare.

Trachoma is a chronic follicular keratoconjunctivitis with neovascularization of the cornea that results from repeated and chronic infection. Blindness secondary to extensive local scarring and inflammation occurs in 1% to 15% of persons with trachoma. Trachoma is rare in the United States.

Pneumonia in young infants is usually an afebrile illness occurring between 2 and 19 weeks after birth. A repetitive staccato cough, tachypnea, and rales are characteristic but not always present. Wheezing is uncommon; however, hyperinflation usually accompanies the infiltrates seen on chest roentgenogram. Nasal stuffiness and otitis media may occur. Untreated disease can linger or recur. Severe chlamydial pneumonia has occurred in infants and some immunocompromised adults.

Urethritis, vaginitis in prepubertal girls, cervicitis, endometritis, salpingitis, and perihepatitis in postpubertal females; epididymitis in males; and Reiter syndrome in either sex also can occur. Infection can persist for months or years. Reinfection is common. In postpubertal females, chlamydial infection can progress to acute or chronic pelvic inflammatory disease and result in ectopic pregnancy or infertility.

Lymphogranuloma venereum is an invasive lymphatic infection with an initial ulcerative lesion on the genitalia accompanied by tender, suppurative, regional lymphadenopathy. Anorectal infection and hemorrhagic proctitis also have been described. The disease has a chronic low-grade course.

ETIOLOGY: *Chlamydia trachomatis* is a bacterial agent with at least 18 serologic variants (serovars) divided between the following 2 biologic variants (biovars): oculogenital (serovars A-K) and LGV (serovars L1, L2, and L3). Trachoma usually is caused by serovars A through C, and genital and perinatal infections are caused by B and D through K.

EPIDEMIOLOGY: *Chlamydia trachomatis* is the most common reportable sexually transmitted infection in the United States with high rates among sexually active adolescents and young adults. Prevalence of the organism in pregnant women varies between 6% and 12% in most populations but can be as low as 2% or as high as 37% in adolescents. Oculogenital serovars of *C trachomatis* can be transmitted from the genital tract of infected mothers to their newborn infants. Acquisition occurs in approximately 50% of infants born vaginally to infected mothers and in some infants delivered by cesarean section with intact membranes. The risk of conjunctivitis is 25% to 50% and that of pneumonia is 5% to 20% in infants who acquire *C trachomatis*. The nasopharynx is the most commonly infected anatomic site.

Genital infection in adolescents and adults is transmitted sexually. Possible sexual abuse should be suspected in prepubertal children beyond infancy who have vaginal, urethral, or rectal chlamydial infection, although asymptomatic infection acquired at birth can persist for as long as 3 years. Infection is not known to be communicable among infants and children. The degree of contagiousness of pulmonary disease is unknown but seems to be low.

Lymphogranuloma venereum biovars are worldwide in distribution but are particularly prevalent in tropical and subtropical areas. Infection is often asymptomatic in women. Perinatal transmission is rare. Lymphogranuloma venereum is infective during active disease, which may last from weeks to many years.

The **incubation period** of chlamydial illness is variable, depending on the type of infection, but is usually at least 1 week.

DIAGNOSTIC TESTS: Definitive diagnosis can be made by isolating the organism in tissue culture. Because *Chlamydia* are obligate intracellular organisms, culture specimens must contain epithelial cells, not just exudate. Nucleic acid amplification methods, such as PCR and ligase chain reaction (LCR) are more sensitive than cell culture and more specific and sensitive than DNA probe, direct fluorescent antibody (DFA) tests, or enzyme immunoassays (EIAs).

Tests for detection of chlamydial antigen or nucleic acid are useful for evaluating urethral specimens from males, cervical specimens from females, and conjunctival specimens from infants. The PCR and LCR tests are useful for evaluating urine specimens from either sex. These tests have not been evaluated adequately for detection of *C trachomatis* in nasopharyngeal specimens. The EIA and DFA tests should not be used for testing rectal, vaginal, or urethral specimens from infants and children, since fecal bacterial flora cross-react with *C trachomatis* antisera.

Positive DFA, EIA, or DNA probe test results should be verified if a false-positive test result is likely to have adverse medical, social, or psychological consequences. Confirmation can be accomplished by culture, a second nonculture test different from the first, or use of a blocking antibody (eg, Chlamydiazyme, Abbott Laboratories, Abbott Park, IL) or competitive probe. When evaluating a child for possible sexual abuse, results of rapid antigen detection or DNA tests are unacceptable, and culture of the organism is the only acceptable method of diagnosis.

In the past, neonatal *C trachomatis* conjunctivitis was diagnosed by Giemsa staining of conjunctival scrapings. The presence of blue-stained intracytoplasmic inclusions within epithelial cells is diagnostic. The sensitivity of the test varies from 22% to 95% depending on the technique of specimen collection and the examiner's expertise.

Serum antibody determinations are difficult to perform and available in only a few clinical laboratories. In children with pneumonia, an acute microimmunofluorescence (MIF) serum titer of *C trachomatis*–specific IgM of 1:32 or greater is diagnostic. A 4-fold rise in MIF titer to LGV antigens or a complement fixation titer of 1:32 or greater is suggestive of LGV in the presence of compatible clinical findings.

Indirect laboratory evidence of chlamydial pneumonia includes hyperinflation and bilateral diffuse infiltrates on roentgenograms, eosinophilia of 0.3 to 0.4 × 10^9/L (300–400/µL) or more in peripheral blood counts, and elevated total serum IgG (≥5 g/L [500 mg/dL]) and IgM (≥1.1 g/L [110 mg/dL]) concentrations. However, the absence of these findings does not exclude the diagnosis. Direct antigen tests and culture are now so widely available that a specific diagnosis should be made based on laboratory tests.

Diagnosis of chlamydial disease in a child, adolescent, or adult should prompt investigation for other sexually transmitted diseases, including syphilis, gonorrhea, hepatitis B virus, and human immunodeficiency virus infection. In the case of an infant, examination of the mother and the infant should be considered.

TREATMENT:

- Young infants with **chlamydial conjunctivitis and pneumonia** are treated with oral erythromycin (50 mg/kg per day in 4 divided doses) for 14 days. Oral sulfonamides may be used after the immediate neonatal period for infants who do not tolerate erythromycin. Topical treatment of conjunctivitis is ineffective and unnecessary. Since the efficacy of erythromycin therapy is approximately 80%, a second course sometimes is required.

  An association between orally administered erythromycin and infantile hypertrophic pyloric stenosis (IHPS) has been reported in infants less than 6 weeks of age. The risk of IHPS after treatment with other macrolides (eg, azithromycin and clarithromycin) is unknown. Since confirmation of erythromycin as a contributor to cases of IHPS will require additional investigation, and since alternative therapies are not as well studied, the AAP continues to recommend use of erythromycin for treatment of diseases due to *C trachomatis.* Physicians who prescribe erythromycin to newborn infants should inform parents about the potential risks of developing IHPS and signs of IHPS. Cases of pyloric stenosis following use of oral erythromycin should be reported to MEDWATCH (see MEDWATCH, p 726). The need for treatment of infants can be avoided by screening pregnant women to detect and treat *C trachomatis* infection prior to delivery. A specific diagnosis of *C trachomatis* infection in an infant should prompt treatment of the mother and her sex partner(s).
- Infants born to mothers known to have untreated chlamydial infection are at high risk for infection; however, prophylactic antibiotic treatment is not indicated because the efficacy of such treatment is unknown. Infants should be monitored to ensure appropriate treatment if infection develops. If adequate follow-up cannot be assured, some experts recommend that prophylaxis be considered.
- Treatment of **trachoma** is more difficult, and recommendations for therapy differ. The most widely used therapy is topical treatment with erythromycin, tetracycline, or sulfacetamide ointment twice a day for 2 months or twice a day for the first 5 days of the month for 6 months. Oral erythromycin or doxycycline for 40 days is given if the infection is severe. Azithromycin (a single dose of 20 mg/kg) also is effective.
- For uncomplicated ***C trachomatis* genital tract infection** in adolescents, oral doxycycline (200 mg/d in 2 divided doses) for 7 days or azithromycin in a single 1-g oral dose is recommended. Alternatives include oral erythromycin base (2.0 g/d in 4 divided doses) for 7 days or erythromycin ethylsuccinate (3.2 g/d in 4 divided doses) for 7 days. Erythromycin or azithromycin is the recommended therapy for children between 6 months and 12 years of age; for infants younger than 6 months of age, erythromycin is recommended. Erythromycin is recommended for pregnant women. Azithromycin, 1 g orally,

is an alternative; preliminary data indicate that azithromycin is safe and effective during pregnancy. Doxycycline is contraindicated during pregnancy. Because the efficacy of erythromycin regimens is approximately 80%, a second course of therapy may be required. If a pregnant woman cannot tolerate erythromycin, half doses daily for 14 days may be given. An alternative but less effective regimen is oral amoxicillin (1.5 g/d in 3 divided doses) for 7 to 10 days.

- For **LGV**, doxycycline (200 mg/d in 2 divided doses) for 21 days is the preferred treatment for children 8 years of age and older. Erythromycin or sulfisoxazole for 21 days (each at a dose of 2 g/d in 4 divided doses) are alternative regimens.

Follow-up Testing. Patients do not need to be retested for *Chlamydia* infection after completing treatment with doxycycline or azithromycin unless symptoms persist or reinfection is suspected. Retesting may be considered at 3 or more weeks after completing regimens with erythromycin or amoxicillin.

Isolation of the Hospitalized Patient: Standard precautions are recommended.

Control Measures:

Pregnancy. The identification and treatment of women with *C trachomatis* genital tract infection during pregnancy can prevent disease in the infant. Pregnant women at high risk for *C trachomatis* infection, in particular women younger than 25 years of age and women with new or multiple sex partners, should be targeted for screening. Some experts advocate routine testing of pregnant women at high risk during the first trimester and again during the third trimester.

Infants born to mothers with untreated chlamydial infection should be treated with oral erythromycin (see Treatment, p 210).

Neonatal Chlamydial Conjunctivitis. The recommended topical prophylaxis with silver nitrate, erythromycin, or tetracycline for all newborns for prevention of gonococcal ophthalmia will not prevent neonatal chlamydial conjunctivitis or extraocular infection (see Prevention of Neonatal Ophthalmia, p 735).

Contacts of Infants With* C trachomatis *Conjunctivitis or Pneumonia. Mothers (and their sexual partners) of infected infants also should be treated for *C trachomatis.*

Gynecologic Examination. Sexually active adolescents should be tested routinely for *Chlamydia* infection during gynecologic examination, even if no symptoms are present. Screening of young adult women aged 20 to 24 years also is desirable, particularly women who do not consistently use barrier contraceptives and who have multiple sex partners.

Management of Sexual Partners. All sexual contacts of patients with *C trachomatis* infection, nongonococcal urethritis, mucopurulent cervicitis, epididymitis, or pelvic inflammatory disease should be evaluated and treated for *C trachomatis* infection if the last sexual contact was within 30 days of a symptomatic index patient's onset of symptoms or within 60 days of an asymptomatic index patient's diagnosis. The most recent sexual contact should be treated regardless of the time elapsed since last contact.

LGV. Nonspecific preventive measures for LGV are the same as measures for sexually transmitted diseases in general and include education, case reporting, and avoidance of sexual contact with infected persons.

Clostridial Infections

Botulism and Infant Botulism

(Clostridium botulinum)

Clinical Manifestations: Botulism is a neuroparalytic disorder that can be classified into the following categories: foodborne, infant, wound, and undetermined. The latter occurs in persons older than 12 months of age in whom no food or wound source is implicated. Except for infant botulism, onset of symptoms occurs abruptly within a few hours or evolves gradually over several days. Symmetric, descending, flaccid paralysis occurs, typically involving the bulbar musculature initially and later affecting the somatic musculature. Symmetric paralysis may progress rapidly. Patients with rapidly evolving illness may have generalized weakness and hypotonia initially. Signs and symptoms in older children or adults can include diplopia, blurred vision, dry mouth, dysphagia, dysphonia, and dysarthria. Classically, infant botulism, which occurs predominantly in infants younger than 6 months of age, is preceded by constipation and is manifest as lethargy, poor feeding, weak cry, diminished gag reflex, subtle ocular palsies, and generalized weakness and hypotonia (eg, "floppy infant"). A spectrum of disease ranging from rapidly progressive (eg, apnea, sudden infant death) to mild (eg, constipation, slow feeding) exists.

Etiology: Seven antigenic toxin types of *Clostridium botulinum* have been identified. Human botulism almost always is caused by neurotoxins A, B, E, and F. Types C and D are associated primarily with botulism in birds and mammals. Almost all cases of infant botulism are caused by types A and B.

Epidemiology: Foodborne botulism (median annual cases, 24) results when a food contaminated with spores of *C botulinum* is preserved or stored improperly under anaerobic conditions that permit germination, multiplication, and toxin production. Restaurant-associated outbreaks from foods such as patty-melts, potato salad, and aluminum foil–wrapped baked potatoes illustrate that not all foodborne botulism results from ingestion of improperly prepared home-canned foods, bottled garlic, and cheese sauce. Illness occurs when the unheated or incompletely reheated food is eaten and preformed botulinum toxin is ingested. Foodborne botulism rarely occurs in infants or children because they are less likely to be exposed to foods that might contain botulinum toxin. Botulism is not transmitted from person to person.

Infant botulism (median annual cases, 71) results after ingested spores of *C botulinum* or related species germinate, multiply, and produce botulinum toxin in the intestine, probably through a mechanism of transient permissiveness of the intestinal microflora. In most cases of infant botulism, the source of spores is not identified (and may be airborne from soil or dust), but honey that has not been certified to be free of *C botulinum* spores is an identified and avoidable source. Light and dark corn syrups are not sterilized when packaged, so they also may be contaminated by *C botulinum* spores.

Wound botulism results when *C botulinum* grows in traumatized tissue and produces toxin. Accidental gross trauma or crush injury may be a predisposing event, but during the last decade, injection of contaminated black tar heroin has resulted in the majority of cases.

Immunity to botulinum toxin does not develop in foodborne botulism, even after severe disease.

The usual **incubation period** for foodborne botulism is 12 to 36 hours (range, 6 hours to 8 days). For wound botulism, it is 4 to 14 days between the time of injury and the onset of symptoms. In infant botulism, the incubation period is estimated at 3 to 30 days from the time of exposure to spore-containing honey.

DIAGNOSTIC TESTS: A toxin neutralization bioassay in mice* is used to identify botulinum toxin in serum, stool, or suspect foods. Enriched and selective media are used to culture *C botulinum* from stool and foods. In infant and wound botulism, the diagnosis is made by demonstrating *C botulinum* organisms or toxin in feces or wound exudate or tissue samples. Toxin has been demonstrated in serum in approximately 1% of infants with botulism. To increase the likelihood of diagnosis, both serum and stool should be obtained from all persons with suspected botulism. In foodborne cases, serum specimens collected more than 3 days after ingestion of toxin usually are negative, at which time stool and gastric aspirates are the best diagnostic specimens for culture. Since obtaining a stool specimen may be difficult because of constipation, an enema using sterile nonbacteriostatic water can be given. The most prominent electromyographic finding is an incremental increase of evoked muscle potentials at high-frequency nerve stimulation (20–50 Hz). In addition, a characteristic pattern of brief, small-amplitude, overly abundant motor action potentials can be seen.

TREATMENT:

Meticulous Supportive Care. The most important aspect of therapy in all forms of botulism is meticulous supportive care, particularly respiratory and nutritional.

Antitoxin. A 5-year, randomized, double-blind, placebo-controlled treatment trial of human-derived botulinum antitoxin (formally known as botulinum immune globulin [BIG]) in infant botulism showed a significant reduction in hospital days, mechanical ventilation, and tube feedings in BIG recipients and a $70 000 reduction in hospital cost per case. The California Department of Health Services (24-hour telephone number, 510-540-2646) should be contacted about procurement of BIG. Treatment with BIG should be started as early in the illness as possible and should not be delayed while awaiting laboratory confirmation. Equine botulinum antitoxin also is obtainable and can be administered to adults after testing for hypersensitivity to equine sera if BIG is not available. Approximately 9% of treated persons experience some degree of hypersensitivity reaction to equine sera. Trivalent antitoxin (types A, B, and E) and bivalent autotoxin (types A and B) can be obtained from

* For information, consult your state health department.

the Centers for Disease Control and Prevention (CDC) through state health departments. If contact cannot be made with the state health department, the CDC Drug Service should be contacted (see Appendix I, Directory of Resources, p 743).

Antimicrobial Agents. In infant botulism, antibiotics are used only to treat secondary infections because lysis of intraluminal *C botulinum* could increase the amount of toxin available for absorption. Aminoglycosides can potentiate the paralytic effects of the toxin and should be avoided.

ISOLATION OF THE HOSPITALIZED PATIENT: Standard precautions are recommended.

CONTROL MEASURES:

- Prophylactic equine antitoxin for asymptomatic persons who have ingested a food known to contain botulinum toxin is not recommended. Because of the danger of hypersensitivity reactions, the decision to administer antitoxin requires careful consideration. Consultation about antitoxin use may be obtained from the state health department or the CDC.
- Elimination of ingested toxin may be facilitated by inducing vomiting and by gastric lavage, rapid purgation, and high enemas. These measures should not be used in infant botulism. Enemas should not be administered to persons with illness except to obtain a stool specimen for diagnostic purposes. Exposed persons should have close medical observation.
- Although most sources of spores for infant botulism are unavoidable, honey should not be given to children younger than 12 months of age.
- Contacts of persons with wound or infant botulism are not at an increased risk of acquiring botulism. Botulinum toxoid (types A, B, C, D, and E) is available from the CDC for immunization of laboratory workers whose regular exposure places them at high risk.
- Education to improve home-canning methods should be promoted, but cases also may be restaurant-acquired. Use of a pressure cooker (at 116°C [240.8°F]) is necessary to kill spores of *C botulinum.* Boiling for 10 minutes will destroy the toxin. Time-temperature-pressure requirements vary with the product being heated. In addition, food containers that appear to bulge may contain gas produced by *C botulinum* and should be discarded. Other foods that appear to be spoiled should not be tasted. Cases of suspected botulism should be reported immediately to local and state health departments.

Clostridium difficile

CLINICAL MANIFESTATIONS: Infections include pseudomembranous colitis and antimicrobial-associated diarrhea. Pseudomembranous colitis generally is characterized by diarrhea, abdominal cramps, fever, systemic toxic effects, abdominal tenderness, and passage of stools containing blood and mucus. The colonic mucosa often contains small (2- to 5-mm), raised, yellowish plaques. Characteristically, disease begins while the patient is in a hospital receiving antimicrobial therapy, but it may occur weeks after discharge from the hospital or after discontinuation of therapy.

Rarely, the onset may not be associated with antimicrobial therapy or hospitalization. Severe or fatal disease is more likely to occur in severely neutropenic children with leukemia, in infants with Hirschsprung disease, and in patients with inflammatory bowel disease. Infection also may result only in mild diarrhea or asymptomatic carriage, especially in newborn infants and in children younger than 1 year of age.

ETIOLOGY: *Clostridium difficile* is a spore-forming, obligately anaerobic, gram-positive bacillus. It is the cause of pseudomembranous colitis and of a high percentage of episodes of antimicrobial-associated diarrhea. Disease is related to the action of toxin(s) produced by these vegetative organisms. Two toxins, A and B, have been characterized.

EPIDEMIOLOGY: *Clostridium difficile* can be isolated from soil and frequently is present in the environment. Spores of *C difficile* are acquired from the environment or by fecal-oral transmission from colonized persons. Intestinal colonization rates in healthy neonates and young infants can be as high as 50% but usually are less than 5% in children older than 2 years of age and in adults. Hospitals and child care facilities are major reservoirs for *C difficile.* Risk factors for disease are those that increase exposure to organisms and those that diminish the barrier effect of the normal intestinal flora, allowing *C difficile* to proliferate and elaborate toxin(s) in vivo. Risk factors for acquisition include having an infected roommate, prolonged hospitalization, and presence of symptomatically infected patients on the same hospital ward. Risk factors for developing disease include antimicrobial therapy, repeated enemas, prolonged nasogastric tube insertion, and gastrointestinal tract surgery. Penicillins, clindamycin, and cephalosporins are the antimicrobial drugs most frequently associated with *C difficile* colitis, but colitis has been associated with almost every antimicrobial agent. Although *C difficile* toxin rarely is recovered from stool specimens from asymptomatic adults, it may be recovered from stool specimens from neonates and infants who have no gastrointestinal tract illness. This finding confounds the interpretation of positive toxin assays in patients younger than 12 to 24 months.

The **incubation period** is unknown.

DIAGNOSTIC TESTS: Endoscopic findings of pseudomembranes and hyperemic, friable, rectal mucosa suggest pseudomembranous colitis. To diagnose *C difficile* disease, stool should be tested for the presence of *C difficile* toxins. Testing for toxin is performed by enzyme immunoassay (EIA) or cell cytotoxin assay, which has been the "gold standard" for toxin B. The EIAs are sensitive and easy to perform. Commercially available EIAs that detect both toxins A and B may be used, or an EIA for toxin A may be used in conjunction with cell culture cytotoxicity assay for toxin B. Latex agglutination tests should not be used.

TREATMENT:

- Antimicrobial therapy should be discontinued as soon as possible in patients in whom clinically significant diarrhea or colitis develops.
- Antimicrobial therapy for *C difficile* disease is indicated for patients with severe toxic effects or in whom diarrhea persists after antimicrobial therapy is discontinued.

- Strains of *C difficile* are susceptible to metronidazole and vancomycin, and both are effective. Metronidazole (30 mg/kg per day in 4 divided doses) is the drug of choice for the initial treatment of most patients with colitis. Oral vancomycin (40 mg/kg per day in 4 divided doses) is an alternative drug, but its use should be discouraged because of the potential for promoting vancomycin-resistant organisms. Vancomycin is indicated for patients who do not respond to metronidazole. Metronidazole is effective when given orally or intravenously. Bacitracin is another therapeutic choice; it is administered orally with minimal intestinal tract absorption. Bacitracin and vancomycin are more costly than metronidazole.
- Antimicrobial agents usually are administered for 7 to 10 days.
- As many as 10% to 20% of patients experience a relapse after discontinuing therapy, but the infection usually responds to a second course of the same treatment.
- Cholestyramine resin, which binds toxin, can relieve symptoms. However, its effect has not been evaluated in children with disease caused by *C difficile.* Because cholestyramine also binds vancomycin, the drugs should not be administered concurrently.
- Drugs that decrease intestinal motility should not be given.

ISOLATION OF THE HOSPITALIZED PATIENT: In addition to standard precautions, contact precautions are recommended for the duration of illness.

CONTROL MEASURES:

- Meticulous hand-washing techniques, proper handling of contaminated waste (including diapers) and fomites, and limiting use of antimicrobial agents are the best available methods for control of *C difficile* disease.
- Thorough cleaning of hospital rooms and bathrooms of patients with *C difficile* colitis is essential. Germicide resistance as a cause of survival of *C difficile* in the environment has not been demonstrated.
- In child care settings, children with *C difficile* colitis should be in a separate protected area or excluded from child care for the duration of diarrhea.

Clostridial Myonecrosis

(Gas Gangrene)

CLINICAL MANIFESTATIONS: The onset is heralded by acute pain at the site of the wound, followed by edema, tenderness, exudate, and progression of pain. Systemic findings initially include tachycardia disproportionate to the degree of fever, pallor, diaphoresis, hypotension, renal failure, and, later, alterations in mental status. Crepitus is suggestive, but not pathognomonic, of *Clostridium* infection and is not always present. Diagnosis is based on clinical manifestations, including the characteristic appearance of necrotic muscle at surgery. Untreated gas gangrene can lead to death within hours.

ETIOLOGY: Gas gangrene is caused by *Clostridium* species, most commonly *Clostridium perfringens*, which are large, gram-positive, anaerobic bacilli with blunt ends. Other *Clostridium* species (ie, *Clostridium sordellii*) also can be associated with gas gangrene. Mixed infection with other gram-positive and gram-negative bacteria is frequent.

EPIDEMIOLOGY: Gas gangrene usually results from contamination of open wounds involving muscle. The sources of *Clostridium* species are soil, contaminated objects, and human and animal feces. Dirty surgical or traumatic wounds with significant devitalized tissue and foreign bodies predispose to disease. Nontraumatic gas gangrene occurs occasionally from *Clostridium* organisms in a person's gastrointestinal tract.

The **incubation period** is 6 hours to 3 weeks, usually 2 to 4 days.

DIAGNOSTIC TESTS: Anaerobic cultures of wound exudate, involved soft tissue and muscle, and blood should be performed. Because *Clostridium* species are ubiquitous, their recovery from a wound is not diagnostic unless the appropriate clinical manifestations are present. A Gram-stained smear of wound discharge demonstrating characteristic gram-positive bacilli and absent or sparse polymorphonuclear leukocytes suggests clostridial infection. Tissue samples and aspirates, but not swabs, are appropriate specimens for anaerobic culture. Inoculation of material into culture media in the operating room or aspiration of material into a capped syringe and rapid transport of samples to the laboratory are essential to ensure recovery of anaerobic organisms. A roentgenogram of the affected site may demonstrate gas in the tissue.

TREATMENT:

- Early and complete surgical excision of necrotic tissue and removal of foreign material is the most important therapeutic measure.
- Management of shock, fluid and electrolyte imbalance, hemolytic anemia, and other complications is essential.
- High-dose penicillin G (250 000–400 000 U/kg per day) should be given intravenously. Clindamycin, metronidazole, imipenem-cilastatin or meropenem, and chloramphenicol are alternative drugs for penicillin-sensitive patients.
- Hyperbaric oxygen may be beneficial, but adequately controlled data are not available.
- Treatment with antitoxin is of no value.

ISOLATION OF THE HOSPITALIZED PATIENT: Standard precautions are recommended.

CONTROL MEASURES: In wound management, prompt and careful débridement, flushing of contaminated wounds, and removal of foreign material with standard aseptic surgical techniques should be performed routinely.

Penicillin G (50 000 U/kg per day) or clindamycin (20–30 mg/kg per day) may be of prophylactic value in patients with grossly contaminated wounds.

Clostridium perfringens Food Poisoning

CLINICAL MANIFESTATIONS: Food poisoning is characterized by a sudden onset of watery diarrhea and moderate to severe, crampy, midepigastric pain. Vomiting and fever are uncommon. Symptoms usually resolve within 24 hours. The absence of fever in most patients differentiates *C perfringens* foodborne disease from shigellosis and salmonellosis, and the infrequency of vomiting and longer incubation period contrast with the clinical features of foodborne disease associated with heavy metals, *Staphylococcus aureus* enterotoxins, and fish and shellfish toxins. Diarrheal illness caused by *Bacillus cereus* enterotoxin may be indistinguishable from that caused by *C perfringens.* Enteritis necroticans (known locally as pigbel) is a cause of severe illness and death due to *C perfringens* food poisoning among children in Papua, New Guinea.

ETIOLOGY: Food poisoning is caused by a heat-labile toxin produced in vivo by *C perfringens* type A; type C causes enteritis necroticans.

EPIDEMIOLOGY: *Clostridium perfringens* is ubiquitous in the environment and frequently is present in raw meat and poultry. Spores of *C perfringens* survive cooking. The spores germinate and multiply during cooling and holding at room temperatures. Once ingested, an enterotoxin produced by the organisms in the lower intestine is responsible for symptoms. Beef, poultry, gravies, and dried or precooked foods are common sources. Infection usually is acquired at banquets or institutions (eg, schools and camps) or from food caterers or restaurants where food is prepared in large quantities and kept warm for prolonged periods. Illness is not transmissible from person to person.

The **incubation period** is 6 to 24 hours, usually 8 to 12 hours.

DIAGNOSTIC TESTS: Because the fecal flora of healthy persons frequently includes *C perfringens,* counts of at least 10^6 *C perfringens* spores per gram of feces obtained within 48 hours of onset of illness are required to support the diagnosis in ill persons. The diagnosis also can be established by detection of *C perfringens* enterotoxin in stool by commercially available kits. To confirm *C perfringens* as the cause, the concentration of organisms should be at least 10^5 per gram in the epidemiologically implicated food. Although *C perfringens* is an anaerobe, special transport conditions are unnecessary because the spores are durable. Stool rather than rectal swabs should be collected.

TREATMENT: Usually no treatment is required. Oral rehydration or, occasionally, intravenous fluid and electrolyte replacement may be indicated for patients with severe dehydration. Antibiotics are not indicated.

ISOLATION OF THE HOSPITALIZED PATIENT: Standard precautions are recommended.

CONTROL MEASURES: Preventive measures depend on limiting proliferation of *C perfringens* in foods by maintaining food warmer than 60°C (140°F) or cooler than 7°C (45°F). Meat dishes should be served hot shortly after cooking. Foods should never be held at room temperature to cool, but should be refrigerated after removal from warming devices or serving tables. Foods should be reheated to at least 74°C (165.2°F) or higher before serving. Roasts, stews, and similar dishes should be divided into small quantities for cooking and refrigeration to limit the time such foods are at temperatures at which *C perfringens* replicates.

Coccidioidomycosis

CLINICAL MANIFESTATIONS: The primary infection is acquired by the respiratory route and is asymptomatic or inapparent in 60% of children. Symptomatic disease may resemble influenza, with malaise, fever, cough, myalgia, headache, and chest pain. A diffuse erythematous maculopapular rash, erythema multiforme, erythema nodosum, and/or arthralgias frequently occur and may be the only clinical manifestations in some children. Chronic pulmonary lesions are rare.

Extrapulmonary infection is rare, usually follows trauma, and includes cutaneous lesions or soft tissue infections with associated regional lymphadenitis.

Disseminated disease occurs in fewer than 1% of infected persons. The skin, bones and joints, central nervous system (CNS), and lungs are the affected sites. Limited dissemination to one or more sites is frequent in children. Meningitis is a serious manifestation of disseminated disease and can be fatal if untreated. Congenital infection is rare.

ETIOLOGY: *Coccidioides immitis* is a dimorphic fungus. In soil, it exists in the hyphal phase. Infectious arthroconidia produced in some of the hyphae subsequently become airborne spores that on inhalation or inoculation infect the host. In tissues of the infected host, spores enlarge to form spherules. Mature spherules release endospores that develop into new spherules and continue the tissue cycle.

EPIDEMIOLOGY: *Coccidioides immitis* is found extensively in soil and is endemic in the southwestern United States, northern Mexico, and certain areas of Central and South America. Climatic conditions (ie, hot summers and infrequent winter freezes) combine with alkaline soil conditions and alternating periods of rain and drought to produce favorable circumstances for propagation of arthroconidia and their dissemination by aerosols. Persons are infected through inhalation of dust-borne arthroconidia. Infection provides lifelong immunity. Person-to-person transmission of coccidioidomycosis does not occur. African Americans, Filipinos, pregnant women, neonates, elderly persons, and immunocompromised persons have an increased risk of dissemination and fatal outcome.

The **incubation period** is 10 to 16 days; the range is from less than 1 week to approximately 1 month.

DIAGNOSTIC TESTS: Serologic tests are useful to confirm diagnoses and provide prognostic information. The immunoglobulin (Ig) M response can be detected by latex agglutination, enzyme immunoassay (EIA), immunodiffusion, or tube precipitin. Latex agglutination is a rapid sensitive test that lacks specificity; hence, positive results should be confirmed by other tests. An IgM response is detectable 1 to 3 weeks after symptoms appear and lasts 3 to 4 months in most cases.

The IgG response can be detected by immunodiffusion, EIA, or complement fixation (CF). Complement fixation antibodies in serum usually are of low titer and transient if the disease is asymptomatic or mild. High (≥1:32) persistent titers occur in severe disease and almost always in disseminated infection. Cerebrospinal fluid (CSF) antibodies also are detectable by CF. The concentration and persistence of antibody titers in serum from patients with disseminated severe disease and in CSF specimens from patients with meningitis are useful prognostically and for guiding treatment. Increasing serum and CSF titers indicate progressive disease, while decreasing titers suggest improvement. Low or nondetectable titers in immunocompromised patients should be interpreted with caution.

Skin tests may be useful for diagnosis. A delayed hypersensitivity reaction to a coccidioidin or spherulin skin test is indicative of past or current infection. The spherule skin test is preferred for general use, and conversion of the result from negative to positive in a patient with a clinically compatible syndrome strongly suggests coccidioidomycosis. A positive skin test can appear from 10 to 45 days after infection, but anergy is common in disseminated disease, and overreliance on skin test results can lead to errors in diagnosis.

Spherules as large as 80 µm in diameter, in selected instances, can be visualized in infected body fluids and biopsy specimens of skin lesions or organs. Culture of the organism is possible but is potentially hazardous to laboratory personnel, since spherules can convert to arthroconidia-bearing mycelia on culture plates. Suspect cultures should be sealed at the outset and thereafter handled only by trained personnel using appropriate safety equipment and procedures. A DNA probe can identify *C immitis* in cultures, thereby reducing the risk of exposure to infectious fungi.

TREATMENT: Antifungal therapy is not indicated for uncomplicated primary infection.

Amphotericin B is the recommended initial therapy for severe progressive disseminated infection not involving the CNS and for immunocompromised patients, such as patients with human immunodeficiency virus (HIV) infection (see Drugs for Invasive and Other Serious Fungal Infections, Table 4.6, p 672). Fluconazole is recommended for CNS infections. Fluconazole and itraconazole also are useful for treatment of less severe disseminated infections. For CNS infections unresponsive to fluconazole, intravenous amphotericin B therapy is augmented by repetitive CSF instillation of this drug. A subcutaneous reservoir can facilitate administration into the cisternal space or lateral ventricle, although technical difficulties are frequent with this route of therapy. Orally administered fluconazole and itraconazole have suppressed coccidioidal meningitis in many patients, but therapy probably must be continued for the lifetime of such patients.

In some localized infections with sinuses, fistulae, or abscesses, amphotericin B has been instilled or used for irrigation.

The duration of amphotericin B therapy is variable and depends on the site(s) of involvement, clinical response, and mycologic and immunologic test results. In general, therapy is continued until clinical and laboratory evidence indicates that the active infection has subsided. The minimum duration of treatment for disseminated coccidioidomycosis is 1 month. The required duration of treatment with azoles is uncertain, except for patients with CNS infection or underlying HIV infection for whom treatment is lifelong.

Surgical débridement or excision of lesions in bone and lung has been advocated for localized, symptomatic, persistent, resistant, or progressive lesions.

Isolation of the Hospitalized Patient: Standard precautions are recommended. Care should be taken in handling, changing, and discarding dressings, casts, and similar materials in which arthroconidial contamination could occur.

Control Measures: Measures to control dust are recommended in endemic areas at construction sites, archaeological projects, or where other activities cause excessive soil disturbance. Immunocompromised persons residing in or traveling to endemic areas should be counseled to avoid exposure to activities that may aerosolize spores in contaminated soil.

Coronaviruses

Clinical Manifestations: Coronaviruses are a common cause of upper respiratory tract infection in adults and children and occasionally have been implicated in lower respiratory tract disease. Coronavirus-like particles, not confirmed as coronavirus, have been associated with several outbreaks of diarrhea in nurseries and, rarely, with neonatal necrotizing enterocolitis in infants.

Etiology: Coronaviruses are RNA viruses that are large (80 to 160 nm), enveloped with lipid-soluble coats, and pleomorphic (spherical or elliptical). At least 2 distinct antigenic groups of respiratory coronaviruses have been identified.

Epidemiology: Human coronaviruses most likely are transmitted via respiratory tract secretions, possibly by small particle and droplet aerosols; transmission is facilitated by close contact. Although several animal coronaviruses have antigens in common with human strains, no evidence implicates animals as reservoirs or vectors for human disease. The distribution of coronaviruses is worldwide. In temperate climates, outbreaks occur in the winter. Young children have the highest infection rate during outbreaks. The period of communicability is unknown but probably persists for the duration of respiratory tract symptoms.

The **incubation period** is usually 2 to 5 days.

Diagnostic Tests: Diagnostic tests, including antibody assays, for human coronavirus infection are not available commercially. Most strains cannot be isolated by the methods commonly used in diagnostic virology laboratories. Viral particles have been visualized by immune electron microscopy and viral antigens detected by immunoassay.

TREATMENT: Supportive.

ISOLATION OF THE HOSPITALIZED PATIENT: In addition to standard precautions, contact isolation is recommended for the duration of symptoms for diapered and incontinent children with possible enteric coronavirus infection.

CONTROL MEASURES: None.

Cryptococcus neoformans Infections

CLINICAL MANIFESTATIONS: Primary infection is acquired by inhalation of aerosolized fungal elements and often is inapparent or mild. Pulmonary disease, when symptomatic, is characterized by cough, hemoptysis, chest pain, and constitutional symptoms. Chest radiographs may reveal a solitary nodule or focal or diffuse infiltrates. Hematogenous dissemination to the central nervous system, bones and joints, skin, and mucous membranes can occur, but dissemination is rare in children without defects in cell-mediated immunity (eg, transplantation, malignant neoplasm, collagen-vascular disease, long-term corticosteroid administration, or sarcoidosis). Usually, several sites are infected, but manifestations of involvement of one site predominate. Cryptococcal meningitis, the most common and serious form of cryptococcal disease, often follows an indolent course. Symptoms are characteristic of meningitis, meningoencephalitis, or space-occupying lesions but may manifest as only behavioral changes. Cryptococcal fungemia, without apparent organ involvement, occurs in patients with human immunodeficiency virus (HIV) infection but is uncommon in children. Cryptococcosis is one of the acquired immunodeficiency syndrome (AIDS)-defining diseases.

ETIOLOGY: *Cryptococcus neoformans,* an encapsulated yeast that grows at 37°C (98°F), is the only species of the genus *Cryptococcus* considered to be a human pathogen.

EPIDEMIOLOGY: *Cryptococcus neoformans* var *neoformans* is isolated primarily from soil contaminated with bird droppings and causes most human infections, especially infections in immunocompromised hosts. *Cryptococcus neoformans* var *gattii* occurs most commonly in tropical and subtropical regions and causes disease primarily in immunocompetent persons. Acquisition begins by inhalation of airborne organisms from contaminated soil. Person-to-person transmission does not occur. *Cryptococcus* species infect 5% to 10% of adults with AIDS, but infection is uncommon in HIV-infected children.

The **incubation period** is unknown.

DIAGNOSTIC TESTS: Encapsulated yeast cells can be visualized by India ink or other stains of cerebrospinal fluid (CSF) containing 10^3 or more colony-forming units of yeast per milliliter. Definitive diagnosis requires isolation of the organism from body fluid or tissue. The lysis-centrifugation method is the most sensitive technique for recovery of *C neoformans* from blood cultures. Media containing cycloheximide, which inhibits growth of *C neoformans,* should not be used. Sabouraud glucose agar is optimal for isolation of *Cryptococcus* from sputum, bronchopulmonary lavage, tissue, or CSF specimens. Few organisms may be present in the CSF, and large quantities of CSF may be needed to recover the organism. The latex agglutination and enzyme immunoassay tests for detection of cryptococcal capsular polysaccharide antigen in serum or CSF are excellent rapid diagnostic tests. Antigen detection in CSF or serum is positive in 90% of patients with cryptococcal meningitis. Cryptococcal antibody testing is useful, but skin testing is of no value.

TREATMENT: Amphotericin B, 0.5 to 0.7 mg/kg per day (see Drugs for Invasive and Other Serious Fungal Infections, p 672), in combination with oral flucytosine is indicated for patients with meningeal and other serious cryptococcal infections. Combination antifungal therapy probably is superior to amphotericin B alone. Flucytosine can induce cytopenia, which often necessitates discontinuation of the medication, especially in HIV-infected patients, as well as hepatic dysfunction, rash, and diarrhea, especially in patients with azotemia. When flucytosine is used, serum concentrations should be monitored. Patients with meningitis should receive combination therapy for at least 2 weeks or until CSF culture results are negative; at least 6 weeks of total treatment should be completed with amphotericin B or fluconazole alone. Patients with HIV infection should be treated for longer periods than non–HIV-infected patients. Patients with less severe disease may be treated with fluconazole or itraconazole, but data on use of these drugs for children with *C neoformans* infection are limited.

Patients infected with HIV who have completed initial therapy for cryptococcosis should receive lifelong maintenance with low-dose fluconazole; adult dosages range from 200 mg to 600 mg/d.

ISOLATION OF THE HOSPITALIZED PATIENT: Standard precautions are recommended.

CONTROL MEASURES: None.

Cryptosporidiosis

CLINICAL MANIFESTATIONS: Frequent, nonbloody, watery diarrhea is the most common presenting symptom, although infection can be asymptomatic. Other symptoms include abdominal cramps, fatigue, vomiting, anorexia, and weight loss. Fever and vomiting are relatively common among children and often lead to a misdiagnosis of viral gastroenteritis. In infected immunocompetent persons, including children, the diarrheal illness is self-limited, usually lasting 1 to 20 days (mean, 10 days). In immunocompromised persons, especially those with human immunodeficiency virus infection, chronic severe diarrhea can develop resulting in malnutrition, dehydration, and death. Pulmonary, biliary tract, or disseminated infection can occur in immunocompromised persons, although infection usually is limited to the gastrointestinal tract.

ETIOLOGY: *Cryptosporidium parvum* is a spore-forming coccidian protozoan.

EPIDEMIOLOGY: *Cryptosporidium parvum* has been found in a variety of hosts, including mammals, birds, and reptiles. Extensive waterborne outbreaks have occurred associated with contamination of municipal water and exposure to contaminated swimming pools. In children, the incidence of cryptosporidiosis is greatest in the summer and early fall, corresponding to the outdoor swimming season. Transmission to humans can occur from farm livestock, particularly young animals such as those found in petting zoos, or pets. Person-to-person transmission occurs and can cause outbreaks in child care centers, with rates of 30% to 60% reported. *Cryptosporidium parvum* also causes traveler's diarrhea. Since the parasite is resistant to chlorine, appropriately functioning water filtration systems are critical for the safety of public water supplies. Most sand filters used for swimming pools are ineffective for removing oocysts from contaminated water.

The median **incubation period** is 7 days, with a range of 2 to 14 days.

Oocysts continue to be detected in stool a mean of 7 days after symptoms resolve. In most people, shedding of *C parvum* stops within 2 weeks, but in a few, shedding continues for up to 2 months.

DIAGNOSTIC TESTS: The finding of oocysts on microscopic examination of stool specimens is diagnostic. Unfortunately, routine laboratory examination of stool for ova and parasites is inadequate to detect *C parvum,* so health care professionals should ask laboratory personnel to test specifically for *C parvum.* The sucrose flotation method or formalin-ethyl acetate method is used to concentrate oocysts in stool before staining with a modified Kinyoun acid-fast stain. Monoclonal antibody–based fluorescein-conjugated stain for oocysts in stool and an enzyme immunoassay (EIA) for detecting antigen in stool are available commercially. With EIA methods, false-positive results may occur, and confirmation by microscopy may be necessary. Since shedding can be intermittent, at least 3 stool specimens collected on separate days should be examined before considering the test results to be negative. Oocysts are small (4–6 µm in diameter) and can be missed in a rapid scan of a slide. Organisms also can be identified in intestinal biopsy tissue or intestinal fluid.

TREATMENT: Other than rehydration and correction of electrolyte abnormalities, definitive therapy has not been established. Paromomycin, azithromycin, or nitazoxanide, an investigational agent with potential benefit, may be beneficial for some persons (see Drugs for Parasitic Infections, p 693). In immunocompromised patients with cryptosporidiosis, orally administered human serum immunoglobulin or bovine colostrum has been beneficial.

ISOLATION OF THE HOSPITALIZED PATIENT: In addition to standard precautions, contact precautions are recommended for diapered or incontinent children.

CONTROL MEASURES: In waterborne outbreaks due to contaminated drinking water, advisories to boil water may be issued to prevent cases until proper water treatment is restored. Persons with diarrhea should not use public recreational water (eg, swimming pools, lakes, ponds), and persons with a diagnosis of cryptosporidiosis should not use recreational waters for 2 weeks after symptoms resolve.

Cutaneous Larva Migrans

CLINICAL MANIFESTATIONS: Nematode larvae produce pruritic, reddish papules at the site of skin entry. As the larvae migrate through the skin and advance several millimeters to a few centimeters a day, intensely pruritic, serpiginous tracks are formed. Larval activity can continue for several weeks or months but eventually is self-limiting. An advancing serpiginous tunnel in the skin with an associated intense pruritus is virtually pathognomonic. Rarely, in infections with a large burden of parasites, pneumonitis (Löeffler syndrome), which can be severe, and myositis may follow skin lesions. Occasionally, the larvae reach the intestine and may cause eosinophilic enteritis.

ETIOLOGY: Infective larvae of cat and dog hookworms, ie, *Ancylostoma braziliense* and *Ancylostoma caninum,* are the usual causes. Other skin-penetrating nematodes are occasional causes.

EPIDEMIOLOGY: Cutaneous larva migrans is a disease of children, utility workers, gardeners, sunbathers, and others who come in contact with soil contaminated with cat and dog feces. In the United States, the disease is most prevalent in the Southeast.

DIAGNOSTIC TESTS: Since the diagnosis usually is made clinically, biopsies are not indicated. Biopsy specimens typically demonstrate an eosinophilic inflammatory infiltrate, but the migrating parasite is not visualized. Eosinophilia occurs in some cases. Larvae have been detected in sputum and gastric washings in patients with the rare complication of pneumonitis. Serologic testing with an enzyme immunoassay or Western blot using antigens of *A caninum* may help detect occult infections. These tests, however, generally are available only in research laboratories and are not warranted routinely.

TREATMENT: The disease usually is self-limited, with spontaneous cure after several weeks or months. Albendazole and ivermectin have been reported to be effective. Thiabendazole given orally or topically relieves cutaneous symptoms.

ISOLATION OF THE HOSPITALIZED PATIENT: Standard precautions are recommended.

CONTROL MEASURES: Skin contact with moist soil contaminated with animal feces should be avoided. In warm climates, beaches should be kept free of dog and cat feces.

Cyclospora Infections

CLINICAL MANIFESTATIONS: Profuse, nonbloody, watery diarrhea is the most common but not always the initial symptom of cyclosporiasis. An influenza-like illness may precede development of diarrhea in some cases. Vomiting, fatigue, anorexia, abdominal bloating or cramping, and weight loss also can occur. Fever occurs in approximately 50% of patients. Infection usually is self-limited, but diarrhea and systemic symptoms can persist for weeks. Relapse of symptoms also is common in untreated patients. Prolonged symptoms may persist in immunocompromised patients.

ETIOLOGY: *Cyclospora cayetanensis* is a coccidian parasite. This organism previously was called "cyanobacteriumlike" or "coccidianlike" in reported outbreaks of diarrhea.

EPIDEMIOLOGY: *Cyclospora cayetanensis* is found throughout the world and is endemic in some countries, such as Nepal, Peru, and Haiti. Outbreaks have been associated with contaminated food and water. Outbreaks in the United States have been associated with imported raspberries and with other fresh produce. Agricultural water used for spraying may contaminate berries, and their delicate surfaces make thorough cleaning difficult. *Cyclospora cayetanensis* has been reported as a cause of traveler's diarrhea and of isolated community-acquired cases of diarrhea.

Direct animal-to-human or person-to-person transmission has not been documented probably because excreted oocysts take days to weeks under certain environmental conditions to sporulate and become infectious.

The **incubation period** is approximately 7 days (range, 1–14 days).

DIAGNOSTIC TESTS: Diagnosis is made by identification of the oocyst in stool. Oocysts are 8 to 10 µm in diameter. The organisms can be seen after modified acid-fast staining, but also can be detected with a safranin-based stain and heating of fecal smears and by autofluorescence.

TREATMENT: Trimethoprim-sulfamethoxazole for 7 days is effective therapy.

ISOLATION OF THE HOSPITALIZED PATIENT: The risk of nosocomial infection is unknown. Standard precautions should be used.

CONTROL MEASURES: Fresh produce should be washed thoroughly before it is eaten. This precaution, however, may not entirely eliminate the risk of transmission.

Cytomegalovirus Infection

CLINICAL MANIFESTATIONS: Manifestations of acquired human cytomegalovirus (CMV) infection vary with the age and immunocompetence of the host. Asymptomatic infections are the most common, particularly in children. An infectious mononucleosis-like syndrome with prolonged fever and mild hepatitis, occurring in the absence of heterophil antibody production, can occur in adolescents and adults. Pneumonia, colitis, and retinitis occur in immunocompromised hosts (particularly those receiving treatment for malignant neoplasms), in human immunodeficiency virus (HIV) infection, or in persons receiving immunosuppressive therapy for organ transplantation.

Congenital infection has a spectrum of manifestations but is usually asymptomatic. Some congenitally infected infants who seem asymptomatic at birth are later found to have a hearing loss or learning disability. Approximately 5% of infants with congenital CMV infection have profound involvement, with intrauterine growth retardation, neonatal jaundice, purpura, hepatosplenomegaly, microcephaly, brain damage, intracerebral calcifications, and retinitis. Approximately 15% of infants born after maternal primary infection will have one or more sequelae of intrauterine infection.

Infection acquired at birth or shortly thereafter from maternal cervical secretions or human milk usually is not associated with clinical illness. Infection resulting from transfusion from CMV-seropositive donors to preterm infants has been associated with lower respiratory tract disease.

ETIOLOGY: Human CMV, a DNA virus, is a member of the herpesvirus group.

EPIDEMIOLOGY: Cytomegalovirus is highly species-specific, and only human strains are known to produce human disease. This virus is ubiquitous and is transmitted horizontally (by direct person-to-person contact with virus-containing secretions), vertically (from mother to infant before, during, or after birth), and via infected blood transfusions (see Blood Safety, p 88). Infections have no seasonal predilection. Cytomegalovirus persists in latent form after a primary infection, and reactivation can occur years later, particularly under conditions of immunosuppression.

Horizontal transmission is probably the result of salivary contamination or sexual transmission, but contact with infected urine also can have a role. Spread of CMV in households and child care centers is well documented. Excretion rates in child care centers can be as high as 70% in children 1 to 3 years of age. Young children can transmit CMV to their parents and other caregivers, such as child care staff (see also Children in Out-of-Home Child Care, p 105). In adolescents and adults, sexual transmission also occurs, as evidenced by virus in seminal and cervical fluids.

Seropositive healthy persons have latent CMV in their leukocytes and tissues; hence, blood transfusions and organ transplantation can result in viral transmission. Severe CMV disease is more likely to occur if the recipient is seronegative or is a premature infant. Latent CMV frequently will reactivate in immunosuppressed persons and can result in disease if the immunosuppression is severe (eg, patients with acquired immunodeficiency syndrome and solid-organ and bone marrow transplant recipients).

Vertical transmission of CMV to an infant occurs by one of the following methods: (1) in utero by transplacental passage of maternal bloodborne virus, (2) at birth by passage through an infected maternal genital tract, or (3) postnatally by ingestion of CMV-positive human milk. Approximately 1% of all live-born infants are infected in utero and excrete CMV at birth. While in utero fetal infection can occur after maternal primary infection or after reactivation of infection during pregnancy, sequelae are far more common in infants after maternal primary infection, with 10% to 20% diagnosed with mental retardation or sensorineural deafness in childhood and 5% having manifestations evident at birth.

Maternal cervical infection is common, resulting in exposure of many infants to CMV at birth. Cervical excretion rates are highest among young mothers in lower socioeconomic groups. Although interstitial pneumonia caused by CMV can develop during the early months of life, most infected infants remain asymptomatic. Similarly, although symptomatic disease can occur in seronegative infants fed CMV-infected milk from milk banks, most infants infected from ingestion of human milk do not develop clinical illness, most likely because of the presence of passively transferred maternal antibody. For infants who acquire infection from maternal cervical secretions or human milk, premature infants are at greater risk of symptomatic disease and sequelae than are term infants.

The **incubation period** for horizontally transmitted CMV infections in households is unknown. Infection usually manifests 3 to 12 weeks after blood transfusions and between 1 and 4 months after tissue transplantation.

DIAGNOSTIC TESTS: The diagnosis of CMV is confounded by the ubiquity of the virus, the high rate of asymptomatic excretion, the frequency of reactivated infections, development of serum immunoglobulin (Ig) M CMV-specific antibody in some episodes of reactivation, and concurrent infection with other pathogens.

Virus can be isolated in cell culture from urine, pharynx, peripheral blood leukocytes, human milk, semen, cervical secretions, and other tissues and body fluids. Examination of cells shed in urine for intranuclear inclusions is an insensitive test.

Recovery of virus from a target organ provides unequivocal evidence that the disease is caused by CMV infection. However, a presumptive diagnosis can be made on the basis of a 4-fold antibody titer rise in paired serum samples or by virus excretion. Techniques for detection of viral DNA in tissues and some fluids, especially cerebrospinal fluid, by polymerase chain reaction or hybridization are available from specialty laboratories. Detection of pp65 antigen in white blood cells is used to detect infection in immunocompromised hosts.

Complement fixation is the least sensitive serologic method for diagnosis of CMV infection and should not be used to establish previous infection or passively acquired maternal antibody. Various immunofluorescence assays, indirect hemagglutination, latex agglutination, and enzyme immunoassays are preferred for this purpose.

Proof of congenital infection requires obtaining specimens within 3 weeks of birth. Virus isolation is considered diagnostic. Differentiation between intrauterine and perinatal infection is difficult later in infancy, unless clinical manifestations of the former, such as chorioretinitis or ventriculitis, are present. A strongly positive test for serum IgM anti-CMV antibody is suggestive during early infancy but not diagnostic and is less useful during later infancy.

TREATMENT: Ganciclovir (see Antiviral Drugs for Non-HIV Infections, p 675) is beneficial for treatment of retinitis caused by acquired or recurrent CMV infection in HIV-infected patients. This drug is approved in the United States for treatment of severe retinitis in immunocompromised adults. Limited data in children suggest that safety and efficacy are similar to those in adults. The combination of oral ganciclovir and intraocular ganciclovir implant is efficacious in adults with CMV retinitis, but data in children are not available. Ganciclovir often is useful in other types of CMV organ involvement. Although ganciclovir has been used to treat some congenitally infected infants, it is not recommended routinely because of insufficient efficacy data. In bone marrow transplant recipients, the combination of CMV Immune Globulin Intravenous (CMV-IGIV) and ganciclovir, given intravenously, has been reported to be synergistic in treatment of CMV pneumonia. Foscarnet also has been approved for treatment of CMV retinitis and is an alternative drug (see Antiviral Drugs for Non-HIV Infections, p 675). This drug is more toxic but may be advantageous for some patients with HIV infection, such as those with disease caused by ganciclovir-resistant virus or those unable to tolerate ganciclovir. Cidofovir is efficacious for treatment of CMV retinitis in adults, but it has not been studied in children. Ganciclovir sustained-release implant is available for adults and adolescents. Cidofovir is nephrotoxic. Formivirsen is an antisense drug recently licensed for intraocular administration.

Cytomegalovirus disease in HIV-infected patients is not cured by currently available antiviral agents. However, treatment with highly active antiretroviral therapy has significantly decreased severity and the need for long-term suppression.

ISOLATION OF THE HOSPITALIZED PATIENT: Standard precautions are recommended. Since CMV is spread by intimate contact with infectious secretions, hand washing after exposure to secretions is particularly important for pregnant personnel.

CONTROL MEASURES:

Care of Exposed Persons. When caring for all children, hand washing, particularly after changing diapers, is advised to reduce the transmission of CMV. Since asymptomatic excretion of CMV is common in persons of all ages, the child with congenital CMV infection should not be treated differently from other children and should not be excluded from school or institutions. Institutional screening programs for CMV-excreting children are not justifiable.

Although unrecognized exposure to persons asymptomatically shedding CMV is likely to be frequent, concern arises when immunocompromised or pregnant patients or health care personnel are exposed to patients with clinically recognizable CMV infection. Serologic testing can be used to identify nonimmune persons. If indicated, follow-up serologic testing can establish whether infection has occurred, but routine serologic screening is not recommended.

Prevention of exposure of severely immunocompromised patients to recognized cases of CMV infection is prudent. Since unrecognized exposure may occur, infection control procedures, such as careful hand washing and other hygienic practices, should be used.

Pregnant personnel who may be in contact with CMV-infected patients should be counseled about the potential risks of acquisition and urged to practice good hygiene, particularly hand washing. Approximately 1% of infants in most newborn nurseries and a higher percentage of older children excrete CMV without clinical manifestations. Risks to the fetus are greatest during the first half of gestation. Amniocentesis has been used in several small series of patients to establish the presence of intrauterine infection.

Child Care (see also Children in Out-of-Home Child Care, p 105). Educational programs about the epidemiology of CMV, its potential risks, and appropriate hygienic measures to minimize occupationally acquired infection should be provided for female workers in child care centers. Risk seems to be greatest for child care personnel who provide care for children younger than 2 years of age. Routine serologic screening of staff at child care centers for antibody to CMV is not recommended.

Immunoprophylaxis. Cytomegalovirus IGIV has been developed for prophylaxis of disease in seronegative transplant recipients. The initial dose is 150 mg/kg and is followed by doses once every 2 weeks at a gradually reduced dose for 16 weeks. Cytomegalovirus IGIV seems to be moderately effective in kidney and liver transplant recipients. Results of studies of its use in the prevention of CMV transmission to newborn infants are inconclusive. Evaluation of investigational vaccines in healthy volunteers and renal transplant recipients is in progress.

Prevention of Transmission by Blood Transfusion. Transmission of CMV by blood transfusion to preterm infants or others has been virtually eliminated by the use of CMV antibody–negative donors, by freezing Red Blood Cells in glycerol before administration, by removal of the buffy coat, or by filtration to remove White Blood Cells.

Prevention of Transmission by Human Milk. Pasteurization or freezing of donated human milk can reduce the likelihood of CMV transmission. If fresh donated milk is needed for infants born to CMV antibody–negative mothers, providing these infants with milk from only CMV antibody–negative women should be considered. For further information on breastfeeding, see Human Milk (p 98).

Prevention of Transmission in Transplant Recipients. Cytomegalovirus antibody–negative persons who receive tissue from CMV-seropositive persons are at high risk for CMV disease. If such circumstances cannot be avoided, administration of CMV-IGIV is beneficial for reducing this risk. Treatment of transplant recipients with acyclovir or ganciclovir at the onset of CMV viremia may prevent serious CMV disease.

Diphtheria

CLINICAL MANIFESTATIONS: Diphtheria usually occurs as membranous nasopharyngitis or obstructive laryngotracheitis. These local infections are associated with a low-grade fever and the gradual onset of manifestations during 1 to 2 days. Less commonly, the disease presents as cutaneous, vaginal, conjunctival, or otic infections. Cutaneous diphtheria is more common in tropical areas and among the homeless. Serious complications of diphtheria include upper airway obstruction caused by extensive membrane formation, myocarditis, and peripheral neuropathies.

ETIOLOGY: *Corynebacterium diphtheriae* is an irregularly staining, gram-positive, non–spore-forming, nonmotile, pleomorphic bacillus with 3 colony types (mitis, intermedius, and gravis). Strains of *C diphtheriae* may be toxigenic or nontoxigenic. Extracellular toxin consisting of an enzymatically active A domain and a binding B domain is mediated by bacteriophage infection of the bacterium and is not related to colony type.

EPIDEMIOLOGY: Humans are the only known reservoir of *C diphtheriae,* with periods of excretion of organisms in discharges from the nose, throat, eye, and skin lesions for 2 to 6 weeks after infection. In patients treated with an appropriate antimicrobial agent, communicability usually lasts less than 4 days. Occasionally, chronic carriage occurs even after administration of antimicrobial therapy. Transmission results primarily from intimate contact with a patient or carrier; rarely, fomites and foodborne sources serve as vehicles of transmission. Illness is most common in groups living in crowded conditions. Infection can occur in immunized and partially immunized persons and in persons who are not immunized; disease is most common and most severe in persons who are not immunized or who are inadequately immunized. The incidence of respiratory diphtheria is greatest in the autumn and winter, but summer epidemics may occur in warm moist climates in which skin infections are prevalent. Since 1990, epidemic diphtheria has occurred throughout the newly independent states of the former Soviet Union, including Russia, the Ukraine, and the central Asian republics. The case-fatality rate has ranged from 3% to 23% in these epidemics.

The **incubation period** usually is 2 to 7 days but occasionally longer.

DIAGNOSTIC TESTS: Specimens for culture should be obtained from the nose, throat, or any mucosal or cutaneous lesion. Material should be obtained from beneath the membrane, or a portion of the membrane itself should be submitted for culture. Because special media are required, laboratory personnel should be notified that *C diphtheriae* is suspected. In remote areas, throat swabs can be placed in silica gel packs or tellurite enrichment medium and sent to a reference laboratory for culture. Direct-stained smears and fluorescent antibody–stained smears are unreliable. When *C diphtheriae* is recovered, the strain should be tested for toxigenicity at a laboratory recommended by state and local authorities. All *C diphtheriae* isolates also should be sent through the state health department to the Diphtheria Laboratory, National Center for Infectious Diseases of the Centers for Disease Control and Prevention (CDC).

TREATMENT:

Antitoxin. Because the condition of patients with diphtheria may deteriorate rapidly, a single dose of equine antitoxin should be administered on the basis of clinical diagnosis, even before culture results are available. To neutralize toxin as rapidly as possible, the preferred route of administration is intravenous. Before intravenous administration, however, tests for sensitivity to horse serum should be performed with a 1:1000 dilution of antitoxin in saline (see Sensitivity Tests for Reactions to Animal Sera, p 48). If the patient is sensitive to equine antitoxin, desensitization is necessary (see Desensitization to Animal Sera, p 49). Although intravenous immunoglobulin preparations contain antibodies to diphtheria toxin, their use for therapy of cutaneous or respiratory tract diphtheria has not been approved, and optimal dosages have not been established. Antitoxin can be obtained from the National Immunization Program of the CDC (see Directory of Resources, p 743). The site and size of the diphtheritic membrane, the degree of toxic effects, and the duration of illness are guides for estimating the dose of antitoxin; the presence of soft, diffuse, cervical lymphadenitis suggests moderate to severe toxin absorption. Suggested dose ranges are the following: pharyngeal or laryngeal disease of 48 hours' duration or less, 20 000 to 40 000 U; nasopharyngeal lesions, 40 000 to 60 000 U; extensive disease of 3 or more days' duration or diffuse swelling of the neck, 80 000 to 120 000 U. Antitoxin probably is of no value for cutaneous disease, but some experts recommend 20 000 to 40 000 U of antitoxin because toxic sequelae have been reported.

Antimicrobial Therapy. Erythromycin given orally or parenterally (40 to 50 mg/kg per day, maximum 2 g/d) for 14 days; or penicillin G given parenterally (aqueous crystalline, 100 000 to 150 000 U/kg per day, in 4 divided doses intravenously; or aqueous procaine penicillin, 25 000 to 50 000 U/kg per day, maximum 1.2 million U, in 2 divided doses intramuscularly) for 14 days, constitutes acceptable therapy. Antimicrobial therapy is required to eradicate the organism and prevent spread; **it is not a substitute for antitoxin.** Elimination of the organism should be documented by 2 consecutive negative cultures after completion of treatment.

Cutaneous Diphtheria. Thorough cleansing of the lesion with soap and water and administration of an appropriate antimicrobial agent for 10 days are recommended.

Carriers. If not immunized, carriers should receive active immunization promptly, and measures should be taken to ensure completion of the immunization schedule. If a carrier has been immunized previously but has not received a booster within 1 year, a booster dose of a preparation containing diphtheria toxoid (DTaP, DT, or dT, depending on age) should be given. Carriers should be given antimicrobial therapy, specifically oral erythromycin or penicillin G for 7 days, or a single intramuscular dose of benzathine penicillin G (600 000 U for those weighing <30 kg and 1.2 million U for children weighing >30 kg and adults). Follow-up cultures should be obtained at least 2 weeks after completion of therapy; if cultures are positive, an additional 10-day course of oral erythromycin should be given. Erythromycin-resistant strains have been identified, but their epidemiologic significance has not been determined. Clindamycin, fluoroquinolones, rifampin, and newer macrolides, clarithromycin and azithromycin, have good in vitro activity and may be better tolerated than erythromycin, but they have not been critically evaluated in clinical infection or in carriers.

ISOLATION OF THE HOSPITALIZED PATIENT: In addition to standard precautions, droplet precautions are recommended for patients and carriers with pharyngeal diphtheria until 2 cultures from both the nose and the throat are negative for *C diphtheriae.* Contact precautions are recommended for patients with cutaneous diphtheria until 2 cultures of skin lesions are negative. Material for these cultures should be taken at least 24 hours apart after cessation of antimicrobial therapy.

Control Measures:

Care of Exposed Persons. Whenever the diagnosis of diphtheria is strongly suspected or proven, local public health officials should be notified promptly. Management of exposed persons is based on individual circumstances, including immunization status and likelihood of compliance with follow-up and prophylaxis. The following is recommended:

- Identification of close contacts of a person suspected to have diphtheria should be initiated promptly. Contact tracing should begin in the household and usually can be limited to household members and other persons with a history of habitual close contact with the person suspected of having the disease.
- For close contacts, *irrespective of their immunization status,* the following measures should be taken: (1) surveillance for 7 days for evidence of disease, (2) culture for *C diphtheriae,* and (3) antimicrobial prophylaxis with oral erythromycin (40 to 50 mg/kg per day for 7 days, maximum 2 g/d) or a single intramuscular injection of benzathine penicillin G (600 000 U for those weighing <30 kg and 1.2 million U for children weighing >30 kg and adults). The efficacy of antimicrobial prophylaxis is presumed but not proven. Repeated pharyngeal cultures should be obtained from contacts proven to be carriers at a minimum of 2 weeks after completion of therapy (see Carriers, p 232).
- Asymptomatic, previously immunized, close contacts should receive a booster dose of a preparation containing diphtheria toxoid (DTaP, DT, or dT, depending on age) if they have not received a booster dose of diphtheria toxoid within 5 years. Children in need of their fourth dose should be immunized.
- For asymptomatic close contacts who are not fully immunized (defined as having had fewer than 3 doses of diphtheria toxoid) or whose immunization status is not known, active immunization should be undertaken with DTaP, DT, or dT, depending on age.
- Contacts who cannot be kept under surveillance should receive benzathine penicillin G, but not erythromycin because adherence to an oral regimen is less likely, and a dose of DTaP, DT, or dT, depending on age and the person's immunization history.

The use of equine diphtheria antitoxin in unimmunized close contacts is not recommended because there is no evidence that it provides additional benefit for contacts who have received antimicrobial prophylaxis and because of the 5% to 20% risk of allergic reactions to horse serum.

Immunization. Universal immunization with diphtheria toxoid is the only effective control measure. For all indications, diphtheria immunization is administered with tetanus toxoid–containing vaccines. The schedules for immunization against diphtheria are presented in the chapter on tetanus (see Tetanus, p 563). The value of diphtheria toxoid is proven by the rarity of disease in countries in which high rates of immunization with diphtheria toxoid have been achieved. Fewer than 5 cases have been reported annually in the United States in recent years. As a result of high immunization rates, exposure to persons with diphtheria or to carriers is much less frequent now than in the past. However, the decreased frequency of exposure to the organism implies decreased maintenance of immunity secondary to community contact. Therefore, assurance of continuing immunity requires regular booster injections of diphtheria toxoid (as dT) every 10 years after completion of the initial immunization series.

Vaccine is given intramuscularly. *Haemophilus influenzae* conjugate vaccines containing diphtheria toxoid (PRP-D) or CRM197 protein (HbOC), a nontoxic variant of diphtheria toxin, are not substitutes for diphtheria toxoid immunization.

Immunization for children from 2 months of age to the seventh birthday (see Fig 1.1 and Table 1.5, p 22 and p 24) should consist of 5 doses of diphtheria and tetanus toxoid–containing vaccine (see Tetanus, p 563).

Immunization against diphtheria and tetanus for children younger than 7 years of age in whom pertussis immunization is contraindicated (see Pertussis, p 435) should be accomplished with DT instead of DTaP (see Tetanus, p 563).

Other recommendations for diphtheria immunization, including those for older children can be found in the chapter on tetanus (see Tetanus, p 563).

- When children and adults require tetanus toxoid for wound management (see Tetanus, p 563), the use of preparations containing diphtheria toxoid (DTaP, DT, or dT as appropriate for age or specific contraindication to pertussis immunization) will help ensure continuing diphtheria immunity.
- Active immunization against diphtheria should be undertaken during convalescence from diphtheria because disease does not necessarily confer immunity.
- Travelers to countries with endemic or epidemic diphtheria should have their diphtheria immunization status reviewed and updated when necessary.

Precautions and Contraindications. See Pertussis (p 435) and Tetanus (p 563).

Ehrlichiosis
(Human)

CLINICAL MANIFESTATIONS: Human ehrlichiosis in North America consists of at least 2 distinct diseases that are referred to as *human monocytic ehrlichiosis* and *human granulocytic ehrlichiosis.* These 2 diseases have different causes but similar signs, symptoms, and clinical course. Both are acute, systemic, febrile illnesses that are similar clinically to Rocky Mountain spotted fever but with more frequent occurrence of leukopenia, anemia, and hepatitis and less frequent occurrence of rash. The febrile illness often is accompanied by headache, chills, malaise, myalgia, arthralgia, nausea, vomiting, anorexia, and acute weight loss. Rash is variable in appearance and location, typically develops about 1 week after onset of illness, and occurs only in approximately 50% of reported cases of human monocytic ehrlichiosis and fewer than 10% of persons with human granulocytic ehrlichiosis. Diarrhea, abdominal pain, and change in mental status occur infrequently. Reported complications of both diseases include pulmonary infiltrates, bone marrow hypoplasia, respiratory failure, encephalopathy, meningitis, disseminated intravascular coagulation, and renal failure. Anemia, hyponatremia, thrombocytopenia, elevated liver enzyme concentrations, and cerebrospinal fluid abnormalities (ie, pleocytosis with a predominance of lymphocytes and elevated total protein concentration) are common. Although both diseases typically last 1 to 2 weeks, and recovery generally occurs without sequelae, reports suggest the occurrence of neurologic complications in some children. Fatal as well as asymptomatic infections have been reported. Secondary or opportunistic infections may occur in severe illness, resulting in possible delayed recognition of ehrlichiosis and appropriate antibiotic treatment.

ETIOLOGY: In the United States, human ehrlichiosis may be caused by 2 distinct species of obligate intracellular bacteria. Human monocytic ehrlichiosis results from infection with *Ehrlichia chaffeensis.* Human granulocytic ehrlichiosis is caused by an unnamed *Ehrlichia* species closely related to *Ehrlichia phagocytophila* and *Ehrlichia equi.* A third human ehrlichial pathogen, *Ehrlichia sennetsu,* causes Sennetsu fever, a self-limited mononucleosis-like illness that occurs in Japan and Malaysia. *Ehrlichia ewingii,* an agent reported as a cause of granulocytic ehrlichiosis in dogs, reportedly causes disease in humans.

EPIDEMIOLOGY: The majority of human monocytic ehrlichiosis infections occur in persons from the southeastern and south central United States, but a small number of cases have been described from other areas. *Ehrlichia chaffeensis* is transmitted by the Lone Star tick *(Amblyomma americanum).* Cases of *E chaffeensis* infection occurring in states beyond the geographic distribution of *A americanum* suggest transmission by additional tick species. Most cases of human granulocytic ehrlichiosis have been reported in Wisconsin, Minnesota, Connecticut, and New York, but cases have been reported in many other states, particularly along the West Coast. Human granulocytic ehrlichiosis is transmitted by the black-legged tick *(Ixodes scapularis),* which also is the vector of *Borrelia burgdorferi* (the agent of Lyme disease). The principal mammalian reservoirs for the agents of human ehrlichiosis remain to be identified, although white-tailed deer and white-footed mice may be infected naturally with *E chaffeensis* and the human granulocytic ehrlichiosis (HGE) agent, respectively. Compared with patients with Rocky Mountain spotted fever (see p 491), persons with symptomatic ehrlichiosis are characteristically older, with age-specific incidences greatest in persons older than 40 years of age. Most human infections occur between April and September; peak occurrence is from May through July. The incidence of reported cases seems to be increasing. Coinfections with other tick-borne diseases, including babesiosis and Lyme disease, are recognized.

The **incubation period** of human ehrlichiosis typically is 7 to 14 days after a tick bite or exposure (median, 10 days).

DIAGNOSTIC TESTS: The Centers for Disease Control and Prevention (CDC) defines a confirmed case of ehrlichiosis as a 4-fold or greater change in antibody titer by indirect immunofluorescence assay (IFA) between acute and convalescent serum samples (ideally collected 3 to 6 weeks apart), polymerase chain reaction (PCR) amplification of ehrlichial DNA from a clinical sample, or detection of intraleukocytoplasmic *Ehrlichia* microcolonies (morulae) and a single IFA titer of more than 64. A probable case is defined as a single IFA titer of more than 64 or the presence of morulae within infected leukocytes. *Ehrlichia chaffeensis* is used as the antigen for the serologic diagnosis of human monocytic ehrlichiosis, and the HGE agent is used as the antigen in assays for the diagnosis of human granulocytic ehrlichiosis. These tests are available in reference laboratories, some commercial laboratories and state health departments, and at the CDC. More than 10 isolates of

E chaffeensis have been obtained from human patients. Examination of peripheral blood smears to detect morulae in peripheral blood monocytes or granulocytes is insensitive, but this test is warranted for patients for whom a high index of suspicion exists. The use of the PCR test to amplify nucleic acid from acute phase peripheral blood of patients with ehrlichiosis seems sensitive, specific, and promising for early diagnosis but currently is available only in research laboratories and at the CDC.

TREATMENT: Doxycycline is the drug of choice for treatment of human ehrlichiosis. The recommended dosage of doxycycline is 3 to 4 mg/kg per day in 2 divided doses. The clinical efficacy of chloramphenicol in the treatment of human ehrlichiosis is uncertain. Ehrlichiosis may be severe or fatal in untreated patients, and initiation of therapy early in the course of the disease helps minimize complications of the illness. Tetracycline drugs ordinarily should not be given to children younger than 8 years of age because of the risk of dental staining (see Antimicrobial Agents and Related Therapy, p 645). However, comparison of the benefits and risks of a single short course of tetracycline with those of chloramphenicol when deciding which antimicrobial agent to give to a child younger than 8 years of age justifies the use of doxycycline. Furthermore, oral chloramphenicol is no longer available in the United States.

Treatment should continue for 3 days after defervescence for a minimum total course of 5 to 7 days. Severe or complicated disease may require longer treatment courses.

The clinical manifestations and geographic distributions of ehrlichiosis and Rocky Mountain spotted fever overlap. If no other cause can be identified by the fourth day of an illness with clinical findings consistent with either of these tick-borne diseases, doxycycline should be started for presumptive treatment of either disease.

ISOLATION OF THE HOSPITALIZED PATIENT: Standard precautions are recommended.

CONTROL MEASURES: Specific measures focus on limiting exposures to ticks and are similar to those for Rocky Mountain spotted fever and other tick-borne diseases (see Prevention of Tick-borne Infections, p 159).

Enterovirus (Nonpolio) Infections

(Group A and B Coxsackieviruses, Echoviruses, and Enteroviruses)

CLINICAL MANIFESTATIONS: Nonpolio enteroviruses are responsible for significant and frequent illnesses in infants and children and result in protean clinical manifestations. The most common presentation is nonspecific febrile illness, which in young infants may lead to evaluation for bacterial sepsis. Neonates who acquire infection without maternal antibody are at risk of severe disease with a high mortality rate. Manifestations can include the following: (1) respiratory—common cold, pharyngitis, herpangina, stomatitis, pneumonia, and pleurodynia; (2) skin—exanthem; (3) neurologic—aseptic meningitis, encephalitis, and paralysis;

(4) gastrointestinal—vomiting, diarrhea, abdominal pain, and hepatitis; (5) eye—acute hemorrhagic conjunctivitis; and (6) heart—myopericarditis. Although each of these findings can be caused by several different enteroviruses, some associations between virus and disease are particularly noteworthy. These associations include coxsackievirus A16 and enterovirus 71 with hand, foot, and mouth syndrome; coxsackievirus A24 variant and enterovirus 70 with acute hemorrhagic conjunctivitis; enterovirus 71 with encephalitis and polio-like paralysis; echovirus 9 with a petechial exanthem and meningitis; and coxsackieviruses B1 to B5 with pleurodynia and myopericarditis.

Immunocompromised patients with humoral deficiencies can have persistent central nervous system infections lasting for several months or more.

ETIOLOGY: The nonpolio enteroviruses are RNA viruses, which include 23 group A coxsackieviruses (types A1-A24, except type A23), 6 group B coxsackieviruses (types B1-B6), 29 echoviruses (types 1-33, except types 10, 22, 23, and 28), and 4 enteroviruses (types 68-71).

EPIDEMIOLOGY: Enterovirus infections are common and are spread by fecal-oral and respiratory routes and from mother to infant in the peripartum period. Enteroviruses may survive on environmental surfaces for periods long enough to allow transmission from fomites. Infections and clinical attack rates typically are highest in young children, and infections occur more frequently in lower socioeconomic groups, in tropical areas, and when hygiene is poor. In temperate climates, enteroviral infections are most common in the summer and early fall, but seasonal patterns are less evident in the tropics. Fecal viral shedding can continue for several weeks after onset of infection, while respiratory tract shedding usually is limited to a week or less. Viral shedding can occur without signs of clinical illness.

The usual **incubation period** is 3 to 6 days, except for acute hemorrhagic conjunctivitis, in which it is 24 to 72 hours.

DIAGNOSTIC TESTS: Specimens providing the highest rate of viral isolation are those obtained from the throat, stool, and rectal swabs. Specimens also should be obtained from any sites of clinical involvement, such as cerebrospinal fluid (CSF). Enteroviruses also may be recovered from blood during the acute febrile phase and, rarely, from biopsy material. Specimens should be sent to the laboratory at 4°C (39°F). Repeated freezing, thawing, and drying of specimens are detrimental to viral recovery. In patients with serious illnesses, viral isolation as a means of diagnosis is particularly important. Viral isolation from any specimen except feces usually can be considered causally related to the patient's illness. Isolation of an enterovirus from stool alone is less specific, because some asymptomatic infected persons may shed virus in feces for as long as 6 to 12 weeks. Most viral diagnostic laboratories use cell culture techniques that are capable of recovering echoviruses, group B coxsackieviruses, and some group A coxsackieviruses. Suckling mouse inoculation, which is not a routine procedure, is required for recovery of certain group A coxsackievirus serotypes. Polymerase chain reaction testing for the presence of enterovirus RNA in CSF, which is available in a few research laboratories, is more sensitive than viral isolation. Serum samples for antibody testing can be collected at the onset of illness and 4 weeks later and stored frozen. The demonstration of a rise in titer of virus-specific neutralizing antibody can be used to confirm infection, particularly when the specific virus has been identified previously during a community outbreak. Serologic screening without a suspected serotype generally is not performed.

TREATMENT: No specific therapy is available, although an antiviral agent, pleconaril, is undergoing clinical evaluation in immunocompetent infants with aseptic meningitis and in immunodeficient children. For chronic enteroviral meningoencephalitis in an immunodeficient patient, Immune Globulin Intravenous (IGIV) containing high antibody titer to the infecting virus may be beneficial for treatment of persistent enterovirus infection. Immune Globulin Intravenous also has been used in life-threatening neonatal infections, although there is no convincing evidence of efficacy for this use. Since IGIV preparations vary in the amount of enteroviral antibody, specific manufacturer information should be consulted.

ISOLATION OF THE HOSPITALIZED PATIENT: In addition to standard precautions, contact precautions are indicated for infants and young children for the duration of hospitalization.

CONTROL MEASURES: Particular attention should be given to hand washing and personal hygiene, especially after diaper changing.

Epstein-Barr Virus Infections

(Infectious Mononucleosis)

CLINICAL MANIFESTATIONS: Infectious mononucleosis is manifested typically by fever, exudative pharyngitis, lymphadenopathy, hepatosplenomegaly, and atypical lymphocytosis. The spectrum of diseases is variable, ranging from asymptomatic to fatal infection. Infections frequently are unrecognized in infants and young children. Rash can occur and is more frequent in patients treated with ampicillin, as well as with penicillin. Central nervous system (CNS) complications include aseptic meningitis, encephalitis, and Guillain-Barré syndrome. Rare complications include splenic rupture, thrombocytopenia, agranulocytosis, hemolytic anemia, hemophagocytic syndrome, orchitis, and myocarditis. Replication of Epstein-Barr virus (EBV) in B lymphocytes and the resulting lymphoproliferation usually is inhibited by natural killer and T-cell responses, but in patients who have congenital or acquired cellular immune deficiencies, fatal disseminated infection or B-cell lymphomas can occur.

Epstein-Barr virus causes several other distinct disorders, including the X-linked lymphoproliferative syndrome (also known as Duncan syndrome), posttransplantation lymphoproliferative disorders, Burkitt lymphoma, nasopharyngeal carcinoma, and undifferentiated B-cell lymphomas of the CNS. The X-linked lymphoproliferative syndrome occurs in persons with an inherited, maternally derived, recessive genetic defect characterized by several phenotypic expressions, including occurrence of infectious mononucleosis early in life among boys, nodular B-cell lymphomas often with CNS involvement, and profound hypogammaglobulinemia.

Epstein-Barr virus–associated lymphoproliferative disorders result in a number of complex syndromes associated with immunosuppression, including human immunodeficiency virus (HIV) infection, and occur in approximately 2% of graft recipients. The highest incidence occurs after heart transplantation.

Other EBV syndromes are of greater importance outside the United States, including Burkitt lymphoma (a B-cell tumor), found primarily in Central Africa, and nasopharyngeal carcinoma, found in Southeast Asia.

The chronic fatigue syndrome is not related specifically to EBV infection. A small group of patients with recurring or persistent symptoms have abnormal serologic test results for EBV, as well as for other viruses.

ETIOLOGY: Epstein-Barr virus, a DNA virus, is a B-lymphotropic herpesvirus and is the most common cause of infectious mononucleosis.

EPIDEMIOLOGY: Humans are the only source of EBV. Close personal contact usually is required for transmission. The virus is viable in saliva for several hours outside the body, but the role of fomites in transmission is unknown. Epstein-Barr virus also is transmitted occasionally by blood transfusion. Infection frequently is contracted early in life, particularly among lower socioeconomic groups, in which intrafamilial spread is common. Endemic infectious mononucleosis is common in group settings of adolescents, such as in educational institutions. No seasonal pattern has been documented. Respiratory tract viral excretion can occur for many months after infection, and asymptomatic carriage is common. Intermittent excretion is lifelong. The period of communicability is indeterminate.

The **incubation period** of infectious mononucleosis is estimated to be 30 to 50 days.

DIAGNOSTIC TESTS: Isolation of EBV from oropharyngeal secretions is possible, but techniques for performing this procedure usually are not available in routine diagnostic laboratories, and viral isolation does not necessarily indicate acute infection. Hence, diagnosis depends on serologic testing. Nonspecific tests for heterophil antibody, including the Paul-Bunnell test and slide agglutination reaction, are most commonly available. The results of these tests are often negative in infants and children younger than 4 years of age with EBV infection, but they identify approximately 90% of cases (proven by EBV-specific serology) in older children and adults. An absolute increase in atypical lymphocytes in the second week of illness with infectious mononucleosis is a characteristic but not specific finding.

Multiple specific serologic antibody tests for EBV are available in diagnostic virology laboratories (see Table 3.4, p 240). The most commonly performed test is for antibody against the viral capsid antigen (VCA). Since immunoglobulin (Ig) G antibody against VCA occurs in high titers early after onset of infection, testing of acute and convalescent serum samples for anti-VCA may not be useful for establishing the presence of infection. Testing for IgM anti-VCA antibody and for antibodies against early antigen is useful for identifying recent infections. Since serum antibody against EBV nuclear antigen (EBNA) is not present until several weeks to months after onset of the infection, a positive anti-EBNA antibody test excludes acute infection.

Table 3.4. Serum Epstein-Barr Virus (EBV) Antibodies in EBV Infection*

Infection	Anti-VCA-IgG	Anti-VCA-IgM	Anti-EA (D)	Anti-EBNA
No previous infection	–	–	–	–
Acute infection	+	+	+/–	–
Recent infection	+	+/–	+/–	+/–
Past infection	+	–	–	+

* Anti-VCA-IgG indicates immunoglobulin (Ig) G class antibody to viral capsid antigen; anti-VCA-IgM, IgM class antibody to VCA; EA (D), early antigen diffuse staining; and EBNA, EBV nuclear antigen.

Serologic tests for EBV are particularly useful for evaluating patients who have heterophil-negative infectious mononucleosis. Testing for other viral agents, especially cytomegalovirus, is indicated for these patients. In research studies, culture of saliva or peripheral blood mononuclear cells for EBV, in situ DNA hybridization, or polymerase chain reaction can determine the presence of EBV or EBV DNA and may implicate EBV with a syndrome, such as lymphoproliferation.

TREATMENT: Supportive therapy should include rest in the acute stages of illness. Contact sports should be avoided until the patient is recovered fully from infectious mononucleosis and the spleen is no longer palpable. Although short-course corticosteroid therapy may have a beneficial effect on acute symptoms, due to long-term concerns about potential negative effects on the normal immune response to EBV, routine use is not recommended. Corticosteroid use is considered only for cases with complications such as marked tonsillar inflammation with impending airway obstruction, massive splenomegaly, myocarditis, hemolytic anemia, and hemophagocytic syndrome. The dosage of prednisone is usually 1 mg/kg per day orally for 7 days with a subsequent tapering. Although acyclovir has in vitro antiviral activity against EBV, the clinical benefits of treatment have not been demonstrated, with the possible exception of HIV-infected patients with hairy leukoplakia. Reducing immunosuppressive therapy is beneficial for patients with EBV-induced lymphoproliferation, such as the posttransplant lymphoproliferative disorders. Therapy for EBV is of no proven value in EBV lymphoproliferative syndromes.

ISOLATION OF THE HOSPITALIZED PATIENT: Standard precautions are recommended.

CONTROL MEASURES: Patients with a recent history of EBV infection or an illness similar to infectious mononucleosis should not donate blood.

Escherichia coli and Other Gram-negative Bacilli

(Septicemia and Meningitis in Neonates)

CLINICAL MANIFESTATIONS: Neonatal septicemia or meningitis caused by *Escherichia coli* and other gram-negative bacilli cannot be differentiated clinically from serious infections caused by other infectious agents. The first signs of sepsis may be minimal and similar to those observed in noninfectious processes. Clinical signs of septicemia include fever, temperature instability, apnea, cyanosis, jaundice, hepatomegaly, lethargy, irritability, anorexia, vomiting, abdominal distention, and diarrhea. Meningitis may be concomitant with septicemia without overt signs attributable to the central nervous system. Some gram-negative bacilli such as *Citrobacter diversus* and *Enterobacter sakazakii* are associated with brain abscesses in infants with meningitis due to these organisms.

ETIOLOGY: *Escherichia coli* strains with the K1 capsular polysaccharide antigen cause approximately 40% of cases of septicemia and 75% of cases of meningitis caused by *E coli.* Other important gram-negative bacilli that can cause neonatal septicemia include non-K1 strains of *E coli* and *Klebsiella, Enterobacter, Proteus, Citrobacter, Salmonella,* and *Pseudomonas* species. Anaerobic gram-negative bacilli are rare causes, as are nonencapsulated strains of *Haemophilus influenzae.*

EPIDEMIOLOGY: The source of *E coli* and other gram-negative bacterial pathogens in neonatal infections usually is the maternal genital tract. In addition, nosocomial acquisition of gram-negative flora through person-to-person transmission among nursery personnel and from nursery environmental sites, such as fluid reservoirs of incubators, has been documented, especially in preterm infants who require prolonged intensive care management. Predisposing host factors in neonatal gram-negative bacterial infections include maternal perinatal infections, low birth weight, prolonged rupture of membranes, and septic or traumatic delivery. Metabolic abnormalities, such as galactosemia, fetal hypoxia, and acidosis also have been implicated as predisposing factors. Neonates with defects in the integrity of skin or mucosa (eg, myelomeningocele) are at increased risk for gram-negative bacterial infections. In intensive care nurseries, sophisticated systems for respiratory and metabolic support, invasive procedures, indwelling vascular lines, and the frequent use of antimicrobial agents enable selection and proliferation of multiply antimicrobial-resistant strains of pathogenic gram-negative bacilli.

The **incubation period** is highly variable; time of onset of infection ranges from birth to several weeks of age.

DIAGNOSTIC TESTS: The diagnosis is established by growth of *E coli* or other gram-negative bacilli from blood, cerebrospinal fluid, or other usually sterile sites.

TREATMENT:

- Initial empiric treatment of a neonate with suspected bacterial septicemia or meningitis is ampicillin and an aminoglycoside. An alternative regimen of ampicillin and a cephalosporin (such as cefotaxime) active against most gram-negative bacilli can be used, but rapid emergence of cephalosporin-resistant strains, especially *Enterobacter cloacae, Klebsiella* species, and *Serratia* species, can occur as a result of routine use of expanded-spectrum cephalosporins in a nursery. Hence, routine use of expanded-spectrum cephalosporins is not recommended unless gram-negative bacterial meningitis is strongly suspected.
- Once the causative agent and its in vitro antimicrobial susceptibility pattern are known, nonmeningeal infections should be treated with ampicillin, an appropriate aminoglycoside, or an expanded-spectrum cephalosporin (such as cefotaxime). Many experts would treat nonmeningeal infections caused by *Enterobacter, Serratia,* and *Pseudomonas* species and some other less frequently occurring gram-negative bacilli with a ß-lactam antibiotic and an aminoglycoside. Meningitis usually is treated with ampicillin or an expanded-spectrum cephalosporin in combination with an aminoglycoside. Expert advice from an infectious disease specialist may be helpful for management of meningitis.
- Duration of therapy is based on the patient's clinical and bacteriologic response; the usual duration of therapy for uncomplicated septicemia is 10 to 14 days, and for meningitis, the minimum duration is 21 days.
- A therapeutic role for immunoglobulin or other adjunctive therapy in septicemia or meningitis caused by *E coli* or other gram-negative organisms has not been established.
- All infants with meningitis should undergo careful follow-up examinations, including testing for hearing loss and neurologic abnormalities.

ISOLATION OF THE HOSPITALIZED PATIENT: Standard precautions are recommended for infants with septicemia or meningitis caused by *E coli* or other enteric gram-negative bacilli. Exceptions include nursery epidemics, infants with *Salmonella* infection, and infants with infection caused by multiply antibiotic-resistant gram-negative bacilli; for these situations, contact precautions in addition to standard precautions are indicated.

CONTROL MEASURES: The physician director of the nursery and infection control personnel should be aware of pathogens causing infections in infants and nursery personnel so that clusters of infections are recognized and investigated appropriately. Several cases of infection caused by the same genus and species of bacteria occurring in infants in physical proximity or caused by an unusual pathogen indicate the need for an epidemiologic investigation (see Infection Control for Hospitalized Children, p 127). Periodic review of the in vitro antimicrobial susceptibility patterns of clinically important bacterial isolates from newborn infants, especially infants in the intensive care nursery, can provide useful epidemiologic and therapeutic information.

Escherichia coli Diarrhea

(Including Hemolytic-Uremic Syndrome)

CLINICAL MANIFESTATIONS: At least 5 pathotypes of diarrhea-producing *Escherichia coli* strains have been identified. Clinical features of disease caused by each pathotype are summarized as follows (see also Table 3.5, below):

- Enterohemorrhagic *E coli* (EHEC), also known as Shiga-toxin producing *E coli* or verotoxin-producing *E coli,* strains are associated with diarrhea, hemorrhagic colitis, hemolytic-uremic syndrome (HUS), and postdiarrheal thrombotic thrombocytopenic purpura (TTP). Enterohemorrhagic *E coli* O157:H7 is the prototype for this class of organisms. Illness caused by EHEC often begins as nonbloody diarrhea but usually progresses to diarrhea with visible or occult blood. Severe abdominal pain is typical; fever occurs in fewer than one third of cases. Hemorrhagic colitis is the most severe intestinal infection.
- Diarrhea caused by enteropathogenic *E coli* (EPEC) is characterized by watery diarrhea that often is severe and can result in dehydration. Enteropathogenic *E coli* is a cause of chronic diarrhea that can lead to growth retardation. Illness occurs almost exclusively in neonates and children younger than 2 years of age and predominantly in developing countries, either sporadically or in epidemics.
- Diarrhea caused by enterotoxigenic *E coli* (ETEC) is a self-limited illness of moderate severity with watery stools and abdominal cramps.

Table 3.5. **Classification of *Escherichia coli* Associated With Diarrhea**

E coli Pathotype	Epidemiology	Type of Diarrhea	Mechanism of Pathogenesis
Enterohemorrhagic	Hemorrhagic colitis and hemolytic uremic syndrome in all ages and postdiarrheal thrombotic thrombocytopenic purpura in adults	Bloody or nonbloody	Adherence and effacement, cytotoxin production
Enteropathogenic	Acute and chronic endemic and epidemic diarrhea in infants	Watery	Adherence, effacement
Enterotoxigenic	Infantile diarrhea in developing countries and traveler's diarrhea in all ages	Watery	Adherence, enterotoxin production
Enteroinvasive	Diarrhea with fever in all ages	Bloody or nonbloody; dysentery	Adherence, mucosal invasion and inflammation
Enteroaggregative	Acute and chronic diarrhea in infants	Watery, occasionally bloody	Adherence, mucosal damage

- Infection caused by enteroinvasive *E coli* (EIEC) is similar clinically and pathogenetically to infection caused by *Shigella* species. Although dysentery can occur, diarrhea usually is watery without blood or mucus. Patients often are febrile, and stools may contain fecal leukocytes.
- Enteroaggregative *E coli* (EAEC) causes watery diarrhea, predominantly in infants and young children in the developing world. Enteroaggregative *E coli* has been associated with persistent diarrhea (>14 days).

Late Sequelae of EHEC Infection. Hemolytic-uremic syndrome is a sequela of enteric infection with EHEC, especially EHEC O157:H7. Hemolytic-uremic syndrome is defined by the triad of microangiopathic hemolytic anemia, thrombocytopenia, and acute renal dysfunction. In many children with diarrhea caused by EHEC O157:H7, mild, self-limited, microangiopathic hematologic changes, thrombocytopenia, and/or nephropathy develop during the 2 weeks after onset of diarrhea. Thrombocytopenic purpura occurs in adults, may follow EHEC infection, includes central nervous system involvement and fever, may have a more gradual onset than HUS, and is part of a disease spectrum often designated as TTP-HUS. While most cases of childhood HUS in the United States are caused by EHEC O157:H7, most cases of TTP in adults are of unknown cause.

ETIOLOGY: Each pathotype of *E coli* strains has a distinct set of somatic (O) and flagellar (H) antigens. Each pathotype has specific virulence characteristics, most often encoded on pathotype-specific plasmids. Microbiologic characteristics are as follows:

- Illness caused by EHEC O157:H7 occurs in a 2-step process. The intestinal phase is characterized by formation of the so-called attaching and effacing lesion, resulting in secretory diarrhea. This phase is followed by elaboration of Shiga toxin, a potent cytotoxin also found in *Shigella dysenteriae* 1. The action of Shiga toxin on intestinal cells results in hemorrhagic colitis, and toxin circulation through the bloodstream is responsible for HUS.
- Strains of EPEC traditionally were defined as members of specific *E coli* serotypes that were incriminated epidemiologically as causes of infantile diarrhea. Enteropathogenic *E coli* belong typically to 12 O serogroups. Strains of EPEC adhere to the small bowel mucosa and, like EHEC O157:H7, produce attaching and effacing lesions. The capacity to form the attaching and effacing lesions in the absence of Shiga toxin production defines EPEC.
- Strains of ETEC colonize the small intestine without invading and produce heat-labile enterotoxin, heat-stable enterotoxin, or both. Heat-stable enterotoxin producers are responsible for most human illness due to ETEC.
- Strains of EIEC are typically lactose nonfermenting and, like *Shigella* species, invade the colonic mucosa, where they spread laterally and induce a local inflammatory response.
- The EAEC organisms are defined by their characteristic "stacked brick" adherence pattern in tissue culture–based assays. These organisms elaborate one or more enterotoxins and elicit damage to the intestinal mucosa.

EPIDEMIOLOGY: Transmission of most diarrhea-associated *E coli* strains is from infected symptomatic persons or carriers or from food or water contaminated with human or animal feces. The only *E coli* pathotype common in the United States is EHEC. Enterohemorrhagic *E coli* O157:H7 is shed in the feces of cattle, deer, and other ruminants and is transmitted by undercooked ground beef, unpasteurized milk, and a wide variety of vehicles contaminated with bovine feces. Infections caused by EHEC O157:H7 are increasingly common in the United States and can occur sporadically or in outbreaks. Outbreaks have been linked to contaminated apple cider, raw vegetables, salami, yogurt, drinking water, and ingestion of recreational water. The infectious dose is low (about 100 organisms), and person-to-person transmission is common in outbreaks. The frequency of HUS as a complication of EHEC O157:H7 infection in children has been estimated to be 5% to 10% but may be higher during outbreaks. Diarrhea and sometimes HUS caused by EHEC strains other than O157:H7 is common outside the United States. The burden of disease from these strains in the United States is unknown.

Non-EHEC pathotypes of *E coli* are associated with disease predominantly in the developing world, where food and water supplies frequently are contaminated and facilities for hand washing are suboptimal. Epidemic EPEC disease in newborn nurseries is uncommon, but EPEC and EHEC O157:H7 have caused numerous outbreaks of diarrhea in child care centers. Diarrhea due to ETEC occurs in persons of all ages but is especially important in infants. Outbreaks have occurred in adults, usually from ingestion of contaminated food or water. Enterotoxigenic *E coli* is the major cause of traveler's diarrhea. Outbreaks of infection due to EIEC and EAEC have occurred, usually secondary to contaminated food, among persons of all ages in developed countries. The period of communicability is for the duration of excretion of the specific pathogen.

The **incubation period** for most *E coli* strains is from 10 hours to 6 days; for EHEC O157:H7, it usually is 3 to 4 days but can be as long as 8 days.

DIAGNOSTIC TESTS: Diagnosis of infection caused by diarrhea-associated *E coli* usually is difficult because most clinical laboratories cannot differentiate diarrhea-associated *E coli* strains from normal *E coli* stool flora. The exceptions are EHEC O157:H7 and EIEC, which can be identified presumptively or specifically. For definitive identification, isolates suspected to be associated with diarrhea should be sent to reference or research laboratories.

Clinical laboratories can screen for EHEC O157:H7 by using MacConkey agar base with sorbitol substituted for lactose. Approximately 90% of human intestinal *E coli* strains rapidly ferment sorbitol, whereas EHEC O157:H7 strains do not. These sorbitol-negative *E coli* then can be serotyped, using commercially available antisera, to determine whether they are O157:H7. DNA probes and polymerase chain reaction (PCR) are available in research and reference laboratories for identification of each *E coli* pathotype and now are considered preferable to serotyping for identification of EPEC. If a case or outbreak due to diarrhea-associated *E coli* other than O157:H7 is suspected, *E coli* isolates should be referred to the state public health laboratory or another reference laboratory for serotyping and identification of pathotypes.

Strains of EHEC should be sought in the following instances: bloody diarrhea (indicated by history or inspection of stool), HUS, postdiarrheal TTP, and any type of diarrhea in contacts of patients with HUS. Persons with presumptive diagnoses of intussusception, inflammatory bowel disease, or ischemic colitis sometimes have disease caused by EHEC O157:H7. Methods for definitive identification of EHEC that are used in reference or research laboratories include DNA probes, PCR, enzyme immunoassay (EIA), and phenotypic testing of strains or stool specimens for Shiga toxin. Serologic diagnosis using an EIA to detect serum antibodies to EHEC O157:H7 lipopolysaccharide is available in reference laboratories.

Hemolytic-Uremic Syndrome. For all patients with HUS, stool specimens should be cultured for EHEC O157:H7 and, if results are negative, for other EHEC serotypes. However, the absence of EHEC in feces does not preclude the diagnosis of EHEC-associated HUS, since HUS typically is diagnosed a week or more after onset of diarrhea when the organism no longer may be detectable. When EHEC infection is considered, a stool culture should be obtained as early as possible in the illness.

TREATMENT: Dehydration and electrolyte abnormalities should be corrected. Orally administered solutions usually are adequate.* Antimotility agents should not be administered to children with inflammatory or bloody diarrhea. Careful follow-up of patients with hemorrhagic colitis (including complete blood cell count with smear, blood urea nitrogen level, and creatinine level) is recommended to detect changes suggestive of HUS. If patients have no laboratory evidence of hemolysis, thrombocytopenia, or nephropathy by 3 days after resolution of diarrhea, their risk of developing HUS is low.

Antimicrobial Therapy. The role of antimicrobial therapy in patients with hemorrhagic colitis caused by EHEC is uncertain. Therapy does not seem to prevent progression to HUS. For infants with mild diarrhea caused by EPEC, nonabsorbable antibiotics, such as neomycin or gentamicin, given orally in 3 to 4 divided doses for 5 days, can be administered, although resistance may develop. These agents should not be used to treat infants with inflammatory or bloody diarrhea. Trimethoprim-sulfamethoxazole should be considered if diarrhea is moderate, severe, or intractable and if the organism is susceptible. If systemic infection is suspected, parenteral antimicrobial therapy should be given. For dysentery caused by EIEC strains and for chronic diarrhea caused by EPEC strains, antimicrobial agents such as trimethoprim-sulfamethoxazole can be given orally. Antimicrobial selection should be based on susceptibility testing of the isolates.

ISOLATION OF THE HOSPITALIZED PATIENT: In addition to standard precautions, contact precautions are indicated for patients with all types of *E coli* diarrhea for the duration of illness. During outbreaks, contact precautions for infants with diarrhea caused by EPEC strains should be maintained until cultures of stool

* For further information and detailed recommendations, see American Academy of Pediatrics Provisional Committee on Quality Improvement, Subcommittee on Gastroenteritis. Practice parameter: the management of acute gastroenteritis in young children. *Pediatrics.* 1996;97:424-435

taken after cessation of antimicrobial therapy are negative for the infecting strain. For patients with HUS, contact precautions should be continued until 2 consecutive stool cultures are negative for EHEC O157:H7.

CONTROL MEASURES:

EHEC O157:H7 Infection. In an outbreak of diarrhea due to EHEC O157:H7 and HUS in a child care center, immediate involvement of public health authorities is critical. Infection caused by EHEC O157:H7 is reportable, and rapid reporting of cases can lead to intervention to prevent further disease. Ill children should not be permitted to reenter the child care center until diarrhea has stopped and 2 stool cultures are negative for *E coli* O157:H7. Strict attention to hand washing and hygiene is important but may be insufficient to prevent continued transmission. A child care center should be closed to new admissions, and care should be exercised to prevent transfer of exposed children to other centers. All ground beef should be cooked thoroughly until no pink meat remains and the juices are clear. Raw milk should not be ingested, and only pasteurized apple juice products should be consumed.

Nursery and Other Institutional Outbreaks. Strict attention to hand-washing techniques is essential for limiting spread. Exposed patients should be observed closely and their stools cultured for the causative organism. Unexposed patients should be separated from infants who have been exposed. In a newborn nursery, management of EPEC infection is based on the number of cases.

Traveler's Diarrhea. Traveler's diarrhea has been associated with many enteropathogens, usually is acquired by ingestion of contaminated food or water, and is a significant problem for persons traveling in developing countries. Travelers should be advised to drink only carbonated beverages and boiled or carbonated (bottled) water; they should avoid ice, salads, and fruit they have not peeled themselves. Foods should be eaten hot. Antimicrobial agents usually are not recommended for prevention of traveler's diarrhea in children. Although several antimicrobial agents, such as trimethoprim-sulfamethoxazole, doxycycline, and ciprofloxacin, are effective prophylactically for decreasing the incidence of traveler's diarrhea, the benefit usually is outweighed by the potential risks, including allergic drug reactions, antibiotic-associated colitis, and the selective pressure of widespread use of antimicrobial agents leading to antimicrobial resistance. If diarrhea occurs, packets of oral rehydration salts can help maintain fluid balance. If diarrhea is moderate or severe or is associated with fever or bloody stools, empiric antimicrobial therapy may be indicated until symptoms resolve; empiric therapy should not be continued for more than 3 days.

Filariasis

(Bancroftian, Malayan, and Timorian)

CLINICAL MANIFESTATIONS: Most filarial infections are asymptomatic. Early in infection, symptoms often are caused by an acute inflammatory response that can lead to dysfunction of the lymphatics where the adult worms develop. Fever, headache, myalgia, and lymphadenitis develop with acute inflammation. The acute disease may manifest as early as 3 months after acquisition. Over time, moderate lymphadenopathy occurs, particularly involving the inguinal lymph nodes. Inflammation of the lymphatics of the extremities and genitalia leads to adenolymphangitis that is characteristically retrograde. Epididymitis, orchitis, and funiculitis also can occur along with fever, chills, and other nonspecific systemic symptoms. Lymphatic dysfunction, with resulting chronically progressive edema of the limbs and genitalia, is relatively infrequent in children. In a few persons, elephantiasis can result from fibrosis caused by chronic dysfunction of the lymphatic channels. Chyluria can occur as a manifestation of bancroftian filariasis.

Cough, fever, marked eosinophilia, and high serum immunoglobulin E concentrations are the manifestations of the tropical pulmonary eosinophilia syndrome.

ETIOLOGY: Filariasis is caused by the following 3 filarial nematodes: *Wuchereria bancrofti, Brugia malayi,* and *Brugia timori.*

EPIDEMIOLOGY: Disease is transmitted by the bite of infected species of various genera of mosquitoes, including *Culex, Aedes, Anopheles*, and *Mansonia. Wuchereria bancrofti* is found in many scattered areas of the Caribbean, Venezuela, Columbia, the Guianas, Brazil, Central America, sub-Saharan Africa, North Africa, Turkey, and Asia, extending into a broad zone from Saudi Arabia through the Indonesian archipelago into Southern China and Oceania. *Brugia malayi* is found mostly in India, Southeast Asia, and the Far East. *Brugia timori* is restricted to certain islands at the eastern end of the Indonesian archipelago. Because the adult worms are long-lived (5–8 years on average), and reinfection is common, microfilariae infective for mosquitoes may remain in the patient's blood for decades; individual microfilaria have a life span up to 1.5 years. The adult worm is not transmissible from person to person or by blood transfusion, but microfilariae may be transmitted by transfusion.

The **incubation period** is not well established; the period from acquisition to the appearance of microfilariae in blood can be 3 to 12 months, depending on the nematode.

DIAGNOSTIC TESTS: Microfilariae can be detected microscopically on routine blood smears obtained at night (10 PM to 4 AM) after concentration of blood preserved in formalin or by membrane filtration. Adult worms can be identified in tissue specimens obtained at biopsy. Serologic enzyme immunoassay tests are available, but interpretation of results is affected by cross-reactions of filarial antibodies with antibodies against other helminths. Assays for circulating parasite antigen of *W bancrofti* are now available commercially. Lymphatic filariasis often must be diagnosed clinically because dependable serologic assays are not uniformly available, and in elephantiasis, the microfilariae may no longer be present. Eosinophilia frequently occurs in the early inflammatory phase of the disease.

TREATMENT: Diethylcarbamazine citrate (DEC) is the drug of choice for early lymphatic filariasis. Because reactions induced by disintegrating microfilariae after treatment occur in heavy infections, beginning treatment with low doses for the first 4 to 5 days may be advantageous. The late obstructive phase of the disease is not affected by chemotherapy. Ivermectin is effective against the microfilariae of *W bancrofti* but has no effect on the adult parasite. Albendazole also has been shown to be effective in *W bancrofti* infections (see Drugs for Parasitic Infections, p 693).

Complex decongestive physiotherapy may be effective for treating elephantiasis. Plastic surgical repair of the genitalia gives variable results. Chyluria originating in the bladder responds to fulguration; chyluria originating in the kidney cannot be corrected. Prompt identification and treatment of superinfections, particularly streptococcal and staphylococcal infections, and careful treatment of intertriginous and ungual infections are important aspects of therapy.

ISOLATION OF THE HOSPITALIZED PATIENT: Standard precautions are recommended.

CONTROL MEASURES: Control measures recently have been instituted based on annual community-wide single-dose DEC (or combinations of DEC and ivermectin or albendazole and ivermectin) to reduce transmission in high-risk areas.

Fungal Diseases

In addition to the mycoses listed by individual agents in Section 3, infants and children can have infections caused by infrequently encountered fungi. Infections caused by these additional agents usually occur in children with immunosuppression or other underlying conditions predisposing to infection. Children who are immunocompetent can acquire infection with these fungi through inhalation via the respiratory tract or direct inoculation following traumatic disruption of cutaneous barriers. A list of these fungal agents and the pertinent underlying host conditions, route of entry, clinical manifestations, diagnostic tests, and treatment for each is found in Table 3.6 (p 250). Taken as a group, a paucity of fungal susceptibility data are available on which to base treatment recommendations for these infections, especially in children. Consultation with a pediatric infectious disease specialist should be considered when caring for a child infected with one of these mycoses.

Table 3.6. **Additional Fungal Diseases**

Disease and Agent	Underlying Condition(s)	Reservoir(s) or Route(s) of Entry	Common Clinical Manifestations	Diagnostic Laboratory Test(s)	Treatment
Fusariosis					
Fusarium species	Granulocytopenia; bone marrow transplantation	Respiratory tract; sinuses; skin	Pulmonary infiltrates; cutaneous lesions; sinusitis; disseminated infection	Culture of blood or tissue specimen	High-dose amphotericin B deoxycholate (AmB) (1–1.5 mg/kg per day)*† and flucytosine
Malassezia species	Prematurity; exposure to parenteral nutrition that includes fat emulsions	Skin	Catheter-associated bloodstream infection; interstitial pneumonitis; urinary tract infection; meningitis	Culture of blood, catheter tip, or tissue specimen; olive oil overlay of Sabouraud dextrose agar is an effective culture medium	Removal of catheters and temporary cessation of lipid infusions; AmB; imidazoles
Penicilliosis					
Penicillium marneffei	Human immunodeficiency virus infection	Respiratory tract	Pneumonitis; invasive dermatitis; disseminated infection	Culture of blood, bone marrow or tissue; histopathologic examination of tissue	Itraconazole or AmB with or without flucytosine
Phaeohyphomycosis					
Bipolaris species	None or organ transplantation	Environment	Sinusitis	Culture and histopathologic examination of tissue	Itraconazole or AmB; surgical excision
Curvularia species	Prematurity; altered skin integrity; asthma or nasal polyps; chronic sinusitis	Environment	Allergic fungal sinusitis; invasive dermatitis; disseminated infection with or without solid organ involvement	Culture and histopathologic examination of tissue	Allergic fungal sinusitis: surgery and corticosteroids Invasive disease: itraconazole‡ or AmB
Exserohilum species	Immunosuppression; altered skin integrity	Environment	Sinusitis; pneumonia; ocular infection; cutaneous lesions	Culture and histopathologic examination of tissue	AmB* or itraconazole; surgical excision

Table 3.6. **Additional Fungal Diseases, continued**

Disease and Agent	Underlying Condition(s)	Reservoir(s) or Route(s) of Entry	Common Clinical Manifestations	Diagnostic Laboratory Test(s)	Treatment
Phaeohyphomycosis, continued					
Pseudallescheria boydii	Immunosuppression	Environment	Pneumonia; disseminated infection; mycetoma (immunocompetent patients)	Culture and histopathologic examination of tissue	Itraconazole§; surgical excision for pulmonary infection, as feasible
Scedosporium species	Immunosuppression	Environment	Pneumonia; disseminated infection; osteomyelitis or septic arthritis (immunocompetent patients)	Culture and histopathologic examination of tissue	Itraconazole‡ or AmB
Trichosporin beigelii	Immunosuppression	Normal flora of skin, stool or urine cultures	Bloodstream infection; endocarditis; pneumonitis	Blood culture; histopathologic examination of tissue	AmB and flucytosine
Zygomycosis					
Rhizopus; Mucormycosis; *Absidia*	Immunosuppression; hematologic malignant neoplasm; renal failure; diabetes mellitus; receipt of multiple antimicrobial agents; exposure to construction activity; use of nonsterile adhesive dressings	Respiratory tract; skin	Rhinocerebral infection; pulmonary infection; disseminated infection; skin and gastrointestinal tract less frequently	Histopathologic examination of tissue	High dose of AmB (1–1.5 mg/kg per day)* and surgical excision, as feasible

* Consider use of a lipid formulation of amphotericin B.

† Infection may be refractory to AmB; use of investigational antifungal compounds may be required.

‡ Itraconazole is the treatment of choice, but data on use in children are limited.

§ Immunocompromised patients may fail to respond. AmB has activity against some strains. Enhanced fungal activity may be observed when AmB is combined with itraconazole or fluconazole.

Giardia lamblia Infections

(Giardiasis)

CLINICAL MANIFESTATIONS: Symptomatic infection causes a broad spectrum of clinical manifestations. Acute watery diarrhea with abdominal pain may develop in patients with clinical illness, or they may experience a protracted, intermittent, often debilitating disease, which is characterized by passage of foul-smelling stools associated with flatulence, abdominal distention, and anorexia. Anorexia combined with malabsorption can lead to significant weight loss, failure to thrive, and anemia. Asymptomatic infection is common.

ETIOLOGY: *Giardia lamblia* is a flagellate protozoan that exists in trophozoite and cyst forms; the infective form is the cyst. Infection is limited to the small intestine and biliary tract.

EPIDEMIOLOGY: Giardiasis has a worldwide distribution. Humans are the principal reservoir of infection, but *Giardia* organisms can infect dogs, cats, beavers, and other animals. These animals can contaminate water with feces containing cysts that are infectious for humans. Persons become infected directly (by hand-to-mouth transfer of cysts from feces of an infected person) or indirectly (by ingestion of fecally contaminated water or food). Many persons who become infected with *G lamblia* remain asymptomatic. Most community-wide epidemics result from a contaminated water supply. Epidemics resulting from person-to-person transmission occur in child care centers and in institutions for mentally retarded persons. Staff and family members in contact with persons in these settings occasionally become infected. Humoral immunodeficiencies predispose to chronic symptomatic *G lamblia* infections. Surveys conducted in the United States have demonstrated prevalence rates of *Giardia* organisms in stool specimens that range from 1% to 20%, depending on geographic location and age. Duration of cyst excretion is variable and may be months. The disease is communicable for as long as the infected person excretes cysts.

The **incubation period** usually is 1 to 4 weeks.

DIAGNOSTIC TESTS: Identification of trophozoites or cysts on direct smear examination or immunofluorescent antibody (IFA) testing of stool specimens or duodenal fluid or detection of *G lamblia* antigens in these specimens by enzyme immunoassay (EIA) is diagnostic. Commercially available EIA techniques for stool specimens have greater sensitivity than microscopy but fail to detect other parasites. One commercially available IFA test allows microscopic detection of *Giardia* and *Cryptosporidium* species in stool with a sensitivity of approximately 75%. A single direct smear examination of stool has a sensitivity of 50% to 75%, which is increased to approximately 95% by testing 3 specimens. To enhance detection, microscopic examination of stool specimens or duodenal fluid should be performed soon after they are obtained, or stool should be mixed, placed in fixative, concentrated, and examined by wet mount and permanent stain. Commercially available stool collection kits containing a vial of 10% formalin and a vial of polyvinyl alcohol fixative in childproof containers are convenient for preserving stool specimens collected at home. Laboratories can reduce reagent and personnel costs by pooling specimens before evaluation by microscopy or EIA. Examination of duodenal contents obtained by direct aspiration or by using a commercially available string test (Entero-Test, HDC Corporation, San Jose, Calif) is a more sensitive procedure than examination of a single stool specimen. Rarely, duodenal biopsy is required for diagnosis.

TREATMENT: Metronidazole is the drug of choice; a 5- to 7-day course of therapy has a cure rate of 80% to 95%. Tinidazole, a nitroimidazole, has a cure rate of 90% to 100% after a single dose, but limited safety and efficacy data are available in children. Furazolidone is 72% to 100% effective when given for 7 to 10 days and has an acceptable flavor for pediatric use. Albendazole has been shown to be as effective as metronidazole for treating giardiasis in children, and it has fewer adverse effects. Albendazole can be formulated into a suspension and has been given to children 2 years of age or older at a dose of 400 mg by mouth daily for 5 days. Paromomycin, a nonabsorbable aminoglycoside that is 50% to 70% effective, is recommended for treatment of symptomatic infection in pregnant women. Quinacrine can be obtained by special order (see Drugs for Parasitic Infections, p 693).

If therapy fails, a course can be repeated with the same drug. Relapse is common in immunocompromised patients who may require prolonged treatment. Some experts recommend combination therapy for giardiasis in immunocompromised patients who are unresponsive to courses of both drugs used separately.

Treatment of asymptomatic carriers generally is not recommended. Possible exceptions to prevent transmission are in households of patients with hypogammaglobulinemia or cystic fibrosis and in pregnant women with toddlers.

ISOLATION OF THE HOSPITALIZED PATIENT: In addition to standard precautions, contact precautions for the duration of illness are recommended for diapered and incontinent children.

CONTROL MEASURES:

- In child care centers, improved sanitation and personal hygiene should be emphasized (see also Children in Out-of-Home Child Care, p 105). Hand washing by staff and children should be emphasized, especially after toilet use or handling of soiled diapers. When an outbreak is suspected, the local health department should be contacted, and an epidemiologic investigation should be undertaken to identify and treat all symptomatic children, child care workers, and family members infected with *G lamblia.* Persons with diarrhea should be excluded from the child care center until they become asymptomatic. Treatment of asymptomatic carriers is not effective for outbreak control. Exclusion of carriers from child care is not recommended.
- Waterborne outbreaks can be prevented by the combination of adequate filtration of water from surface water sources (eg, lakes, rivers, streams), chlorination, and maintenance of water distribution systems.
- Backpackers, campers, and persons likely to be exposed to contaminated water should avoid drinking directly from streams. Boiling of water will kill the infective cysts and other waterborne pathogens.

Gonococcal Infections

CLINICAL MANIFESTATIONS: Gonococcal infections in children occur in 3 distinct age groups.

- Infection in the **newborn infant** usually involves the eyes. Other sites of infection include scalp abscess (which can be associated with fetal monitoring), vaginitis, and disseminated disease with bacteremia, arthritis, meningitis, or endocarditis.
- In **prepubertal children** beyond the newborn period, gonococcal infection may occur in the genital tract and is almost always sexually transmitted. Rarely, transmission from household contact can occur. Vaginitis is the most common manifestation; pelvic inflammatory disease (PID) and perihepatitis can occur but are rare. Gonococcal urethritis in the prepubertal male is uncommon. Anorectal and tonsillopharyngeal infection also can occur in prepubertal children.
- In **sexually active adolescents,** as in adults, gonococcal infection of the genital tract in females is most frequently asymptomatic, and common clinical syndromes are urethritis, endocervicitis, and salpingitis. In males, infection usually is symptomatic, and the primary site is the urethra. Infection of the rectum and pharynx can occur alone or can accompany genitourinary tract infection in either sex. Rectal and pharyngeal infections often are asymptomatic. Extension from primary genital mucosal sites can lead to epididymitis, bartholinitis, PID, and perihepatitis. Even asymptomatic infection can progress to PID with tubal scarring that can result in ectopic pregnancy or infertility. Infection involving other mucous membranes can produce conjunctivitis, pharyngitis, or proctitis. Hematogenous spread can involve skin and joints (arthritis-dermatitis syndrome) and occurs in up to 3% of untreated persons with mucosal gonorrhea. Bacteremia causes a maculopapular rash with necrosis, tenosynovitis, and migratory arthritis. Arthritis can occur as a reactive (sterile) or septic arthritis. Meningitis and endocarditis occur rarely. Dissemination is more common in females infected within 1 week of menstruation.

ETIOLOGY: *Neisseria gonorrhoeae* is a gram-negative oxidase-positive diplococcus.

EPIDEMIOLOGY: Gonococcal infections occur only in humans. The source of the organism is exudate and secretions from infected mucous surfaces; *N gonorrhoeae* is communicable as long as a person harbors the organism. Transmission results from intimate contact, such as sexual acts, parturition, and, rarely, household exposure in prepubertal children. Sexual abuse should be strongly considered when genital, rectal, or pharyngeal colonization or infections are diagnosed in children beyond the newborn period and before puberty and in adolescents who deny that they are sexually active. An estimated 1 million new cases of gonococcal infection occur annually in the United States. Adolescents between 15 and 19 years of age have the highest reported incidence of infection, followed by persons 20 to 24 years of age. Concurrent infection with *Chlamydia trachomatis* is common.

The **incubation period** is usually 2 to 7 days.

DIAGNOSTIC TESTS: Microscopic examination of Gram-stained smears of exudate from the eyes, the endocervix of postpubertal females, the vagina of prepubertal girls, male urethra, skin lesions, synovial fluid, and, when clinically warranted, cerebrospinal fluid (CSF) is useful in the initial evaluation. Identification of gram-negative intracellular diplococci in these smears can be helpful, particularly if the organism is not recovered in culture. Gram stains of material obtained from the endocervix of postpubertal females are less sensitive than culture for detection of infection, but they can be of immediate help in the differential diagnosis of a patient with acute abdominal pain or when immediate therapy is indicated. Other *Neisseria* species and gram-negative cocci may be present in the female genital tract, but these organisms are seldom observed within polymorphonuclear leukocytes. In prepubertal girls, vaginal specimens are adequate for diagnosis, and endocervical specimens are unnecessary.

Neisseria gonorrhoeae can be cultured from normally sterile sites, such as blood, CSF, or synovial fluid, using nonselective chocolate agar with incubation in 5% to 10% carbon dioxide or specialized culture media. Selective media that inhibit normal flora and nonpathogenic *Neisseria* organisms are used for culture from nonsterile sites, such as the cervix, vagina, rectum, urethra, and pharynx. Specimens for *N gonorrhoeae* culture from mucosal sites should be inoculated immediately onto the appropriate agar or placed in transport medium because *N gonorrhoeae* is extremely sensitive to drying and temperature changes.

Caution should be exercised when interpreting the significance of the isolation of *Neisseria* organisms, as *N gonorrhoeae* can be confused with other *Neisseria* species that colonize the genitourinary tract or pharynx. At least 2 confirmatory bacteriologic tests involving different principles (eg, biochemical, enzyme substrate, or serology) should be performed. Interpretation of culture results as *N gonorrhoeae* from the pharynx of young children necessitates particular caution because of the high carriage rate of nonpathogenic *Neisseria* species.

During the last few years, nucleic acid amplification methods by polymerase chain reaction or ligase chain reaction have become clinically available. They are highly sensitive and specific when used on urethral and cervicovaginal swabs. They also can be used with good sensitivity and specificity on first-void urine specimens, which has led to increased compliance with testing and follow-up in hard-to-access populations, such as adolescents. These techniques also permit dual testing of urine for *C trachomatis* and *N gonorrhoeae.*

Sexual Abuse.* In all prepubertal children beyond the newborn period and in nonsexually active adolescents who have gonococcal infection, sexual abuse must be considered to have occurred unless proven otherwise. Genital, rectal, and pharyngeal cultures should be obtained from all patients before antibiotic treatment. All gonococcal isolates from such patients should be preserved. Nonculture gonococcal tests including Gram stain, DNA probes, or enzyme immunoassay tests of oropharyngeal, rectal, or genital tract specimens in children cannot be relied on for diagnosis of gonococcal infection for this purpose, since false-positive results can occur. Appropriate cultures should be obtained from persons who have had contact with

* American Academy of Pediatrics Committee on Child Abuse and Neglect. Guidelines for the evaluation of sexual abuse of children: subject review [published correction appears in *Pediatrics.* 1999;103:1049]. *Pediatrics.* 1999;103:186–191

a child suspected to have been sexually abused. Children in whom sexual abuse is suspected because of detection of gonorrhea should be evaluated for other sexually transmitted diseases, such as *C trachomatis* infection, syphilis, hepatitis B virus, and human immunodeficiency virus (HIV) infection (for further information, see Sexual Abuse, p 255).

TREATMENT: Because of the prevalence of penicillin-resistant *N gonorrhoeae,* an extended-spectrum cephalosporin (eg, ceftriaxone) is recommended as initial therapy for children and either an extended-spectrum cephalosporin or quinolone for adults. High-level resistance to tetracycline is becoming more common, and quinolone-resistant *N gonorrhoeae* has been reported in many parts of the United States but is still at a low level. Resistance to spectinomycin is still uncommon.

Parenteral cephalosporins are recommended for use in young children; ceftriaxone is approved for all gonococcal indications in children, and cefotaxime is approved only for gonococcal ophthalmia. Antimicrobial agents administered orally that have been demonstrated to be effective for treating gonococcal urethritis and cervicitis in adults and older adolescents include cefixime, cefuroxime axetil, azithromycin, ciprofloxacin, ofloxacin, and the newer fluoroquinolones. Although azithromycin, 2 g orally, is effective for uncomplicated gonorrhea, it is expensive and may cause gastrointestinal tract upset. While data to support the use of cefixime to treat gonorrhea in young children are not available, experience in adults indicates that this agent may be considered for uncomplicated infections, provided that follow-up is assured. Fluoroquinolones generally are not recommended for persons younger than 18 years of age (see Antimicrobial Agents and Related Therapy, p 645) and are contraindicated in pregnant or nursing women.

All patients with presumed or proven gonorrhea should be evaluated for concurrent syphilis, hepatitis B virus, HIV, and *C trachomatis* infections. Patients beyond the neonatal period should be treated presumptively for *C trachomatis* infection (see *Chlamydia trachomatis,* p 208).

Culture for a test of cure need not be performed for adolescents and adults with uncomplicated gonorrhea who are asymptomatic after treatment with one of the recommended antibiotic regimens. Children treated with ceftriaxone do not require follow-up cultures, but if treated with other regimens, follow-up is indicated.

Specific recommendations for management and antimicrobial therapy are as follows:

Neonatal Disease. Infants with clinical evidence of ophthalmia neonatorum, scalp abscess, or disseminated infections should be hospitalized. Cultures of blood, eye discharge, or other sites of infection, such as CSF, should be obtained from the infant to confirm the diagnosis and determine antimicrobial susceptibility. Tests for concomitant infection with *C trachomatis* also should be performed as should tests to rule out congenital syphilis and HIV infection. The mother and her partner(s) also need appropriate examination and management for *N gonorrhoeae.*

Nondisseminated Infections. Recommended antimicrobial therapy, including that for ophthalmia neonatorum, is ceftriaxone (25 to 50 mg/kg intravenously or intramuscularly, not to exceed 125 mg) given once. A single dose of cefotaxime (100 mg/kg given intravenously or intramuscularly) is an alternative treatment for ophthalmia neonatorum.

Infants with gonococcal ophthalmia should receive eye irrigations with saline immediately and at frequent intervals until the discharge is eliminated. Topical antibiotic treatment alone is inadequate and is unnecessary when recommended systemic antibiotic treatment is given.

Disseminated Infections. Recommended therapy for arthritis and septicemia is ceftriaxone (25 to 50 mg/kg intravenously or intramuscularly, given once a day) for 7 days or cefotaxime (50 mg/kg per day given intravenously or intramuscularly in 2 divided doses) for 7 days. Cefotaxime is recommended for hyperbilirubinemic infants. If meningitis is documented, treatment should be continued for a total of 10 to 14 days.

Gonococcal Infections in Children Beyond the Neonatal Period and in Adolescents. Recommendations for treatment of gonococcal infections, by age and weight, are given in Tables 3.7 and 3.8 (p 258 and p 259).

Presumptive Treatment for* C trachomatis *Infection. Patients with gonococcal infection also should be treated for presumptive *C trachomatis* infection (see Tables 3.7 and 3.8, p 258 and p 259) and *C trachomatis* (p 208). They also should be evaluated for coinfection with syphilis and other sexually transmitted diseases.

Approximately half of recurrent *C trachomatis* infections occurring after treatment with the recommended schedules are caused by reinfection and indicate the need for improved partner notification, treatment, and patient education.

Special Problems in Treatment of Children (Beyond the Neonatal Period) and Adolescents. Patients with uncomplicated endocervical infection, urethritis, or proctitis who are allergic to cephalosporins should be treated with spectinomycin (40 mg/kg, maximum 2 g, given intramuscularly) if they are not old enough to receive a fluoroquinolone. Patients for whom doxycycline, tetracycline, and azithromycin are contraindicated or who are unable to tolerate these drugs can be given erythromycin base or stearate (2 g/d orally in 4 divided doses for adults) or erythromycin ethyl succinate (3.2 g/d orally in 4 divided doses for adults) for the concurrent treatment of presumptive *C trachomatis* infection.

Patients with uncomplicated pharyngeal gonococcal infection should be treated with ceftriaxone (125 mg, intramuscularly) in a single dose. Those who cannot tolerate ceftriaxone should be treated with ciprofloxacin or ofloxacin (see Antimicrobials and Related Therapy, p 645). Trimethoprim-sulfamethoxazole (720 to 3600 mg) given orally once a day for 5 days may be effective. Spectinomycin is not effective for the treatment of pharyngeal gonorrhea.

Patients who have concurrent infection with syphilis are not effectively treated with a single dose of ceftriaxone (see Syphilis, p 547). Fluoroquinolones and spectinomycin are not active against *Treponema pallidum.*

Children or adolescents with HIV infection should receive the same treatment for gonococcal infection as those without such infection.

Acute PID. *Neisseria gonorrhoeae* and *C trachomatis* are implicated in most cases, and many cases have a polymicrobial cause. No reliable clinical criteria distinguish gonococcal from nongonococcal PID. Hence, broad-spectrum treatment regimens are recommended (see Pelvic Inflammatory Disease, p 431).

Acute Epididymitis. Sexually transmitted organisms, such as *N gonorrhoeae* or *C trachomatis,* can cause acute epididymitis in sexually active adolescents and young adults but rarely cause acute epididymitis in prepubertal children.

Table 3.7. **Uncomplicated Gonococcal Infection: Treatment of Children Beyond the Newborn Period and Adolescents***

Disease†	Prepubertal Children Who Weigh <100 lb (45 kg)	Disease†	Patients Who Weigh ≥100 lb (45 kg) and Who Are 8 Years or Older
Uncomplicated vulvovaginitis, cervicitis, urethritis, proctitis, or pharyngitis	Ceftriaxone, 125 mg IM in a single dose *or* Spectinomycin,‡ 50 mg/kg (maximum, 2 g) IM in a single dose **PLUS** Erythromycin, 50 mg/kg per day (maximum, 2 g/d) in 4 divided doses for 7 d *or* Azithromycin, 20 mg/kg (maximum, 1 g) in a single dose	Uncomplicated endocervicitis, urethritis, epididymitis, proctitis, or pharyngitis§	Ceftriaxone, 125 mg IM in a single dose *or* Cefixime, 400 mg orally in a single dose *or* Ciprofloxacin,‖ 500 mg orally in a single dose *or* Ofloxacin,‖ 400 mg orally in a single dose **PLUS¶** Doxycycline (100 mg orally twice a day for 7 days) *or* Azithromycin (1 g orally in a single dose)

* In addition to the recommended treatment for gonococcal infection, therapy for *Chlamydia trachomatis* is recommended on the presumption that the patient has concomitant infection. IM indicates intramuscularly.

† Hospitalization should be considered, especially for persons treated as outpatients whose infection has failed to respond and for persons who are unlikely to adhere to treatment regimens.

‡ Spectinomycin is not recommended for treatment of pharyngeal infections; in persons who cannot take a cephalosporin or a fluoroquinolone, a 5-day oral regimen of trimethoprim-sulfamethoxazole may be given.

§ Alternative regimens include spectinomycin (2 g IM in a single dose), ceftizoxime, cefotaxime, cefotetan, and cefoxitin. Spectinomycin is not recommended for pharyngitis.

‖ Fluoroquinolones are contraindicated for pregnant women, nursing women, and usually for persons younger than 18 years of age (see Antimicrobial Agents and Related Therapy, p 645).

¶ In all cases, in addition to the recommended treatment for gonococcal infection, doxycycline or azithromycin is recommended on the presumption that the patient has concomitant infection with *C trachomatis*.

Table 3.8. **Complicated Gonococcal Infection: Treatment of Children Beyond the Newborn Period and Adolescents***

Disease†	Prepubertal Children Who Weigh <100 lb (45 kg)	Disease	Patients Who Weigh ≥100 lb (45 kg) and Who Are 8 Years of Age or Older
Disseminated gonococcal infection (eg, arthritis-dermatitis syndrome)	Ceftriaxone, 50 mg/kg per day (maximum, 1 g/d) IV or IM once a day for 7 d **PLUS*** Erythromycin, doxycycline, or azithromycin	Disseminated gonococcal infections§	Ceftriaxone, 1 g IV or IM given once a day for 7 d‖ ***or*** Cefotaxime, 1 g IV every 8 hours for 7 d‖ **PLUS** Doxycycline, 100 mg orally twice a day for 7 days ***or*** Azithromycin, 1 g orally in a single dose*
Meningitis or endocarditis	Ceftriaxone, 50 mg/kg per day (maximum, 2 g/d) IV or IM given every 12 h; for meningitis, duration is 10–14 d; for endocarditis, duration is at least 28 d **PLUS*** Erythromycin, 40 mg/kg per day (maximum, 2 g/d) in 4 divided doses for 7 d	Meningitis or endocarditis†	Ceftriaxone, 1–2 g IV every 12 h; for meningitis, duration is 10–14 d; for endocarditis, duration is at least 28 d
		Conjunctivitis‡	Ceftriaxone, 1 g IM in a single dose
Conjunctivitis‡	Ceftriaxone, 50 mg/kg (maximum, 1 g) IM in a single dose	Pelvic inflammatory disease	See Table 3.42 (p 434)

* In addition to the recommended treatment for gonococcal infection, therapy for *Chlamydia trachomatis* is recommended on the presumption that the patient has concomitant infection. IV indicates intravenously, and IM, intramuscularly.

† Hospitalization is required; follow-up cultures are necessary to ensure that treatment has been effective.

‡ Eyes should be lavaged with saline to clear accumulated secretions.

§ For persons allergic to ß-lactam drugs: ciprofloxacin (500 mg IV every 12 h) *or* ofloxacin (400 mg IV every 12 h) *or* spectinomycin (2 g IM every 12 h). Spectinomycin is not recommended for treatment of pharyngeal gonococcal infection. Hospitalization recommended.

‖ Alternatively, parenteral therapy can be discontinued 24 to 48 hours after improvement occurs and a 7-day course completed with an appropriate oral antimicrobial such as cefixime, 400 mg orally twice a day; or ciprofloxacin, 500 mg orally twice a day; or ofloxacin, 400 mg orally twice a day. Both ciprofloxacin and ofloxacin are contraindicated for pregnant women, nursing women, and usually for persons younger than 18 years of age (see Antimicrobial Agents and Related Therapy, p 645). Some experts advise a 10- to 14-day course of therapy.

The recommended regimen for sexually transmitted epididymitis is ceftriaxone and erythromycin, azithromycin, or doxycycline, depending on the patient's age (see Table 3.7, p 258).

ISOLATION OF THE HOSPITALIZED PATIENT: Standard precautions are recommended, including for newborn infants with ophthalmia.

CONTROL MEASURES:

Neonatal Ophthalmia. For routine prophylaxis of infants immediately after birth, a 1% solution of silver nitrate, or 1% tetracycline, or 0.5% erythromycin ophthalmic ointment, or 2.5% povidone-iodine solution is instilled into each eye; subsequent irrigation should not be performed (see Prevention of Neonatal Ophthalmia, p 735). Prophylaxis may be delayed for as long as 1 hour after birth to facilitate parent-infant bonding. Topical antibiotics are less likely to cause a chemical irritation than silver nitrate; all are ineffective against *C trachomatis*, since topical ophthalmic treatment does not eradicate this organism from the nasopharynx.

Infants Born to Mothers With Gonococcal Infections. When prophylaxis is administered correctly, infants born to mothers with gonococcal infection infrequently develop gonococcal ophthalmia. However, since gonococcal ophthalmia or disseminated infection occasionally can occur in this situation, infants born to mothers with gonorrhea should receive a single dose of ceftriaxone, 125 mg intravenously or intramuscularly; for premature and low-birth-weight infants, the dose is 25 to 50 mg/kg to a maximum of 125 mg. Cefotaxime in a single dose (100 mg/kg given intravenously or intramuscularly) is an alternative.

Children and Adolescents With Sexual Exposure to a Patient Known to Have Gonorrhea. Exposed persons should undergo examination, culture, and treatment the same as those known to have gonorrhea.

Education. Sustained educational efforts are necessary to control sexually transmitted diseases among adolescents (see Sexually Transmitted Diseases, p 663).

Pregnancy. All pregnant females should have an endocervical culture for gonococci as an integral part of their prenatal care at the first visit. A second culture late in the third trimester is recommended for women at high risk of exposure to gonococcal infection. Recommended therapeutic regimens for patients found to be infected are those previously described for uncomplicated gonorrhea, except that a tetracycline or fluoroquinolone should not be used because of the potential toxic effects on the fetus. Women who are allergic to cephalosporins should be treated with spectinomycin.

Case Reporting and Management of Sex Partners. All cases of gonorrhea must be reported to public health officials (see Appendix VIII, Nationally Notifiable Infectious Diseases in the United States, p 777). Cases in prepubertal children must be investigated to determine the source of infection. Ensuring that sexual contacts are treated and counseled is essential for community control, prevention of reinfection, and prevention of complications in the contact.

Granuloma Inguinale

(Donovanosis)

CLINICAL MANIFESTATIONS: Initial lesions are single or multiple subcutaneous nodules that progress to form painless, friable, granulomatous ulcers. Lesions usually involve the genitalia, but anal infections occur in 5% to 10% of patients; lesions at distant sites (eg, face, mouth, or liver) are rare. Subcutaneous extension into the inguinal area results in induration that can mimic inguinal adenopathy, ie, the "pseudobubo" of granuloma inguinale. Fibrosis manifests as sinus tracts, adhesions, and lymphedema, resulting in extreme genital deformity.

ETIOLOGY: The disease is caused by *Calymmatobacterium granulomatis*, a gram-negative bacillus.

EPIDEMIOLOGY: Indigenous granuloma inguinale no longer occurs in the United States and most developed countries. Cases that occur in the United States are imported. Donovanosis is common in New Guinea and parts of India, Africa, and, to a much lesser extent, the Caribbean and parts of South America, most notably, Brazil. The highest incidence of disease occurs in tropical and subtropical environments. The incidence of infection seems to correlate strongly with sustained high temperatures and high relative humidity. Infection usually is acquired by sexual intercourse, most commonly with a person with active infection, but possibly also from a person with asymptomatic rectal infection. Granuloma inguinale is mildly contagious, and repeated exposure may be necessary for development of disease. Young children can acquire infection by contact with infected secretions. The period of communicability extends throughout the duration of active lesions or rectal colonization.

The **incubation period** is 8 to 80 days.

DIAGNOSTIC TESTS: The microscopic demonstration of intracytoplasmic Donovan bodies on Wright or Giemsa staining of a crush preparation from subsurface scrapings of a lesion or tissue is diagnostic. The microorganism also can be detected by histologic examination of biopsy specimens. Culture of *C granulomatis* has been accomplished using Hep-2 cells, but this technique is not available routinely. Lesions, however, should be cultured for *Haemophilus ducreyi* to exclude chancroid (pseudogranuloma inguinale). Granuloma inguinale frequently is misdiagnosed as carcinoma, which can be excluded by histologic examination of tissue or by response of the lesion to antibiotics. Diagnosis by polymerase chain reaction and serology is available, although only on a research basis.

TREATMENT: Doxycycline (which ordinarily should not be given to children younger than 8 years of age) at a dosage of 100 mg orally twice a day and trimethoprim-sulfamethoxazole have been reported to be effective. Gentamicin and ciprofloxacin, which is not recommended for use in pregnant women or children younger than 18 years of age, are effective but reserved for resistant cases. Erythromycin has been used in treatment of pregnant patients. Antimicrobial therapy is continued for at least 3 weeks or until the lesions have resolved. If antimicrobial therapy is effective, partial healing usually is noted within 7 days. Relapse can occur, especially if the antibiotic is stopped before the primary lesion has healed completely.

Patients should be evaluated for other sexually transmitted diseases, such as gonorrhea, syphilis, and infection with *Chlamydia trachomatis*, hepatitis B virus, and human immunodeficiency virus.

ISOLATION OF THE HOSPITALIZED PATIENT: Standard precautions are recommended.

CONTROL MEASURES: Sexual partners should be examined, counseled to use condoms, and given antimicrobial therapy.

Haemophilus influenzae Infections

CLINICAL MANIFESTATIONS: *Haemophilus influenzae* causes otitis media, sinusitis, epiglottitis, septic arthritis, occult febrile bacteremia, cellulitis, meningitis, pneumonia, and empyema. Other *H influenzae* infections include purulent pericarditis, endocarditis, conjunctivitis, endophthalmitis, osteomyelitis, peritonitis, epididymo-orchitis, glossitis, uvulitis, and septic thrombophlebitis. Occasionally, nonencapsulated strains cause neonatal septicemia, pneumonia, and meningitis.

ETIOLOGY: *Haemophilus influenzae* is a pleomorphic gram-negative coccobacillus. Isolates are classified into 6 antigenically distinct capsular types (a through f) and nonencapsulated, nontypeable strains. Most cases of invasive diseases in children, before the introduction of *H influenzae* type b (Hib) conjugate vaccination, were caused by type b. Type f is the most common other serotype causing invasive infections. Nonencapsulated strains cause upper respiratory tract infection, including otitis media, sinusitis, tracheitis, and bronchitis, and may cause pneumonia.

EPIDEMIOLOGY: The source of the organism is the upper respiratory tract. The mode of transmission presumably is person-to-person, by direct contact or through inhalation of droplets of respiratory tract secretions containing the organism, or in the neonate by intrapartum aspiration of amniotic fluid or genital tract secretions containing the organism. Asymptomatic colonization by *H influenzae* strains is common; nonencapsulated strains are recovered from the throat of 60% to 90% of children. Colonization by type b organisms is infrequent, ranging from 2% to 5% of children in the prevaccine era; widespread use of Hib conjugate vaccines has resulted in even lower colonization rates. The exact period of communicability is unknown.

Before introduction of effective vaccines, Hib was the most common cause of bacterial meningitis in children in the United States. Meningitis and other invasive infections due to Hib were most common in children 3 months to 3 years of age. In contrast with most other invasive Hib disease, epiglottitis is rare in infants younger than 12 months of age. In the prevaccine era, the peak age for epiglottitis occurred at 2 to 4 years of age; epiglottitis can occur in older unimmunized children and adults.

Invasive disease has been more frequent in boys, African Americans, Alaskan Eskimos, Apache and Navajo Indians, child care center attendees, children living in overcrowded conditions, and children who were not breastfed. Unimmunized children, particularly those younger than 4 years of age who are in prolonged close contact (such as in a household setting) with a child with invasive Hib disease, are at an increased risk for invasive Hib disease. Other factors predisposing to invasive disease include sickle cell disease, asplenia, human immunodeficiency virus (HIV) infection, certain immunodeficiency syndromes, and malignant neoplasms.

Since 1988 when Hib conjugate vaccines were introduced, the incidence of invasive Hib disease in infants and young children has declined by 99%. The incidence of invasive infections caused by all other encapsulated types combined now is similar to that caused by type b. As a result of this success, the US Public Health Service has targeted Hib disease in children younger than 5 years of age for elimination in this country. Invasive Hib disease occurs now primarily in underimmunized children and among infants too young to have completed the primary immunization series.

The **incubation period** is unknown.

DIAGNOSTIC TESTS: Cerebrospinal fluid (CSF), blood, synovial fluid, pleural fluid, and middle ear aspirates should be cultured on a medium such as chocolate agar enriched with X and V cofactors. A Gram stain of an infected body fluid can disclose the organism and allows a presumptive diagnosis to be made. Latex particle agglutination for detection of type b capsular antigen in CSF may be helpful when antimicrobial therapy was initiated before cultures were obtained. However, antigen testing of serum and of urine is not recommended since antigen can be detected as a result of asymptomatic nasopharyngeal carriage of Hib, recent immunization with an Hib conjugate vaccine, or contamination of urine specimens by cross-reacting fecal organisms. All *H influenzae* isolates associated with an invasive infection should be serotyped to determine whether the strain is type b. If testing is not available, isolates should be submitted to the state health department, to the Centers for Disease Control and Prevention, or to a reference laboratory for testing.

TREATMENT:

- Initial therapy for children with meningitis possibly caused by Hib is cefotaxime, ceftriaxone, or ampicillin in combination with chloramphenicol. Ampicillin alone should not be used as initial therapy since 10% to 40% of Hib isolates are ampicillin-resistant.
- For patients with uncomplicated meningitis whose infection responds rapidly, therapy for 7 to 10 days administered intravenously in a high dose usually is satisfactory. Therapy for more than 10 days may be indicated in complicated cases.
- For treatment of other invasive *H influenzae* infections, including non–type b capsular types, recommendations are similar but primarily are based on empiric experience.
- Dexamethasone is recommended for treatment of infants and children with Hib meningitis.
- Epiglottitis is a medical emergency. An airway must be established promptly by endotracheal tube or tracheostomy.

- Infected synovial, pleural, or pericardial fluid should be drained.
- For empiric therapy of acute otitis media, most experts recommend oral amoxicillin (see details in Pneumococcal Infections, p 452). Duration of therapy is 5 to 10 days. The 5-day course is considered for children 2 years of age and older. Approximately 35% of *H influenzae* isolates in the United States produce ß-lactamase, necessitating a ß-lactamase–resistant agent, such as an oral cephalosporin, a newer macrolide, or amoxicillin-clavulanate. In vitro susceptibility testing of isolates from middle ear fluid specimens may help guide therapy in complicated or persistent cases.

ISOLATION OF THE HOSPITALIZED PATIENT: In addition to standard precautions, droplet precautions are recommended for 24 hours after initiation of antimicrobial therapy for invasive Hib disease.

CONTROL MEASURES (FOR INVASIVE HIB INFECTIONS):

Care of Exposed Persons.

Careful observation of exposed unimmunized or incompletely immunized household, child care, or nursery contacts is essential. Exposed children in whom a febrile illness develops should receive prompt medical evaluation. If indicated, antimicrobial therapy appropriate for invasive Hib infection should be initiated.

Chemoprophylaxis. The risk of invasive Hib disease among unimmunized household contacts younger than 4 years of age is increased. Asymptomatic colonization with Hib also is more frequent in household contacts of all ages than in the general population. Rifampin eradicates Hib from the pharynx in approximately 95% of carriers. Limited data indicate that rifampin prophylaxis also decreases the risk of secondary invasive illness in exposed household contacts. Nursery and child care center contacts also may be at increased risk of secondary disease, but experts disagree about the magnitude of the risk. The risk of secondary disease in children attending child care centers seems to be lower than that observed for age-susceptible household contacts, and secondary disease in child care contacts is rare when all contacts are older than 2 years of age. Moreover, the efficacy of rifampin in preventing disease in child care groups is not established.

Indications and guidelines for chemoprophylaxis in different circumstances are summarized in Table 3.9 (p 265).

- ***Household.*** Chemoprophylaxis is not recommended for occupants of households with no children younger than 48 months of age other than the index case and when all household contacts younger than 48 months of age have completed their Hib immunization series (see Table 3.9, p 265). In households with at least 1 contact younger than 48 months of age who is unimmunized or incompletely immunized against Hib, rifampin prophylaxis is recommended for all household contacts, irrespective of age. The exception to this recommendation is that all members of households with a fully immunized but immunocompromised child, regardless of age, should receive rifampin because of concern that the immunization series may not have been effective. Although the risk of secondary disease is low in an infant who has completed the primary 2- or 3-dose series, all members of a household with a child younger

Table 3.9. Indications and Guidelines for Rifampin Chemoprophylaxis for Contacts of Index Cases of Invasive *Haemophilus influenzae* Type b (Hib) Disease

Chemoprophylaxis Not Recommended

- Occupants of households with no children younger than 4 years of age other than the index patient
- Occupants of households when all household contacts younger than 48 months of age have completed their Hib immunization series*
- Nursery and child care center contacts of 1 index case, especially those older than 2 years of age
- Pregnant women

Chemoprophylaxis Recommended

- All household contacts (except pregnant women),† irrespective of age, with at least 1 contact younger than 4 years of age who is unimmunized or incompletely immunized* The index patient also should receive chemoprophylaxis
- All members of a household with a child younger than 12 months of age, even if the primary series has been given
- All occupants of a household with an immunocompromised child, irrespective of the child's Hib immunization status
- Nursery and child care center contacts, irrespective of age, when 2 or more cases of invasive disease have occurred within 60 days
- Index case, if treated with regimens other than cefotaxime or ceftriaxone. Chemoprophylaxis usually is provided just before discharge

* Complete immunization is defined as having had at least 1 dose of conjugate vaccine at 15 months of age or older; 2 doses between 12 and 14 months of age; or a 2- or 3-dose primary series when younger than 12 months with a booster dose at 12 months of age or older.

† Defined as persons residing with the index patient or nonresidents who spent 4 or more hours with the index case for at least 5 of the 7 days preceding the day of hospital admission of the index case.

than 12 months of age (ie, who has not yet received the booster vaccine dose) should receive rifampin prophylaxis.

When indicated, prophylaxis should be initiated as soon as possible since the majority of secondary cases in households occur during the first week after hospitalization of the index patient. The time of occurrence of the remaining secondary cases after the first week suggests that prophylaxis of household contacts initiated 7 days or more after hospitalization of the index patient, although not optimal, may still be of benefit.

- ***Child care and nursery school.*** When 2 or more cases of invasive disease have occurred within 60 days and unimmunized or incompletely immunized children attend the child care facility, administration of rifampin to all attendees and supervisory personnel is indicated. When a single case has occurred, the advisability of rifampin prophylaxis in exposed child care groups with unimmunized or incompletely immunized children is controversial, but many experts recommend no prophylaxis.

In addition to these recommendations for chemoprophylaxis, unimmunized or incompletely immunized children should receive a dose of vaccine and should be scheduled for completion of the recommended age-specific immunization schedule (see Immunization, below).

- ***Index case.*** The index patient also should receive rifampin prophylaxis only if ampicillin or chloramphenicol was used for treatment.
- ***Dosage.*** Rifampin should be given orally once a day for 4 days (in a dose of 20 mg/kg; maximum dose, 600 mg). The dose for infants younger than 1 month of age is not established; some experts recommend lowering the dose to 10 mg/kg. For adults, each dose is 600 mg.

Immunization.

Four Hib conjugate vaccines have been licensed in the United States (see Table 3.10, p 267). These vaccines consist of the Hib capsular polysaccharide (ie, polyribosylribotol phosphate [PRP] or PRP oligomers) covalently linked to a carrier protein directly or via an intervening spacer molecule. Protective antibodies are directed against PRP. Conjugate vaccines differ in composition and immunogenicity, and, as a result, recommendations for their use differ. In Native American and Alaskan Native children, because of their increased risk for disease in early infancy, it may be advantageous to use PRP-OMP (outer membrane protein) for the first dose in a series because of the substantial antibody response after 1 dose.*

A primary series consisting of 3 doses given at 2, 4, and 6 months of age or 2 doses given at 2 and 4 months of age, depending on the vaccine product, is recommended (see Recommendations for Immunization, p 268, and Table 3.11, p 268). The recommended doses may be given as combination vaccines. The regimens in Table 3.11 are likely to be equivalent in protection after completion of the recommended primary series.

After administration of the primary series, serum antibody concentrations decline rapidly. Therefore, an additional booster dose of any conjugate vaccine licensed by the US Food and Drug Administration is recommended at 12 to 15 months of age, regardless of which regimen was used for the primary series. This dose may be given as a combination vaccine.

Vaccine Interchangeability. These products are considered interchangeable for primary as well as booster immunization. If PRP-OMP is administered in a primary series, the recommended number of doses to complete the series is determined by the other Hib conjugate vaccine.

Dosage and Route of Administration. The dose of each Hib conjugate vaccine is 0.5 mL, given intramuscularly.

Children With Immunologic Impairment. Children at increased risk of Hib disease may have impaired anti-PRP antibody responses to conjugate vaccines. Examples of such children include those with HIV infection, immunoglobulin deficiency, anatomic or functional asplenia, and sickle cell disease, as well as recipients of bone marrow transplants and those receiving chemotherapy for a malignant neoplasm. Some children with immunologic impairment may benefit from more doses of conjugate vaccine than usually indicated (see Recommendations for Immunization, p 268).

---

* American Academy of Pediatrics Committee on Native American Child Health and Committee on Infectious Diseases. Immunizations for Native American children. *Pediatrics.* 1999;104:564–567

Table 3.10. Licensed *Haemophilus influenzae* Type b Conjugate Vaccines Available in the United States*

Manufacturer	Abbreviation	Trade Name	Carrier Protein
Lederle Laboratories, Pearl River, NY (distributed by Wyeth-Lederle Vaccines, Wyeth-Ayerst Laboratories, Philadelphia, Pa)	HbOC	HibTITER	CRM_{197} (a nontoxic mutant diphtheria toxin)
Merck & Co, Inc, West Point, Pa†	PRP-OMP	PedvaxHIB	OMP (an outer membrane protein of *Neisseria meningitidis*)
Pasteur Mérieux Sérums & Vaccins, SA, Lyon, France (distributed by Connaught Laboratories, Swiftwater, Pa, and by SmithKline Beecham Pharmaceuticals, Philadephia, Pa)	PRP-T	ActHIB, OmniHIB	Tetanus toxoid
Pasteur Mérieux Connaught, Swiftwater, Pa	PRP-D	ProHIBiT	Diphtheria toxoid

* HbOC (diphtheria CRM_{197} protein conjugate), PRP-OMP (polyribosylribotol phosphate–outer membrane protein), and PRP-T are recommended for infants beginning at approximately 2 months of age. PRP-D is recommended only for children 12 months of age or older. The US Food and Drug Administration (FDA), however, has approved labeling for PRP-D for booster administration beginning at 12 months of age and for primary administration at 15 months of age. These vaccines may be given in combination products or as reconstituted products with DTaP (diphtheria and tetanus toxoids and acellular pertussis) or DTP (diphtheria and tetanus toxoids and pertussis), provided the combination or reconstituted vaccine is approved by the FDA for the child's age and administration of the other vaccine component(s) also is justified.

† A combination of *H influenzae* (PRP-OMP) and hepatitis B (Recombivax, 5 µg) vaccine is licensed for use at 2, 4, and 12 to 15 months of age (Comvax).

Vaccine Failure. Despite receiving immunization with a conjugate vaccine, Hib disease can occur. Since serum antibody responses do not occur for 1 to 2 weeks after immunization, recipients are not expected to be protected during this immediate postimmunization period. The interval after immunization when protection can be anticipated is unknown. Health care professionals should be aware of this uncertainty and should not expect protection simultaneously with vaccine administration.

Adverse Reactions. Adverse reactions to the Hib conjugate vaccines are few. Pain, redness, and swelling at the injection site occur in approximately 25% of recipients, but these symptoms typically are mild and last less than 24 hours. Systemic reactions are infrequent. When conjugate vaccines are administered during the same visit that diphtheria and tetanus toxoid and acellular pertussis (DTaP) vaccine is given, the rates of systemic reactions do not differ from those observed when only DTaP vaccine is administered.

Table 3.11. **Currently Recommended Regimens for Routine *Haemophilus influenzae* Type b Conjugate Immunization for Children Immunized Beginning at 2 to 6 Months of Age***

Vaccine Product at Initiation	Total No. of Doses To Be Administered	Recommended Regimen
HbOC or PRP-T	4	3 doses at 2-mo intervals initially; fourth dose at 12 to 15 mo of age; any conjugate vaccine for dose 4†
PRP-OMP	3	2 doses at 2-mo interval initially; when feasible, same vaccine for doses 1 and 2; third dose at 12–15 mo of age; any conjugate vaccine for dose 3†

* See text and Table 3.10 for further information about specific vaccines and for explanation of the abbreviations. These vaccines may be given in combination products or as reconstituted products with DTaP or DTP, provided the combination or reconstituted vaccine is approved by the US Food and Drug Administration for the child's age and administration of the other vaccine component(s) also is justified.

† The safety and efficacy of PRP-OMP, PRP-T, HbOC, and, PRP-D are likely to be equivalent for children 12 months of age and older. If a different product is given for dose 2, then the recommendations for that product (eg, HbOC or PRP-T) apply.

Recommendations for Immunization.

Indications and Schedule

- All children should be immunized with an Hib conjugate vaccine beginning at approximately 2 months of age or as soon as possible thereafter (see Table 3.11, above). Other generic recommendations are as follows:
  - Immunization can be initiated as early as 6 weeks of age.
  - Vaccine may be given during visits when vaccines for diphtheria, tetanus, pertussis (DTaP), polio, hepatitis B, MMR (measles, mumps, rubella), and varicella are given (see Simultaneous Administration of Multiple Vaccines, p 26). No known contraindications exist to simultaneous administration of Hib conjugate vaccine with pneumococcal or meningococcal vaccine when given in separate syringes at different sites.
- For routine immunization of children younger than 7 months of age, the following guidelines are recommended:
  - *Primary series.* A 3-dose regimen of HbOC (diphtheria CRM_{197} protein conjugate) or PRP-T or a 2-dose regimen of PRP-OMP should be administered (see Table 3.11, above). Doses are given at approximately 2-month intervals. When sequential doses of different vaccine products are given or uncertainty exists about which products previously were administered, 3 doses of any conjugate vaccine are considered sufficient to complete the primary series, irrespective of the regimen used.
  - *Booster immunization at 12 to 15 months of age.* For children who have completed a primary series, an additional dose of conjugate vaccine is recommended at 12 to 15 months of age or as soon as possible thereafter. Any

Table 3.12. **Recommendations for *Haemophilus influenzae* Type b Conjugate Immunization for Children in Whom Initial Immunization Is Delayed Until 7 Months of Age or Older***

Age at Initiation of Immunization, mo	Vaccine Product at Initiation	Total No. of Doses To Be Administered	Recommended Vaccine Regimens
7–11	HbOC, PRP-T, P or PRP-OM	3	2 doses at 2-mo intervals; third dose at 12–15 mo of age, given at 2 mo after dose 2; any conjugate vaccine for dose 3†
12–14	HbOC, PRP-T, PRP-OMP, or PRP-D	2	2-mo interval between doses
15–59	HbOC, PRP-T, PRP-OMP, or PRP-D	1‡	Any conjugate vaccine
60 and older§	HbOC, PRP-T, PRP-OMP, or PRP-D	1 or 2‡	Any conjugate vaccine

* See text and Table 3.10 for further information about specific vaccines and for explanation of the abbreviations. These vaccines may be given in combination products or as reconstituted products with DTaP or DTP, provided the combination or reconstituted vaccine is approved by the US Food and Drug Administration for the child's age and administration of the other vaccine component(s) also is justified.

† The safety and efficacy of PRP-OMP, PRP-T, HbOC or PRP-D are likely to be equivalent for use as a booster dose for children 12 months or older.

‡ Two doses separated by 2 months are recommended by some experts for children with certain underlying diseases associated with increased risk of disease and impaired antibody responses to *H influenzae* type b conjugate vaccination (see text).

§ Only for children with chronic illness known to be associated with an increased risk for *H influenzae* type b disease (see text).

conjugate vaccine (HbOC, PRP-OMP, PRP-T, or PRP-D) is acceptable for this dose.

- Children younger than 5 years of age who did not receive Hib conjugate vaccine during the first 6 months of life should be immunized according to the recommended schedules (see Table 3.12, above). For accelerated immunization, a minimum of a 1-month (4-week) interval between doses may be used.
  - For children in whom immunization is initiated at 7 to 11 months of age, the recommended schedules for HbOC, PRP-OMP, and PRP-T are identical and require 3 doses. The first 2 doses are given at 2-month intervals. The third (booster) dose should be given at 12 to 18 months of age, preferably 2 months after the second dose. For the third dose, any licensed conjugate vaccine is acceptable.

   - For children in whom immunization is initiated at 12 to 14 months of age, the recommended regimens for HbOC, PRP-OMP, and PRP-T are identical and require 2 doses given at a 2-month interval. PRP-D can be given as the second dose.
   - For children in whom immunization is initiated at 15 months of age or older and who have not yet reached their fifth birthday (ie, 59 months of age or younger), the recommended regimen is a single dose of any licensed conjugate vaccine.
   - Circumstances may suggest a need for more rapid catch-up immunization, in which case 1 month (4 weeks) is the recommended accelerated interval between doses.
- Special circumstances are as follows:
   - *Lapsed immunizations.* Recommendations for children who have had a lapse in the schedule of immunizations are based on limited data. The current recommendations are summarized in Table 3.13 (p 271).
   - *Premature infants.* For infants born prematurely, immunization should be based on chronologic age and initiated at 2 months of age according to recommendations in Table 3.11 (p 268). This recommendation is based on available data suggesting that even very-low-birth-weight (ie, premature) infants have adequate antibody responses to these vaccines, although the serum concentrations of antibody may be decreased in chronically ill infants in comparison with those in full-term infants.
   - *Children who may be at increased risk of invasive Hib disease resulting from immunologic or other host defense abnormalities (eg, sickle cell disease and postsplenectomy).* Children with decreased or absent splenic function who have received a primary series of Hib immunizations and a booster dose at 12 months of age or older need not be immunized further. Children who complete a primary series followed by a booster dose who are undergoing scheduled splenectomy (eg, for Hodgkin disease, spherocytosis, immune thrombocytopenia, or hypersplenism) may benefit from an additional dose of any licensed conjugate vaccine. This dose should be provided at least 7 to 10 days before the procedure. Patients with HIV infection or immunoglobulin (Ig) G2 subclass deficiency and those receiving chemotherapy for malignant neoplasms also are at increased risk for invasive Hib disease. Whether these children will benefit from additional doses after completion of the primary series of immunizations and the booster dose at 12 months of age or later is unknown. Every effort should be made to ensure completion of the primary immunization and booster series.

     For children 12 to 59 months of age with an underlying condition predisposing to Hib disease who are not immunized or have received only 1 dose of conjugate vaccine before 12 months of age, 2 doses of any conjugate vaccine, separated by 2 months, are recommended. For children in this age group who received 2 doses before 12 months of age, 1 additional dose of conjugate vaccine is recommended.
   - *Unimmunized children with an underlying disease possibly predisposing to Hib disease who are older than 59 months of age.* These children should be immu-

Table 3.13. **Recommendations for *Haemophilus influenzae* Type b Conjugate Immunization in Children With a Lapse in Administration***

Age at Presentation, mo	Previous Immunization History	Recommended Regimen
7–11	1 dose of HbOC or PRP-T	1 or 2 doses of conjugate vaccine at 7–11 mo of age (depending on age), with a booster dose given at least 2 mo later, at 12–15 mo of age
	2 doses of HbOC or PRP-T or 1 dose of PRP-OMP	1 dose of conjugate vaccine at 7–11 mo of age with a booster dose given at least 2 mo later at 12–15 mo of age
12–14	2 doses before 12 mo of age†	A single dose of any licensed conjugate vaccine‡
12–14	1 dose before 12 mo of age†	2 additional doses of any licensed conjugate vaccine, separated by 2 mo‡
15–59	Any incomplete schedule	A single dose of any licensed conjugate vaccine‡

* See text and Table 3.10 for further information about specific vaccines and for explanation of abbreviations. These vaccines may be given in combination products or as reconstituted products with DTaP or DTP, provided the combination or reconstituted vaccine is approved by the US Food and Drug Administration for the child's age and the administration of the other vaccine component(s) also is justified.

† PRP-OMP, PRP-T, or HbOC.

‡ The safety and efficacy of PRP-OMP, PRP-T, or HbOC or PRP-D are likely to be equivalent when used for children 12 months of age or older.

nized with any licensed conjugate vaccine. Based on limited data, 2 doses separated by 1 to 2 months are suggested for children with HIV infection or IgG2 deficiency.

- Haemophilus influenzae *type b invasive infection.* Children who had invasive disease when younger than 24 months of age frequently have low anticapsular antibody concentrations in convalescent serum samples and may remain at risk of developing a second episode of disease. Immunization in these patients should be administered according to the age-appropriate schedule for unimmunized children and as if they had received no prior Hib vaccine doses (see Tables 3.11, p 268 and 3.13, above). Immunization should be initiated 1 month after onset of disease or as soon as possible thereafter. Children whose disease occurred at 24 months of age or older do not need immunization because the disease most likely induced a protective immune response and second episodes of disease at this age are rare.

  Immunologic evaluation should be performed for children who experience invasive Hib disease after 2 to 3 doses of vaccine administered before 12 months of age or in children with a history of recurrent infection. Immunized infants and children who contract invasive *H influenzae* non–type b infection have a high likelihood of underlying immune deficiency. These children should undergo immunologic evaluation.

Reporting. *Haemophilus influenzae* invasive disease, including type b and non–type b infection and cases in fully or partially immunized children, should be reported to the Centers for Disease Control and Prevention through the local and state public health departments.

Hantavirus Cardiopulmonary Syndrome

CLINICAL MANIFESTATIONS: The prodromal illness of 3 to 7 days is characterized by fever; chills; headache; myalgias of the shoulders, lower back, and thighs; nausea; vomiting; diarrhea; and dizziness. Respiratory tract symptoms or signs do not occur for the first 3 to 7 days until pulmonary edema and severe hypoxemia appear abruptly and progress over a few hours. In severe cases, persistent hypotension caused by myocardial dysfunction is present, hence the name, hantavirus cardiopulmonary syndrome (HPS).

The extensive bilateral interstitial and alveolar pulmonary edema and pleural effusions are the result of a diffuse pulmonary capillary leak and seem to be immune-mediated. Intubation usually is required for only 2 to 4 days, with resolution heralded by the onset of diuresis and rapid clinical improvement. Full recovery can be expected since there are no necrotic pulmonary parenchymal changes.

The severe myocardial depression is different from that of septic shock; the cardiac indices and the stroke volume index are low, the pulmonary wedge pressure is normal, and the systemic vascular resistance is increased. Poor prognostic indicators include persistent hypotension, marked hemoconcentration, a cardiac index of less than 2, and the abrupt onset of lactic acidosis with a serum lactate of greater than 4 mmol/L (36 mg/dL).

The mortality rate for patients with cardiopulmonary disease is 45%. Asymptomatic and mild disease are rare in adults, but limited information suggests they may be more common in children. Permanent sequelae are uncommon.

ETIOLOGY: Hantaviruses are RNA viruses of the Bunyaviridae family that in humans cause HPS or hemorrhagic fever with renal syndrome (HFRS) (see Hemorrhagic Fevers and Related Syndromes, p 278). Within the hantavirus genus, the viruses associated with HPS in the Americas include Sin Nombre virus (SNV), a major cause of HPS in the United States, and Bayou virus, Black Creek Canal virus, and the New York virus, sporadic causes in Louisiana, Florida, and New York, respectively. In recent years, new hantavirus serotypes, including Andes virus associated with an HPS-like syndrome, have been isolated in South America.

EPIDEMIOLOGY: Rodents, the natural hosts for the hantaviruses, acquire a lifelong, asymptomatic, chronic infection with persistent viremia, viruria, and virus in saliva. Humans acquire infection through direct contact with infected rodents, rodent droppings, nests, or inhalation of aerosolized virus particles from rodent urine, droppings, or saliva. Rarely, infection may be acquired from rodent bites or contamination of broken skin with excreta. Despite thorough investigation, person-to-person transmission of the viruses in the United States has not been demonstrated, but cases of person-to-person spread of Andes virus have been reported from Patagonia in South America. At-risk activities include handling or trapping rodents, cleaning or entering closed, rarely used rodent infested structures, cleaning feed storage or animal shelter areas, hand plowing, peridomestic cleaning, and living in a home with an increased density of mice in or around the home. For hikers, sleeping in a structure also inhabited by rodents has been associated with HPS. Weather conditions resulting in exceptionally heavy rainfall and, therefore, improved rodent food supplies can result in an increase in the rodent population by 10- to 20-fold. The increased rodent population results in a closer interaction between humans and infected mice and seems to account for recently recognized outbreaks. Most cases occur during spring and summer, and the geographic location is determined by the habitat of the rodent carrier.

The SNV, responsible for most HPS cases, is transmitted by the deer mouse *Peromyscus maniculatus*. The Black Creek Canal virus is transmitted by the cotton rat, *Sigmodon hispidus*, the Bayou virus by the rice rat, *Oryzomys palustris*, and the New York virus by the white-footed mouse, *Peromyscus leucopus*.

The **incubation period** may be 1 to 6 weeks after exposure to infected rodents, their saliva, or excreta, but the period has not been established definitely.

DIAGNOSTIC TESTS: Characteristic laboratory values include a neutrophilic leukocytosis with immature granulocytes, more than 10% immunoblasts (basophilic cytoplasm, prominent nucleoli, and an increased nuclear-cytoplasmic ratio), thrombocytopenia, and elevated hematocrit. In fatal cases, SNV has been identified by immunohistochemical staining in capillary endothelial cells in almost every organ in the body. The SNV RNA has been detected uniformly by the reverse transcriptase–polymerase chain reaction in peripheral blood mononuclear cells and other clinical specimens from the first few days of hospitalization up to 10 to 21 days after symptom onset. Viral RNA is not detected readily in bronchoalveolar lavage fluids, and the duration of viremia is unknown.

Hantavirus-specific immunoglobulin (Ig) G and IgM antibodies are present when the cardiopulmonary manifestations begin. A rapid diagnostic test can facilitate early transfer to a tertiary care facility, result in immediate appropriate supportive therapy, and permit early enrollment in antiviral trials. The rapid immunoblot assay is a simple dipstick-like assay that takes 5 hours, requires minimal equipment, and can be used in rural laboratories.

Enzyme immunoassay (available through many state health departments and the Centers for Disease Control and Prevention) and Western blot are assays that use recombinant antigens and have a high degree of specificity for detection of IgG and IgM heterologous and homologous antiviral antigens.

Viral culture is available only in research laboratories that have specialized facilities to protect laboratory workers.

TREATMENT: Patients with suspected HPS should be rapidly transferred to a tertiary care facility. Supportive management of the pulmonary edema, severe hypoxemia, and hypotension during the first 24 to 48 hours is complex and critical for recovery. A flow-directed pulmonary catheter for monitoring fluid administration and the use of inotropic support, vasopressors, and careful ventilatory control are important.

Extracorporeal membrane oxygenation (ECMO) may provide particularly important short-term support for the severe capillary leak syndrome in the lungs. Venoarterial ECMO, which also can provide circulatory support, has provided encouraging early results with rapid and dramatic hemodynamic improvement in patients after only 12 hours and a total duration of only 4 to 5 days using ECMO.

Ribavirin is active in vitro against previously isolated hantaviruses and SNV. In a controlled trial, intravenous ribavirin reduced the mortality of HFRS.

ISOLATION OF THE HOSPITALIZED PATIENT: Standard precautions are recommended. Hantavirus cardiopulmonary syndrome has not been associated with nosocomial or person-to-person transmission.

CONTROL MEASURES:

Care of Exposed Persons. Serial clinical examinations and serologic testing could be used to monitor patients assessed to be at high risk for infection after a high-risk exposure (see Epidemiology, p 272).

Environmental Control. Hantavirus infections of humans occur primarily in adults and are associated with domestic, occupational, or leisure activities bringing humans into contact with infected rodents, usually in a rural setting. Eradicating the host reservoir is neither feasible nor desirable. The best currently available approach for disease control and prevention is risk reduction through environmental hygiene practices that discourage rodents from colonizing the home and work environment and that minimize aerosolization and contact with virus in saliva and excreta. The hantavirus lipid envelope is susceptible to most disinfectants, including dilute bleach solutions, detergents, and most general household disinfectants.

Measures to decrease exposure in the home and workplace include eliminating food sources available to rodents in structures used by humans, limiting possible nesting sites, sealing holes and other possible entrances for rodents in homes, and using "snap traps" and rodenticides. Other methods include using a 10% bleach solution to disinfect dead rodents and wearing rubber gloves before handling trapped or dead rodents. Gloves and traps should be disinfected after use. Before entering areas with potential rodent infestations, doors and windows should be opened to ventilate the enclosure. Persons entering these areas should avoid stirring up or breathing potentially contaminated dust. Dusty or dirty areas or articles should be moistened with a 10% bleach or other disinfectant solution before being cleaned. Brooms and vacuum cleaners should not be used to clean rodent-infested areas.

Efficacious chemoprophylaxis measures or vaccines are not available.

Public Health Reporting. Confirmed cases should be reported to the local public health authorities immediately.

Helicobacter pylori Infections

CLINICAL MANIFESTATIONS: Acute infection is manifested by epigastric pain, nausea, vomiting, hematemesis, and guaiac-positive stools. Symptoms usually resolve within a few days despite persistence of infection for years or life. *Helicobacter pylori* causes chronic-active gastritis and duodenal ulcer and is associated less frequently with gastric ulcer; chronic infection has a high attributable risk of gastric cancer. *Helicobacter pylori* infection is not associated with autoimmune or chemical gastritis.

ETIOLOGY: *Helicobacter pylori* is a gram-negative and spiral, curved, or U-shaped microaerophilic bacillus that has 2 to 6 polar sheathed flagella at one end.

EPIDEMIOLOGY: *Helicobacter pylori* have been isolated only from humans and other primates. An animal reservoir for human transmission has not been demonstrated. The routes by which organisms are transmitted from infected humans are unknown, but fecal-oral transmission may occur. Infection rates are low in children, but prevalence rises until age 60 years. Most carriage is asymptomatic, but almost all infected persons have chronic gastritis. Infection is acquired at a younger age in developing countries, in persons in lower socioeconomic groups, and among Latino, African, Asian, and Native Americans.

The **incubation period** is unknown.

DIAGNOSTIC TESTS: *Helicobacter pylori* infection can be diagnosed by culture of gastric biopsy tissue on nonselective media (eg, chocolate agar) or selective media (eg, Skirrow) at 37°C (98°F) under microaerobic conditions for 2 to 5 days. Organisms usually can be visualized on histologic sections with Warthin-Starry silver, Steiner, Giemsa, or Genta staining. Infection with *H pylori* can be diagnosed but not excluded on the basis of hematoxylin-eosin stains. Because of production of urease by the organisms, urease testing of a gastric specimen can give a rapid and specific microbiologic diagnosis. Each of these tests requires endoscopy and biopsy. Noninvasive, commercially available tests include the breath test, which detects labeled carbon dioxide in expired air after oral administration of isotopically labeled urea, and serology for the presence of immunoglobulin G to *H pylori.* Each of the diagnostic tests has a sensitivity and specificity of 95% or more.

TREATMENT: Treatment is recommended only for infected patients who have peptic ulcer disease, gastric mucosa-associated lymphoid tissue type lymphoma, or early gastric cancer. *Helicobacter pylori* is susceptible to a variety of antimicrobial agents, including amoxicillin, tetracycline, metronidazole, clarithromycin, and bismuth salts, but none have proven therapeutic effectiveness as single agents. Therapy for *H pylori* infection consists of 2 weeks of 1 or 2 effective antimicrobial agents plus ranitidine, bismuth citrate, bismuth subsalicylate, or a proton pump inhibitor (lansoprazole or omeprazole). These regimens are effective for eliminating the organism, healing the ulcer, and avoiding recurrence. The tolerance and efficacy of regimens other than a proton pump inhibitor plus an antibiotic in children are unknown. Such therapies result in eradication rates ranging from 61% to 94% in adults depending on the regimen used. Triple-drug therapy regimens are more effective for eradication than are 2-drug therapy regimens.

ISOLATION OF THE HOSPITALIZED PATIENT: Standard precautions are recommended.

CONTROL MEASURES: Disinfection of gastroscopes prevents transmission of the organism between patients.

Hemorrhagic Fevers Caused By Arenaviruses

CLINICAL MANIFESTATIONS: These zoonotic diseases range in severity from mild, acute, febrile infections to severe illnesses in which shock is a prominent feature. Fever, headache, myalgia, conjunctival suffusion, and abdominal pain are common early symptoms in all infections. Axillary petechiae are usual in Argentine (AHF), Bolivian (BHF), and Venezuelan (VHF) hemorrhagic fevers, and exudative pharyngitis often occurs in Lassa fever. Mucosal bleeding occurs in severe cases as a consequence of vascular damage, thrombocytopenia, and platelet dysfunction. Proteinuria is common, but renal failure is unusual. Elevated serum concentrations of aspartate aminotransferase can indicate an adverse or fatal outcome of Lassa fever. Shock develops 7 to 9 days after onset of the illness in more severely ill patients with these infections. Upper and lower respiratory tract symptoms can develop in persons with Lassa fever in whom sensorineural hearing loss is a common sequela. Encephalopathic signs with tremor, alterations in consciousness, and seizures can occur in the South American hemorrhagic fevers and in severe cases of Lassa fever.

ETIOLOGY: Arenaviruses are RNA viruses. The major New World arenavirus hemorrhagic fevers occurring in the Western hemisphere, AHF, BHF, and VHF, are caused by Junin, Machupo, and Guanarito viruses, respectively. A fourth arenavirus associated with a single naturally occurring hemorrhagic fever, Sabia virus, has been isolated in Brazil. The Old World complex of arenaviruses includes Lassa virus, which causes Lassa fever, a disease occurring in West Africa, and lymphocytic choriomeningitis virus (see Lymphocytic Choriomeningitis, p 380), which produces the least severe infection of the arenaviruses.

EPIDEMIOLOGY: Arenaviruses are maintained in nature by association with specific rodent hosts in which they produce chronic viremia and viruria. Inhalation and mucous membrane and skin contact (eg, through cuts, scratches, or abrasions) with urine and salivary secretions from these persistently infected rodents are the principal routes of infection. All arenaviruses are infectious as aerosols; those causing hemorrhagic fever should be considered highly hazardous to laboratory workers. The geographic distribution and habitats of the specific rodents that serve as reservoir hosts largely determine the endemic area and groups of persons at risk. Before immunization became available, several hundred cases of AHF occurred yearly in agricultural workers and inhabitants of the Argentine pampas. Epidemics of BHF occurred from 1962 to 1964; sporadic disease activity has continued since then. Venezuelan hemorrhagic fever was first identified in 1989 and occurs in rural north-central Venezuela. Lassa fever is highly endemic in most of West Africa, where its rodent host lives in proximity with humans, causing thousands of infections annually. Lassa fever has been reported in the United States in travelers from West Africa and Sabia virus in travelers from Brazil, and, in addition, a case has been reported after a laboratory accident.

The **incubation periods** are from 6 to 17 days.

DIAGNOSTIC TESTS: Diagnosis is made by demonstrating virus-specific serum immunoglobulin (Ig) M, an increase in virus-specific IgG antibody titers in serial serum specimens, viral isolation, or by identifying viral antigen in blood or tissues. Early detection of antigen and IgM antibodies by enzyme immunoassay is replacing immunofluorescence and plaque neutralization assays. These viruses may be recovered from the blood of acutely ill patients, as well as from various tissues obtained postmortem, but isolation should only be attempted under biosafety level-4 conditions.

TREATMENT: Plasma from convalescent patients has proven effective in reducing the mortality associated with AHF from 15% to 30% in untreated patients to less than 1% in those receiving appropriate quantities (based on neutralizing antibody content) within the first 8 days of illness. Intravenous ribavirin reduces mortality significantly in patients with severe Lassa fever, particularly if they are treated during the first week of illness, and is probably beneficial in treating South American arenavirus infections.

ISOLATION OF THE HOSPITALIZED PATIENT: In addition to standard precautions, contact and droplet precautions, including careful prevention of needle-stick injuries, and management of clinical specimens are recommended for all the hemorrhagic fevers caused by arenaviruses for the duration of the illness. Respiratory precautions also may be required in certain circumstances. Because of the risk of nosocomial transmission, the state health department and the Centers for Disease Control and Prevention (CDC) should be contacted for specific advice about management and diagnosis of suspected cases.

CONTROL MEASURES:

Care of Exposed Persons. No specific measures are warranted for exposed persons unless direct contamination with blood, excretions, or secretions from an infected patient has occurred. If such contamination has occurred, daily temperature recordings for 21 days during this interval are recommended, with prompt reporting of fever. Recommendations are similar for those who have had unprotected sexual contact, both immediately before illness and for 6 weeks afterward.

Immunoprophylaxis. An investigational live-attenuated Junin vaccine protects against AHF and probably against BHF. The vaccine is associated with minimal side effects in adults; similar findings have been obtained from limited safety studies in children 4 years of age and older.

Environmental. In town-based outbreaks of BHF, rodent control has proven successful. Rodent control is not practical for control of AHF or VHF because the reservoirs are more ubiquitous in relationship to the site of exposure. Intensive rodent control efforts have modestly reduced periodomestic Lassa virus infection, but rodents eventually reinvade human dwellings, and infection still occurs in rural occupational settings.

Public Health Reporting. Because of the risk of nosocomial transmission, the state health department and the CDC should be contacted for specific advice about management and diagnosis of suspected cases.

Hemorrhagic Fevers and Related Syndromes, Excluding Hantavirus Cardiopulmonary Syndrome, Caused By Viruses of the Family Bunyaviridae

CLINICAL MANIFESTATIONS: These zoonotic infections are severe febrile diseases in which shock and bleeding can be significant, and multisystem involvement can occur. In the United States, one of these infections causes an illness marked by acute respiratory and cardiovascular failure (see Hantavirus Cardiopulmonary Syndrome, p 272).

Hemorrhagic fever with renal syndrome (HFRS) is a complex multiphasic disease characterized by vascular instability and varying degrees of renal insufficiency. Fever, flushing, conjunctival injection, abdominal pain, and lumbar pain are followed by hypotension, oliguria, and, subsequently, polyuria. Petechiae and more serious bleeding manifestations are common. Shock and acute renal insufficiency may occur. Nephropathia epidemica, the clinical syndrome of HFRS in Europe, is a milder disease characterized by a grippe-like illness with abdominal pain and proteinuria. Acute renal dysfunction also occurs, but hypotensive shock or a requirement for dialysis is infrequent.

Hantavirus pulmonary syndrome (HPS) is an acute febrile illness with high case-fatality that progresses to acute respiratory failure and shock (see Hantavirus Cardiopulmonary Syndrome, p 272).

Crimean-Congo hemorrhagic fever (CCHF) is a multisystem disease characterized by hepatitis and, often, profuse bleeding. Fever, headache, and myalgia are followed by signs of a diffuse capillary leak syndrome, such as facial suffusion, conjunctivitis, and proteinuria. Petechiae and purpura frequently appear on the skin and mucous membranes. A hypotensive crisis often occurs after the appearance of frank hemorrhage from the gastrointestinal tract, nose, mouth, or uterus.

Rift Valley fever (RVF), in most cases, is a self-limited febrile illness. Occasionally, hemorrhagic fever with shock and icterus, encephalitis, or retinitis develops.

ETIOLOGY: Bunyaviridae are single-stranded RNA viruses with different geographic distributions depending on their vector. Hemorrhagic fever syndromes are associated with viruses from 3 genera: hantaviruses, nairoviruses (CCHF virus), and phleboviruses (RVF virus). Old World hantaviruses (Hantaan, Seoul, Dobrava, and Puumala) cause HFRS, and New World hantaviruses (Sin Nombre and related viruses) cause HPS.

EPIDEMIOLOGY: The epidemiology of these diseases is mainly a function of the distribution and behavior of their reservoirs and vectors. All genera except hantaviruses are associated with arthropod vectors, while hantaviruses are associated with exposure to infected rodents. Classic HFRS occurs throughout much of Asia, Eastern and Western Europe, and the Balkans and may cause up to 100 000 cases per year. The most severe form of the disease is due to the prototype Hantaan virus and Dobrava viruses in rural Asia and the Balkans; Puumala virus is associated with milder disease (nephropathia epidemica) in Europe. Seoul virus is distributed worldwide in association with *Rattus* species and often causes an urban disease of variable severity. Person-to-person transmission has never been reported with HFRS.

Crimean-Congo hemorrhagic fever occurs in much of sub-Saharan Africa, the Middle East, areas in West and Central Asia, and Eastern Europe. The CCHF virus is transmitted by ticks and, occasionally, at the slaughter of domestic animals. Nosocomial transmission of CCHF is a serious hazard.

Rift Valley fever occurs throughout sub-Saharan Africa and has caused epidemics in Egypt in 1977 and 1993 to 1995. The virus is arthropod-borne and is transmitted from domestic livestock to humans by mosquitoes. It also can be transmitted by aerosol and by direct contact with infected fresh animal carcasses. Person-to-person transmission has not been reported.

The **incubation periods** for CCHF and RVF range from 2 to 10 days; for HFRS, incubation periods usually are longer, ranging from 7 to 42 days.

DIAGNOSTIC TESTS: The CCHF and RVF but not hantaviruses are cultivated readily from blood and tissues of infected patients. Detection of viral antigen is a useful alternative for diagnosis of CCHF and RVF, but it has been unsuccessful for HFRS. Serum immunoglobulin (Ig) M and IgG virus-specific antibodies typically develop early in convalescence in CCHF and RVF. In HFRS, IgM and IgG antibodies usually are detectable at the time of onset of illness or within 48 hours. Immunoglobulin M antibodies or rising IgG titers in paired serum samples, as demonstrated by enzyme immunoassay, are diagnostic; neutralizing antibody tests provide greater virus-strain specificity. Immunofluorescent and complement-fixing antibody tests also are used for serologic diagnosis.

TREATMENT: Ribavirin given intravenously to patients with HFRS within the first 4 days of illness seems effective in reducing renal dysfunction, vascular instability, and mortality. Supportive therapy for HFRS should include the following: (1) avoidance of transporting patients, (2) supportive care for shock, (3) prevention of overhydration (particularly with crystalloid solutions), (4) dialysis for complications of renal failure, (5) control of hypertension during the oliguric phase, and (6) early recognition of possible myocardial failure with appropriate therapy.

Ribavirin given to patients with CCHF has resulted in clinical responses, although no controlled studies have been performed. Experimental animal data suggest the potential for use of ribavirin in treatment of hemorrhagic RVF as well.

ISOLATION OF THE HOSPITALIZED PATIENT: In addition to standard precautions, contact and droplet precautions, including careful prevention of needlestick injuries and management of clinical specimens, are indicated for patients with CCHF for the duration for their illness. Respiratory precautions also may be required in certain circumstances. Rift Valley fever and HFRS have not been demonstrated to be contagious, but standard precautions should be followed.

CONTROL MEASURES:

Care of Exposed Persons. Persons having direct contact with blood or other secretions from patients with CCHF should be monitored for fever daily for 14 days and closely observed, and immediate therapy with intravenous ribavirin should be considered at the first sign of disease, in consultation with appropriate experts.

Environmental Immunoprophylaxis. Monitoring of laboratory rat colonies and urban rodent control may be effective for rat-borne HFRS.

CCHF. Arachnicides for tick control generally have limited benefit but should be used in stockyard settings. Personal protective measures (eg, physical tick removal and protective clothing with permethrin sprays) may be effective.

RVF. Immunization of domestic animals is important for limiting or preventing RVF outbreaks and protecting humans. Mosquito control usually is not effective.

Public Health Reporting. Because of the risk of nosocomial transmission of CCHF and diagnostic confusion with other viral hemorrhagic fevers, the state health department and the Centers for Disease Control and Prevention should be contacted about management and diagnosis of any person with suspected viral hemorrhagic fever.

Hepatitis A

CLINICAL MANIFESTATIONS: Hepatitis A characteristically is an acute self-limited illness associated with fever, malaise, jaundice, anorexia, and nausea. Symptomatic hepatitis occurs in approximately 30% of infected children younger than 6 years of age; few of these children will have jaundice. Among older children and adults, infection usually is symptomatic and typically lasts several weeks, with jaundice occurring in approximately 70%. Prolonged or relapsing disease lasting as long as 6 months can occur. Fulminant hepatitis is rare but is more frequent in persons with underlying liver disease. Chronic infection does not occur.

ETIOLOGY: Hepatitis A virus (HAV) is an RNA virus classified as a member of the picornavirus group.

EPIDEMIOLOGY: The most common mode of transmission is person-to-person, resulting from fecal contamination and oral ingestion, ie, the fecal-oral route. Age of infection varies with socioeconomic status and associated living conditions. In developing countries, where infection is endemic, most persons are infected during the first decade of life; in developed countries, infection may occur at an older age. In the United States, hepatitis A is one of the most frequently reported vaccine-preventable diseases; in 1998, more than 23 000 clinical cases were reported to the Centers for Disease Control and Prevention (CDC). The highest rates have occurred in children 5 to 14 years of age and the lowest rates among adults older than 40 years of age. During the past several decades, reported cases of hepatitis A have had an unequal geographic distribution, with the highest rates of disease occurring in a limited number of states and communities. While yearly rates in these areas may fluctuate, they consistently remain above the US national average.

Among cases of hepatitis A reported to the CDC, the identified sources of infection included close personal contact with a person infected with hepatitis A, household or personal contact with a child care center, international travel, a recognized foodborne or waterborne outbreak, male homosexual activity, and use of injection drugs. Transmission by blood transfusion or from mother to newborn infant (ie, vertical transmission) is rare. Infection has been contracted rarely from nonhuman primates not born in captivity. In approximately 50% of reported cases, the source cannot be determined. Fecal-oral spread from persons with asymptomatic infections, particularly young children, likely accounts for many of these cases with an unknown source.

Most HAV infection and illness occurs in the context of community-wide epidemics, in which infection primarily is transmitted in households and extended family settings. Common-source foodborne outbreaks occur; waterborne outbreaks are rare. Nosocomial transmission is unusual, but outbreaks caused by transmission from hospitalized patients to health care professionals have been reported. In addition, outbreaks have occurred in neonatal intensive care units from neonates infected through transfused blood who subsequently transmitted HAV to other neonates and staff.

In child care centers, in contrast with most other infectious diseases in this setting, recognized symptomatic (icteric) illness occurs primarily among adult contacts of children in child care. Most infected children in child care are asymptomatic or have nonspecific manifestations. Hence, spread of HAV infection in and from a child care center frequently occurs before recognition of the index case(s). Outbreaks occur most commonly in large child care centers and those that enroll children in diapers.

In most infected persons, the highest titers of HAV in stool occur during the 1 to 2 weeks before the onset of illness, when patients are most likely to transmit HAV. The risk subsequently diminishes and is minimal by 1 week after the onset of jaundice. However, HAV can be detected in stool for longer periods, especially in neonates and young children.

The **incubation period** is 15 to 50 days, with an average of 25 to 30 days.

DIAGNOSTIC TESTS: Serologic tests for HAV-specific total and immunoglobulin (Ig) M antibody are available commercially. Serum IgM is present at the onset of illness and usually disappears within 4 months but may persist for 6 months or longer. Presence of serum IgM indicates current or recent infection, although false-positive results can occur. Anti-HAV IgG is detectable shortly after the appearance of IgM. The presence of total anti-HAV without IgM anti-HAV indicates past infection and immunity.

TREATMENT: Supportive.

ISOLATION OF THE HOSPITALIZED PATIENT: In addition to standard precautions, contact precautions are recommended for diapered and incontinent patients for 1 week after the onset of symptoms.

CONTROL MEASURES:

General Measures. The major methods for prevention of HAV infections are improved sanitation (eg, of water sources and in food preparation) and personal hygiene (eg, hand washing after diaper changes in child care settings).

Schools, Child Care, and Work. Children and adults with acute HAV infection who work as food handlers or attend or work in child care settings should be excluded for 1 week after onset of the illness.

Immune Globulin. Immune Globulin (IG) for intramuscular administration, when given within 2 weeks after exposure to HAV, is greater than 85% effective in preventing symptomatic infection. Recommended preexposure and postexposure IG doses and duration of protection are given in Table 3.14 (below) and Table 3.15 (p 283). Pregnant women and infants should receive a preparation that does not contain thimerosal.

Hepatitis A Vaccine. Two inactivated hepatitis A vaccines, Havrix (manufactured by SmithKline Beecham Biologicals, Rixensart, Belgium; distributed by SmithKline Beecham Pharmaceuticals, Philadelphia, Pa) and Vaqta (Merck & Co, Inc, West Point, Pa), currently are available in the United States. The vaccines are prepared from cell culture–adapted HAV, which is propagated in human fibroblasts, purified from cell lysates, formalin inactivated, and adsorbed to an aluminum hydroxide adjuvant. Havrix is formulated with the preservative 2-phenoxyethanol; Vaqta is formulated without a preservative.

Administration, Dosages, and Schedules (see Table 3.16, p 283). Both hepatitis A vaccines are approved for persons older than 2 years of age and have pediatric and adult formulations that are given in a 2-dose schedule. The adult formulation

Table 3.14. Recommendations for Preexposure Immunoprophylaxis of Hepatitis A Virus Infection for Travelers*

Age, y	Likely Exposure, mo	Recommended Prophylaxis
<2	<3	IG 0.02 mL/kg[†]
	3–5	IG 0.06 mL/k[†]
	Long-term	IG 0.06 mL/kg at departure and every 5 mo if exposure to HAV continues[†]
≥2	<3[‡]	Hepatitis A vaccine[§‖] **OR** IG 0.02 mL/kg[†]
	3–5[‡]	Hepatitis A vaccine[§‖] **OR** IG 0.06 mL/kg[†]
	Long-term	Hepatitis A vaccine[§‖]

* IG indicates immune globulin; HAV, hepatitis A virus.

† IG should be administered deep into a large muscle mass. Ordinarily no more than 5 mL should be administered in 1 site in an adult or large child; lesser amounts (maximum, 3 mL) should be given to small children and infants.

‡ Vaccine is preferable, but IG is an acceptable alternative.

§ To ensure protection in travelers whose departure is imminent, IG also may be given (see text).

‖ Dose and schedule of hepatitis A vaccine as recommended according to age in Table 3.16, p 283.

Table 3.15. **Recommendations for Postexposure Immunoprophylaxis of Hepatitis A Infection**

Time Since Exposure, wk	Future Exposure Likely, or Immunization Recommended	Age of Patient, y	Recommended Prophylaxis
≤2	No	All ages	IG (0.02 mL/kg)*
	Yes	≥2	IG (0.02 mL/kg)* **AND** Hepatitis A vaccine†
>2	No	All ages	No prophylaxis
	Yes	≥2	Hepatitis A vaccine†

* Immune globulin (IG) should be administered deep into a large muscle mass. Ordinarily no more than 5 mL should be administered in 1 site in an adult or large child; lesser amounts (maximum, 3 mL) should be given to small children and infants.

† Dosage and schedule of hepatitis A vaccine as recommended according to age in Table 3.16, below.

Table 3.16. **Recommended Doses and Schedules for Inactivated Hepatitis A Vaccines***

Age, y	Vaccine	Antigen Dose	Volume per Dose, mL	No. of Doses	Schedule
2–18	Havrix†	720 ELU	0.5	2	Initial and 6–12 mo later
2–17	Vaqta	25 U‡	0.5	2	Initial and 6–18 mo later
19 and older	Havrix	1440 ELU	1.0	2	Initial and 6–12 mo later
18 and older	Vaqta	50 U‡	1.0	2	Initial and 6 mo later

* Havrix is manufactured by SmithKline Beecham Biologicals, Rixensart, Belgium, and distributed by SmithKline Beecham Pharmaceuticals, Philadelphia, Pa; Vaqta is manufactured and distributed by (Merck & Co, Inc, West Point, Pa. ELU indicates enzyme-linked immunoassay units.

† A formulation consisting of 360 ELU per 0.5 mL dose given as a 3-dose schedule, was available for children and adolescents until 1997. Children who received a single dose of 360 ELU should receive 2 doses of 720 ELU to complete the schedule.

‡ Antigen units (each unit is equivalent to approximately 1 µg of viral protein).

of Havrix is recommended for persons 19 years of age and older and the adult formulation of Vaqta for persons 18 years of age and older. All currently licensed vaccines are given intramuscularly. Recommended doses and schedules for these different products and formulations are given in Table 3.16 (above).

Detection of Anti-HAV After Immunization. The concentrations of anti-HAV resulting from hepatitis A immunization are 10- to 100-fold lower than those produced after natural infection and may be below the detection level of commercially available assays. The lower levels of antibody induced by immunization are measured by modified immunoassays, expressed as milli-international units (mIU) per milliliter. The lower limit of antibody needed to confer immunity has not been defined. In most studies conducted with Havrix, concentrations of 20 mIU/mL or greater as measured with a modified enzyme immunoassay, were considered to be protective; studies with Vaqta have been based on levels of greater than 10 mIU/mL, measured using a modified radioimmunoassay.

IgM Anti-HAV After Immunization. Immunoglobulin M anti-HAV occasionally is detectable by standard assays in adults 2 weeks after receiving hepatitis A vaccine. No data are available for children at 2 weeks after immunization; in 1 study, none had detectable IgM anti-HAV 1 month after immunization.

Immunogenicity. The different vaccine formulations are similarly immunogenic when given in their respective recommended schedules and doses. One dose of Havrix induced seroconversion by 15 days in 88% to 93% of children, adolescents, and adults and by 1 month in 95% to 99%; 1 month after a second dose, administered 6 months after the first dose, 100% had protective serum antibody concentrations with high geometric mean titers. Similar results were achieved with Vaqta. One month after the first dose of vaccine, 95% to 100% of children, adolescents, and adults had protective levels of antibody. One month after a second dose, administered 6 months after the first dose, 100% had seroconverted.

Limited data on immunogenicity of hepatitis A vaccine in infants indicate high rates of seroconversion, but the geometric mean serum antibody titers are significantly less in infants with passively acquired maternal anti-HAV in comparison with vaccine recipients lacking anti-HAV. Further studies of the immunogenicity of hepatitis A vaccine in infants are in progress.

Efficacy. In double-blind, controlled, randomized trials, the protective efficacy in preventing clinical hepatitis A was 94% to 100%.

Duration of Protection. The need for booster doses cannot be determined because hepatitis A vaccines have been under evaluation for only a short time and long-term efficacy has not been established. Detectable antibody, however, persists for at least 8 years after a 3-dose series in adults. Kinetic models suggest that protective antibody levels will persist for at least 20 years.

Vaccine in Immunocompromised Patients. The immune response in immunocompromised persons, including persons with human immunodeficiency virus, may be suboptimal.

Effect of IG on Vaccine Immunogenicity. Seroconversion rates are not impaired by simultaneous administration of IG and the first vaccine dose, but lower serum antibody concentrations may be achieved. This reduced immunogenicity is not likely to be clinically significant. If rapid protection is needed (ie, in <2 weeks) after the first dose of vaccine, concomitant administration of IG is indicated.

Vaccine Interchangeability. Vaqta and Havrix, when given as recommended, seem to be similarly effective. Studies among adults have found no difference in the immunogenicity of a vaccine series that mixed the 2 currently available vaccines compared with using the same vaccine throughout the licensed schedule. Therefore, completion of the immunization regimen with the same product is preferable, but vaccination with either product is acceptable.

Administration With Other Vaccines. Limited data from studies among adults indicate that hepatitis A vaccine may be administered simultaneously with other vaccines. Vaccines should be given in a separate syringe and at a separate site (see Simultaneous Administration of Multiple Vaccines, p 26).

Adverse Events. Adverse reactions are mild and include local pain and, less frequently, induration at the injection site. No serious adverse events attributed definitively to hepatitis A vaccine have been reported.

Precautions and Contraindications. The vaccine should not be administered to persons with a hypersensitivity to any of the vaccine components, such as alum or, in the case of Havrix, phenoxyethanol. Safety data in pregnant women are not available, but the risk is considered to be low or nonexistent because the vaccine contains inactivated, purified, viral proteins.

Preimmunization Serologic Testing. Preimmunization testing for anti-HAV generally is not recommended for children. Testing may be cost-effective for persons who have a high likelihood of immunity from prior infection, such as those whose early childhood was in areas of high endemicity, those with a history of jaundice potentially caused by HAV, and those older than 40 years of age.

Postimmunization Serologic Testing. Postimmunization testing for anti-HAV is not indicated because of the high seroconversion rates in adults and children. In addition, commercially available anti-HAV tests may not detect low but protective concentrations of antibody induced by vaccine.

RECOMMENDATIONS FOR IMMUNOPROPHYLAXIS:

Preexposure Prophylaxis (see Table 3.14, p 282).

Foreign Travel. For susceptible persons traveling to or working in countries with intermediate or high endemic rates of HAV infection, immunoprophylaxis before departure is indicated. Such countries include those other than Australia, Canada, Japan, New Zealand, and those in Western Europe and Scandinavia. For persons 2 years of age and older, vaccine is preferable, but IG is an acceptable alternative. Factors to consider in choosing active and/or passive prophylaxis include the interval before departure, the relative costs and availability of IG and hepatitis A vaccine, the duration of the stay, and the likelihood of repeated exposure during subsequent travel (see Table 3.14, p 282).

Immune globulin is considered protective against hepatitis A immediately after administration, whereas the precise time required from receiving 1 dose of vaccine to onset of protection has not been established but likely requires 2 to 4 weeks. To ensure protection in travelers whose departure is imminent, both IG (see Table 3.14, p 282) and the first dose of vaccine (see Effect of IG on Vaccine Immunogenicity, p 284) can be administered simultaneously. However, the additional benefit of administration of IG with the first dose of vaccine has not been evaluated in field trials and may be marginal.

Children younger than 2 years of age should receive only IG because vaccine is not yet approved for this age group (see Table 3.14, p 282).

Other Indications for Vaccination. Hepatitis A vaccination is recommended routinely for the following:

- ***Children living in communities with consistently elevated hepatitis A rates.*** Areas with consistently elevated rates of hepatitis A can be considered to include states, counties, and communities in which the average annual reported hepatitis A incidence during 1987–1997 was equal to or greater than twice the national average. The national average is approximately 10 cases per 100 000 population. States in this category include Arizona, Alaska, Oregon, New Mexico, Utah, Washington, Oklahoma, South Dakota, Idaho, Nevada, and California. Routine immunization of children living in these areas is recommended to achieve a sustained reduction in hepatitis A incidence. In addition, routine immunization can be considered for children living in states, counties, and communities where reported hepatitis A rates were less than twice but at least at the national average during this time (eg, ≥10 but <20 cases per 100 000 population). These states include Missouri, Texas, Colorado, Arkansas, Montana, and Wyoming. Because hepatitis A vaccine is not licensed for children younger than 2 years of age, immunization of older children is necessary. In addition, hepatitis A immunization programs can be considered to control ongoing community-wide epidemics. However, in general, available data suggest the effect of such programs may be limited, and efforts might be better focused on ongoing routine immunization to prevent future epidemics.

Widespread use of IG during community-wide epidemics, other than for contacts of hepatitis A cases, generally has been ineffective because unrecognized transmission is common and protection is of limited duration.

- ***Persons with chronic liver disease.*** Because persons with chronic liver disease are at increased risk for fulminant hepatitis A, susceptible patients with chronic liver disease should be immunized. The reported incidence of adverse events after hepatitis A immunization of persons with chronic liver disease has not been higher than that reported among healthy immunized adults.
- ***Homosexual and bisexual men.*** Hepatitis A outbreaks among men who have sex with men have been reported frequently, including in urban areas in the United States, Canada, and Australia. Therefore, sexually active men who have sex with men (adolescents and adults) should be immunized. Preimmunization serologic testing may be warranted for older adults in this group.
- ***Users of injection and noninjection illegal drugs.*** Periodic outbreaks among injecting and noninjecting drug users have been reported during the past decade in many parts of the United States and in Europe. Adolescents and adults who use illegal drugs should be immunized. Preimmunization serologic testing may be cost-effective for older persons in this group.
- ***Patients with clotting-factor disorders.*** Outbreaks of hepatitis A in patients with hemophilia receiving solvent-detergent–treated factor VIII and factor IX concentrates have been reported primarily in Europe, but also in one instance in the United States. Therefore, susceptible patients who receive clotting factor concentrates, especially those receiving solvent-detergent–treated preparations, should be vaccinated. Preimmunization testing for anti-HAV may be cost-effective.
- ***Persons at risk of occupational exposure (eg, handlers of nonhuman primates and persons working with HAV in a research laboratory setting).*** Outbreaks of hepatitis A have been reported among persons working with nonhuman primates that are susceptible to hepatitis A infection. Infected primates were those born in the wild, not those that had been born and raised in captivity.

Hepatitis A Immunization in Other Settings.

- ***Child care center staff and attendees.*** Hepatitis A outbreaks at child care centers may be the source of outbreaks in a community, but disease in child care centers more commonly reflects extended transmission from the community. In addition to the recommended postexposure prophylaxis (see below), hepatitis A immunization can be considered in child care settings with ongoing or recurrent outbreaks, especially in communities where routine immunization of children is recommended. In the absence of ongoing outbreaks, immunization in child care centers also can be used to implement routine hepatitis A immunization, particularly in communities where cases in the child care centers contribute substantially to the total number of hepatitis A cases and seem to have a role in sustaining community-wide outbreaks.
- ***Custodial care institutions.*** Epidemic hepatitis A was reported in custodial care institutions during the 1970s and 1980s, but few cases have been reported recently. However, hepatitis A vaccine, in addition to IG as indicated for postexposure prophylaxis (see below), may be considered for staff and residents in institutions in which a hepatitis A outbreak is occurring.
- ***Hospital personnel.*** Usually nosocomial hepatitis A in hospital personnel has occurred through spread from patients with acute infection in whom the diagnosis of HAV infection was not recognized. Careful hygienic practices should be emphasized when a patient with hepatitis A infection is admitted to the hospital. When outbreaks occur, IG is recommended for persons in close contact with infected patients (see below). The role of hepatitis A vaccine in these settings has not been studied. Routine preexposure use of hepatitis A vaccine for hospital personnel is not recommended.
- ***Food handlers.*** Recognized foodborne outbreaks of hepatitis A are relatively uncommon in the United States and usually are associated with contamination of uncooked food during preparation by a food handler who is infected with HAV. The most important means of preventing these outbreaks is by careful hygienic practices during food preparation. Routine hepatitis A immunization of food handlers is not warranted.
- ***Other.*** In addition, any healthy person at least 2 years of age may receive hepatitis A vaccine at the discretion of the physician and the patient or patient's family.

Postexposure Prophylaxis (see Table 3.15, p 283). Use of IG is recommended as follows (see Table 3.15 for dosages):

- ***Household and sexual contacts.*** All previously unimmunized persons with close personal contact with a hepatitis A case, such as household and sexual contacts, should receive IG within 2 weeks after last exposure. Serologic testing of contacts is not recommended because it adds unnecessary cost and may delay administration of IG. The use of IG more than 2 weeks after the last exposure is not indicated.
- ***Newborn infants of HAV-infected mothers.*** Perinatal transmission of HAV is rare in this circumstance. Some experts advise giving IG (0.02 mL/kg) to the infant if the mother's symptoms began between 2 weeks before and 1 week

after delivery. Efficacy in this circumstance has not been established. Severe disease in healthy infants seems rare.

- ***Child care center staff, employees, children, and their household contacts.*** Serological testing for IgM anti-HAV to confirm HAV infection in suspected cases is indicated. When a hepatitis A case is identified in an employee or child enrolled in a center in which all children are toilet trained, IG is recommended for previously unimmunized employees in contact with the index case and for unimmunized children in the same room as the index case.

  When an HAV infection is identified in an employee or a child or in the household contacts of 2 or more of the enrolled children in a child care center in which children are not toilet trained, IG is recommended for all previously unimmunized employees and children in the facility. During the 6 weeks after the last case is identified, unimmunized new employees and children also should receive IG.

  Hepatitis A vaccine can be given with IG to previously unimmunized children if routine vaccination is recommended for children in the community (see p 28).

  If recognition of a hepatitis A outbreak in a child care center is delayed by 3 or more weeks from the onset of the index case or if illness has occurred in 3 or more families, the infection is likely to have already spread widely. In these circumstances, IG also should be considered for household members of center attendees in diapers.

  Children and adults with acute HAV infection should be excluded from the center until 1 week after onset of the illness, until the IG prophylaxis program has been initiated, or until directed by the responsible health department. Although precise data concerning the onset of protection after a dose of IG are not available, allowing IG recipients to return to the child care center setting immediately following receipt of the IG dose seems reasonable.

  Further study is needed about the effectiveness of hepatitis A vaccine alone in controlling outbreaks in child care centers. Vaccines alone can be considered as an alternative option for prophylaxis of new employees if the risk of exposure is considered to be low during their initial 2 weeks of employment.
- ***Schools.*** Schoolroom exposure generally does not pose an appreciable risk of infection, and IG administration is not indicated when a single case occurs. However, IG could be used if transmission within the school setting is documented. Hepatitis A vaccine can be given in addition to IG if routine immunization of children in the community is recommended.
- ***Institutions and hospitals.*** In institutions for custodial care with an outbreak of HAV infection, residents and staff in close personal contact with infected patients should receive IG. Administration of IG to hospital personnel caring for patients with hepatitis A is not indicated routinely, unless an outbreak among patients or between patients and staff is documented. The addition of hepatitis A vaccine can be considered if repeated exposure is anticipated.
- ***Common-source exposure.*** These outbreaks often are recognized too late for IG to be effective in preventing hepatitis A in exposed persons, and IG administration usually is not recommended. Immune Globulin can be con-

sidered if it can be administered to exposed persons within 2 weeks of the last exposure to the HAV-contaminated water or food.

- ***Hepatitis A vaccine for postexposure prophylaxis.*** Available data are insufficient to recommend hepatitis A vaccine alone for postexposure prophylaxis. Clinical trials are needed to determine the effectiveness of hepatitis A vaccine compared with IG after exposure.

Hepatitis B

CLINICAL MANIFESTATIONS: Hepatitis B virus (HBV) causes a wide spectrum of manifestations, ranging from asymptomatic seroconversion, subacute illness with nonspecific symptoms (eg, anorexia, nausea, or malaise) or extrahepatic symptoms, and clinical hepatitis with jaundice, to fulminant fatal hepatitis. Anicteric or asymptomatic infection is most common in young children. Arthralgias, arthritis, or macular rashes can occur early in the course of the illness. Chronic HBV infection with persistence of hepatitis B surface antigen (HBsAg) occurs in as many as 90% of infants infected by perinatal transmission, in an average of 30% of children 1 to 5 years of age infected after birth, and in 2% to 6% of older children, adolescents, and adults with HBV infection. Although fewer than 10% of new HBV infections occur in children, approximately one third of the 1.25 million Americans with chronic HBV infection are estimated to acquire their infection as infants or young children based on the higher risk of chronic infection during childhood. Chronically infected persons are at increased risk for developing chronic liver disease (eg, cirrhosis, chronic active hepatitis, or chronic persistent hepatitis) or primary hepatocellular carcinoma in later life. The risk of death due to HBV-related liver cancer or cirrhosis is approximately 25% for persons who become chronically infected during early childhood.

ETIOLOGY: Hepatitis B virus is a DNA-containing, 42-nm hepadnavirus. Important components include HBsAg, hepatitis B core antigen, and hepatitis B e antigen (HBeAg).

EPIDEMIOLOGY: Hepatitis B virus is transmitted through blood or body fluids, such as wound exudates, semen, cervical secretions, and saliva of people who are HBsAg-positive. Blood and serum contain the highest concentrations of virus; saliva contains the lowest. Persons with chronic HBV infection (defined as a person who is HBsAg-positive for 6 months or who is immunoglobulin [Ig] M anti–HBc [antibody to hepatitis B core antigen] negative and HBsAg-positive) are the primary reservoirs for infection. Modes of transmission include transfusion of blood or blood products, which is now rare in the United States because of routine screening of blood donors and viral inactivation of certain blood products (see Blood Safety, p 88), sharing or reusing nonsterilized needles or syringes, percutaneous or mucous membrane exposure to blood or body fluids, and homosexual and heterosexual activity. Person-to-person spread of HBV can occur in settings involving interpersonal contact over extended periods, such as when a chronically infected person resides in a household. In household settings, nonsexual transmission occurs primarily from child to child, and young children are at highest risk for infection. The precise mechanisms of transmission from child to child are unknown; however, frequent interpersonal contact of nonintact skin or mucous membranes with blood-containing secretions or, perhaps, saliva are the most likely means of transmission. Transmission from sharing inanimate objects, such as wash cloths, towels, or toothbrushes, also may occur because HBV can survive at ambient temperatures in the environment for 1 week or longer. Hepatitis B virus is not transmitted by the fecal-oral route.

Persons with chronic HBV infection, especially persons infected as infants and young children, are at increased risk of ultimately dying of chronic liver disease (ie, chronic active hepatitis or cirrhosis) or primary hepatocellular carcinoma. The risk of chronic infection with HBV is related inversely to the age at infection. Transmission from mother to infant during the perinatal period (ie, transmission from HBsAg-positive mothers) results in chronic infection in 70% to 90% of the infants if the mother is HBeAg-positive. If not infected during the perinatal period, infants of HBsAg-positive mothers remain at high risk of acquiring chronic HBV infection by person-to-person (ie, horizontal) transmission during the first 5 years of life.

Multiple studies have documented high rates of HBV transmission among children born in the United States to HBsAg-negative mothers. When race-ethnicity–specific infection rates from these studies are applied to the childhood population in the United States, estimates are that about 33 000 children (younger than 10 years of age) born to HBsAg-negative mothers were infected each year before implementation of routine childhood hepatitis B immunization. The highest risk of early childhood transmission is among children born to HBsAg-negative mothers who immigrated to the United States from countries where HBV infection is highly endemic (eg, Southeast Asia, China), but the majority of early childhood HBV infections occur among African American and white children.

Other young children at risk for infection include the following: (1) household contacts of persons with chronic HBV infection, (2) residents of institutions for the developmentally disabled, (3) patients undergoing hemodialysis, and (4) patients with clotting disorders and others receiving blood products. In child care facilities in the United States, the risk of transmission seems to be small and should become negligible with universal infant immunization.

Most infected persons in the United States acquire HBV infection as adolescents or adults. Groups at highest risk include users of injection drugs, persons with multiple heterosexual partners, and men who have sex with men. Others at increased risk include those with occupational exposure to blood or body fluids, staff of institutions and nonresidential child care programs for the developmentally disabled, patients undergoing hemodialysis, and sexual or household contacts of persons with an acute or chronic infection. However, approximately one third of infected persons do not have a readily identifiable risk factor. The prevalence of infection among adolescents and adults in the general population is 3 to 4 times greater for African Americans than for whites. Infection with HBV in adolescents and adults is associated with other sexually transmitted diseases, including syphilis.

The frequency of HBV infection and patterns of transmission vary markedly throughout the world. In most areas of the United States, Canada, Western Europe, Australia, and southern South America, the infection is of low endemicity and occurs primarily in adolescents and adults; 5% to 8% of the total population has been infected, and 0.2% to 0.9% of the population has a chronic infection. However, populations with a high endemicity of infection are present in these countries, including Alaskan natives, Asian-Pacific Islanders, and immigrants from countries with a high endemicity of infection. In contrast, HBV infection is highly endemic in China, Southeast Asia, eastern Europe, the Central Asian republics of the former Soviet Union, most of the Middle East, Africa, the Amazon Basin, some Caribbean islands, and the Pacific Islands. In these areas, most infections occur in infants or children younger than 5 years of age, 70% to 90% of the adult population has been infected, and 8% to 15% have a chronic infection. In the rest of the world, HBV infection is of intermediate endemicity with chronic HBV carriage occurring in 2% to 7% of the population. Worldwide, HBV is a major cause of chronic liver disease and primary hepatocellular carcinoma.

The **incubation period** for acute infection is 45 to 160 days with an average of 90 days.

DIAGNOSTIC TESTS: Commercial serologic antigen tests are available to detect HBsAg and HBeAg. Assays also are available for detection of antibody to HBsAg (anti-HBs), total antibody to hepatitis B core antigen (anti-HBc), IgM anti-HBc, and antibody to HBeAg (see Table 3.17, below). In addition, hybridization assays and gene amplification techniques (eg, polymerase chain reaction, branched DNA methods) are available to detect and quantitate HBV DNA. Hepatitis B surface antigen is detectable during acute infection. If the infection is self-limited, HBsAg

Table 3.17. Diagnostic Tests for Hepatitis B Virus (HBV) Antigens and Antibodies

Factor To Be Tested	Hepatitis B Virus Antigen or Antibody	Use
HBsAg	Hepatitis B surface antigen	Detection of acutely or chronically infected persons; antigen used in hepatitis B vaccine
Anti-HBs	Antibody to HBsAg	Identification of persons who have resolved infections with HBV; determination of immunity after immunization
HBeAg	Hepatitis B e antigen	Identification of infected persons at increased risk for transmitting HBV
Anti-HBe	Antibody to HBe	Identification of infected persons with lower risk for transmitting HBV
Anti-HBc	Antibody to HBcAg*	Identification of persons with acute, resolved, or chronic HBV infection (not present after immunization)
IgM anti-HBc	IgM antibody to HBcAg	Identification of acute or recent HBV infections (including those in HBsAg-negative persons during the "window" phase of infection)

* No test is available commercially to measure hepatitis B core antigen (HBcAg). Ig indicates immunoglobulin.

disappears in most patients before serum anti-HBs can be detected (termed the *window phase* of infection). The IgM anti-HBc is highly specific for establishing the diagnosis of acute infection because it is present early in the infection and during the window phase in older children and adults. However, IgM anti-HBc usually is not present in infants infected perinatally. Persons with chronic HBV infection have circulating HBsAg and anti-HBc; on rare occasions, anti-HBs also is present. Both anti-HBs and anti-HBc are detected in persons with resolved infection, whereas anti-HBs alone is present in persons immunized with hepatitis B vaccine. The presence of HBeAg in serum correlates with higher titers of HBV and greater infectivity. In addition, tests for HBeAg and HBV DNA are useful in the selection of candidates to receive antiviral therapy and to monitor the response to therapy.

TREATMENT: No specific therapy for acute HBV infection is available. In chronic infection with liver disease in adults, interferon alfa has been demonstrated to induce a long-term remission in 25% to 40% of treated patients. The drug has been less effective for chronic infections acquired during early childhood. Lamivudine also is licensed for treatment of chronic HBV infection in adults, but no data are available for use in children.

Children and adolescents who have chronic HBV infection are at risk for development of serious liver disease, including primary hepatocellular carcinoma, with advancing age. While most cases of primary hepatocellular carcinoma do not occur until adulthood, with a peak incidence in the fifth decade of life, primary hepatocellular carcinoma occasionally can occur in children. The primary risk factor for serious liver disease is acquisition of chronic infection at birth or during early childhood. Children with chronic HBV infection should be screened periodically for hepatic complications using serum liver transaminase tests, α-fetoprotein concentration, and abdominal ultrasonography, but definitive recommendations on the frequency and the indications for specific tests are not yet available because of a lack of data on efficacy and cost-effectiveness. Patients with persistently elevated serum transaminase concentrations (exceeding twice the upper limits of normal) and patients with an elevated serum α-fetoprotein concentration or abnormal findings on abdominal ultrasonography should be referred to a gastroenterologist for further management.

ISOLATION OF THE HOSPITALIZED PATIENT: Standard precautions are indicated for patients with acute or chronic HBV infection.

For infants born to HBsAg-positive mothers, no special care other than removal of maternal blood by a gloved attendant and standard precautions is necessary.

CONTROL MEASURES:

Hepatitis B Immunoprophylaxis. Preexposure immunization of susceptible persons with hepatitis B vaccine is the most effective means to prevent HBV transmission. To reduce and eventually eliminate transmission of HBV as soon as possible, universal immunization is necessary. Accordingly, hepatitis B immunization is recommended for all infants as part of the routine childhood immunization schedule, and all children who have not received the vaccine previously should be immunized by or before 11 to 12 years of age. Immunization before 11 years of age (for children not previously immunized) can be advantageous because of more likely compliance with routine medical visits to complete the 3-dose schedule.

Postexposure immunoprophylaxis with either hepatitis B vaccine and Hepatitis B Immune Globulin (HBIG) or hepatitis B vaccine alone effectively can prevent infection after exposure to HBV. Serologic testing of all pregnant women for HBsAg is essential for identifying infants who require postexposure immunoprophylaxis beginning at birth to prevent perinatal HBV infections (see Care of Exposed Persons, p 298).

Two types of products are available for immunoprophylaxis. Hepatitis B Immune Globulin provides temporary protection and is indicated only in specific postexposure circumstances (see Care of Exposed Persons, p 298). Hepatitis B vaccine is used for both preexposure and postexposure protection and provides long-term protection.

Hepatitis B Immune Globulin.* Hepatitis B Immune Globulin is prepared from hyperimmunized donors whose plasma is known to contain a high titer of anti-HBs and to be negative for antibodies to human immunodeficiency virus (HIV) and hepatitis C virus (HCV). The process used to prepare HBIG inactivates or eliminates HIV and HCV. Standard immune globulin is not effective for postexposure prophylaxis against HBV infection since titers of anti-HBs are too low.

Hepatitis B Vaccine. Two highly effective and safe hepatitis B vaccines produced by recombinant DNA technology have been licensed in the United States. The original plasma-derived vaccine is no longer produced in the United States, but plasma-derived vaccines are used widely in other countries. The recombinant vaccines contain 10 to 40 µg of HBsAg protein per milliliter adsorbed to aluminum hydroxide, and some contain thimerosal as a preservative. While the concentration of HBsAg protein differs in the two recombinant vaccine products, equal rates of seroconversion are achieved with both vaccines when given to healthy infants, children, adolescents, or young adults in the doses recommended (see Table 3.18, p 294).

Hepatitis B vaccine can be given concurrently with other vaccines (see Simultaneous Administration of Multiple Vaccines, p 26).

Vaccine Interchangeability. The immune response using 1 or 2 doses of a vaccine produced by one manufacturer followed by 1 or more subsequent doses from a different manufacturer has been demonstrated to be comparable to a full course of immunization with a single product.

Routes of Administration. Vaccine is administered intramuscularly in the anterolateral thigh or deltoid area depending on the age of the recipient (see Vaccine Administration, p 16). Immunogenicity of hepatitis B vaccine in adults is diminished when given in the buttock. In patients with a bleeding diathesis, the risk of bleeding after intramuscular vaccine injection can be minimized by administration immediately after the patient receives replacement factor, use of a 23-gauge needle (or smaller), and application of direct pressure to the immunization site for at least 2 minutes.

Since low doses of hepatitis B vaccine given by the intradermal route result in lower seroconversion rates and concentrations of anti-HBs, intradermal immunization should not be used for infants or children and is not recommended for adults.

* Dosages recommended for postexposure prophylaxis are for products licensed in the United States. Because the concentration of anti-HBs in other products may vary, different dosages may be recommended in other countries.

Table 3.18. Recommended Dosages of Hepatitis B Vaccines*

	Vaccine†	
	Recombivax HB‡ Dose, µg (mL)	Engerix-B§ Dose, µg (mL)
Infants of HBsAg-negative mothers, children and adolescents younger than 20 y of age	5 (0.5)	10 (0.5)
Infants of HBsAg-positive mothers (HBIG [0.5 mL] also is recommended)	5 (0.5)	10 (0.5)
Adults 20 y of age or older	10 (1.0)	20 (1.0)
Patients undergoing dialysis and other immunosuppressed adults	40 (1.0)‖	40 (2.0)¶

* HBsAg indicates hepatitis B surface antigen; HBIG, Hepatitis B Immune Globulin.

† Vaccines should be stored at 2°C to 8°C (36°F–46°F). Freezing destroys effectiveness. Both vaccines are administered in a 3-dose schedule. A 2-dose schedule, administered at 0 and 4 to 6 mo later, is available for adolescents 11–15 years of age using the adult dose of Recombivax HB (10 µg).

‡ Available from Merck and Co, Inc, West Point, Pa. A combination of hepatitis B (Recombivax, 5 µg) and *Haemophilus influenzae* b (PRP-OMP) vaccine is licensed for use at 2, 4, and 12 to 15 months of age (Comvax).

§ Available from SmithKline Beecham Pharmaceuticals, Philadelphia, Pa. The US Food and Drug Administration has approved this vaccine for use in an optional 4-dose schedule at 0, 1, 2, and 12 mo.

‖ Special formulation for dialysis patients.

¶ Two 1.0-mL doses given in 1 site in a 4-dose schedule at 0, 1, 2, and 6 to 12 mo.

Efficacy and Duration of Protection. Hepatitis B vaccines licensed in the United States have a 90% to 95% efficacy for preventing HBV infection and clinical hepatitis B among susceptible children and adults. Protection seems to be durable. Long-term studies of adults and children indicate that immune memory remains intact for 12 years or more and protects against chronic HBV infection, even though anti-HBs concentrations may become low or undetectable.

Booster Doses. For children and adults with normal immune status, routine booster doses of vaccine are not recommended currently. For hemodialysis patients, the need for booster doses should be assessed by annual anti-HBs testing. A booster dose should be given if the anti-HBs concentration is less than 10 mIU/mL.

Adverse Reactions. Pain at the injection site and a temperature greater than 37.7°C (99.8°F) are the most frequently reported side effects in adults and children, with fever occurring in 1% to 6% of recipients and pain at the injection site in 3% to 29%.

Allergic reactions after hepatitis B immunization have been reported infrequently. Anaphylaxis seems to be uncommon, occurring in approximately 1 in 600 000 recipients according to passive reporting of vaccine adverse events, and has been reported rarely in children and adolescents.

Cases of Guillain-Barré syndrome, rheumatoid arthritis, and demyelinating diseases of the central nervous system rarely have been reported after hepatitis B immunization. However, evidence for a causal link to immunization has not been found. Data show no association between hepatitis B vaccine and sudden infant death syndrome, multiple sclerosis, autoimmune disease, or chronic fatigue syndrome.

Immunization During Pregnancy or Lactation. No adverse effect on the developing fetus has been observed when pregnant women have been immunized. Because HBV infection may result in severe disease in the mother and chronic infection in the newborn, pregnancy should not be considered a contraindication to immunization of women. Lactation also is not a contraindication.

Serologic Testing. Susceptibility testing before immunization is not indicated routinely for children or adolescents. Testing for previous infection may be considered for adults in risk groups with high rates of HBV infection, such as users of injection drugs, homosexually or bisexually active men, and household contacts of HBsAg-positive persons, provided it does not delay or impede vaccine uptake.

Routine postimmunization testing for anti-HBs is not necessary. Testing is advised 1 to 2 months after the third vaccine dose for the following: (1) hemodialysis patients, (2) persons with HIV infection, (3) those at occupational risk of exposure from sharps injuries, (4) immunocompromised patients at risk of exposure to HBV, (5) regular sexual contacts of HBsAg-positive persons, and (6) infants born to HBsAg-positive mothers.

Management of Nonresponders. Vaccine recipients who do not develop a serum anti-HBs-antibody response (≥10 mIU/mL) after a primary vaccine series should be reimmunized (unless they are determined to be HBsAg-positive). Reimmunization consists of 1 to 3 doses; those who remain anti-HBs-negative after a reimmunization series of 3 doses are unlikely to respond to additional doses of vaccine.

Altered Doses and Schedules. Larger vaccine doses, an increased number of doses, or both may be required to induce protective anti-HBs concentrations in adult hemodialysis patients (Table 3.18, p 294). Additional or larger doses also may be necessary for immunocompromised persons, including HIV-seropositive persons. However, few data exist for adults and none for children concerning the response to higher doses of vaccine in these patients. Specific recommendations thus cannot be made. For children with progressive chronic renal failure, hepatitis B vaccine is recommended early in the disease course to provide protection and potentially decrease the need for larger doses once dialysis is initiated.

Preexposure Universal Immunization. Routine preexposure immunization is recommended for all infants at or soon after birth (0 to 2 months), for all children by 11 to 12 years of age, and older persons in certain high-risk groups (see Table 3.19, p 296).

High seroconversion rates and protective concentrations of anti-HBs (≥10 mIU/mL) are achieved when hepatitis B vaccine is administered in any of the various 3-dose schedules, including those begun soon after birth in term infants. Guidelines for minimum scheduling time between vaccine doses for infants are as follows: (1) dose 1, at or soon after birth; (2) dose 2, at least 1 month after dose 1; and (3) dose 3, the infant must be at least 6 months old, and the third dose must be at least 2 months after dose 2 and at least 4 months after dose 1. The choice of schedule should be used to facilitate high rates of compliance with the 3-dose primary vaccine series. The 3-dose schedule for infants born to HBsAg-negative mothers should be completed by 18 months of age. For immunization of older children and adolescents, doses may be given in a schedule of 0, 1, and 6 months or of 0, 2, and 4 months; for adolescents, spacing at 0, 12, and 24 months results in equivalent immunogenicity.

Table 3.19. Persons Who Should Receive Preexposure Hepatitis B Immunization*

All infants
Children at high risk for early childhood HBV infection†
Adolescents‡: Hepatitis B vaccination should be given by or before 11 to 12 years of age. Special efforts should be made to vaccinate **all** adolescents, not only those at high risk.
Injection drug users
Sexually active heterosexual persons with more than one sex partner during the previous 6 months or who have a sexually transmitted disease
Sexually active men who have sex with men
Household contacts and sexual partners of HBsAg-positive persons
Health care personnel and others at occupational risk of exposure to blood or blood-contaminated body fluid
Residents and staff of institutions for developmentally disabled persons
Staff of nonresidential child care and school programs for developmentally disabled persons if the program is attended by a known HBsAg-positive person
Patients undergoing hemodialysis
Patients with bleeding disorders who receive clotting factor concentrates
Members of households with adoptees who are HBsAg-positive
International travelers to areas in which HBV infection is of high or intermediate endemicity
Inmates of juvenile detention and other correctional facilities

* HBV indicates hepatitis B virus; HBsAg, hepatitis B surface antigen.
† Alaskan Native and Asian-Pacific Islander children and children born to first-generation immigrants from HBV-endemic areas.
‡ Immunization can be initiated before children reach adolescence.

The recommended schedule for routine hepatitis B immunization of infants born to HBsAg-negative mothers is given in Fig 1.1 (p 22). Age-specific vaccine dosages are given in Table 3.18 (p 294). Combination products containing hepatitis B vaccine may be given, provided they are approved by the US Food and Drug Administration for the child's current age, and administration of the other vaccine component(s) also is justified.

Lapsed Immunizations. For infants with lapsed immunizations (ie, the interval between doses is longer than that in one of the recommended schedules), the 3-dose series can be completed, regardless of the interval from the last dose of vaccine (see Lapsed Immunizations, p 27).

SPECIAL CONSIDERATIONS:

Immunization of Children and Youth. Since the initiation of routine immunization of infants, many children and adolescents are unimmunized and remain at risk for HBV infection. For most, the risk of HBV infection is low until adolescence, and immunization at or before adolescence will provide protection. However, without immunization during early childhood, high rates of HBV infection would be expected to continue to occur among Alaskan Native and Asian-Pacific Islander children and among children residing in households of first-generation immigrants from countries where HBV infection is endemic. As a result, targeted efforts are needed to achieve high immunization coverage among these children.

Preterm Infants. For preterm infants weighing less than 2 kg at birth and born to HBsAg-negative women, initiation of immunization should be delayed until just before hospital discharge if the infant weighs 2 kg or more, or until approximately 2 months of age when other routine immunizations are given to improve response. These infants do not need to have serologic testing for anti-HBs performed routinely after the third dose if immunized according to this recommendation.

All preterm infants born to HBsAg-positive mothers should receive immunoprophylaxis (HBIG and vaccine) beginning as soon as possible after birth, followed by appropriate postimmunization testing (see Prevention of Perinatal HBV Infection, p 298).

Immunization of High-Risk Groups (see Table 3.19, p 296).

Sexually Active Heterosexual Adolescents and Adults. Persons diagnosed with a sexually transmitted disease or have had more than one sex partner in the previous 6 months should be immunized.

Household Contacts and Sexual Partners of HBV Carriers. Household and sexual contacts of HBV carriers identified through prenatal screening, blood donor screening, or diagnostic or other serologic testing should be immunized.

Health Care Personnel and Others With Occupational Exposure to Blood. The risk to a health care worker for HBV exposure depends on the tasks the worker performs. Personnel with contact with blood or blood-contaminated body fluids should be immunized. Because the risks for occupational HBV infection are often highest during the training of health care personnel, immunization should be completed during training and before contact with blood.

Residents and Staff of Institutions for the Developmentally Disabled. Susceptible children in institutions for the developmentally disabled and the staff who work closely with the children should be immunized. Susceptible children and staff who live or work in smaller (group) residential settings where other staff members or residents are known to be HBsAg-positive also should be immunized. Children discharged from residential institutions into community programs should be screened for HBsAg to allow appropriate measures to prevent HBV transmission.

Staff of nonresidential child care programs (eg, schools and other group settings) attended by known HBsAg-positive persons have a risk of infection comparable to that of health care personnel and should be immunized. Immunization of staff and attendees in these programs should be considered and is strongly encouraged if an attendee who is HBsAg-positive behaves aggressively or has special medical problems (eg, exudative dermatitis or open skin lesions) that increase the risk of exposure to that attendee's blood or secretions.

Hemodialysis Patients. Immunization is recommended for susceptible hemodialysis patients. Identification of patients with renal disease for immunization early in the course of their disease is encouraged since response is better than in advanced disease.

Adoptees and Their Household Contacts From Countries Where HBV Infection is Endemic. Adoptees from countries where HBV infection is endemic should be screened for HBsAg at the time of adoption. Before adoption, for adoptees found to be HBsAg positive, previously unimmunized family members and other household contacts should be immunized. Adoptees found to be HBsAg negative should be immunized.

Inmates in Juvenile Detention and Other Correctional Facilities. Immunization is recommended when the length of stay is sufficient to administer at least 2 vaccine doses or when follow-up mechanisms are established to complete the immunization series.

Patients With Bleeding Disorders Who Receive Clotting Factor Concentrates. Although the risk from currently manufactured products is low, the potential risk of HBV transmission remains; thus, immunization is recommended as soon as the specific clotting disorder is diagnosed.

International Travelers. Persons traveling to areas in which HBV infection is of high or intermediate endemicity (see Epidemiology, p 289) who will have close contact with the local population or who likely will have contact with blood (eg, in a medical setting) or sexual contact with residents should be immunized. Immunization should begin at least 4 to 6 months before travel, so that a 3-dose regimen can be completed (see Preexposure Universal Immunization, p 295). For persons in whom immunization is initiated at less than 4 months before departure, the alternative 4-dose schedule of 0, 1, 2, and 12 months (see Table 3.18, p 294) should provide protection if the first 3 doses can be administered before travel. If departure is within less than 2 months, an incomplete 2-dose regimen that is completed on return or a 0-, 1-, 3-week schedule with a fourth dose at 6 to 12 months will provide protection (see Lapsed Immunizations, p 27).

These and additional indications for immunization of high-risk persons are given in Table 3.19, p 296.

Care of Exposed Persons (Postexposure Immunoprophylaxis) (see also Table 3.20, p 299).

Prevention of Perinatal HBV Infection. Transmission of perinatal HBV infection can be prevented in approximately 95% of infants born to HBsAg-positive mothers by early active and passive immunoprophylaxis of the infants, ie, immunization and HBIG administration. Immunization subsequently should be completed during the first 6 months of life. Hepatitis B immunization only, initiated at or shortly after birth, also is highly effective for preventing perinatal HBV infections.

Serologic Screening of Pregnant Women. Prenatal HBsAg testing of all pregnant women is recommended to identify newborns who require immediate post-exposure prophylaxis and because selective testing fails to detect more than 50% of women who are HBsAg-positive. Testing should be accomplished during an early prenatal visit in each pregnancy and should be repeated late in pregnancy for HBsAg-negative women who are at high risk for HBV infection (eg, intravenous drug users and those with intercurrent sexually transmitted diseases) or who have had clinical hepatitis. Household contacts and sexual partners of HBsAg-positive women identified through prenatal screening should be immunized if susceptible or judged likely to be susceptible to infection.

Management of Infants Born to HBsAg-Positive Women. Infants born to HBsAg-positive mothers, including preterm infants, should receive the initial dose

Table 3.20. **Guide to Postexposure Immunoprophylaxis for Hepatitis B Virus Infection***

Type of Exposure	Immunoprophylaxis†	Refer to:
Percutaneous or permucosal exposure to blood	Immunization ± HBIG	p 302 (see Table 3.22)
Household contact HBsAg-positive person	Immunization	p 297
Household contact acute case with identifiable blood exposure	Immunization + HBIG	p 300
Perinatal	Immunization + HBIG	p 298
Sexual, partner has acute infection	Immunization + HBIG	p 301
Sexual, partner has chronic infection	Immunization	p 301

* HBIG indicates Hepatitis B Immune Globulin; HBsAg, hepatitis B surface antigen.
† For susceptible patients (eg, previously unimmunized).

of hepatitis B vaccine within 12 hours of birth (see Table 3.18, p 294, for appropriate dosages), and HBIG (0.5 mL) should be given concurrently at a different site. Subsequent doses of vaccine should be given as recommended in Table 3.21 (p 300). For preterm infants who weigh less than 2 kg at birth, the initial vaccine dose should not be counted in the required 3-dose schedule, and the subsequent 3 doses should be given in accordance with schedule for immunization of preterm infants (see Preterm Infants, p 54). Thus, a total of 4 doses are recommended in this circumstance.

These infants should be tested serologically for anti-HBs and HBsAg 1 to 3 months after completion of the immunization series. Testing for HBsAg will identify infants who become chronically infected and will aid in their long-term medical management. Infants with anti-HBs concentrations of less than 10 mIU/mL and who are HBsAg-negative should receive 3 additional doses of vaccine in a 0-, 1-, and 6-month schedule followed by testing for anti-HBs 1 month after the third dose. Alternatively, additional doses (1–3) of vaccine can be administered, followed by testing for anti-HBs 1 month after each dose to determine whether subsequent doses are needed.

Term Infants Born to Mothers Not Tested During Pregnancy for HBsAg. Pregnant women whose HBsAg status is unknown at delivery should undergo blood testing as soon as possible. While awaiting results, the infant should receive the first hepatitis B vaccine dose within 12 hours of birth in the dose recommended for infants born to HBsAg-positive mothers (see Table 3.18, p 294). Because hepatitis B vaccine when given at birth is highly effective for preventing perinatal infection in term infants, the possible added value and the cost of HBIG do not warrant its use when the mother's HBsAg status is not known. If the woman is found to be HBsAg-positive, the infant should receive HBIG (0.5 mL) as soon as possible, but within 7 days of birth, and be immunized subsequently as recommended (see Table 3.18, p 294). If HBIG is unavailable, the infant still should receive the 2 subsequent

Table 3.21. **Recommended Schedule of Hepatitis B Immunoprophylaxis to Prevent Perinatal Transmission***

Vaccine Dose† and HBIG	Age
Infant Born to Mother Known To Be HBsAg Positive‡	
First	Birth (within 12 h)
HBIG§	Birth (within 12 h)
Second	1–2 mo
Third	6 mo
Infant Born to Mother Not Screened for HBsAg‖	
First	Birth (within 12 h)
HBIG§	If mother is HBsAg-positive, give 0.5 mL as soon as possible, not later than 1 wk after birth‖
Second	1–2 mo
Third	6 mo¶

* HBsAg indicates hepatitis B surface antigen; HBIG, Hepatitis B Immune Globulin.
† See Table 3.18 (p 294) for appropriate vaccine dose.
‡ See text (p 298) for recommendations for subsequent serologic testing.
§ HBIG (0.5 mL) given intramuscularly at a site different from that used for vaccine.
‖ See text (below) for immunization recommendations for preterm infants.
¶ Infants of HBsAg-negative mothers should receive third dose at 6–18 months of age.

doses of hepatitis B vaccine at 1 to 2 and 6 months of age (see Table 3.21, above). If the mother is HBsAg-negative, hepatitis B immunization in the dose and routine schedule for infants should be completed (see Table 3.18, p 294).

Preterm Infants Born to Mothers Not Tested During Pregnancy for HBsAg. The maternal HBsAg status should be determined as soon as possible, and the infant should receive hepatitis B vaccine, as recommended for term infants in this category. For preterm infants who weigh less than 2 kg at birth, HBIG (0.5 mL) should be given if the mother's HBsAg status cannot be determined within the initial 12 hours of birth because of the poor immunogenicity of vaccine in these infants. The initial vaccine dose should not be counted in the required 3 doses to complete the immunization series. The subsequent 3 doses (for a total of 4 doses) are given in accordance with the recommendations for the immunization of preterm infants with birth weights less than 2 kg born to HBsAg-negative women (see Preterm Infants, p 54). For preterm infants of HBsAg-positive mothers, follow-up testing on completion of immunization series is recommended (see Management of Infants Born to HBsAg-Positive Women, p 298).

Breastfeeding. Breastfeeding of the infant by an HBsAg-positive mother poses no additional risk for acquisition of HBV infection by the infant (see Human Milk, p 98).

Household Contacts of Persons With Acute HBV Infection. Infants (ie, younger than 12 months of age) who have close contact with primary caregivers with acute infection and who have begun the immunization series should complete the series on schedule. If immunization has not been initiated, the infant should receive HBIG (0.5 mL), and hepatitis vaccine should be given in accordance with the routinely recommended 3-dose schedule (see Preexposure Universal Immunization, p 295).

Prophylaxis with HBIG for other unimmunized household contacts of persons with acute HBV infection is not indicated unless they have identifiable blood exposure to the index patient, such as by sharing of toothbrushes or razors. Such exposures should be treated as in sexual exposures to a person with acute HBV infection. All such persons, however, should be immunized as soon as possible against hepatitis B because of the possibility of future household exposures.

Sexual Partners of Persons With Acute HBV Infection. Susceptible sex partners should receive a single dose of HBIG (0.06 mL/kg) and should begin the hepatitis B vaccine series. Sexual partners of persons with acute HBV infection are at increased risk for infection, and HBIG is 75% effective for preventing these infections. The period after sexual exposure during which HBIG is effective is unknown, but is unlikely to exceed 14 days.

Exposure to Blood That Contains (or Might Contain) HBsAg. For inadvertent percutaneous (eg, needle stick, laceration, or bite) or permucosal (eg, ocular or mucous membrane) exposure to blood, the decision to give HBIG prophylaxis and to immunize the exposed person includes consideration of whether the HBsAg status of the person who was the source of the exposure is known and the hepatitis B immunization and response status of the exposed person. Immunization is recommended for any person exposed but not previously immunized. If possible, a blood sample from the person who was the source of the exposure should be tested for HBsAg and appropriate prophylaxis administered according to the hepatitis B immunization status and anti-HBs response status (if known) of the exposed person (see Table 3.22, p 302, and Injuries From Discarded Needles in the Community, p 153).

Detailed guidelines for the management of health care personnel and other persons exposed to blood that is or might be HBsAg-positive is provided in the recommendations of the Advisory Committee of the Immunization Practices of the Centers for Disease Control and Prevention* (see also Table 3.22, p 302).

Child Care. All children, including those in child care, should receive hepatitis B vaccine as part of their routine immunization schedule. Immunization not only will reduce the potential for transmission after bites, but also will allay anxiety about transmission from attendees who may be HBsAg-positive.

Children who are HBsAg-positive and who have no behavioral or medical risk factors, such as unusually aggressive behavior (eg, biting), generalized dermatitis, or a bleeding problem, should be admitted to child care without restrictions. Under these circumstances, the risk of HBV transmission in child care settings seems negligible. Routine screening for HBsAg is not warranted. Admission of HBsAg-positive children with behavioral or medical risk factors should be assessed on an individual basis by the child's physician, the program director, and the responsible public health authorities (for further discussion, see Children in Out-of-Home Child Care, p 105).

---

* Centers for Disease Control and Prevention. Hepatitis B virus infection: a comprehensive immunization strategy to eliminate transmission in the United States—1999 update: recommendations of the Advisory Committee on Immunization Practices (ACIP). *MMWR Morb Mortal Wkly Rep.* In press

Table 3.22. **Recommendations for Hepatitis B Prophylaxis After Percutaneous Exposure to Blood That Contains (or Might Contain) HBsAg***

	Treatment When Source Is		
Exposed Person	**HBsAg-Positive**	**HBsAg-Negative**	**Unknown or Not Tested**
Unimmunized	Administer HBIG,† 1 dose and initiate hepatitis B vaccine	Initiate hepatitis B vaccine series	Initiate hepatitis B vaccine series
Previously immunized			
Known responder	No treatment	No treatment	No treatment
Known nonresponder	HBIG, 2 doses or HBIG, 1 dose **and** initiate immunization‡	No treatment	If known high-risk source, treat as if source were HBsAg-positive
Response unknown	Test exposed person for anti-HBs§ • If inadequate HBIG,† 1 dose **and** vaccine booster dose‖ • If adequate, no treatment	No treatment	Test exposed person for anti-HBs§ • If inadequate, vaccine booster dose‖ • If adequate, no treatment

* Modified from the Centers for Disease Control and Prevention. Immunization of health-care workers: recommendations of the Advisory Committee on Immunization Practices (ACIP) and the Hospital Infection Control Committee (HICPAC). *MMWR Morb Mortal Wkly Rep.* 1997;46(RR-18):22–23. HBsAg indicates hepatitis B surface antigen; HBIG, hepatitis B immune globulin; anti-HBs, antibody to HBsAg.

† Dose of HBIG, 0.06 mL/kg, intramuscularly.

‡ Persons known NOT to have responded to a 3-dose vaccine series and to reimmunization with 3 additional doses should be given 2 doses of HBIG (0.06 mL/kg), one dose as soon as possible after exposure and the second 1 mo later.

§ Adequate anti-HBs is ≥10 mIU/mL.

‖ The person should be evaluated for antibody response after the vaccine booster dose. For persons who received HBIG, anti-HBs testing should be done when passively acquired antibody from HBIG is no longer detectable (eg, 4–6 mo); if they did not receive HBIG, anti-HBs testing should be done 1–2 months after the vaccine booster dose. If anti-HBs is inadequate (<10 mIU/mL) after the vaccine booster dose, 2 additional doses should be administered to complete a 3-dose reimmunization series.

Hepatitis C

CLINICAL MANIFESTATIONS: The signs and symptoms of hepatitis C virus (HCV) infection usually are indistinguishable from those of hepatitis A or B. Acute disease tends to be mild and insidious in onset, and in children most infections are asymptomatic. Jaundice occurs in 25% of patients, and abnormalities in liver function tests generally are less pronounced than those in patients with hepatitis B virus (HBV) infection. Persistent infection with HCV occurs in 75% to 85% of infected persons, even in the absence of biochemical evidence of liver disease. Most children with chronic infection are asymptomatic. Chronic hepatitis develops in approximately 60% to 70% of chronically infected patients, and cirrhosis develops in 10% to 20%; primary hepatocellular carcinoma can occur in these patients. Infection with HCV is the leading reason for liver transplantation in the United States.

ETIOLOGY: Hepatitis C virus is a small, single-stranded RNA virus and is a member of the Flavivirus family. Multiple HCV genotypes exist that fail to elicit cross-neutralizing antibodies in animal models.

EPIDEMIOLOGY: The prevalence of HCV infection in the general population of the United States is estimated at 1.8%. In children and adolescents, the seroprevalence rate is 0.2% for children younger than 12 years of age and 0.4% for those 12 to 19 years of age. Seroprevalence rates vary among individuals according to their associated risk factors.

Infection is spread primarily by parenteral exposure to blood and blood products from HCV-infected persons. The current risk of HCV infection after blood transfusion in the United States is estimated at 0.001% per unit transfused because of the exclusion of high-risk donors and by the HCV screening of units (see Blood Safety, p 88). Outbreaks of HCV-associated contaminated Immune Globulin Intravenous (IGIV) product have occurred. Currently, all intravenous and intramuscular immunoglobulin products available commercially in the United States undergo an inactivation procedure for HCV or are documented to be HCV RNA-negative before release.

The highest seroprevalence rates of infection (60% to 90%) occur in persons with large or repeated direct percutaneous exposure to blood or blood products, such as injection drug users and persons with hemophilia who were treated with clotting factor concentrates produced before 1987. Rates are moderately high among those with frequent but smaller direct percutaneous exposures, such as patients receiving hemodialysis (10% to 20%). Lower rates are found among persons with inapparent percutaneous or mucosal exposures, such as persons with high-risk sexual behaviors (1% to 10%), or among persons with sporadic percutaneous exposures, such as health care personnel (1%).

Other body fluids contaminated with infected blood also can be sources of infection. Sexual transmission among monogamous couples is uncommon, with infection found only in 1.5% of spouses without other risk factors. Transmission among family contacts also is uncommon but could occur from direct or inapparent percutaneous or mucosal exposure to blood. In persons with no risk factors, seroprevalence rates are less than 0.5%. For most infected children and adolescents, no specific source of infection can be identified.

Seroprevalence among pregnant women in the United States has been estimated at 1% to 2%, but maternal-infant (perinatal) transmission is only 5% (range, 0% to 25%). Maternal coinfection with human immunodeficiency virus (HIV) has been associated with increased risk of perinatal transmission of HCV and may depend in part on the HCV genotype and the serum titer of maternal HCV RNA. Serum anti-HCV antibody and HCV RNA have been detected in colostrum, but HCV transmission by breastfeeding to infants in the limited number of patients studied has not been demonstrated. The rate of transmission among breastfed infants has been the same as that among bottle-fed infants.

All persons with HCV antibody or HCV-RNA in their blood are considered to be infectious.

The **incubation period** for HCV infection averages 6 to 7 weeks with a range of 2 weeks to 6 months.

DIAGNOSTIC TESTS: The 2 major types of tests available for the laboratory diagnosis of HCV infections are (1) antibody assays for anti-HCV and (2) assays to detect HCV nucleic acid (RNA). Diagnosis by antibody assays involves an initial screening enzyme immunoassay (EIA); repeated positive results are confirmed by a recombinant immunoblot assay (RIBA), analogous to testing for HIV infection. Both assays detect immunoglobulin (Ig) G antibody; no IgM assays are available. The current EIA and RIBA assays are at least 97% sensitive and more than 95% specific. False-negative results early in the course of acute infection result from the prolonged interval between exposure or onset of illness and seroconversion that may occur. Within 15 weeks after exposure and within 5 to 6 weeks after the onset of hepatitis, 80% of patients will have positive test results for serum HCV antibody.

Highly sensitive polymerase chain reaction (PCR) assays for detection of HCV RNA are available from several commercial laboratories for investigational testing. Hepatitis C virus RNA can be detected in serum or plasma within 1 to 2 weeks after exposure to the virus and weeks before onset of liver enzyme abnormalities or appearance of anti-HCV. Although not approved by the US Food and Drug Administration (FDA), PCR assays for HCV infection are used commonly in clinical practice in the early diagnosis of infection, for identifying infection in infants early in life (ie, perinatal transmission) when maternal serum antibody interferes with the ability to detect antibody produced by the infant, and for monitoring patients receiving antiviral therapy. However, false-positive and false-negative results can occur from improper handling, storage, and contamination of the test samples. Viral RNA may be detected intermittently, and, thus, a single negative PCR assay result is not conclusive. Quantitative assays for measuring the concentration of HCV RNA also are available for investigational testing but are not standardized, and the clinical value of these assays is not yet established.

TREATMENT: Interferon-∝ alone or in combination with ribavirin is FDA-approved for treatment of chronic HCV infection in adults. Given alone, interferon results in a sustained response in 15% to 25% of patients treated; combination therapy results in a sustained response in about 40%. Lower sustained response rates are observed with both therapy regimens in patients with genotype 1, the most common strain in the United States. There are no FDA-approved therapies for persons younger than 18 years of age. Limited experience in children with interferon-alfa therapy suggests efficacy similar to that observed in adults. Children with severe disease or histologically advanced pathologic features (bridging necrosis or active cirrhosis) should be referred to a specialist in the management of chronic hepatitis C.

Persons with HCV-related chronic liver disease should be immunized against hepatitis A, and all children should be immunized against HBV unless they have been demonstrated to be nonsusceptible.

Management of Chronic HCV Infection. Persons who have chronic HCV infection are at risk for development of chronic hepatitis and its complications with advancing age, including cirrhosis and primary hepatocellular carcinoma. However, primary hepatocellular carcinoma from chronic hepatitis C has been reported only in adults. Children with chronic infection should be screened periodically for chronic hepatitis with serum liver function tests because of their potential long-term risk for chronic liver disease. Definitive recommendations on frequency of screening have not been established. Children with persistently elevated serum transaminase concentrations (exceeding twice the upper limits of normal) should be referred to a gastroenterologist for further management. The need for testing for alpha-fetoprotein concentration and of abdominal ultrasonography in children has not been determined.

ISOLATION OF THE HOSPITALIZED PATIENT: Standard precautions are recommended.

CONTROL MEASURES:

Care of Exposed Persons.

Immunoprophylaxis. Based on lack of clinical efficacy in humans and on data from studies using animals, the use of Immune Globulin for postexposure prophylaxis against HCV infection is not recommended. Furthermore, Immune Globulin is manufactured currently from plasma documented to be negative for anti-HCV antibodies.

Breastfeeding. Mothers infected with HCV should be advised that transmission of HCV by breastfeeding has not been documented. According to current guidelines of the Centers for Disease Control and Prevention (CDC), maternal HCV infection is not a contraindication to breastfeeding. The decision to breastfeed should be based on an informed discussion between the mother and the health care professional. Mothers who are HCV-positive and choose to breastfeed should consider abstaining if their nipples are cracked or bleeding.

Child Care. Exclusion of children with HCV infection from out-of-home child care is not indicated.

Serologic Testing for HCV Infection.

Persons Who Have Risk Factor(s) for HCV Infection. Routine serologic testing is recommended for current or former injection drug users, recipients of 1 or more units of blood or blood products before July 1992, recipients of a solid organ transplant before July 1992, patients receiving long-term hemodialysis, persons who received clotting factor concentrates produced before 1987, and persons with persistently abnormal alanine aminotransferase (ALT) levels.

Screening of Pregnant Women. Routine serologic testing of pregnant women for HCV infection is not recommended. Testing should be reserved for persons whose history suggests an increased risk for HCV infection.

Children Born to Women With HCV Infection. Children born to women previously identified to be HCV-infected should be tested for HCV infection because approximately 5% will acquire the infection. The duration of passive maternal antibody in infants is unknown but is unlikely to be more than 12 months in most cases. Therefore, testing for anti-HCV should not be performed until after 12 months of age. If earlier diagnosis is desired, PCR for HCV RNA may be performed at or after the infant's first well-child visit at 1 to 2 months of age.

Adoptees. Routine serologic testing of adoptees, either domestic or international, is not recommended. Testing is indicated, however, if the biological mother has an increased risk of HCV infection (see Medical Evaluation of Internationally Adopted Children for Infectious Diseases, p 148).

Recipients of IGIV. The US Public Health Service recommends that persons who received Gammagard (produced by Baxter Healthcare Corporation) between April 1, 1993, and February 23, 1994, should be offered serologic testing for ALT concentrations and for anti-HCV. Because of concerns that anti-HCV may not be detectable in persons who are immunocompromised, PCR testing for HCV RNA is recommended for persons with elevated ALT concentrations who are negative for anti-HCV on repeated testing. Screening of children who have received other IGIV products is not indicated.

Counseling of Patients With HCV Infection. All persons with HCV infection should be considered infectious, be informed of the possibility of transmission to others, and refrain from donating blood, organs, tissues, or semen and sharing toothbrushes and razors.

Infected persons should be counseled on how to avoid hepatotoxic agents, including medications, particularly if given for prolonged periods, and on the risks of alcohol ingestion. Patients with chronic liver disease, if susceptible, should be immunized against HBV.

Changes in sexual practices of infected persons with a steady partner currently are not recommended; however, they should be informed of the possible risks and use of precautions to prevent transmission. Persons with multiple partners should be advised to reduce the number of partners and to use condoms to prevent transmission. No data exist to support counseling a woman against pregnancy.

The Hepatitis Branch of the Division of Viral and Rickettsial Diseases at the CDC has implemented a toll-free number to allow access to information on viral hepatitis, 1-888-4HEPCDC, and maintains a Web site (http://www.cdc.gov/ncidod/diseases/hepatitis/) with information on hepatitis for health care professionals and the public, which includes specific information for persons who have received blood transfusions before 1992.

Hepatitis D

CLINICAL MANIFESTATIONS: Hepatitis D virus (HDV) infection causes hepatitis only in persons with acute or chronic hepatitis B virus (HBV) infection; the HDV requires HBV as a helper virus and cannot produce infection in the absence of HBV. The importance of HDV infection lies in its ability to convert an asymptomatic or mild chronic HBV infection into a fulminant or more severe or rapidly progressive disease. Acute coinfection with HBV and HDV usually causes an acute illness indistinguishable from acute HBV infection alone, except that the likelihood of fulminant hepatitis can be as high as 5%.

ETIOLOGY: The HDV is a 36- to 43-nm particle consisting of an RNA genome and a delta protein antigen (HDAg), both of which are coated with hepatitis B surface antigen (HBsAg).

Epidemiology: The HDV can cause an infection at the same time as the initial HBV infection (coinfection), or it can infect a person already chronically infected (superinfection). Acquisition of HDV is similar to that of HBV, ie, by parenteral, percutaneous, or mucous membrane inoculation. The HDV can be transmitted by blood or blood products, injection drug use, or sexual contact, as long as HBV also is present in the patient. Transmission from mother to newborn infant is uncommon. Intrafamilial spread can occur among HBsAg carriers. High-prevalence areas include southern Italy and parts of Eastern Europe, South America, Africa, and the Middle East. In contrast with HBV, HDV infection is uncommon in the Far East. In the United States, HDV infection is found most frequently in parenteral drug abusers, persons with hemophilia, and persons immigrating from endemic areas.

The **incubation period** for HDV superinfection, estimated from inoculation of animals, is approximately 2 to 8 weeks. When HBV and HDV viruses infect simultaneously, the incubation period is similar to that of hepatitis B (45–160 days; average, 90 days).

Diagnostic Tests: Radioimmunoassay and enzyme immunoassay for anti-HDV antibody are available commercially, usually at referral laboratories. Tests for immunoglobulin (Ig) M–specific anti-HDV antibody and HDAg are research procedures at present. If markers for HDV infection exist, coinfection with HBV usually can be differentiated from superinfection of an established HBsAg carrier by testing for IgM hepatitis B core antibody; absence of this core antibody suggests that the person is an HBsAg carrier. Methods for detection of HDV RNA are available.

Treatment: Supportive.

Isolation of the Hospitalized Patient: Standard precautions are recommended.

Control Measures: The same control and preventive measures as for HBV infection are indicated. Because HDV cannot be transmitted in the absence of HBV infection, hepatitis B immunization protects against HDV infection. Carriers of HBsAg should take extreme care to avoid exposure to HDV because no currently available immunobiologic exists for prevention of HDV superinfection.

Hepatitis E

Clinical Manifestations: Hepatitis E is an acute illness with jaundice, malaise, anorexia, fever, abdominal pain, and arthralgia. Subclinical infection also occurs.

Etiology: The hepatitis E virus (HEV) is a spherical, nonenveloped, positive-strand RNA virus and is the only known agent of enterically transmitted non-A, non-B hepatitis. Hepatitis E virus formerly was classified in the family Caliciviridae, genus *Calicivirus*; however, HEV has been reassigned to an unassigned genus of "hepatitis E-like" viruses because certain characteristics distinguish HEV from typical caliciviruses.

EPIDEMIOLOGY: Transmission of HEV is by the fecal-oral route. Disease is more common among adults than among children, and it has an unusually high case-fatality rate among pregnant women. Cases have been reported in epidemics or sporadically in parts of Asia, Africa, and Mexico. Outbreaks usually have been associated with contaminated water. Hepatitis E rarely is reported in the United States, and most reported cases have occurred among travelers to endemic regions. However, acute hepatitis E cases, verified by isolation of a "US strain" of HEV, have been reported among persons with no recent history of travel outside the United States. The discovery of a swine virus in the United States that is related closely to human HEV raises the possibility of a zoonotic reservoir for HEV. The period of communicability after acute infection is unknown, but fecal shedding of the virus and viremia occur commonly for at least 2 weeks. Chronic infection does not seem to occur.

DIAGNOSTIC TESTS: The diagnosis of acute HEV infection can be made by detecting immunoglobulin (Ig) M antibody to HEV (anti-HEV) in serum or by detecting HEV RNA by polymerase chain reaction (PCR) in serum or feces. Serologic and PCR-based assays for the diagnosis of acute HEV infection are available in research and commercial laboratories. However, none of these assays are approved by the US Food and Drug Administration. Health care professionals who require information about HEV diagnostic tests may contact the Hepatitis Branch, Centers for Disease Control and Prevention (CDC) at 404-639-3048; fax, 404-639-1538. The CDC criteria for considering whether an acute phase serum specimen should be tested for evidence of HEV infection include a discrete onset of illness with jaundice or with a serum alanine aminotransferase level at least 2.5 times the upper limit of normal and negative results for IgM antibody to hepatitis A virus, IgM antibody to hepatitis B core antigen, and antibody to hepatitis C virus.

TREATMENT: Supportive.

ISOLATION OF THE HOSPITALIZED PATIENT: In addition to standard precautions, contact precautions are recommended.

CONTROL MEASURES: Good sanitation and not ingesting potentially contaminated food and water are the most effective measures. Passive immunoprophylaxis against HEV infection with immune globulin prepared in the United States has not proven effective.

Hepatitis G

CLINICAL MANIFESTATIONS: Although hepatitis G virus (HGV) can cause chronic infection and viremia, it is a rare cause of hepatic inflammation, and most infected persons are asymptomatic. Histologic evidence of HGV infection is rare, and serum aminotransferase concentrations usually are normal. Although high levels of HGV RNA are found in blood, the liver is not a significant site of replication. Currently, no conclusive evidence indicates that HGV causes fulminant or chronic disease, and coinfection does not seem to worsen the course or severity of concurrent infection with hepatitis B virus (HBV) or hepatitis C virus (HCV).

ETIOLOGY: The HGV is a single-stranded RNA virus that is included in the Flaviviridae family and shares a 27% homology with HCV. The name HGV actually denotes 2 independent viruses, HGV and GBV-C. The HGV has not yet been isolated.

EPIDEMIOLOGY: The HGV has been reported in adults and children throughout the world and is found in about 1.5% of blood donors in the United States. Infection has been reported in 10% to 20% of adults with chronic HBV or HCV infection, indicating that coinfection is a common occurrence. The primary route of spread is thought to be through transfusions, but HGV also can be transmitted by organ transplantation. Other important risk factors for infection include injection drug use, hemodialysis, and homosexual and bisexual relationships, indicating that sexual transmission also may occur. Transplacental transmission seems to be rare and has been associated with high-titer maternal viremia; when it occurs, infection usually becomes persistent in infants.

The **incubation period** is unknown.

DIAGNOSTIC TESTS: Currently, HGV infection can be diagnosed only by identifying viral genomes by using polymerase chain reaction assay, which is not widely available. No serologic test is available.

TREATMENT: No treatment is indicated for this virus that causes mild, if any, disease.

ISOLATION OF THE HOSPITALIZED PATIENT: Standard precautions are recommended.

CONTROL MEASURES: No method to prevent infection with HGV is known.

Herpes Simplex

CLINICAL MANIFESTATIONS:

Neonatal. In newborns, herpes simplex virus (HSV) infection can manifest as the following: (1) disseminated disease involving multiple organs, most prominently the liver and lungs; (2) localized central nervous system (CNS) disease; or (3) disease localized to the skin, eyes, and mouth. Approximately 25% of cases are disseminated, 35% are CNS disease, and 40% affect the skin, eyes, and mouth, although there may be clinical overlap among disease types. In many neonates with disseminated or CNS disease, skin lesions do not develop, or the lesions appear late. In the absence of skin lesions, the diagnosis of neonatal HSV infection is difficult. Disseminated infection should be considered in neonates with sepsis syndrome, negative bacterial culture results, and severe liver dysfunction. Herpes simplex virus also should be considered as a causative agent in neonates with fever, irritability, and abnormal cerebrospinal fluid (CSF) findings, especially in the presence of seizures. Although asymptomatic HSV infection is common in older children, it rarely, if ever, occurs in infected neonates.

Neonatal herpetic infections often are severe, with attendant high mortality and morbidity rates, even when antiviral therapy is administered. Recurrent skin lesions are frequent in surviving infants and may be associated with CNS sequelae if they occur frequently during the first 6 months of life.

Initial symptoms of HSV infection can occur anytime between birth and approximately 4 weeks of age. Disseminated disease has the earliest age of onset, often during the first week of life; CNS disease presents latest, usually between the second and third weeks of life.

Children and Infants Beyond the Neonatal Period. Most primary HSV infections are asymptomatic. Gingivostomatitis, which is the most common clinical manifestation in this age group, usually is caused by HSV type 1 (HSV-1). Gingivostomatitis is characterized by fever, irritability, tender submandibular adenopathy, and an ulcerative enanthem involving the gingiva and mucous membranes of the mouth, often with perioral vesicular lesions.

Genital herpes, which is the most common manifestation of HSV infection in adolescents and adults, is characterized by vesicular or ulcerative lesions of the male or female genital organs, perineum, or both. Genital herpes usually is caused by HSV type 2 (HSV-2).

Eczema herpeticum with vesicular lesions concentrated in the areas of eczematous involvement can develop in patients who are infected with HSV.

In immunocompromised patients, severe local lesions and, less commonly, disseminated HSV infection with generalized vesicular skin lesions and visceral involvement can occur.

After primary infection, HSV persists for life in a latent form. The site of latency for virus causing herpes labialis is the trigeminal ganglion, and the usual site of latency for genital herpes is the sacral ganglia, although any sensory ganglia can be involved depending on the site of primary infection. Reactivation of latent virus most commonly occurs in the absence of symptoms. When symptomatic, recurrent herpes labialis HSV-1 is manifested by single or grouped vesicles in the perioral region, usually on the vermilion border of the lips (cold sores). Symptomatic recurrent genital herpes is manifested by vesicular lesions on the penis, scrotum, vulva, cervix, buttocks, perianal areas, thighs, or back.

Conjunctivitis and keratitis can result from primary or recurrent HSV infection. Herpetic whitlow consists of single or multiple vesicular lesions on the distal parts of fingers. Herpes simplex virus infection has been implicated as a precipitating factor in erythema multiforme.

Herpes simplex virus encephalitis can result from primary or recurrent infection and usually is associated with fever, alterations in the state of consciousness, personality changes, seizures, and focal neurologic findings. Encephalitis frequently has an acute onset with a fulminant course, leading to coma and death in untreated patients. Cerebrospinal fluid pleocytosis with a predominance of lymphocytes and, occasionally, erythrocytes is usual. Herpes simplex virus infection also can cause meningitis with nonspecific clinical manifestations that usually are mild and self-limited. Such episodes of meningitis usually are associated with genital HSV-2 infection. A number of unusual CNS manifestations of HSV have been described, including Bell palsy, atypical pain syndromes, trigeminal neuralgia, ascending myelitis, and postinfectious encephalomyelitis.

ETIOLOGY: Herpes simplex viruses are enveloped, double-stranded, DNA viruses. Infections with HSV-1 usually involve the face and skin above the waist; however, an increasing number of genital herpes cases are attributable to HSV-1. Infections with HSV-2 usually involve the genitalia and skin below the waist in sexually active adolescents and adults; HSV-2 is the most common cause of disease in neonates. Either type of virus can be found in either site, depending on the source of infection.

EPIDEMIOLOGY:

Neonatal. The incidence of neonatal HSV infection is estimated to range from 1 per 3000 to 20 000 live births. Infants in whom HSV infection develops are significantly more likely to be born prematurely. Herpes simplex virus is transmitted to an infant most frequently during birth through an infected maternal genital tract or by an ascending infection, sometimes through apparently intact membranes. In the United States, about 75% of neonatal infections are caused by HSV-2, and 25% are caused by HSV-1. Intrauterine infections causing congenital malformations have been implicated in rare cases. Other less common sources of neonatal infection include postnatal transmission from a parent or other caregiver, most often from a nongenital infection (eg, mouth or hands), or from another infected infant or caregiver in the nursery, probably via the hands of personnel attending the infants. Postnatal transmission from nursery personnel with oral lesions (fever blisters or cold sores) is rare.

The risk of HSV infection at delivery in an infant born vaginally to a mother with primary genital infection is estimated to be 33% to 50%. The risk to an infant born to a mother shedding HSV as a result of reactivated infection is much lower, in the range of 0% to 5%. Distinguishing between primary and recurrent HSV infections in women by history or physical examination may be impossible. Both primary and recurrent infections may be asymptomatic or associated with non-specific findings (eg, vaginal discharge, genital pain, or shallow ulcers). More than three quarters of infants who contract HSV infection have been born to women with no history or clinical findings suggestive of active HSV infection during pregnancy.

Children and Infants Beyond the Neonatal Period. Herpes simplex virus infections are ubiquitous and are transmitted from persons who are symptomatic or asymptomatic with primary or recurrent infections. Infection with HSV-1 usually results from direct contact with infected oral secretions or lesions. Infection with HSV-2 usually results from direct contact with infected genital secretions or lesions through sexual activity. Genital infections caused by HSV-1 in children can result from autoinoculation of virus from the mouth, whereas sexual abuse always should be considered in prepubertal children with genital HSV-2 infections. Genital HSV isolates from children should be typed to differentiate between HSV-1 and HSV-2.

Usually, HSV-1 is contracted during the first few years of life by persons from lower socioeconomic groups. Infection typically occurs later in life among persons from higher socioeconomic groups. The frequency of HSV-2 infection correlates with the number of sexual partners and with the acquisition of other sexually transmitted diseases.

Inoculation of skin occurs from direct contact with HSV-containing oral or genital secretions. This contact can result in herpes gladiatorum among wrestlers, herpes rugbiaforum among rugby players, or herpetic whitlow of the fingers in any exposed person.

Herpes simplex virus frequently is transmitted by infected persons who are shedding the virus asymptomatically. Patients with primary gingivostomatitis or genital herpes usually shed virus for at least 1 week and occasionally for several weeks. Patients with recurrent infection shed virus for a much shorter period, typically 3 to 4 days. Intermittent asymptomatic reactivation of oral and genital herpes is common and persists for life, occurring on 1% of days among previously infected persons. The greatest concentration of virus is shed during symptomatic primary infections and the least during asymptomatic recurrent infections.

Genital HSV-2 infection usually results from sexual intercourse, whereas genital infection with HSV-1 usually results from oral-genital contact. Following primary genital infection, which often is asymptomatic, some persons experience frequent clinical recurrences, while others have no recurrences. Genital HSV-2 infection is more likely to recur than is genital infection caused by HSV-1.

The **incubation period** for HSV infection occurring beyond the neonatal period ranges from 2 days to 2 weeks.

DIAGNOSTIC TESTS: Herpes simplex virus grows readily in cell culture. Special transport media are available for specimens that cannot be inoculated immediately onto susceptible cell culture media. Cytopathogenic effects typical of HSV usually are observed 1 to 3 days after inoculation. Methods for culture confirmation include fluorescent antibody staining and enzyme immunoassays. Cultures that remain negative by day 15 are likely to continue to remain negative. Rapid diagnostic techniques also are available, such as direct fluorescent antibody staining of vesicle scrapings or enzyme immunoassay detection of HSV antigens. These techniques are as specific but slightly less sensitive than culture. Typing HSV strains differentiates between HSV-1 and HSV-2 isolates. Polymerase chain reaction (PCR) is a sensitive method for detecting HSV DNA and is of particular value for evaluating CSF specimens from cases of suspected herpes encephalitis. Histologic examination of lesions for the presence of multinucleated giant cells and eosinophilic intranuclear inclusions typical of HSV (eg, Tzanck preparation) has low sensitivity and is not recommended as a rapid diagnostic test.

For the diagnosis of neonatal HSV infection, specimens for culture should be obtained from skin vesicles, mouth or nasopharynx, eyes, urine, blood, stool or rectum, and CSF. Positive cultures obtained from any of these sites more than 48 hours after birth indicate viral replication, suggestive of infant infection rather than colonization after intrapartum exposure.

Serologic tests generally are not helpful for the diagnosis of acute HSV infections. Serum samples often are obtained late in the clinical course, and an increase in antibody titers may be missed. Furthermore, recurrent infections may boost preexisting antibody titers. An additional problem with serologic diagnosis is the extensive cross-reaction between antibodies against HSV-1 and HSV-2; despite claims to the contrary, most commercial assays for HSV antibody generally cannot differentiate between HSV-1 and HSV-2 infection. A new assay based on the type-specific glycoprotein G has substantially improved determination of the type and is becoming more widely available. Immunoglobulin M HSV antibody assays are poorly standardized and are not helpful for diagnosing acute HSV infection.

Herpes simplex virus DNA in CSF frequently can be detected by PCR in patients with HSV encephalitis and is the diagnostic method of choice when performed by experienced laboratory personnel. Histologic examination and viral culture of brain tissue obtained by biopsy is the most definitive method for confirming the diagnosis of encephalitis caused by HSV. Cultures of CSF for HSV usually are negative.

TREATMENT: For recommended antiviral dosages and duration of therapy with acyclovir, valaciclovir, famciclovir, and penciclovir for different HSV infections, see Antiviral Drugs for Non-HIV Infections (p 675). Neither valaciclovir nor famciclovir is approved by the US Food and Drug Administration (FDA) for use in children.

Neonatal. Parenteral acyclovir is the treatment of choice for neonatal HSV infections. Acyclovir should be administered to all neonates with HSV infection, irrespective of presenting clinical findings. The best outcome in terms of morbidity and mortality is observed among infants with disease limited to the skin, eyes, and mouth. Although most neonates treated for HSV encephalitis survive, the majority suffer substantial neurologic sequelae. Approximately 50% of neonates with disseminated disease die despite antiviral therapy. The dosage of acyclovir is 60 mg/kg per day in 3 divided doses, given intravenously for 14 days if disease is limited to the skin, eye, and mouth and for 21 days if disease is disseminated or involves the CNS. Relapse of skin, eyes, and mouth and CNS disease can occur after cessation of treatment. The optimal management of these recurrences is not established. The value of long-term suppressive or intermittent acyclovir therapy for neonates with disease of the skin, eyes, and mouth is being evaluated.

Infants with ocular involvement due to HSV infection should receive a topical ophthalmic drug (1% to 2% trifluridine, 1% iododeoxyuridine, or 3% vidarabine), as well as parenteral antiviral therapy.

Genital Infection.

Primary. In adults, acyclovir, famciclovir, and valaciclovir reduce the duration of symptoms and viral shedding in primary genital herpes. Oral acyclovir therapy, initiated within 6 days of onset of disease, shortens the duration of illness and viral shedding by 3 to 5 days. Valaciclovir and famciclovir do not seem to be more effective than acyclovir, but they offer the advantage of less frequent dosing. No pediatric formulation of valaciclovir or famciclovir is available. Intravenous acyclovir is indicated for patients with a severe or complicated primary infection that requires hospitalization. Topical acyclovir (5%) ointment for primary genital herpes infection has minimal effects on the duration of viral shedding and symptoms and is not recommended. Systemic or topical treatment of primary herpetic lesions does not affect the subsequent frequency or severity of recurrences.

Recurrent. Antiviral therapy has minimal effect on recurrent genital herpes. Oral acyclovir therapy initiated within 2 days of the onset of symptoms shortens the mean clinical course by approximately 1 day. Valaciclovir and famciclovir are licensed for treatment of adults with recurrent genital herpes; however, no data exist for treatment of pediatric disease. Topical acyclovir is not beneficial for immunocompetent hosts.

In adults, daily oral acyclovir suppressive therapy is effective for decreasing the frequency of symptomatic recurrences in persons with frequent genital HSV recurrences (6 or more episodes per year). After approximately 1 year of continuous daily therapy, acyclovir should be discontinued and the recurrence rate assessed. If recurrences are observed, additional suppressive therapy should be considered. Acyclovir seems to be safe for adults receiving the drug for more than 10 years, but long-term effects are unknown. Data also support suppressive therapy in adults with valaciclovir or famciclovir.

Data on the use of acyclovir for suppressive therapy in children are not available. Acyclovir is not recommended for pregnant women unless disease is life-threatening.

Mucocutaneous and Other HSV Infections.

Immunocompromised Hosts. Intravenous acyclovir is effective for the treatment and prevention of mucocutaneous HSV infections. Topical acyclovir also may accelerate healing of lesions in immunocompromised patients.

Acyclovir-resistant strains of HSV have been isolated from immunocompromised persons receiving prolonged treatment with acyclovir. Under these circumstances, progressive disease may be observed despite acyclovir therapy. Foscarnet is the drug of choice for disease caused by acyclovir-resistant HSV isolates.

Immunocompetent Hosts. Limited data are available on the effects of acyclovir on the course of primary or recurrent nongenital mucocutaneous HSV infections in immunocompetent hosts. Therapeutic benefit has been noted in a limited number of children with primary gingivostomatitis treated with oral acyclovir. Minimal therapeutic benefit of oral acyclovir therapy has been demonstrated among adults with recurrent herpes labialis. Topical acyclovir is ineffective.

In a small controlled study in adults with recurrent herpes labialis (6 or more episodes per year), prophylactic acyclovir given in a dosage of 400 mg twice a day was effective for reducing the frequency of recurrent episodes. Although no studies of prophylactic therapy have been performed in children, children with frequent recurrences may benefit from continuous oral acyclovir therapy (20 mg/kg every 6 hours); reevaluation should be performed after 1 year of continuous therapy.

Central Nervous System. Patients with HSV encephalitis should be treated for 21 days with intravenous acyclovir. Therapy is less effective in older adults than in children and patients who are comatose or semicomatose at initiation of therapy. For persons with Bell palsy, the combination of acyclovir and prednisone should be considered.

Ocular. Treatment of eye lesions should be undertaken in consultation with an ophthalmologist. Several DNA inhibitor drugs, such as 1% to 2% trifluridine, 1% iododeoxyuridine, and 3% vidarabine, have proven efficacy for topical therapy of superficial keratitis. Topical corticosteroids are contraindicated in suspected HSV conjunctivitis; however, ophthalmologists may choose to use corticosteroids in conjunction with antiviral drugs to treat locally invasive infections. For children with recurrent ocular lesions, oral suppressive therapy with acyclovir (20 mg/kg every 6 hours) may be of benefit.

Isolation of the Hospitalized Patient: In addition to standard precautions, the following recommendations should be followed.

Neonates With HSV Infection. Neonates with HSV infection should be hospitalized in a private room and managed with contact precautions for the duration of the illness.

Neonates Exposed to HSV During Delivery. Infants born to women with active HSV lesions should be managed with contact precautions during the incubation period. Some experts believe that contact precautions are unnecessary if exposed infants were born by cesarean delivery, provided membranes were ruptured for less than 4 to 6 hours. The risk of HSV infection in possibly exposed infants (eg, those born to a mother with a history of recurrent genital herpes) is low.

One method of infection control for neonates with documented perinatal exposure to HSV is continuous rooming-in with the mother in a private room.

Women in Labor and Postpartum Women With HSV Infection. Women with active HSV lesions should be managed during labor, delivery, and the postpartum period with contact precautions. These women should be instructed about the importance of careful hand washing before and after caring for their infants. A clean covering gown may be used to help avoid contact of the infant with lesions or infectious secretions. A mother with herpes labialis (cold sores) or stomatitis should wear a disposable surgical mask when touching her newborn infant until the lesions have crusted and dried. She should not kiss or nuzzle her newborn until the lesions have cleared. Herpetic lesions on other skin sites should be covered.

Breastfeeding is acceptable if no lesions are present on the breasts and if active lesions elsewhere on the mother are covered (see Human Milk, p 98).

Children With Mucocutaneous HSV Infection. Contact precautions are recommended for patients with severe mucocutaneous HSV infection. Patients with localized recurrent lesions should be managed with standard precautions.

Patients With CNS HSV Infection. Standard precautions are recommended for patients with infection limited to the CNS.

Control Measures:

Prevention of Neonatal Infection. Expert opinion on the appropriate management of pregnant women to minimize the risk of neonatal HSV infection has changed considerably. Cultures for HSV obtained weekly during pregnancy are no longer recommended. Women with a history of genital HSV infection and women whose sexual partners have genital HSV infection are recognized to be at low risk of transmitting HSV to their infants (see Epidemiology, p 311).

Management of infants exposed to HSV during delivery differs according to the status of the mother's infection, mode of delivery, and expert opinion (see Care of Newborn Infants Whose Mothers Have Active Genital Lesions, p 316). Current recommendations for management of pregnant women for the prevention of HSV infection include the following:

- ***During pregnancy.*** During prenatal evaluations, all pregnant women should be asked about past or current signs and symptoms consistent with genital herpes infection in themselves and their sexual partners.
- ***Women in labor.*** During labor, all women should be asked about recent and current signs and symptoms consistent with genital herpes infection, and they should be examined carefully for evidence of genital infection. Cesarean delivery of women who have clinically apparent HSV infection may reduce the risk of neonatal HSV infection if performed within 4 to 6 hours of membrane rupture but is less likely to reduce neonatal infection if performed later. However, many experts recommend cesarean delivery whenever the birth canal is infected, even if membranes have been ruptured for 6 hours or more. In the absence of genital lesions, a maternal history of genital HSV is not an indication for cesarean delivery. Scalp monitors should be avoided when possible in infants of women suspected of having active genital herpes infection.

  A cesarean delivery should be performed immediately on a woman who presents with ruptured membranes and active genital lesions at term. The appropriate management of delivery is not established if membranes rupture in the presence of active genital lesions at a time when the fetal lung is immature. Some experts recommend that intravenous acyclovir (15 mg/kg in 3 divided doses) should be administered to the mother if labor and delivery are delayed. The value and risks of acyclovir in this situation are unknown. Use of acyclovir in this circumstance is not approved by the FDA.

Care of Newborn Infants Whose Mothers Have Active Genital Lesions.*

By Vaginal Delivery. Because the risk to infants exposed to HSV lesions during delivery varies in different circumstances from less than 5% to 50% or more, the decision to treat the asymptomatic exposed infant empirically with intravenous acyclovir is controversial. Since the infection rate of infants born to mothers with active recurrent genital herpes infections is less than 5%, most experts would not treat these infants empirically with acyclovir. The infant's parents or caregivers, however, should be educated about the signs and symptoms of neonatal HSV infection.

For infants born to mothers with a primary genital infection, the risk of infection may exceed 50%. Because of this high infection rate, some experts recommend empiric acyclovir treatment at birth after HSV cultures have been obtained, while others would obtain HSV cultures 24 to 48 hours after delivery and initiate acyclovir therapy only if HSV is recovered from these cultures. However, if the infant has symptoms suggestive of HSV infection, such as skin or scalp rashes (especially vesicular lesions), or unexplained clinical manifestations (such as those of sepsis), cultures should be obtained, irrespective of age, and acyclovir therapy should be initiated immediately.

Differentiating primary genital infection from recurrent HSV infection in the mother would be helpful for assessing the risk of HSV infection for the exposed infant, but the distinction may be difficult. First-episode clinical infections are not

* For further information and recommendations of the Infectious Disease Society of America, see Prober CG, Corey L, Brown ZA, et al. The management of pregnancies complicated by genital infections with herpes simplex virus. *Clin Infect Dis.* 1992;15:1031–1038

always primary infections. Often, primary infections are asymptomatic, in which case the first symptomatic episode will represent a reactivated recurrent infection. In selected instances, serologic testing can be useful. For example, if a woman with herpetic lesions has no detectable HSV antibodies, she is experiencing a primary infection. Assessment of seropositive women necessitates differentiation of HSV-1 from HSV-2 antibodies. Currently, most available commercial assays cannot make this distinction reliably. Newer assays based on type-specific glycoprotein G, may be helpful.

Recommendations. The management of exposed asymptomatic infants who were delivered vaginally of mothers with active genital lesions can be categorized according to the type of maternal infection as follows:

- Mother with primary first-episode infection
- Mother with known recurrent lesions
- Mother whose status (primary vs recurrent) is unknown

For infants in each category, cultures should be obtained for HSV at 24 to 48 hours after birth. Samples for cultures should include swabs or specimens of urine, stool or rectum, mouth, and nasopharynx (see Diagnostic Tests, p 312). For infants whose mothers have presumed or proven primary infection, some experts recommend empiric acyclovir treatment at birth, although no data exist to support the efficacy of such an approach. Other experts would await positive HSV culture results or clinical manifestations of infection before starting therapy.

The infant whose mother has known, recurrent, genital lesions should be observed carefully for signs of infection, including vesicular lesions of the skin, respiratory distress, seizures, or signs of sepsis. Education of parents and caregivers about the signs and symptoms of neonatal HSV infection is prudent. An infant with any of these manifestations should be evaluated immediately for possible HSV infection (as well as for bacterial infection). Specimens for HSV culture should be obtained from skin lesions, conjunctiva, nasopharynx, mouth, stool or rectum, urine, blood buffy coat, and CSF. Testing of CSF by PCR also is recommended. Acyclovir therapy should be initiated if any of the culture results are positive, CSF or PCR findings are abnormal, or HSV infection is otherwise strongly suspected.

Infants born by cesarean delivery to mothers with herpetic lesions should be observed carefully, with cultures performed as recommended for the potentially exposed infants born by vaginal delivery. Antiviral therapy should be initiated if culture results from the infant are positive or if HSV is strongly suspected for other reasons.

Other Recommendations.

- The length of in-hospital observation for infants at increased risk for neonatal HSV is variable and based on factors specific to the infant and local resources, such as the family's ability to observe the infant at home, availability of follow-up care, and clinical assessment.
- Neonatal HSV infection can occur as late as 4 to 6 weeks after delivery; parents and physicians must be vigilant and carefully evaluate any rash or other symptoms that may be caused by HSV.

Infected Hospital Personnel. Transmission of HSV in newborn nurseries from infected personnel to newborns rarely has been documented. The risk of transmission to infants by personnel who have labial HSV infection (cold sores) or who are asymptomatic oral shedders of the virus is low. Compromising patient care by excluding personnel with cold sores who are essential for the operation of the nursery must be weighed against the potential risk of infecting newborns. Personnel with cold sores who have contact with infants should cover and not touch their lesions and should comply with hand-washing policies. Transmission of HSV infection from personnel with genital lesions is not likely as long as personnel comply with hand-washing policies. Personnel with an active herpetic whitlow should not have responsibility for direct care of neonates or immunocompromised patients.

Household Contacts of Infected Persons With Newborns. Intrafamilial transmission of HSV to newborn infants has been described but is rare. Household members with herpetic skin lesions (eg, herpes labialis or herpetic whitlow) should be counseled about the risk and avoid contact of their lesions with newborn infants by taking the same measures as recommended for infected hospital personnel, as well as avoiding kissing and nuzzling the infant while they have active lesions.

Care of Persons With Extensive Dermatitis. Patients with dermatitis are at risk of developing eczema herpeticum. If these patients are hospitalized, special care should be taken to avoid exposure to HSV. They should not be kissed by persons with cold sores or touched by people with herpetic whitlow.

Care of Children With Mucocutaneous Infections Who Are in Child Care or School. Oral HSV infections are common among children who are in child care or school. Most of these infections are asymptomatic, with shedding of virus in saliva occurring in the absence of clinical disease. Only children with HSV gingivostomatitis (ie, primary infection) who do not have control of oral secretions should be excluded from child care. Exclusion of children with cold sores (ie, recurrent infection) from child care or school is not indicated.

Children with uncovered lesions on exposed surfaces pose a small potential risk to contacts. If children are certified by a physician to have recurrent HSV infection, covering the active lesions with clothing, a bandage, or an appropriate dressing when they attend child care or school is sufficient.

HSV Infections Among Wrestlers and Rugby Players. Infection with HSV-1 has been transmitted during athletic competition involving close physical contact and frequent skin abrasions, such as wrestling (herpes gladiatorum) and rugby (herpes rugbiaforum or scrum pox). Competitors often do not recognize or may deny possible infection. Transmission of these infections can be limited or prevented by the following: (1) examination of wrestlers and rugby players for vesicular or ulcerative lesions on exposed areas of their bodies and around their mouths or eyes before practice or competition by a person familiar with the appearance of different mucocutaneous infections (including HSV, herpes zoster, and impetigo); (2) exclusion of athletes with these conditions from competition or practice until healing occurs or a physician's written statement declaring their condition noninfectious is obtained; and (3) cleaning wrestling mats with a freshly prepared solution of household bleach (¼ cup of bleach in 1 gallon of water) applied for a minimum contact time of 15 seconds at least daily and, preferably, between matches. Despite these precautions, HSV spread during wrestling and other sports involving close personal contact still can occur through contact with asymptomatic persons.

Histoplasmosis

CLINICAL MANIFESTATIONS: Histoplasmosis encompasses a spectrum of clinical manifestations in the fewer than 5% of infected persons who are symptomatic. Clinical manifestations may be classified according to site (pulmonary, extrapulmonary, or disseminated), duration of infection (acute, chronic), and pattern of infection (primary vs reactivation). Acute pulmonary histoplasmosis is an influenza-like illness with nonpleuritic chest pain, pulmonary infiltrates, and hilar adenopathy; symptoms persist for 2 or 3 days to 2 weeks. Erythema nodosum can occur in adolescents, but erythema nodosum and chronic pulmonary histoplasmosis are uncommon in children. Primary cutaneous infections can occur after trauma.

Acute disseminated histoplasmosis is most frequent in children with impaired cell-mediated immunity, including patients with human immunodeficiency virus (HIV) infection and solid-organ transplant recipients, and infants younger than 1 year of age. Features include prolonged fever, failure to thrive, cough, hepatosplenomegaly, adenopathy, pneumonia, skin lesions, and pancytopenia. Central nervous system (CNS) involvement is common. Chronic disseminated infection is rare. Histoplasmosis may reactivate years after primary infection in isolated tissues, particularly in the CNS, adrenal glands, and mucocutaneous surfaces, as well as in other sites. Disseminated or extrapulmonary histoplasmosis is an acquired immunodeficiency syndrome–defining condition in an HIV-infected person.

ETIOLOGY: *Histoplasma capsulatum* var *capsulatum* is a dimorphic fungus. In soil, it grows as a spore-bearing mold with macroconidia, but it converts to a yeast phase at body temperature (37°C [98°F]).

EPIDEMIOLOGY: *Histoplasma capsulatum* is encountered in many parts of the world and is endemic in the eastern and central United States, particularly the Mississippi, Ohio, and Missouri river valleys. The source of the organism is soil or dust in barnyards and other locations high in nitrogen concentrations, especially soil containing droppings of bats, chickens, and starlings. Infection is acquired through inhalation of airborne spores (conidia). The quantity of inoculum inhaled, strain virulence, and the immune status of the host affect the degree of illness. Reinfection is possible but requires a large inoculum. Histoplasmosis is not transmitted from person to person.

The **incubation period** is variable but usually is 1 to 3 weeks from the time of exposure.

DIAGNOSTIC TESTS: Culture is the definitive method of diagnosis. *Histoplasma capsulatum* from bone marrow, blood, sputum, and biopsy specimens grows on standard mycologic media, but growth usually requires 2 to 6 weeks. The lysis-centrifugation method is preferred for blood cultures. A DNA probe for *H capsulatum* significantly shortens the time required for identification in cultures. This procedure can be applied to nonsporulating cultures, thereby reducing the risk of exposure of laboratory personnel to infectious spores.

Direct demonstration of intracellular yeast by Gomori methenamine silver or other stains in smears of bone marrow or biopsy material from infected tissues is helpful for diagnosing disseminated or chronic histoplasmosis.

Detection of *H capsulatum* polysaccharide antigen in serum, urine, and bronchoalveolar lavage fluid by radioimmunoassay is a specific, sensitive, and rapid method for the diagnosis of disseminated histoplasmosis, and it can be used to monitor treatment response. Cross-reacting antigens have been detected in persons with disseminated infection due to blastomycosis, paracoccidioidomycosis, and *Penicillium marneffei.*

Both mycelial-phase (histoplasmin) and yeast-phase antigens are used in serologic testing for complement-fixing antibodies to *H capsulatum.* A 4-fold increase in yeast-phase titers or a single titer of 1:32 or greater is presumptive evidence of active infection. Cross-reacting antibodies can result from *Blastomyces dermatiditis* and *Coccidioides immitis* infections. In the immunodiffusion antibody test, H bands, although rarely encountered, are highly suggestive of active infection. The immunodiffusion test is more specific than the complement fixation test, but the complement fixation test is more sensitive.

The histoplasmin skin test is not recommended for diagnostic purposes but is useful for epidemiologic studies.

TREATMENT: Immunocompetent children with uncomplicated, primary pulmonary histoplasmosis rarely require antifungal therapy. Indications for therapy include progressive disseminated infection in infants and acute infection in immunocompromised patients. Other manifestations of histoplasmosis in immunocompetent children for which antifungal therapy should be considered include pulmonary disease with symptoms persisting more than 4 weeks, seriously ill patients with intense exposures, and adenopathy that obstructs critical structures (ie, bronchi, blood vessels).

Amphotericin B is effective and recommended for disseminated disease (see Drugs for Invasive and Other Serious Fungal Infections, p 672). In other circumstances in which antifungal therapy is warranted, itraconazole and fluconazole also have been effective. The safety and efficacy of itraconazole for use in children have not been established, but in adults, itraconazole is preferred over fluconazole and has negligible toxic effects. Itraconazole also has proven effective in the treatment of mild disseminated histoplasmosis in HIV-infected patients.

The duration of treatment for disseminated disease with amphotericin B is 4 weeks except in HIV-infected patients. Mild infections in HIV-infected patients can be treated with itraconazole for 3 months; moderate or severe infections should be treated with 2 weeks of amphotericin B followed by 10 weeks of itraconazole. Patients with HIV infection require lifelong suppressive therapy with itraconazole or, if not tolerated, fluconazole.

ISOLATION OF THE HOSPITALIZED PATIENT: Standard precautions are recommended.

CONTROL MEASURES: In outbreaks, investigation for the common source of infection is indicated. Exposure to soil and dust from areas with significant accumulations of bird and bat droppings should be avoided, especially by immunocompromised persons, or, if unavoidable, controlled through the use of masks, gloves, and disposable clothing. Guidelines for preventing histoplasmosis designed for health and safety professionals, environmental consultants, and persons supervising workers involved in activities in which contaminated materials are disturbed are available. Additional information about the guidelines (publication No. 97-146) is available from the National Institute for Occupational Safety and Health (NIOSH), Publications Dissemination, 4676 Columbia Parkway, Cincinnati, OH 45226-1998; telephone (800) 356-4674; the National Center for Infectious Diseases, telephone (404) 639-3158; and the NIOSH Web site on the World Wide Web (http://www.cdc.gov/niosh/homepage.html or http://www.cdc.gov/niosh/97-146.html).

Hookworm Infections

(*Ancylostoma duodenale* and *Necator americanus*)

CLINICAL MANIFESTATIONS: After contact with contaminated soil, initial skin penetration of larvae, usually involving the feet, causes stinging or burning followed by pruritus and a papulovesicular rash persisting for 1 to 2 weeks. The pathogenesis of hookworm infection is directly related to worm burden. Pneumonitis associated with migrating larvae is uncommon and usually mild, except in heavy (≥25 eggs per glass coverslip on direct fecal smear) infections. Disease after oral ingestion of infectious *Ancylostoma duodenale* larvae can manifest with pharyngeal itching, hoarseness, nausea, and vomiting shortly after ingestion. Colicky abdominal pain with diarrhea and marked eosinophilia can develop 29 to 38 days after exposure. Chronic infection is a common cause of hypochromic microcytic anemia in persons living in tropical developing countries, and heavy infection can cause hypoproteinemia and edema secondary to blood loss.

ETIOLOGY: Infection usually is caused by *Ancylostoma duodenale* and *Necator americanus,* two roundworms (nematodes) with similar life cycles.

EPIDEMIOLOGY: Humans are the major reservoir. Well-nourished, lightly (<5 eggs per glass coverslip on direct fecal smear) infected persons are often asymptomatic. Hookworms are prominent in rural, tropical, and subtropical areas where soil contamination with human feces is common. Larvae and eggs survive in loose, sandy, moist, shady, well-aerated, warm soil (optimal temperature 23°C [73°F]to 33°C [91°F]). Although both worms are equally prevalent in many areas, *A duodenale* is the predominant species in Europe, the Mediterranean region, northern Asia, and the west coast of South America. *Necator americanus* is predominant in the Western hemisphere, sub-Saharan Africa, southeast Asia, and a number of Pacific islands. Hookworm eggs in stool hatch in soil in 1 to 2 days as rhabditoid larvae. These larvae develop into infective filariform larvae in soil within 5 to 7 days and can persist for weeks to months. Percutaneous infection occurs after exposure to infectious larvae. Peroral and possibly transmammary infection can occur with *A duodenale.* Untreated infected patients who do not become reinfected can harbor worms for 5 to 15 years, but a reduction in worm burden of at least 70% generally occurs within 1 to 2 years.

The **incubation period,** the time from exposure to development of symptoms, is 4 to 12 weeks.

DIAGNOSTIC TESTS: Microscopic demonstration of hookworm eggs in feces is diagnostic. Adult worms or larvae are seen rarely. Approximately 8 to 12 weeks are required following infection for eggs to appear in feces. A direct stool smear with potassium iodide saturated with iodine is adequate for diagnosis of heavy hookworm infection; light infections require concentration techniques. Quantification techniques may be available from state or reference laboratories to determine the clinical significance of infection and the response to treatment (eg, Beaver direct smear method; Stoll egg-counting technique).

TREATMENT: Mebendazole, pyrantel pamoate, and albendazole all are effective (see Drugs for Parasitic Infections, p 693). In children younger than 2 years of age, in whom experience with these drugs is limited, the World Health Organization (WHO) recommends one half the adult dose of albendazole or mebendazole in cases of heavy hookworm infections. The dose of pyrantel is determined by weight. In cases of heavy hookworm infection in pregnancy, deworming treatment is recommended by WHO during the second or third trimester. Albendazole, mebendazole, or pyrantel may be used. Adequate protein and iron nutrition also should be maintained throughout pregnancy. A repeated stool examination, using a concentration technique, should be performed 2 weeks after treatment, and, if positive, retreatment is indicated. Nutritional supplementation, including iron, is important when anemia is present. Severely affected children may require blood transfusion.

ISOLATION OF THE HOSPITALIZED PATIENT: Standard precautions are recommended.

CONTROL MEASURES: Sanitary disposal of feces to prevent contamination of soil, particularly in endemic areas, is necessary but rarely accomplished. Treatment of all known infected patients and screening of high-risk groups (ie, children and agricultural workers) in endemic areas can help reduce environmental contamination. Wearing shoes also is helpful.

Human Herpesvirus 6 (Including Roseola) and 7

CLINICAL MANIFESTATIONS: Major clinical manifestations of primary infection with human herpesvirus (HHV) 6 are variable in children younger than 3 years of age. These manifestations include roseola (exanthem subitum, sixth disease) in approximately 20% of children, undifferentiated febrile illness without rash or localizing signs, and other acute febrile illnesses, often accompanied by cervical and postoccipital lymphadenopathy, gastrointestinal or respiratory tract signs, and inflamed tympanic membranes. Fever is characteristically high (>39.5°C [103.0°F]) and persists for 3 to 7 days. In roseola, fever is followed by an erythematous maculopapular rash lasting hours to days. Seizures, which result in emergency department visits, occur during the febrile period in approximately 10% to 15% of primary infections. A bulging anterior fontanelle and encephalopathy occur occasionally.

The virus persists and may reactivate. The clinical circumstances and manifestations of reactivation in healthy persons are unclear. Illness associated with reactivation has been described primarily in immunosuppressed hosts in association with manifestations such as fever, hepatitis, bone marrow suppression, pneumonia, and encephalitis. Recognition of the varied clinical manifestations of HHV-7 infection is evolving. Many, if not most, primary infections with HHV-7 may be asymptomatic or mild; some may present as typical roseola and may account for second or recurrent cases of roseola. Febrile illnesses associated with seizures also have been reported. Some investigators suggest that the association of HHV-7 with these clinical manifestations results from the ability of HHV-7 to reactivate HHV-6 from latency, particularly variant B that causes roseola and other primary HHV-6 infections.

ETIOLOGY: Human herpesvirus 6 and HHV-7 are members of the family Herpesviridae, which contains a large, double-stranded, DNA genome. Strains of HHV-6 belong to 1 of 2 major groups, variants A and B. Almost all primary infections in children are caused by variant B strains. Human herpesvirus 7 is a member of the betaherpesviruses subfamily and is closely related to human cytomegalovirus and HHV-6.

EPIDEMIOLOGY: Humans are the only known natural hosts for HHV-6 and HHV-7. Transmission of HHV-6 to an infant most likely occurs via the asymptomatic shedding of persistent virus in secretions of a family member, caregiver, or other close contact. During the febrile phase of primary infection, HHV-6 can be isolated from peripheral blood lymphocytes in which the virus may persist subsequently, as well as from other sites, including saliva and cerebrospinal fluid. The attack rate is highest in children between the ages of 6 and 24 months. Infection within the first few months of age also occurs but is relatively uncommon before 3 months or after 3 years of age. Virus-specific maternal antibody is present uniformly in the serum of infants at birth and provides some protection. As the level of maternal antibody declines during the first year of life, the rate of infection increases rapidly, and almost all children are seropositive by 2 years of age. Infections occur throughout the year without a distinct seasonal pattern. Secondary cases rarely are identified, although occasional outbreaks of roseola have been reported.

Like HHV-6, HHV-7 is a ubiquitous agent, with infection occurring during early childhood, usually after HHV-6 infection. Lifelong persistent infection is established, and HHV-7 DNA may be detected in cerebrospinal fluid, cervical secretions, and saliva, with infectious virus present in more than three fourths of saliva specimens obtained from healthy adults. Like HHV-6, HHV-7 transmission to young children is likely to occur from contact with infected respiratory tract secretions of healthy persons. Most children show serologic evidence of infection by the age of 4 years. By adulthood, 85% or more of persons have serologic evidence of HHV-7 infection.

The mean **incubation period** for HHV-6 seems to be 9 to 10 days. The incubation period for HHV-7 is unknown.

DIAGNOSTIC TESTS: The diagnosis of primary HHV-6 infection currently necessitates use of research techniques to isolate the virus from peripheral blood, as well as for demonstration of seroconversion. A 4-fold increase in serum antibody alone does not necessarily indicate new infection, as an increase in titer also may occur with reactivation and in association with other infections. Commercial assays for antibody and antigen detection and polymerase chain reaction for detecting HHV-6 DNA are in development, but so far, none of these assays can differentiate reliably between primary infection and viral persistence or reactivation.

Diagnostic tests for HHV-7 are limited to research laboratories, and reliable differentiation between primary infection and reactivated is problematic. Serodiagnosis of HHV-7 is confounded by serologic cross-reactivity with HHV-6 and by the potential ability of HHV-6 to be reactivated by HHV-7 and possibly other infections.

TREATMENT: Supportive. For immunocompromised patients with serious HHV-6 disease, some experts recommend a course of ganciclovir.

ISOLATION OF THE HOSPITALIZED PATIENT: Standard precautions are recommended.

CONTROL MEASURES: None.

Human Herpesvirus 8

CLINICAL MANIFESTATIONS: For children, the clinical implications of the most recently discovered member of the herpesvirus family, human herpesvirus 8 (HHV-8), are unknown. In adults, HHV-8 is the probable etiologic agent of Kaposi sarcoma. The HHV-8 DNA sequences have been detected in all forms of Kaposi sarcoma from all parts of the world in patients with and without human immunodeficiency virus (HIV) infection, in primary effusion lymphomas of the abdominal cavity, in the lymphoproliferative syndrome (although less commonly than Epstein-Barr virus [EBV]), and in multicentric Castleman disease. Evidence of HHV-8 infection in children thus far seems rare, and no clinical associations are known.

ETIOLOGY: Human herpesvirus 8 is a member of the family Herpesviridae, the gammaherpesvirus subfamily closely related to herpesvirus saimiri of monkeys and EBV.

EPIDEMIOLOGY: Little is known about the epidemiology and transmission of HHV-8. However, HHV-8 has been reported to be latent in peripheral blood mononuclear cells and lymphoid tissue from immunocompromised patients and some healthy persons, suggesting that transmission could be via blood or secretions. In the United States in patients with HIV, detection of HHV-8 infection does not seem to occur until after adolescence.

The **incubation period** of HHV8 is unknown.

DIAGNOSTIC TESTS: Diagnostic tests for detection of HHV-8 infections are limited to research laboratories, and reliable differentiation of primary vs latent infection is problematic.

TREATMENT: No effective treatment is known for HHV-8.

ISOLATION OF THE HOSPITALIZED PATIENT: Standard precautions are recommended.

CONTROL MEASURES: None.

Human Immunodeficiency Virus Infection*

CLINICAL MANIFESTATIONS: Human immunodeficiency virus (HIV) infection in children and adolescents causes a broad spectrum of disease and a varied clinical course. Acquired immunodeficiency syndrome (AIDS) represents the most severe end of the clinical spectrum. The current surveillance definitions of the Centers for Disease Control and Prevention (CDC) for AIDS in adults and adolescents (see Table 3.23, p 326) and the pediatric classification system of CDC for children younger than 13 years of age who are born to HIV-infected mothers or who are known to be infected with HIV are given in Tables 3.24 (p 327) and 3.25 (p 329).[†‡] This pediatric classification system, which was established for surveillance of HIV infection, emphasizes the importance of the CD4+ T-lymphocyte count as an immunologic surrogate and prognosis marker but does not use information on viral load as quantitated by RNA polymerase chain reaction (PCR).

The manifestations of HIV infection include generalized lymphadenopathy, hepatomegaly, splenomegaly, failure to thrive, oral candidiasis, recurrent diarrhea, parotitis, cardiomyopathy, hepatitis, nephropathy, central nervous system (CNS) disease (including developmental delay, which can be progressive), lymphoid interstitial pneumonia, recurrent invasive bacterial infections, opportunistic infections,[§] and specific malignant neoplasms:

Pneumocystis carinii pneumonia (PCP) is one of the most commonly reported serious opportunistic infections in children with AIDS and is associated with high mortality (see *Pneumocystis carinii* Infections, p 460). Although PCP occurs most frequently in infants between 3 and 6 months of age who acquired HIV infection before or at birth, PCP can occur in younger infants, beginning as early as 4 to 6 weeks of age, or in older children whose immunologic status has deteriorated. Other common opportunistic infections in children include *Candida* species esophagitis, disseminated cytomegalovirus (CMV) infection, and chronic or disseminated herpes simplex and varicella-zoster virus infections and, less commonly, *Mycobacterium tuberculosis, Mycobacterium avium* complex (MAC) infection, and

* For a complete listing of current AAP guidelines, see American Academy of Pediatrics. *Pediatric Human Immunodeficiency Virus (HIV) Infection — A Compendium of AAP Guidelines on Pediatric HIV Infection.* Elk Grove Village, IL: American Academy of Pediatrics; 1999; this publication is available from the AAP at: 888-227-1770 in the United States and Canada, and 847-228-5005 elsewhere.

† Centers for Disease Control and Prevention. 1993 revised classification system for HIV infection and expanded case surveillance definition for AIDS among adolescents and adults. *MMWR Morb Mortal Wkly Rep.* 1992;41(RR-17):1–19

‡ Centers for Disease Control and Prevention. 1994 revised classification system for human immunodeficiency virus infection in children less than 13 years of age: official authorized addenda: human immunodeficiency virus infection codes and official guidelines for coding and reporting ICD-9-CM. *MMWR Morb Mortal Wkly Rep.* 1994;43(RR-12):1–19

§ Centers for Disease Control and Prevention. 1999 USPHS/IDSA guidelines for the prevention of opportunistic infections in persons infected with human immunodeficiency virus. *MMWR Morb Mortal Wkly Rep.* 1999;48(RR-10):1–59, 61–66

Table 3.23. **1993 Revised Case Definition of AIDS-Defining Conditions for Adults and Adolescents 13 Years of Age and Older***

- Candidiasis of bronchi, trachea, or lungs
- Candidiasis, esophageal
- Cervical cancer, invasive
- Coccidioidomycosis, disseminated or extrapulmonary
- Cryptococcosis, extrapulmonary
- Cryptosporidiosis, chronic intestinal (>1 mo duration)
- Cytomegalovirus disease (other than liver, spleen, or nodes)
- Cytomegalovirus retinitis (with loss of vision)
- Encephalopathy, HIV-related
- Herpes simplex: chronic ulcer(s) (>1 mo duration); or bronchitis, pneumonitis, or esophagitis
- Histoplasmosis, disseminated or extrapulmonary
- Isosporiasis, chronic intestinal (>1 mo duration)
- Kaposi sarcoma
- Lymphoma, Burkitt (or equivalent term)
- Lymphoma, immunoblastic (or equivalent term)
- Lymphoma, primary or brain
- *Mycobacterium avium* complex or *Mycobacterium kansasii,* disseminated or extrapulmonary
- *Mycobacterium tuberculosis,* any site, pulmonary or extrapulmonary
- *Mycobacterium,* other species or unidentified species, disseminated or extrapulmonary
- *Pneumocystis carinii* pneumonia
- Pneumonia, recurrent
- Progressive multifocal leukoencephalopathy
- *Salmonella* septicemia, recurrent
- Toxoplasmosis of brain
- Wasting syndrome due to HIV
- CD4+ T-lymphocyte count less than 200/µL (0.20×10^9/L) or CD4+ percentage less than 15%

* Modified from Centers for Disease Control and Prevention. 1993 revised classification system for HIV infection and expanded case surveillance definition for AIDS among adolescents and adults. *MMWR Morb Mortal Wkly Rep.* 1992;41(RR-17):1–19. AIDS indicates acquired immunodeficiency syndrome; HIV, human immunodeficiency virus.

chronic enteritis caused by *Cryptosporidium, Isospora,* or other agents. Rarely, disseminated or CNS cryptococcal or *Toxoplasma gondii* infections occur in children.

The occurrence of malignant neoplasms in children with HIV infection has been relatively uncommon, but leiomyosarcomas and certain lymphomas, including those of the CNS and non-Hodgkin B-cell lymphomas of the Burkitt type, occur much more frequently in children with HIV infection than in nonimmunocompromised children. Kaposi sarcoma is rare in children in the United States.

The development of opportunistic infections, particularly PCP, progressive neurologic disease, and severe wasting is associated with a poor prognosis. The prognosis for survival also is poor in perinatally infected children when viral load exceeds 100 000 copies per milliliter and the CD4 count is decreased and in children who become symptomatic during the first year of life. With earlier and more effective

Table 3.24. **Clinical Categories for Children Younger Than 13 Years of Age With Human Immunodeficiency Virus (HIV) Infection***

Category N: Not Symptomatic
Children who have no signs or symptoms considered to be the result of HIV infection or have only one 1 of the conditions listed in Category A.

Category A: Mildly Symptomatic
Children with 2 or more of the conditions listed but none of the conditions listed in Categories B and C.

- Lymphadenopathy (≥0.5 cm at more than 2 sites; bilateral at 1 site)
- Hepatomegaly
- Splenomegaly
- Dermatitis
- Parotitis
- Recurrent or persistent upper respiratory tract infection, sinusitis, or otitis media

Category B: Moderately Symptomatic
Children who have symptomatic conditions other than those listed for Category A or C that are attributed to HIV infection.

- Anemia (hemoglobin, <8 g/dL [<80 g/L]), neutropenia (white blood cell count, <1000/µL [$<1.0 \times 10^9$/L]), and/or thrombocytopenia (platelet count, $<100 \times 10^3$/µL [$<100 \times 10^9$/L]) persisting for ≥30 d
- Bacterial meningitis, pneumonia, or sepsis (single episode)
- Candidiasis, oropharyngeal (thrush), persisting (>2 mo) in children older than 6 mo of age
- Cardiomyopathy
- Cytomegalovirus infection, with onset before 1 mo of age
- Diarrhea, recurrent or chronic
- Hepatitis
- Herpes simplex virus (HSV) stomatitis, recurrent (>2 episodes within 1 year)
- HSV bronchitis, pneumonitis, or esophagitis with onset before 1 mo of age
- Herpes zoster (shingles) involving at least 2 distinct episodes or more than 1 dermatome
- Leiomyosarcoma
- Lymphoid interstitial pneumonia or pulmonary lymphoid hyperplasia complex
- Nephropathy
- Nocardiosis
- Persistent fever (lasting >1 mo)
- Toxoplasmosis, onset before 1 mo of age
- Varicella, disseminated (complicated chickenpox)

Category C: Severely Symptomatic

- Serious bacterial infections, multiple or recurrent (ie, any combination of at least 2 culture-confirmed infections within a 2-y period), of the following types: septicemia, pneumonia, meningitis, bone or joint infection, or abscess of an internal organ or body cavity (excluding otitis media, superficial skin or mucosal abscesses, and indwelling catheter–related infections)
- Candidiasis, esophageal or pulmonary (bronchi, trachea, lungs)
- Coccidioidomycosis, disseminated (at site other than or in addition to lungs or cervical or hilar lymph nodes)
- Cryptococcosis, extrapulmonary
- Cryptosporidiosis or isosporiasis with diarrhea persisting >1 mo

Table 3.24. **Clinical Categories for Children Younger Than 13 Years of Age With Human Immunodeficiency Virus (HIV) Infection,* continued**

Category C: Severely Symptomatic, continued

- Cytomegalovirus disease with onset of symptoms after 1 mo of age (at a site other than liver, spleen, or lymph nodes)
- Encephalopathy (at least one of the following progressive findings present for at least 2 mo in the absence of a concurrent illness other than HIV infection that could explain the findings): (1) failure to attain or loss of developmental milestones or loss of intellectual ability, verified by standard developmental scale or neuropsychological tests; (2) impaired brain growth or acquired microcephaly demonstrated by head circumference measurements or brain atrophy demonstrated by computed tomography or magnetic resonance imaging (serial imaging required for children younger than 2 y of age); (3) acquired symmetric motor deficit manifested by 2 or more of the following: paresis, pathologic reflexes, ataxia, or gait disturbance
- HSV infection causing a mucocutaneous ulcer that persists for greater than 1 mo; or bronchitis, pneumonitis, or esophagitis for any duration affecting a child older than 1 mo of age
- Histoplasmosis, disseminated (at a site other than or in addition to lungs or cervical or hilar lymph nodes)
- Kaposi sarcoma
- Lymphoma, primary, in brain
- Lymphoma, small, noncleaved cell (Burkitt), or immunoblastic; or large-cell lymphoma of B-cell or unknown immunologic phenotype
- *Mycobacterium tuberculosis,* disseminated or extrapulmonary
- *Mycobacterium,* other species or unidentified species, disseminated (at a site other than or in addition to lungs, skin, or cervical or hilar lymph nodes)
- *Pneumocystis carinii* pneumonia
- Progressive multifocal leukoencephalopathy
- *Salmonella* (nontyphoid) septicemia, recurrent
- Toxoplasmosis of the brain with onset at after 1 mo of age
- Wasting syndrome in the absence of a concurrent illness other than HIV infection that could explain the following findings: (1) persistent weight loss >10% of baseline OR (2) downward crossing of at least 2 of the following percentile lines on the weight-for-age chart (eg, 95th, 75th, 50th, 25th, 5th) in a child 1 y of age or older OR (3) <5th percentile on weight-for-height chart on 2 consecutive measurements, ≥30 d apart PLUS (1) chronic diarrhea (ie, at least 2 loose stools per day for >30 d) OR (2) documented fever (for >30 d, intermittent or constant)

* Modified from Centers for Disease Control and Prevention. 1994 revised classification system for human immunodeficiency virus infection in children less than 13 years of age: official authorized addenda: human immunodeficiency virus infection codes and official guidelines for coding and reporting ICD-9-CM. *MMWR Morb Mortal Wkly Rep.* 1994;43(RR-12):1–19

Table 3.25. **Pediatric Human Immunodeficiency Virus (HIV) Classification for Children Younger Than 13 Years of Age***

	Clinical Classifications†				Immunologic Categories: Age-Specific CD4+ T-Lymphocyte Count and Percentage of Total Lymphocytes‡					
					<12 mo		1–5 y		6–12 y	
Immunologic Definitions	N: No Signs or Symptoms	A: Mild Signs and Symptoms	B: Moderate Signs and Symptoms§	C: Severe Signs and Symptoms§	µL	%	µL	%	µL	%
1: No evidence of suppression	N1	A1	B1	C1	≥1500	≥25	≥1000	≥25	≥500	≥25
2: Evidence of moderate suppression	N2	A2	B2	C2	750–1499	15–24	500–999	15–24	200–499	15–24
3: Severe suppression	N3	A3	B3	C3	<750	<15	<500	<15	<200	<15

* Modified from Centers for Disease Control and Prevention. 1994 revised classification system for human immunodeficiency virus infection in children less than 13 years of age: official authorized addenda: human immunodeficiency virus infection codes and official guidelines for coding and reporting ICD-9-CM. *MMWR Morb Mortal Wkly Rep*. 1994;43(RR-12):1–19

† Children whose HIV infection status is not confirmed are classified by using this grid with a letter E (for perinatally exposed) placed before the appropriate classification code (eg, EN2).

‡ To convert values in microliters to Système International units ($\times 10^9$/L), multiply by 0.001.

§ Lymphoid interstitial pneumonitis in category B or category C is reportable to state and local health departments as acquired immunodeficiency syndrome (see Table 3.24, p 327, for further definition of clinical categories).

treatment, survival has improved. Median survival to 9 years of age was reported before the availability of more potent combination antiretroviral therapy.

ETIOLOGY: Infection is caused by human RNA retroviruses, HIV type 1 (HIV-1) and, less commonly, HIV-2, a related virus that is extremely uncommon in the United States but more common in West Africa.

EPIDEMIOLOGY: Humans are the only known reservoir of HIV, although related viruses, perhaps genetic ancestors, have been identified in chimpanzees and monkeys. Since retroviruses integrate into the target cell genome as proviruses and the viral genome is copied during cell replication, the virus persists in infected persons for life. Present data demonstrate the persistence of latent virus in peripheral blood mononuclear cells from the time of acquisition even when no viral RNA is detectable in blood. Human immunodeficiency virus has been isolated from blood (including lymphocytes, macrophages, and plasma) and from other body fluids, such as cerebrospinal fluid, pleural fluid, human milk, semen, cervical secretions, saliva, urine, and tears. Only blood, semen, cervical secretions, and human milk, however, have been implicated epidemiologically in transmission of infection.

The established modes of HIV transmission in the United States are the following: (1) sexual contact (homosexual and heterosexual), (2) percutaneous (from needles or other sharp instruments) or mucous membrane exposure to contaminated blood or other body fluids with high titers of HIV, (3) mother-to-infant (ie, vertical) transmission before or around the time of birth, and (4) breastfeeding. Transfusion of blood, blood components, or clotting factor concentrates is now rarely a mode of HIV transmission in the United States because of exclusion of infected donors, viral inactivation treatment of clotting factor concentrates, and the availability of recombinant clotting factors (see Blood Safety, p 88). In the absence of documented parenteral, mucous membrane, or skin contact with blood or blood-containing body fluids, transmission of HIV rarely has been demonstrated to occur in families or households or with routine care in hospitals or clinics. Transmission of HIV has not been demonstrated to occur in schools or child care settings.

Cases of AIDS in children have accounted for 2% of all reported cases in the United States. The total number of reported cases of AIDS in children decreased 66% in 1998 compared with 1993. The decrease is greatest in children younger than 5 years of age and most likely reflects diagnosis and treatment of women during pregnancy and chemoprophylaxis during labor and for the newborn with a resultant decrease in perinatal transmission. To the extent that trimethoprim-sulfamethoxazole (TMP-SMX) prophylaxis prevents PCP and with the use of more potent combination antiretroviral therapy, the clinical progression of AIDS can be delayed. Acquisition of HIV during adolescence continues to increase and contributes to the large number of cases in young adults. Transmission of HIV among adolescents primarily is due to sexual exposure. Among adolescents, the incidence of HIV infection in females is surpassing that in males. The majority of HIV-infected adolescents are asymptomatic and are not aware that they are infected.

More than 90% of infected children in the United States acquired their infection from their mothers; hence, the substantial decrease in recent perinatal AIDS is due to the successful intervention with zidovudine administered to HIV-infected pregnant women. The remainder, including patients with hemophilia or other coagulation disorders, received contaminated blood, its components, or clotting factor concentrates. A few cases of HIV infection in children have resulted from sexual abuse by an HIV-seropositive person. Fewer than 5% of cases have been reported to have no identifiable risk factor, and after careful investigation, most are reclassified into one of the established risk factor groups. Vertically acquired infection now accounts for almost all new infections in preadolescent children.

The risk of infection for an infant born to an HIV-seropositive mother who did not receive antiretroviral therapy during pregnancy is estimated to be between 13% and 39%. The exact timing of transmission from an infected mother to her infant is uncertain, but evidence suggests that approximately 30% of transmission occurs before birth and 70% occurs around the time of delivery. Available evidence suggests that two thirds of the infections occurring before delivery are due to transmission of virus within the last 14 days before delivery. Small studies have suggested higher rates of perinatal transmission by women who seroconvert during pregnancy or during the postpartum period if they breastfeed. Advanced maternal HIV disease also is associated with an increased risk of perinatal transmission. Higher viral loads are best reflected by the HIV RNA concentration. Other indications of advanced disease that have been associated with increased transmission include lower CD4 counts and repeatedly positive blood cultures for HIV. In vaginal deliveries, a first-born twin is at greater risk of HIV infection than a second-born twin. Prolonged rupture of membranes even in the presence of antiretroviral therapy is associated with an increased risk of transmission and must be considered when evaluating the mode of delivery and transmission.

Postpartum transmission occurs through breastfeeding. Worldwide, an estimated one third to one half of mother-to-child transmission of HIV may be through breastfeeding. Human immunodeficiency virus genomes have been detected in cellular and cell-free fractions of human milk, and breastfeeding has been implicated in transmission of HIV infection. The basic biology of transmission via human milk is not known. In the United States, it is possible to provide safe alternative feeding for infants. A means to diminish HIV transmission and continue safe feeding practices for infants born to HIV-infected women in the developing world is needed (see Human Milk, p 98).

INCUBATION PERIOD: Although the median age of onset of symptoms is estimated to be 12 to 18 months for untreated perinatally infected infants, increasing numbers of children are being identified who have remained asymptomatic for more than 5 years. Two patterns of progression of infection based on symptoms have been recognized. Approximately 15% to 20% of untreated children die before 4 years of age, with a median age at death of 11 months, whereas the majority of children survive beyond 5 years of age. Adults develop serum antibody to HIV by 6 to 12 weeks after infection. Infants born to HIV-infected women have transplacentally acquired antibody and, therefore, "test seropositive" from the time of birth.

DIAGNOSTIC TESTS: The laboratory diagnosis of HIV infection during infancy depends on detection of virus or virus nucleic acid. The transplacental transfer of antibody complicates the serologic diagnosis of infant infection.

Human immunodeficiency virus nucleic acid detection by PCR of DNA extracted from peripheral blood mononuclear cells is the preferred test for diagnosis

Table 3.26. **Laboratory Diagnosis of HIV Infection***

Test	Comment
HIV DNA PCR	Preferred test to diagnose HIV infection in infants and children younger than 18 months of age; highly sensitive and specific by 2 weeks of age and available; performed on peripheral blood mononuclear cells
HIV p24 Ag	Less sensitive, false-positive results during first month of life, variable results; not recommended
ICD p24 Ag	Commonly available; negative test result does not rule out infection; not recommended
HIV culture	Expensive, not easily available, requires up to 4 wk to do test
HIV RNA PCR	Not recommended for routine testing of infants and children younger than 18 months of age because a negative result cannot be used to exclude HIV infection

* HIV indicates human immunodeficiency virus; PCR, polymerase chain reaction; Ag, antigen; and ICD, immune complex dissociated.

of HIV infection in infants, and results can be available within 24 hours of obtaining a sample of anticoagulated whole blood (see Table 3.26, above). Approximately 30% of infants with HIV infection will have a positive DNA PCR result from samples obtained before 48 hours of age. The test can detect 1 to 10 DNA copies routinely. Approximately 93% of infected infants have detectable HIV DNA by 2 weeks of age, and almost all infants are HIV positive by 1 month of age. A single DNA PCR assay has a sensitivity of 95% and a specificity of 97% on samples collected from 1 to 36 months of age. DNA PCR is more sensitive on a single assay than is virus culture, and virus need not be replication competent to be detected.

Virus isolation by culture is expensive, available only in a few laboratories, and requires up to 28 days for positive results. This test essentially has been replaced by DNA PCR.

Detection of the p24 antigen (including immune complex dissociated) is specific but significantly less sensitive than DNA PCR or culture. An additional drawback is the occurrence of false-positive test results in samples obtained from infants younger than 1 month of age.

Plasma HIV RNA PCR may be used to diagnose HIV infection if the result is positive. However, this test result may be negative in HIV-infected persons. The test is licensed by the US Food and Drug Administration only in quantitative format and currently is used for quantifying the amount of virus present as a measurement of disease progression, not for diagnosis of HIV infection in infants.

Infants born to HIV-infected women should be tested by HIV DNA PCR during the first 48 hours of life. Because of possible contamination with maternal blood, umbilical cord blood should not be used for this determination. A second test should be performed at 1 to 2 months of age. Obtaining the sample as early as 14 days of age may enable decisions to be made about antiretroviral therapy at an earlier age. A third test is recommended at 3 to 6 months of age. Any time an infant tests positive, testing is repeated on a second blood sample as soon as possible to confirm the diagnosis. An infant is infected if 2 separate samples are positive (see Table 3.27, p 333). Infection can be excluded reasonably when 2 HIV DNA PCR assays

Table 3.27. Revised Surveillance Case Definition for HIV Infection*

This revised definition of HIV infection, which applies to any HIV (eg, HIV-1 or HIV-2), is intended for public health surveillance only.

I. In adults, adolescents, or children ≥18 months† of age, a reportable case of HIV infection must meet at least one of the following criteria:

Laboratory Criteria

- Positive result on a screening test for HIV antibody (eg, repeatedly reactive enzyme immunoassay), followed by a positive result on a confirmatory (sensitive and more specific) test for HIV antibody (eg, Western blot or immunofluorescence antibody test)

OR

- Positive result or report of a detectable quantity on any of the following HIV virologic (nonantibody) tests:
  - HIV nucleic acid (DNA or RNA) detection (eg, DNA polymerase chain reaction [PCR] or plasma HIV-1 RNA)‡
  - HIV p24 antigen test, including neutralization assay
  - HIV isolation (viral culture)

OR

Clinical or Other Criteria (if the above laboratory criteria are not met)

- Diagnosis of HIV infection, based on the laboratory criteria above, that is documented in a medical record by a physician

OR

- Conditions that meet criteria included in the case definition for AIDS (Table 3.23, p 326, and Table 3.24, p 327)

II. In a child aged <18 months, a reportable case of HIV infection must meet at least one of the following criteria:

Laboratory Criteria

Definitive

- Positive results on 2 separate specimens (excluding cord blood) using one or more of the following HIV virologic (nonantibody) tests:
  - HIV nucleic acid (DNA or RNA) detection
  - HIV p24 antigen test, including neutralization assay, in a child ≥1 month of age
  - HIV isolation (viral culture)

OR

Presumptive

A child who does not meet the criteria for definitive HIV infection but who has:

- Positive results on only 1 specimen (excluding cord blood) using the above HIV virologic tests and no subsequent negative HIV virologic or negative HIV antibody tests

OR

Table 3.27. **Revised Surveillance Case Definition for HIV Infection,* continued**

Clinical or Other Criteria (if the above definitive or presumptive laboratory criteria are not met)

- Diagnosis of HIV infection, based on the laboratory criteria above, that is documented in a medical record by a physician

OR

- Conditions that meet criteria included in the 1987 pediatric surveillance case definition for AIDS (Table 3.23, p 326, and Table 3.24, p 327)

III. A child aged <18 months born to an HIV-infected mother will be categorized for surveillance purposes as "not infected with HIV" if the child does not meet the criteria for HIV infection but meets the following criteria:

Laboratory Criteria

Definitive

- At least 2 negative HIV antibody tests from separate specimens obtained at ≥6 months of age

OR

- At least 2 negative HIV virologic tests[§] from separate specimens, both of which were performed at ≥1 month of age and 1 of which was performed at ≥4 months of age

AND

No other laboratory or clinical evidence of HIV infection (ie, has not had any positive virologic tests, if performed, and has not had an AIDS-defining condition)

OR

Presumptive

A child who does not meet the above criteria for definitive "not infected" status but who has:

- One negative EIA HIV antibody test performed at ≥6 months of age and NO positive HIV virologic tests, if performed

OR

- One negative HIV virologic test[§] performed at ≥4 months of age and NO positive HIV virologic tests, if performed

OR

- One positive HIV virologic test with at least 2 subsequent negative virologic tests,[§] at least 1 of which is at ≥4 months of age; or negative HIV antibody test results, at least 1 of which is at ≥6 months of age

AND

No other laboratory or clinical evidence of HIV infection (ie, has not had any positive virologic tests, if performed, and has not had an AIDS-defining condition).

OR

Clinical or Other Criteria (if the above definitive or presumptive laboratory criteria are not met)

- Determined by a physician to be "not infected," and a physician has noted the results of the preceding HIV diagnostic tests in the medical record

AND

Table 3.27. **Revised Surveillance Case Definition for HIV Infection,* continued**

NO other laboratory or clinical evidence of HIV infection (ie, has not had any positive virologic tests, if performed, and has not had an AIDS-defining condition)

IV. A child aged <18 months born to an HIV-infected mother will be categorized as having perinatal exposure to HIV infection if the child does not meet the criteria for HIV infection (II) or the criteria for "not infected with HIV" (III).

* Centers for Disease Control and Prevention. CDC guidelines for national human immunodeficiency virus case surveillance, including monitoring for human immunodeficiency virus infection and acquired immunodeficiency syndrome. *MMWR Morb Mortal Wkly Rep.* 1999;48(RR-13):29–31

† Children aged ≥18 months but <13 years of age are categorized as "not infected with HIV" if they meet the criteria in III.

‡ In adults, adolescents, and children infected by other than perinatal exposure, plasma viral RNA nucleic acid tests should **NOT** be used in lieu of licensed HIV screening tests (eg, repeatedly reactive enzyme immunoassay). In addition, a negative (ie, undetectable) plasma HIV-1 RNA test result does not rule out the diagnosis of HIV infection.

§ HIV nucleic acid (DNA or RNA) detection tests are the virologic methods of choice to exclude infection in children aged <18 months. Although HIV culture can be used for this purpose, it is more complex and expensive to perform and is less well standardized than nucleic acid detection tests. The use of p24 antigen testing to exclude infection in children aged <18 months is not recommended because of its lack of sensitivity.

performed at or beyond 1 month of age are negative and at least 1 assay was performed on a sample obtained at 4 months of age or older. Alternatively, an infant with 2 blood samples negative for HIV antibody obtained after 6 months of age and at an interval of at least 1 month also can be considered not infected.

Enzyme immunoassays (EIAs) are used most widely as the initial test for serum HIV antibody. These tests are highly sensitive and specific. Repeated EIA testing of initially reactive specimens is required to reduce the small likelihood of laboratory error. Western blot or immunofluorescent antibody tests should be used for confirmation, which will overcome the problem of a false-positive EIA result. A positive HIV antibody test result in a child 18 months of age or older usually indicates infection (see Table 3.27, p 333).

Serum antibodies to HIV are present in almost all infected persons, with the exception of a small minority who are hypogammaglobulinemic and the few persons with AIDS who become seronegative late in disease. Some infants who receive combination antiretroviral therapy within 2 to 3 months of age also lose detectable antibody but remain infected.

The most notable finding is a high viral load (as measured by RNA PCR) that does not decline rapidly during the first year of life unless combination antiretroviral therapy is initiated. As the disease progresses, there is an increasing loss of cell-mediated immunity. The peripheral blood lymphocyte count at birth and during the first years of infection can be normal, but eventually lymphopenia develops because of a decrease in the total number of circulating CD4 lymphocytes. The T-suppressor CD8+ lymphocyte count usually increases initially, and cells are not depleted until late in the course of the infection. These changes in cell populations result in a decrease of the normal CD4+ to CD8+ cell ratio. This nonspecific finding, although characteristic of HIV infection, also occurs with other acute viral infections, including infections caused by CMV and Epstein-Barr virus. The normal values for peripheral CD4+ lymphocyte counts and percentages are age-related, and the lower limits of normal are given in Table 3.25 (p 329).

Although the B-lymphocyte count remains normal or is increased somewhat, humoral immune dysfunction may precede and accompany cellular dysfunction. Elevated serum immunoglobulin (Ig) concentrations, particularly IgG and IgA, are manifestations of the humoral immune dysfunction. Specific antibody responses to antigens to which the patient has not been exposed can be abnormal, and, later in disease, recall antibody responses are slow and diminish in magnitude. Measuring the serum antibody response to measles vaccine administered to children 12 months of age or older or to tetanus after 3 doses of diphtheria and tetanus toxoids and acellular pertussis (DTaP) vaccine can be useful for assessing humoral responsiveness. A minority (<10%) of patients will develop panhypogammaglobulinemia.

Perinatal HIV Serologic Testing. The American Academy of Pediatrics (AAP) recommendations include the following*:

- On the basis of recent advances in effective prophylaxis to reduce the rate of perinatal HIV transmission, AAP recommends routinely offering counseling and testing with consent for all pregnant women in the United States. Consent for maternal HIV testing may be obtained in a variety of ways, including by right of refusal, ie, with testing to take place unless rejected in writing by the patient. The AAP supports use of consent procedures that facilitate rapid incorporation of HIV education and testing into routine medical care settings. For women who are examined by a health care professional for the first time in labor and have not been tested for HIV infection during the current pregnancy, counseling and immediate testing should be considered because administration of antiretroviral therapy during labor is recommended and may diminish transmission. Careful attention to further education about HIV infection is recommended during the perinatal period.
- Routine education about HIV infection and testing should be a part of a comprehensive program of health care for women.
- For newborn infants whose mother's HIV antibody status was not determined during pregnancy or the postpartum period, the infant's health care professional should inform the mother about the potential benefits of HIV testing for her infant and the possible risks and benefits to herself of knowing the child's serostatus and recommend immediate HIV testing for the newborn.
- In the absence of known maternal HIV antibody status and parental availability for consent to test the newborn for HIV antibody, procedures should be established to facilitate rapid evaluation and testing of the infant.
- The health care professional for the infant should be informed of maternal HIV serostatus so that appropriate care and testing of the infant can be accomplished. Similarly, if the infant is found to be seropositive, but maternal HIV infection was unknown, the child's health care professional should ensure that this information and its significance be provided to the mother and, with her

* American Academy of Pediatrics, American College of Obstetricians and Gynecologists. Human Immunodeficiency virus screening: joint statement of the American Academy of Pediatrics and the American College of Obstetricians and Gynecologists. *Pediatrics.* 1999;104:128

consent, to her health care professional. The mother should be referred to an appropriate HIV-related service for adults.

- Comprehensive HIV-related medical services should be accessible to all infected mothers, their infants, and other family members.
- The AAP supports legislation and public policy directed toward eliminating any form of discrimination based on HIV serostatus.

Informed Consent for HIV Serologic Testing. Testing for HIV infection is unlike most routine blood testing because risks for discrimination in jobs, school, and child care can be incurred. The parents or other primary caregivers and the patient, if old enough to comprehend, should be counseled about the possible risks and benefits of testing a child and the consequences of HIV infection. The necessity of counseling and consent should not deter efforts to undertake appropriate diagnostic testing for HIV infection. Consent should be obtained from the parent or legal guardian and recorded in the patient's medical chart. State and local laws and hospital regulations should be considered when deciding whether written consent is required and under what circumstances testing can be done without consent. Refusal of parents or patients to give consent does not relieve physicians of professional and legal responsibilities to their patients. If the physician believes that testing is essential to the child's health, authorization for testing may be possible through local laws and can be obtained by other means. The results of serologic tests should be discussed in person with the family, primary caregiver, and, if appropriate according to age, the patient. In many states, minor adolescents can provide their own consent for testing, but the involvement of a supportive adult should be sought. Appropriate counseling and subsequent follow-up care must be provided. Maintaining confidentiality in all cases is essential to preserving patient and parent trust and consent.

TREATMENT: (See Table 4.9, p 678, for a list of antiretroviral drugs and their recommended dosages.) Primary care physicians are encouraged to participate actively in the care of HIV-infected patients in consultation with specialists who have expertise in the care of HIV-infected children and adolescents. Expert opinions and knowledge about diagnostic and therapeutic strategies are changing rapidly (see http://www.hivatis.org). In areas of the United States in which enrollment into clinical trials is possible, enrollment of an HIV-infected child into available clinical trials should be encouraged. Information about trials for adolescents and children can be obtained by contacting the AIDS Clinical Trials Information Service.*

Antiretroviral therapy is indicated for most HIV-infected children. Initiation of antiretroviral therapy depends on virologic, immunologic, and clinical criteria.† This is a rapidly changing area; consultation with an expert in pediatric HIV is suggested. Antiretroviral therapy should be initiated for all HIV-infected children younger than 12 months of age or with more than 100 000 copies of HIV RNA per milliliter of plasma regardless of age. Currently, many experts recommend therapy for all infected infants and children with at least 3 antiretroviral drugs because of demonstrable reduction in viral load and the better prognosis associated with

---

* See Appendix I, Directory of Resources, p 645: AIDS Clinical Trials Information Service at http://www.actis.org/.

† Centers for Disease Control and Prevention. Guidelines for the use of antiretroviral agents in pediatric HIV infection. *MMWR Morb Mortal Wkly Rep.* 1998;47(RR-4):1–43

lower viral load. Other experts would elect not to initiate therapy for children older than 1 year of age who are at low risk for disease progression (eg have low viral load, are asymptomatic, and have normal CD4 lymphocyte counts).

Combination antiretroviral therapy has been shown to be more effective than monotherapy. Data indicate good viral suppression can be achieved with triple therapy including a protease inhibitor or a nonnucleoside reverse transcriptase inhibitor. Based on the principles of therapy,* 3 new antiretroviral drugs should be given whenever possible. Suppression of virus to undetectable levels is the goal to which therapy should aspire. A change in antiretroviral therapy should be considered if there is evidence of disease progression (virologic, immunologic, or clinical), toxic effects or intolerance of drugs, or data suggesting a superior regimen (see Table 4.12, p 692).

Routine Immune Globulin Intravenous (IGIV) therapy is recommended in combination with antiviral agents for children with humoral immunodeficiency only for the following: (1) hypogammaglobulinemia (IgG <250 mg/dL [2.5 g/L]); (2) recurrent, serious, bacterial infections (defined as 2 or more serious bacterial infections such as bacteremia, meningitis, or pneumonia during a 1-year period), although IGIV may not provide additional benefit to children who are receiving daily TMP-SMX; (3) children who fail to form antibodies to common antigens; (4) treatment of parvovirus B19 infections; (5) treatment of thrombocytopenia; and (6) a single dose for children exposed to measles. The dose of IGIV is 400 mg/kg per dose given every 4 weeks or once after exposure to measles. Rh_o (D) Immune Globulin or IGIV also may be useful for treatment of HIV-associated thrombocytopenia in a dose of 500 to 1000 mg/kg per day for 3 to 5 days. In addition, children with bronchiectasis may benefit from adjunctive IGIV therapy at 600 mg/kg per dose, given monthly.

Early diagnosis and aggressive treatment of opportunistic infections may prolong survival. Since PCP can be an early complication of perinatally acquired HIV infection and mortality is high, chemoprophylaxis should be given to HIV-exposed children at risk for PCP.† For infants younger than 12 months of age with possible or proven HIV infection, PCP prophylaxis should be administered beginning at 4 to 6 weeks of age and continued for the first year of life unless HIV infection is excluded reasonably on the basis of 2 or more negative virologic diagnostic assays for HIV (ie, HIV DNA PCR or culture, both of which are performed at 1 month of age or older and one of which is performed at 4 months of age or older). The need for PCP prophylaxis for HIV-infected children 1 year of age and older is determined by CD4+ T-lymphocyte counts (see *Pneumocystis carinii* Infections, p 460).

Guidelines for prevention and treatment of opportunistic infections in children, adolescents, and adults provide appropriate indications for administration of drugs for MAC, CMV, toxoplasmosis, and other organisms.† Of note, the more potent antiretroviral therapies for adults that successfully suppress virus replication to undetectable levels have altered the occurrence of opportunistic infections; CMV retinitis, MAC, toxoplasmosis, and cryptosporidiosis have diminished dramatically. Fewer

* See http://www.hivatis.org for periodic updates of new drugs and new treatment recommendations.

† Centers for Disease Control and Prevention. 1999 USPHS/IDSA guidelines for the prevention of opportunistic infections in persons infected with human immunodeficiency virus. *MMWR Morb Mortal Wkly Rep.* 1999;48(RR-10):1–59, 61–66

such infections have occurred even when CD4 counts failed to rise to levels indicative of functional immunity. It has been postulated that cell-mediated immunity to pathogens other than HIV persists, and, with virus suppression, the T cells again multiply, providing immune function to the host. Data on the safety of discontinuing prophylaxis in HIV-infected children receiving highly active antiretroviral therapy are not yet available; recommendations are expected to continue to evolve to guide physicians in stopping prophylaxis in children with successful virus suppression as more data become available.

Immunization Recommendations (see also Immunocompromised Children, p 56, and Table 3.28, p 340).

Children with HIV infection should be immunized as soon as possible with routine inactivated vaccines (DTaP, inactivated poliovirus vaccine [IPV], *Haemophilus influenzae* type b, and hepatitis B virus), as well as with pneumococcal and influenza vaccines. The suggested schedule for administration of these immunogens is in the Recommended Childhood Immunization Schedule (Fig 1.1, p 22). Oral poliovirus vaccine is no longer recommended routinely for use in any child in the United States, including HIV-infected children or members of their households.

Measles, mumps, rubella (MMR) vaccine should be administered to HIV-infected children at 12 months of age unless they are severely immunocompromised. Based on the case report of an HIV-infected adolescent with severe immunocompromise who developed severe pneumonitis associated with measles vaccine virus, MMR vaccine is contraindicated for severely immunocompromised (category 3, Table 3.25, p 329) persons with HIV infection (see Measles, p 385).* The second dose of MMR may be administered as soon as 4 weeks after the first in an attempt to induce seroconversion as early as possible. Children receiving routine IGIV prophylaxis may not respond to MMR. If an outbreak of measles is in progress and exposure is likely, immunization should begin as early as 6 to 9 months.

In general, children with symptomatic HIV infection have poor immunologic responses to vaccines. Hence, such children, when exposed to a vaccine-preventable disease such as measles or tetanus, should be considered susceptible regardless of the history of immunization and should receive, if indicated, passive immunoprophylaxis (see Passive Immunization of Children With HIV Infection, p 341). Immune globulin (IG) also should be given to any unimmunized household member who is exposed to measles infection.

Children infected with HIV may be at increased risk of morbidity from varicella and herpes zoster. Limited data on immunization of HIV-infected children in CDC class 1 indicate that the vaccine is safe, immunogenic, and effective. Weighing potential risks and benefits, varicella vaccine should be considered for HIV-infected children in CDC class N1 and A1 (no or mild signs or symptoms of disease).

Hepatitis A vaccine is recommended for children living in communities with consistently elevated hepatitis A rates and for persons with chronic liver disease (see Hepatitis A, p 280).

* American Academy of Pediatrics Committee on Infectious Diseases and Committee on Pediatric AIDS. Measles immunization in HIV-infected children. *Pediatrics.* 1999;103:1057–1060

Table 3.28. Recommendations for Routine Immunization of HIV-Infected Children in the United States*

Vaccines	Known Asymptomatic HIV Infection	Symptomatic HIV Infection
Hepatitis B	Yes	Yes
DTaP	Yes	Yes
IPV†	Yes	Yes
MMR	Yes	Yes‡
Hib	Yes	Yes
Pneumococcal§	Yes	Yes
Influenza‖	Yes	Yes
Varicella¶	Consider	Consider
BCG	No	No
Hepatitis A#	See text	See text

* See Fig 1.1 (p 22) and disease-specific chapters for age at which specific vaccines are indicated. HIV indicates human immunodeficiency virus; DTaP, diphtheria and tetanus toxoids and acellular pertussis; IPV, inactivated poliovirus; MMR, live-virus measles, mumps, and rubella; Hib, *Haemophilus influenzae* type b conjugate; and BCG, bacille Calmette-Guérin.

† Only IPV vaccine should be used for HIV-infected children, HIV-exposed infants whose status is indeterminate, and household contacts of HIV-infected persons.

‡ Severely immunocompromised HIV-infected children should not receive MMR vaccine (see text).

§ Pneumococcal vaccine should be administered to all age-appropriate HIV-infected children. Children who are older than 2 months of age should receive pneumococcal vaccine at the time of diagnosis. Reimmunization after 3 to 5 years is recommended in either circumstance.

‖ Influenza vaccine should be provided each autumn and repeated annually for HIV-exposed infants 6 months of age and older, HIV-infected children and adolescents, and household contacts of HIV-infected persons.

¶ Consider for HIV-infected children in Centers for Disease Control and Prevention class N1 and A1 (see Varicella-Zoster Infections, p 624).

Also see Hepatitis A (p 280).

In the United States and in areas of low prevalence of tuberculosis, bacille Calmette-Guérin (BCG) vaccine is not recommended. However, in developing countries where the prevalence of tuberculosis is high, the World Health Organization recommends that BCG be given to all infants at birth if they are asymptomatic, regardless of maternal HIV infection. Disseminated BCG infection has occurred in HIV-infected infants immunized with BCG.

Seronegative Children Residing in the Household of a Patient With Symptomatic HIV Infection. In a household with an adult or child immunocompromised as the result of HIV infection, as in all households, all children should receive IPV vaccine, and MMR vaccine may be given because these vaccine viruses are not transmitted. To reduce the risk of transmission of influenza to patients with symptomatic HIV infection, yearly influenza immunization is indicated for them and for their household contacts (see Influenza, p 351).

Varicella immunization of siblings and susceptible adult caregivers of patients with HIV infection is encouraged to prevent acquisition of wild-type varicella-zoster infection, which can cause severe disease in immunocompromised hosts. Varicella vaccine virus transmission from an immunocompetent host is rare.

Passive Immunization of Children With HIV Infection.

- **Measles** (see Measles, p 385). Symptomatic HIV-infected children who are exposed to measles should receive IG prophylaxis (0.5 mL/kg, maximum 15 mL), regardless of immunization status. Exposed, asymptomatic, HIV-infected patients also should receive IG; the recommended dose is 0.25 mL/kg. Children who have received IGIV within 2 weeks of exposure do not require additional passive immunization.
- **Tetanus.** In the management of wounds classified as tetanus prone (see Tetanus, p 563, and Table 3.58, p 566), children with HIV infection should receive tetanus immune globulin regardless of immunization status.
- **Varicella.** Children infected with HIV who are exposed to varicella or zoster should receive Varicella-Zoster Immune Globulin (VZIG) (see Varicella-Zoster Infections, p 624). Children who have received IGIV or VZIG within 2 weeks of exposure do not require additional passive immunization.

ISOLATION OF THE HOSPITALIZED PATIENT: Standard precautions should be followed by all hospital personnel. The risk to health care personnel of acquiring HIV infection from a patient is minimal, even after accidental exposure from a needle-stick injury (see Epidemiology, p 330). Every effort, nevertheless, should be made to avoid exposures to blood and other body fluids that could contain HIV.

CONTROL MEASURES:

Reduction of Perinatal HIV Transmission.* Oral administration of zidovudine to pregnant women beginning at 14 to 34 weeks' gestation and continuing throughout pregnancy, intravenous administration of zidovudine during labor until delivery (ie, intrapartum), and oral administration of zidovudine to the newborn infant for the first 6 weeks of life reduced the risk of perinatal HIV transmission by two thirds (see Table 3.29, p 342) in a controlled clinical trial. In the United States, nationwide reduction of perinatal AIDS by 66% has occurred since 1993. Current guidelines for use of antiretroviral drugs in pregnant HIV-infected women are the same as those for nonpregnant adults.[†] Therefore, many HIV-infected pregnant women will be receiving combination antiretroviral therapy for treatment of their HIV disease; use of zidovudine prophylaxis alone is reserved for the rare woman with a normal CD4 count and low or undetectable viral load who otherwise would not require therapy. However, the potential effect of antiretroviral drugs, particularly when used in combination, on the fetus and infant is unknown, and decisions about use of any antiretroviral drug during pregnancy requires a discussion of the known benefits and unknown risks to the woman and her fetus. Long-term follow-up is recommended for all infants born to women who have received antiretroviral drugs during pregnancy.

---

* For further information, see Centers for Disease Control and Prevention. Public Health Service Task Force recommendations for the use of antiretroviral drugs in pregnant women infected with HIV-1 for maternal health and for reducing perinatal HIV transmission in the United States. *MMWR Morb Mortal Wkly Rep.* 1998;47(RR-2):1–30.

† Centers for Disease Control and Prevention. Report of the NIH Panel to Define Principles of Therapy of HIV Infection and guidelines for the use of antiretroviral agents in HIV-infected adults and adolescents. *MMWR Morb Mortal Wkly Rep.* 1998;47(RR-5):1–82

Table 3.29. **Zidovudine Regimen for the Reduction of Perinatal Transmission of Human Immunodeficiency Virus (HIV)***

Period of Time	Route	Dosage
During pregnancy, initiate anytime after 14 wk of gestation	Oral	200 mg 3 times a day or 300 mg 2 times a day
During labor and delivery	Intravenous	2 mg/kg during the first hour, then 1 mg/kg per hour until delivery
For the newborn, beginning 8–12 h after birth until 6 wk of age	Oral	2 mg/kg 4 times per day

* Centers for Disease Control and Prevention. Public Health Service Task Force recommendations for the use of antiretroviral drugs in pregnant women infected with HIV-1 for maternal health and for reducing perinatal HIV-1 transmission in the United States. *MMWR Morb Mortal Wkly Rep.* 1998;47(RR-2):1–30. Information about other antiretroviral drugs for reduction of perinatal transmission of HIV can be found at http://www.hivatis.org/.

A trial in Thailand demonstrated that zidovudine administered starting at 36 weeks' gestation and given orally during labor without administration to the infant reduced transmission by more than 50%, from 19% to 9%. This "short-course" regimen supports administration of zidovudine even to women diagnosed late in pregnancy. However, the short-course regimen seems less effective than the full 3-part zidovudine regimen. The goal should be to diagnose HIV infection early in pregnancy to allow initiation of zidovudine prophylaxis and whatever other drugs are needed to treat maternal infection.

A trial in Africa demonstrated that zidovudine and lamivudine initiated during labor and continued for 1 week in the woman and infant reduced transmission by 38%. A trial in Uganda demonstrated that a single 200-mg oral dose of nevirapine given to the mother at the onset of labor combined with a single 2-mg/kg oral dose given to her infant at 72 hours of age reduced transmission by almost 50% compared with a regimen of zidovudine given orally during labor and to the infant for 1 week. These two studies provide potential effective intrapartum and postpartum interventions for women in whom the diagnosis of HIV infection is not made until the time of delivery.

In the United States, the standard of perinatal intervention should not be reduced to 4 weeks. Antiretroviral drugs should be administered to the HIV-infected woman during pregnancy, labor, and delivery. Zidovudine should be offered for all newborns if exposure is recognized before 7 days of age even if their mothers did not receive zidovudine. The pregnant woman and her health care professional should consider the possible benefits and risks of specific antiretroviral agents in the absence of efficacy data for combinations of drugs, pharmacokinetic data in pregnancy for many of the newer agents, and data about toxic effects during pregnancy and to the newborn.

A large meta-analysis has shown transmission decreased by 50% in the absence of zidovudine when delivery was by elective cesarean section before rupture of membranes and onset of labor. The transmission rate was reduced further, to 2%, if the mother received antiretroviral therapy and underwent elective cesarean section before onset of labor and before rupture of membranes. Vaginal delivery and antiretroviral therapy were associated with transmission rates of 7.3%. However, transmission rates for women receiving combination antiretroviral therapy in whom viral load is reduced to levels below assay detection may be lower than in those receiving zidovudine monotherapy. The additional benefit of cesarean section for further reducing transmission risk in women with a low risk of transmission is unknown and may not outweigh the potential risk of operative delivery for the infected mother. Thus, management of delivery without artificial rupture of membranes is wise, and women should be informed of the current state of knowledge about cesarean section.

Breastfeeding (see also Human Milk, p 98). Transmission of HIV by breastfeeding, especially from mothers who acquire infection during the postpartum period, has been demonstrated. In the United States, where safe and alternative sources of feeding are readily available and affordable, HIV-infected women should be counseled not to breastfeed their infants or donate to milk banks. The AAP guidelines for women in the United States are as follows*:

- Women and their health care professionals need to be aware of the potential risk of transmission of HIV infection to infants during pregnancy and the peripartum period, as well as through human milk.
- Routine HIV testing with consent should be part of prenatal care for all women. Each woman should know her HIV status and the methods available to prevent the acquisition and transmission of HIV and to determine whether breastfeeding is appropriate.
- During labor, all women whose HIV status during the current pregnancy is unknown are strongly recommended to be counseled and tested as rapidly as possible. Each woman should understand the benefits to herself and her infant of knowing her serostatus. Antiretroviral drugs can be administered during labor and to the infant if the woman is HIV-positive with the hope that transmission of virus will be decreased. Knowledge of her HIV infection status is important for subsequent decisions about breastfeeding. Hopefully, education will encourage behaviors that would decrease the likelihood of acquisition and transmission of HIV.
- Women who are known to be HIV infected must be counseled not to breastfeed or provide their milk for the nutrition of their own or other infants.
- In general, women who are known to be HIV-seronegative should be encouraged to breastfeed. However, women who are HIV-seronegative and known to have HIV-positive sexual partners or to be active drug users should be counseled further about the potential risk of transmitting HIV through human milk and about methods to reduce the risk of acquiring HIV infection.
- Each woman whose HIV status is unknown should be informed of the potential for HIV-infected women to transmit HIV during the peripartum period and through human milk and the potential benefits to her and her infant of knowing her HIV status and how HIV is acquired and transmitted. It is recommended that all women be tested to learn their HIV status. The health care professional should make an individualized recommendation to assist the woman to decide whether to breastfeed.

* American Academy of Pediatrics Committee on Pediatric AIDS. Human milk, breastfeeding, and transmission of human immunodeficiency virus in the United States. *Pediatrics*. 1995;96:977–979

- Neonatal intensive care units should develop policies that are consistent with these recommendations for use of expressed human milk for neonates. Current standards of the Occupational Safety and Health Administration do not require use of gloves for routine handling of expressed human milk. Gloves, however, should be worn by health care personnel when exposure to human milk might be frequent or prolonged, such as in milk banking.
- Human milk banks should follow the guidelines developed by the US Public Health Service, which include screening all donors for HIV infection, assessing risk factors that predispose to infection, and pasteurizing all donated milk.

Adolescent Education. Adolescents who are sexually active or using illicit drugs are at risk for HIV infection. All adolescents should be educated about this disease and have access to HIV testing and knowledge of their serostatus. Particular efforts should be made to provide access for adolescents who may not have a regular health care professional. Informed consent for testing or release of information about serostatus is necessary.

Specific AAP recommendations for pediatricians caring for adolescents are as follows*:

- Information about HIV infection and AIDS and the availability of HIV testing should be regarded as an important component of anticipatory guidance provided by pediatricians to all adolescent patients. This guidance should include information about prevention, transmission, and the implications of infection.
- Prevention guidance should include helping adolescents understand and reduce their risk. Information should be provided on abstinence and behavior that places them at risk for unplanned pregnancy and sexually transmitted infections, including HIV. All adolescents should be counseled about the correct and consistent use of condoms and other safer sex practices to reduce their risk of infection if they are sexually active.
- The availability of HIV testing should be discussed with all adolescents, and testing with consent should be encouraged for those who are sexually active, substance users, or both. In many states, minor adolescents can provide their own consent for testing, but the involvement of a supportive adult should be sought. Barriers to testing and care should be addressed.
- Youth with HIV infection need specialized medical and psychosocial care to help them with such complex issues as treatment adherence. In general, the course of HIV infection in adolescents follows that of adults, but adolescents frequently require additional support. Medication dosing should be based on Tanner staging of pubertal development and not age. Perinatally infected teens usually present with later stage illness, multisystem disease, or both. The development of support networks is important, as are issues related to disclosure of HIV status to family and sexual partners. The maintenance of confidentiality about HIV status is of great importance. Disclosure of HIV status to sexual partners should be encouraged, and local health departments may provide useful assistance with partner notification. Consent of the adolescent alone

* For further information, see American Academy of Pediatrics Task Force on Pediatric AIDS. Adolescents and human immunodeficiency virus infection: the role of the pediatrician in prevention and intervention. *Pediatrics.* 1993;92:626–630

should be sufficient to provide evaluation and treatment for suspected or confirmed HIV infection in accordance with local laws.

School Attendance and Education of Children With HIV Infection.* In the absence of blood exposure, HIV infection is not acquired through the types of contact that usually occur in a school setting, including contact with saliva or tears. Hence, children with HIV infection should not be excluded from school for the protection of other children or personnel, and disclosure of infection should not be required. Specific recommendations about school attendance of children and adolescents with HIV infection are the following:

- Most school-age children and all adolescents infected with HIV should be allowed to attend school without restrictions, provided the child's physician gives approval. The need for a more restricted school environment for the unusual infected children who might have an increased likelihood of exposing others should be evaluated on a case-by-case basis by the physician. Exudative skin lesions or aggressive biting behavior are examples of conditions in which a theoretical increased risk of exposure occurs.
- Only the child's parents, other guardians, and physician have an absolute need to know that the child is HIV-infected. The number of personnel aware of the child's condition should be kept to the minimum needed to ensure proper care of the child. The family has the right, but is not obligated, to inform the school. Persons involved in the care and education of an infected student must respect the student's right to privacy.
- All schools should adopt routine procedures for handling blood or blood-contaminated fluids, including disposal of sanitary napkins, regardless of whether students with HIV infection are known to be in attendance. School health care personnel, teachers, administrators, and other employees should be educated about procedures (see Housekeeping Procedures for Blood and Body Fluids, p 347).
- Children infected with HIV may be at increased risk of experiencing severe complications from infections such as varicella, tuberculosis, measles, CMV, and herpes simplex virus. Schools should develop procedures for notification of all parents of communicable diseases, such as varicella or measles.
- Routine screening of school children for HIV infection is not recommended.

As the life expectancy of HIV-infected children and adolescents increases, the school population of children and adolescents with this disease also will increase. An understanding of the effect of chronic illness and the recognition of neurodevelopmental problems in some of these children are essential to provide appropriate educational programs. The AAP recommendations about the education of children with HIV infection are as follows[†]:

- All children with HIV infection should receive an appropriate education that is adapted to their evolving special needs. The spectrum of needs differs with the stage of the disease.

---

* American Academy of Pediatrics Committee on Pediatric AIDS and Committee on Infectious Diseases. Issues related to human immunodeficiency virus transmission in schools, child care, medical settings, the home, and community. *Pediatrics.* 1999;104:318–324

† American Academy of Pediatrics Task Force on Pediatric AIDS. Education of children with human immunodeficiency virus infection. *Pediatrics.* In press

- Infection with HIV should be treated like other chronic illnesses that require special education and other related services.
- Continuity of education must be assured, whether at school or at home.
- Because of the stigmata associated with this disease, maintaining confidentiality is essential. Disclosure of information should be only with the informed consent of the parents or legal guardians and age-appropriate assent of the student.

Human Immunodeficiency Virus in the Athletic Setting. Athletes and staff of athletic programs can be exposed to blood during athletic activity. Recommendations have been developed by the AAP for prevention of transmission of HIV and other bloodborne pathogens in the athletic setting (see School Health, Infections Spread by Blood and Body Fluids, p 124).

Child Care and Foster Care.* Current AAP recommendations are as follows[†‡]:

- No reason exists to restrict foster care or adoptive placement of children who have HIV infection to protect the health of other family members. The risk of transmission of HIV infection in family environments is negligible.
- No need exists to restrict the placement of HIV-infected children in child care settings to protect personnel or other children because the risk of transmission of HIV in these settings is negligible.
- Child care personnel need not be informed of the HIV status of a child to protect the health of caregivers or other children in the child care environment. In some jurisdictions, the child's diagnosis cannot be divulged without the written consent of the parent or legal guardian. Parents may choose to inform the child care provider of the child's diagnosis to support a request that the caregiver observe the child closely for signs of illness that may require medical attention and assist the parents with the child's special emotional and social needs.
- The recommended standard precautions should be followed in all child care settings when blood or blood-containing body fluids are handled to minimize the possibility of transmission of bloodborne disease (see Housekeeping Procedures for Blood and Body Fluids, p 347).
- All preschool child care programs routinely should inform all families whenever a highly contagious illness, such as varicella or measles, occurs in any child in that setting. This process will help families protect their immunocompromised children.
- Ascertainment of HIV status is recommended for all pregnant women and newborn infants. This knowledge may help facilitate foster care or adoptive placement.

---

* For additional discussion of recommendations for child care, see Children in Out-of-Home Child Care, p 105.

† American Academy of Pediatrics Committee on Pediatric AIDS and Committee on Infectious Diseases. Issues related to human immunodeficiency virus transmission in schools, child care, medical settings, the home, and community. *Pediatrics*. 1999;104:318–324

‡ Adapted from American Academy of Pediatrics Task Force on Pediatric AIDS. Human immunodeficiency virus (HIV) infection and foster care. *Pediatrics*. In press

Adults With HIV Infection Working in Child Care or Schools. Asymptomatic HIV-infected adults may care for children in school or child care settings provided that they do not have exudative skin lesions or other conditions that would allow contact with their body fluids. No data indicate that HIV-infected adults have transmitted HIV during routine child care or school responsibilities.

Adults with symptomatic HIV infection are immunocompromised and at increased risk from infectious diseases of young children. They should consult their physicians about the safety of their continuing work.

Housekeeping Procedures for Blood and Body Fluids. In general, routine housekeeping procedures using a commercially available cleaner (detergent, disinfectant-detergent, or chemical germicide) compatible with most surfaces is satisfactory for cleaning spills of vomitus, urine, and feces. Nasal secretions can be removed with tissues and discarded in routine waste containers. For spills involving blood or other body fluids, organic material should be removed, and the surface should be disinfected with freshly diluted bleach (1:10). Reusable rubber gloves should be used for cleaning large spills to avoid contamination of the hands of the person cleaning the spill, but gloves are not essential for cleaning small amounts of blood that can be contained easily by the material used for cleaning. Persons involved in cleaning contaminated surfaces should avoid exposure of open skin lesions or mucous membranes to blood or bloody fluids. Whenever possible, disposable towels or tissues should be used and properly discarded, and mops should be rinsed in disinfectant. After clean-up and after removal of gloves, hands should be washed thoroughly with soap and water. Note, gloves are not indicated for routine cleaning tasks not in contact with body secretions, such as sweeping the floor or dusting.

Management and Counseling of Families.* Infection acquired by children before or during birth is a disease of the family. Serologic screening of siblings and parents is recommended. In each case, the physician should provide education and ongoing counseling about HIV and its transmission and outline precautions to be taken within the household and the community to prevent spread of this virus.

Infected women need to be made aware of the risk of having an infected child if they become pregnant, and they should be referred for family planning counseling. Infected persons should not donate blood, plasma, sperm, organs, corneas, bone, other tissues, or human milk.

The infected child should be taught appropriate hygiene and behavior. How much the child is told about the illness depends on age and maturity. Older children and adolescents should be made aware that the disease can be transmitted sexually, and they should be counseled appropriately. Many families are not willing to tell others about the diagnosis because it can create social isolation.

Sexual Abuse. After sexual abuse by a person with or at risk for HIV infection, the child should be tested serologically as soon as possible after the abuse and periodically for 6 months (eg, at 4-6 weeks, 12 weeks, and 6 months) after sexual contact (see Sexually Transmitted Diseases, p 138). Serologic evaluation of the perpetrator

* Centers for Disease Control and Prevention. *HIV Counseling, Testing, and Referral Standards and Guidelines.* Atlanta, GA: US Dept of Health and Human Services; 1994; this publication can be obtained from the CDC Web site: http://www.cdc.gov/publications.htm

for HIV usually cannot be obtained in proximity to the abuse and often is not possible until indictment has occurred. Counseling of the child and family needs to be provided (see Sexually Transmitted Diseases, p 138).

Postexposure Prophylaxis for Possible Sexual or Other Nonoccupational Exposure to HIV. * The US Public Health Service does not recommend for or against the use of antiretroviral agents to reduce HIV transmission after a possible nonoccupational exposure because of a lack of efficacy data.

Considerations related to use of antiretroviral prophylaxis in such circumstances include the probability that the source is HIV infected, the likelihood of transmission by the particular exposure, the interval between exposure and initiation of therapy, the efficacy of the drug(s) used, and the patient's adherence to the drug(s).

The estimated risk of transmission per episode of percutaneous exposure (needle stick in a nonoccupational exposure) to HIV-infected blood is 0.49% (upper limit of 95% confidence interval [CI] = 0.8%). The estimated risk for HIV transmission per episode of receptive penile-anal sexual exposure is 0.1% to 3%; the estimated risk per episode of receptive vaginal exposure is 0.1% to 0.2%. The actual risks to an infant or child after a needle stick or sexual abuse are unknown. However, to date there are no known transmissions of HIV from accidental nonoccupational needle sticks.

In 1995, surveillance data from health care personnel were used in a case-control study that suggested zidovudine use was associated with an 81% (95% CI = 48%–94%) decrease in risk for HIV infection after percutaneous exposure to HIV-infected blood. This may be an overestimate of the benefits because of the methodologic constraints but continues to be the only data available.

Decisions to provide antiretroviral agents to persons after possible nonoccupational HIV exposure must balance the potential benefits and risks. It is probable that the HIV status of the perpetrator (in the case of sexual abuse) or the person using the needle will be unknown. The nature of the exposure, including forced, traumatic intercourse, may increase transmission risk.

All antiretroviral agents have side effects. The most common are mild, and 24% to 36% of adults discontinued drugs used in combination because of side effects. Severe toxic effects, such as nephrolithiasis, pancytopenia, or hepatitis, are possible.

Antiretroviral agents generally should not be used if the risk of transmission is low (eg, needle stick from unknown nonoccupational source) or if care is sought greater than 72 hours after reported exposure. The physician and patient or parent should decide when risk for infection is high, intervention is prompt, and adherence is likely. Consultation with an experienced pediatric HIV care professional is essential.

Blood, Blood Components, and Clotting Factors. Screening blood and plasma for HIV antibody has reduced dramatically the risk of infection through transfusion (see Blood Safety, p 88). Nevertheless, careful scrutiny of the requirements of each patient for blood, its components, or clotting factors is important.

Human Immunodeficiency Virus–Exposed Health Care Personnel. Accidental exposure of health care personnel to HIV, such as from needle-stick injuries or

* Centers for Disease Control and Prevention. Management of possible sexual, injecting-drug-use, or other nonoccupational exposure to HIV, including considerations related to antiretroviral therapy: Public Health Service statement. *MMWR Morb Mortal Wkly Rep.* 1998;47:(RR-17):1–14

HIV-infected blood, rarely has resulted in HIV infection. The risk of infection varies according to the severity and type of exposure. The risk of infection after a percutaneous exposure to HIV-infected blood is 0.3%. The risks after mucous membrane contact and skin exposure to HIV-infected blood are 0.1% and less than 0.1%, respectively. Many of the known cases could have been prevented by careful adherence to infection control measures (see Control Measures, p 341). A health care worker who has had a percutaneous or mucous membrane exposure to blood or bloody secretions from an HIV-seropositive patient should receive counseling and medical evaluation as soon as possible after the exposure. A baseline HIV antibody test should be performed, and the HIV status of the blood source should be investigated. A health care worker who is seronegative should be retested 4 to 6 weeks, 12 weeks, and 6 months after exposure to determine whether transmission has occurred. Most exposed persons who have been infected will seroconvert during the first 3 months after exposure.

Recommendations for postexposure prophylaxis were issued by the US Public Health Service in 1998* (see Table 3.30, p 350). Several antiretroviral agents from at least 3 classes of drugs are available for the treatment of HIV disease. These include the nucleoside analogue reverse transcriptase inhibitors (NRTIs), nonnucleoside reverse transcriptase inhibitors, and protease inhibitors (see Antiretroviral Therapy, Tables 4.9, 4.10, and 4.11, pp 678–691). Among these drugs, zidovudine (an NRTI) is the only agent shown to prevent HIV transmission in humans. Although there are theoretical concerns that the increased prevalence of resistance to zidovudine may diminish its usefulness for postexposure prophylaxis, no data are available to assess whether this is a factor for consideration. Clinical data from the AIDS Clinical Trials Group protocol 076 study documented that despite genotypic evidence of maternal zidovudine resistance, zidovudine prevented perinatal transmission. Thus, based on the available information, it is still reasonable that zidovudine should continue to be the first drug of choice for postexposure prophylaxis regimens. There are no data to directly support the addition of other antiretroviral drugs, such as lamivudine, indinavir, or nelfinavir, to zidovudine to enhance the effectiveness of the postexposure prophylaxis regimen. Theoretically, a combination of drugs with activity at different stages in the viral replication cycle could offer an additive preventive effect in postexposure prophylaxis.

Reporting of Cases. Cases meeting the criteria for AIDS (see Tables 3.24, p 327, and 3.25, p 329) must be reported to the appropriate public health department in all states. In many states, HIV infection or perinatal exposure to HIV also must be reported. The AAP recommends routine reporting of perinatal HIV exposure, infection, and AIDS.

* Centers for Disease Control and Prevention. Public Health Service guidelines for the management of health-care worker exposures to HIV and recommendations for postexposure prophylaxis. *MMWR Morb Mortal Wkly Rep.* 1998;47(RR-7):1–33

Table 3.30 **Provisional Public Health Service Recommendations for Chemoprophylaxis After Occupational Exposure to HIV, by Type of Exposure and Source Material—1998***

Type of Exposure	Source Materials†	Antiretroviral Prophylaxis‡	Antiretroviral Regimen§
Percutaneous	Blood		
	Highest risk	Recommend	Zidovudine plus lamivudine plus either indinavir or nelfinavir
	Increased risk	Recommend	Zidovudine plus lamivudine with or without either indinavir or nelfinavir
	No increased risk	Offer	Zidovudine plus lamivudine
	Fluid containing visible blood, other potentially infectious fluid,‖ or tissue	Offer	Zidovudine plus lamivudine
	Other body fluid (eg, urine)	Not offer	
Mucous membrane	Blood	Offer	Zidovudine plus lamivudine with or without either indinavir or nelfinavir
	Fluid containing visible blood, other potentially infectious fluid,‖ or tissue	Offer	Zidovudine with or without lamivudine
	Other body fluid (eg, urine)	Not offer	
Skin, increased risk¶	Blood	Offer	Zidovudine plus lamivudine with or without either indinavir or nelfinavir
	Fluid containing visible blood, other potentially infectious fluid,‖ or tissue	Offer	Zidovudine with or without lamivudine
	Other body fluid (eg, urine)	Not offer	

* Centers for Disease Control and Prevention. Public Health Service guidelines for the management of health-care worker exposures to HIV and recommendations for postexposure prophylaxis. *MMWR Morb Mortal Wkly Rep.* 1998;47(RR-7):1–33. HIV indicates human immunodeficiency virus; AIDS, acquired immunodeficiency syndrome.

† Any exposure to concentrated HIV (eg, in a research laboratory or production facility) is treated as percutaneous exposure to blood with highest risk. *Highest risk,* exposure that involves BOTH a larger volume of blood (eg, deep injury with large diameter hollow needle previously in source patient's vein or artery, especially involving an injection of source-patient's blood) AND blood containing a high titer of HIV (eg, source with acute retroviral illness or end-stage AIDS; viral load measurement may be considered, but its use in relation to postexposure prophylaxis has not been evaluated). *Increased risk,* EITHER exposure to a larger volume of blood OR blood with a high titer of HIV. *No increased risk,* NEITHER exposure to larger volume of blood NOR blood with a high titer of HIV (eg, solid suture needle injury from source patient with asymptomatic HIV infection).

‡ *Recommend,* postexposure prophylaxis should be recommended to the exposed worker with counseling. *Offer,* postexposure prophylaxis should be offered to the exposed worker with counseling. *Not offer,* postexposure prophylaxis should not be offered because it is not an occupational exposure to HIV.

§ Regimens for adults: zidovudine, 200 mg 3 times a day; lamivudine, 150 mg twice a day; indinavir, 800 mg 3 times a day (if indinavir is not available, ritonavir, 600 mg twice a day, or saquinavir, 600 mg 3 times a day, may be used); nelfinavir, 750 mg 3 times a day. Prophylaxis is given for 4 weeks. For full prescribing information, see package inserts. Possible toxic effects from indinavir or nelfinavir may not be warranted (see text).

‖ Includes semen; vaginal secretions; cerebrospinal, synovial, pleural, peritoneal, pericardial, and amniotic fluids.

¶ For skin, risk is increased for exposures involving a high titer of HIV, prolonged contact, an extensive area, or an area in which skin integrity is visibly compromised. For skin exposures without increased risk, the risk for toxic effects of the drug outweigh the benefit of postexposure prophylaxis.

Influenza

CLINICAL MANIFESTATIONS: Influenza is characterized by the sudden onset of fever, frequently with chills or rigors, headache, malaise, diffuse myalgia, and a nonproductive cough. Subsequently, the respiratory tract signs of sore throat, nasal congestion, rhinitis, and cough become more prominent. Conjunctival injection, abdominal pain, nausea, and vomiting can occur. In some children, influenza can appear as a simple upper respiratory tract infection or as a febrile illness with few respiratory tract signs. In young infants, influenza can produce a sepsis-like picture and occasionally can cause croup or pneumonia. Acute myositis characterized by calf tenderness and refusal to walk may develop after several days of influenza illness, particularly with type B infection. Reye syndrome has been associated with influenza infection, primarily with influenza B. Influenza can alter the metabolism of certain medications, especially theophylline, possibly resulting in the development of toxic effects from high serum concentrations.

ETIOLOGY: Influenza viruses are orthomyxoviruses of 3 antigenic types (A, B, and C). Epidemic disease is caused by influenza virus types A and B. Influenza A viruses are subclassified by 2 surface antigens, hemagglutinin (H) and neuraminidase (N). Three immunologically distinct hemagglutinin subtypes (H1, H2, and H3) and 2 neuraminidase types (N1 and N2) have been recognized as causing global human epidemics. H5N1 and H9N2 avian-related strains have caused localized disease in Asia. Specific antibodies to these various antigens are important determinants of immunity. Major changes in the predominant strain in either of these antigens, such as H1 to H2, are called *antigenic shifts;* minor variations within the same subtypes are called *antigenic drifts.* Antigenic shift has occurred only with influenza A, usually at irregular intervals of 10 or more years. Antigenic drift occurs almost annually in influenza A and B viruses. Although influenza A and B viruses continually undergo antigenic change, influenza B viruses change more slowly and are not divided into subtypes.

EPIDEMIOLOGY: Influenza is spread from person to person by inhalation of small particle aerosols, by direct contact, by large droplet infection, or by contact with articles recently contaminated by nasopharyngeal secretions. During an outbreak of influenza, the highest attack rates occur among school-age children. Secondary spread to adults and other children within the family is common. The attack rates depend in part on immunity developed by previous experience (either by natural disease or immunization) with the circulating strain or a related strain. Antigenic shift or major drift in the circulating strain is most likely to result in widespread epidemics or even pandemics. In temperate climates, epidemics usually occur during the winter months and, within a community, peak within 2 weeks of onset and last 4 to 8 weeks or longer. Activity of 2 or 3 types or subtypes of influenza virus in a community may be associated with a prolongation of the influenza season to 3 months or more. Influenza is highly contagious, especially among institutionalized populations. Patients are most infectious during the 24 hours before the onset of symptoms and during the most symptomatic period. Viral shedding in the nasal secretions usually ceases within 7 days of the onset of illness but can be more prolonged in young children and immunodeficient patients.

The effect of influenza on immunocompetent children and children with underlying high-risk conditions is appreciable during interepidemic years and during epidemic years. Attack rates in healthy children have been estimated at 10% to 40% each year, with approximately 1% resulting in hospitalization. The risk of lower respiratory tract disease complicating influenza infection in children, primarily pneumonia, croup, wheezing, and bronchiolitis, has ranged from 0.2% to 25%. A wide spectrum of complications, such as Reye syndrome, myositis, and central nervous system (CNS) manifestations, can occur. The risk of Reye syndrome, which occurs primarily in school-age children, has decreased during recent years. Respiratory tract viruses other than influenza (eg, respiratory syncytial virus and parainfluenza viruses) produce life-threatening illness more commonly in young children than in adults, and, as a result, morbidity and mortality rates in children for influenza and the effect of control measures are more difficult to determine.

Excess rates of hospitalization have been documented for children with influenza, including neonates and children up to 5 years of age and children who have hemoglobinopathies, bronchopulmonary dysplasia, asthma, cystic fibrosis, malignant neoplasms, diabetes mellitus, or chronic renal disease. Pulmonary complications, such as bronchitis and pneumonia, seem to be more common among these children. Influenza in neonates has been associated with considerable morbidity, including a sepsis-like syndrome, apnea, and lower respiratory tract disease. Studies have shown that children younger than 5 years of age have the second highest rate of hospitalization with influenza, only exceeded by persons older than 65 years of age.

Influenza Pandemics. When the circulating strain of virus is substantially different from that occurring in other years (ie, antigenic shift), more severe epidemics or pandemics can occur with excess morbidity and mortality. During the 20th century, there were 3 influenza pandemics, including the one in 1918 that killed more than 20 million people worldwide, many of whom were young adults. The mortality rates with the more recent pandemics of 1957 and 1968 were reduced, in part, through the use of antimicrobial therapy for secondary bacterial infections and more aggressive supportive care. Experience indicates that these pandemics occur at irregular intervals and have the potential to be true public health emergencies. Dealing with the next influenza pandemic will require extensive use of vaccine and antiviral and antibacterial agents and development of triage policies for hospital and intensive care utilization. An interagency group, which includes members of the American Academy of Pediatrics, is preparing a plan for the public health response to the next pandemic.

The **incubation period** usually is 1 to 3 days.

DIAGNOSTIC TESTS: When viral cultures are performed, specimens should be obtained during the first 72 hours of illness because the quantity of virus shed subsequently decreases rapidly. Nasopharyngeal secretions obtained by swab or aspirate should be placed in appropriate transport media for culture. After inoculation into eggs or cell culture, virus usually can be isolated within 2 to 6 days. Rapid diagnostic tests for identification of influenza A and B antigens in nasopharyngeal specimens are available commercially, although their sensitivity and specificity have been variable. Serologic diagnosis can be established retrospectively by a significant change in antibody titer between acute and convalescent serum samples, as determined by complement fixation, hemagglutination inhibition, neutralization, or enzyme immunoassay tests.

TREATMENT: Amantadine and rimantadine are approved for treatment of influenza A in adults, but only amantadine is approved for treatment in children. Studies evaluating the efficacy of amantadine and rimantadine in children are limited, but they indicate that treatment with either drug diminishes the severity of influenza A infection when administered within 48 hours of onset of illness. Neither amantadine nor rimantadine is effective against influenza B infections. Two products from a new class of antiviral drugs have been approved for treatment of influenza A and B.* These neuraminidase inhibitors decrease release of virus from infected cells. Zanamivir is approved for persons 12 years of age and older. It is inhaled twice a day for 5 days with a special breath-activated plastic inhaler. Oseltamivir is approved for persons 18 years of age and older. It is administered orally twice a day for 5 days.

Therapy for influenza virus infection should be considered for the following: (1) patients in whom amelioration of clinical symptoms may be particularly beneficial, such as those at increased risk for severe or complicated influenza infection; (2) otherwise healthy children with severe illness; and (3) persons with special environmental, family, or social situations, such as examinations in school and athletic competitions. Although influenza A virus may become resistant to amantadine and rimantadine during treatment, this does not seem to affect clinical benefits. Resistant virus has not been demonstrated to spread more easily or cause more serious disease and thus far has not been shown to persist in the population in the absence of antiviral drug therapy. Nevertheless, the epidemiologic implications of influenza A antiviral drug resistance are unclear. Any influenza A isolate obtained from a patient receiving prophylactic amantadine or rimantadine should be submitted for antiviral susceptibility testing to the Centers for Disease Control and Prevention (CDC) through the state health department. Development of resistance to zanamivir and oseltamivir during treatment has been identified but does not appear to be frequent.

If antiviral therapy is indicated, treatment should be started as soon as possible after the onset of symptoms and, in immunocompetent patients, continued for 2 to 5 days or for 24 to 48 hours after the person becomes asymptomatic. Immunocompromised patients may require a longer course of therapy. The recommended dosages for amantadine and rimantadine in children are given in Table 3.31 (p 354). Patients with any degree of renal insufficiency should be monitored for adverse events. Dosage should be reduced for persons with severe renal insufficiency. Either amantadine or rimantadine, but especially amantadine, may cause CNS symptoms, which resolve with discontinuation of the drug. An increased incidence of seizures has been reported in children with epilepsy who receive amantadine and, to a lesser extent, in children who receive rimantadine.

The role of zanamivir in the treatment of children with influenza virus infection will require further evaluation. Oseltamivir is not approved for use in children.

Control of fever with acetaminophen or other appropriate antipyretics may be important in young children because the fever and other symptoms of influenza

* Centers for Disease Control and Prevention. Neuraminidase inhibitors for treatment of influenza A and B infections. *MMWR Morb Mortal Wkly Rep.* 1999;48(RR-14):1–9

Table 3.31. **Dosage Recommendations for Children and Adolescents for Treatment and Prophylaxis of Influenza A by Amantadine and Rimantadine***

	Age, y		
	1–9	≥10	
		Weight <40 kg	Weight ≥ 40 kg
Treatment	5 mg/kg per day, maximum 150 mg/d, in 1 or 2 divided doses	5 mg/kg per day in 1 or 2 divided doses	200 mg/d in 1 or 2 divided doses
Prophylaxis	Dosages are the same as those for treatment. An alternative and equally acceptable dosage is 100 mg/d for children weighing >20 kg and adults. For either regimen, the total daily dosage may be given in 1 or 2 divided doses.		

* Amantadine and rimantadine are not approved by the US Food and Drug Administration (FDA) for use in children younger than 1 year of age. Rimantadine is FDA-approved for prophylaxis but not for treatment of children. Patients with any degree of renal insufficiency should be monitored for adverse effects and the dosage reduced or the drug discontinued as necessary (see product label for further information). See text for recommendations for zanamivir and oseltamivir.

could exacerbate underlying chronic conditions. Children and teenagers with influenza should not receive salicylates because of the resulting increased risk of developing Reye syndrome.

Isolation of the Hospitalized Patient: In addition to standard precautions, droplet precautions are recommended for children hospitalized with influenza or an influenza-like illness for the duration of the illness. Respiratory tract secretions should be considered infectious, and strict hand-washing procedures should be used.

Control Measures:

Influenza Vaccine. The inactivated influenza vaccines produced in embryonated eggs are immunogenic and associated with minimal side effects. These multivalent vaccines contain 3 virus strains (usually 2 type A and 1 type B) with composition changed periodically in anticipation of the prevalent influenza strains expected to circulate in the United States in the upcoming winter. Vaccines include inactivated whole-virus vaccine prepared from the intact purified virus particles, the subvirion vaccine prepared by the additional step of disrupting the lipid-containing membrane of the virus, and purified surface-antigen vaccine. Only the subvirion or purified surface-antigen vaccines, ie, those termed "split-virus" vaccines, should be administered to children younger than 13 years of age. The whole-virus vaccines are associated with higher rates of adverse effects than split-virus vaccines in young children but not in adolescents and adults.

Immunogenicity in Children. Children younger than 9 years of age who have little experience with influenza require 2 doses of vaccine administered 1 month apart to produce a satisfactory antibody response (see Table 3.32, p 355). Children previously primed with a related strain of influenza by infection or immunization exhibit a brisk antibody response to 1 dose of the vaccine.

Table 3.32. **Schedule for Influenza Vaccine Dosage by Age***

Age	Recommended Vaccine†	Dose, mL‡	No. of Doses
6–35 mo	Split virus only	0.25	1–2§
3–8 y	Split virus only	0.5	1–2§
9–12 y	Split virus only	0.5	1
>12 y	Whole or split virus	0.5	1

* Vaccine is administered intramuscularly.

† Split-virus vaccine may be termed *split, subvirion,* or *purified surface-antigen* vaccine.

‡ Dosages are those recommended in recent years. Physicians should refer to the product circular each year to ensure that the appropriate dosage is given.

§ Two doses administered at least 1 month apart are recommended for children who are receiving influenza vaccine for the first time.

Vaccine Efficacy. The effect of influenza immunization on acute respiratory tract illness is less likely to be evident in pediatric than adult populations because of the frequency of upper respiratory tract infections and influenza-like illness caused by other viral agents in young children. Protection in healthy subjects usually is 70% to 80%, with a range of 50% to 95% varying with the closeness of vaccine strain match to the wild strain. The duration of protection is brief, usually presumed to be less than 1 year. Efficacy has not been evaluated in infants immunized during the first 6 months of life.

A cold-adapted, live, attenuated influenza vaccine that is administered intranasally and prepared by viral reassortment is under consideration for licensure by the US Food and Drug Administration (FDA).

Special Considerations, Killed Influenza Vaccine.

- In children receiving immunosuppressive chemotherapy, influenza immunization with a new vaccine antigen results in a poor response. The optimal time to immunize children with malignant neoplasms who must undergo chemotherapy is 3 to 4 weeks after chemotherapy has been discontinued, when the peripheral granulocyte and lymphocyte counts are greater than 1000/µL (1.0×10^9/L). Children who are no longer receiving chemotherapy generally have high rates of seroconversion.
- Children with hemodynamically unstable cardiac disease constitute a large group of children potentially at high risk for complications of influenza. The immune response and safety of influenza vaccine in these children are comparable to those in healthy children.
- Corticosteroids administered for brief periods or every other day seem to have only a minimal effect on antibody response to influenza vaccine. Prolonged administration of high doses of corticosteroids (ie, a dose equivalent to either 2 mg/kg or greater or a total of 20 mg/d of prednisone) may impair antibody response. Influenza immunization can be deferred temporarily during the time of receipt of high-dose corticosteroids, provided deferral does not compromise the likelihood of immunization before the start of the influenza season (see Vaccine Administration, p 16).

- Infants younger than 6 months of age with high-risk conditions (see Recommendations for Influenza Immunization, below), especially those with cardiopulmonary compromise, may have the same or greater risk as older children. Neither influenza vaccine nor prophylaxis with rimantadine, amantadine, or zanamivir is recommended for this age group. Immunization and chemoprophylaxis of adults who are in close contact with high-risk infants are important means of protection of infants (see Recommendations for Influenza Immunization, below, and Indications for Chemoprophylaxis, p 358).
- Studies indicate that influenza vaccine may reduce the incidence of acute otitis media in children in child care centers.

Recommendations for Influenza Immunization.

Annual influenza vaccine can be given to infants older than 6 months of age, children, adolescents, and adults to reduce the impact of influenza. Priority should be given to targeted high-risk groups.

Targeted High-Risk Children and Adolescents. Yearly influenza immunization, administered during the autumn (see Vaccine Administration, p 16), is recommended for children 6 months of age and older with one or more specific risk factors:

- Asthma or other chronic pulmonary diseases, such as cystic fibrosis
- Hemodynamically significant cardiac disease
- Immunosuppressive disorders or therapy (see Special Considerations, p 355)
- Human immunodeficiency virus infection (see HIV Infection, p 325)
- Sickle cell anemia and other hemoglobinopathies
- Diseases requiring long-term aspirin therapy, such as rheumatoid arthritis or Kawasaki disease, which may increase the risk for development of Reye syndrome following influenza
- Chronic renal dysfunction
- Chronic metabolic disease, including diabetes mellitus
- ***Pregnancy.*** Women who will be in the second or third trimester of pregnancy during influenza season should receive influenza vaccine during the autumn since pregnancy increases the risk of complications and hospitalization from influenza. Because the current intramuscularly administered influenza vaccine is not a live virus vaccine and only rarely is associated with major systemic reactions, some experts consider the vaccine safe during any stage of pregnancy. Because spontaneous abortion is common during the first trimester of pregnancy and unnecessary exposures during this time generally are avoided, some experts prefer immunization only during the second and third trimesters.

Close Contacts of High-Risk Patients. Immunization and chemoprophylaxis of persons who are in close contact with high-risk children are important means of protection for these children. In addition, immunization of pregnant women may be beneficial to their unborn infants because transplacentally acquired antibody seems to protect the infants from infection with influenza A virus. Immunization is recommended for the following:

- All health care personnel in contact with pediatric patients in hospital and outpatient care settings

- Household contacts, including siblings and primary caregivers of high-risk children
- Children who are members of households with high-risk adults, including those with symptomatic HIV infection
- Providers of home care to children and adolescents in high-risk groups

Foreign Travel. Persons traveling to foreign areas where influenza outbreaks are or may be occurring should be considered for immunization. The decision to immunize will depend on the person's destination, duration of travel, risk of acquiring influenza (such as the season of the year and other factors), and potential for severe illness. In temperate climate zones of the northern and southern hemispheres, travelers also can be exposed to influenza during the summer, especially when traveling as part of large organized tourist groups that include persons from areas of the world where influenza viruses may be circulating.

Other Children. Immunization should be considered for any child or adolescent with an underlying condition that may compromise the child's resistance to influenza, including young age, and for groups of persons whose close contact facilitates rapid transmission and spread of infection that may result in disruption of routine activities. These groups include students in colleges, schools, and other institutions of learning, particularly persons who reside in dormitories or who are members of athletic teams, and persons living in residential institutions.

Influenza vaccine may be administered to any healthy child or adolescent who wishes to reduce the chance of becoming infected with influenza. The morbidity from influenza among healthy children can be appreciable. Influenza vaccine does not adversely affect the safety of breastfeeding for mothers or infants; therefore, breastfeeding is not a contraindication for immunization.

Vaccine Administration. Influenza vaccine should be administered during the autumn of each year before the start of the influenza season at the time specified in the yearly recommendations of the CDC Advisory Committee on Immunization Practices. The optimal time in recent years has been from the beginning of October through mid-November. However, persons may be immunized in September when the vaccine for the forthcoming influenza season becomes available. Vaccine should be offered up to and even after influenza activity is documented in a community. The recommended vaccine, dose, and schedule for different age groups are given in Table 3.32 (p 355).

Annual immunization is recommended because of declining immunity during the year after immunization and because in most years, at least one of the antigens is changed to increase the antigenic similarity between the vaccine and circulating strains.

Influenza vaccine may be administered simultaneously (but at a separate site and with a different syringe) with other routine immunizations in children.

Reactions, Adverse Effects, and Contraindications. Inactivated influenza vaccine contains only noninfectious viruses and cannot cause influenza. In children younger than 13 years of age, febrile reactions are infrequent, especially after administration of split-virus vaccine. Fever occurs primarily 6 to 24 hours after immunization in children younger than 24 months of age. For children older than 12 years of age and for adults, the adverse effects and immunogenicity of the whole- and split-virus vaccines are similar when used at the recommended doses (see Table 3.32, p 355). Local reactions are infrequent in children younger than 13 years of age. In children 13 years of age or older, local reactions occur in approximately 10% after immunization with whole- or split-virus vaccine.

Influenza vaccines have been associated with a slightly increased frequency of Guillain-Barré syndrome (GBS). Estimating the precise risk for a rare condition such as GBS is difficult, but a study conducted during 1992–1994 showed a small increase may have occurred in the number of GBS cases in immunized adults. This represented an excess of approximately 1 GBS case per million persons immunized. No cases were observed in persons younger than 45 years of age. Even if GBS were a causally related adverse effect, the very low estimated risk of GBS is less than that of severe influenza that could be prevented by immunization. In addition, GBS has not been associated with influenza immunization of children.

Immunization of children who have asthma or cystic fibrosis with the currently available influenza vaccines is not associated with a detectable increase in adverse reactions or exacerbations.

Children demonstrating severe anaphylactic reaction to chickens or egg protein can experience, on rare occasions, a similar type of reaction to killed influenza vaccines. Although influenza vaccine has been administered safely to such children after skin testing and even desensitization, these children generally should not receive influenza vaccine because of their risk of reactions, the likely need for yearly immunization, and the availability of chemoprophylaxis against influenza infection.

Chemoprophylaxis: An Alternative Method of Protecting Children Against Influenza.

The currently licensed antiviral drugs, amantadine, and rimantadine are important adjuvants to influenza vaccine for control and prevention of influenza disease. Efficacy studies against influenza A infection in adults have demonstrated 70% to 90% effectiveness in preventing clinical illness, but asymptomatic infection can occur. Studies in children have indicated a similar beneficial effect in diminishing spread of influenza A among institutionalized children and family members and in pediatric hospitals. Amantadine and rimantadine are FDA-approved for prophylaxis in children older than 1 year of age and in adults but are effective only against influenza A. The usual recommended doses of rimantadine and amantadine for prophylaxis are the same as those for treatment. A dosage of 100 mg/d in 1 or 2 divided doses for prophylaxis in adults and in children weighing more than 20 kg is as effective as the recommended dosage of 200 mg/d for treatment and may be associated with fewer adverse effects. The prophylactic dosages for children are given in Table 3.31 (p 354). Zanamivir and oseltamivir are not approved for prophylaxis.

Indications for Chemoprophylaxis

- Amantadine and rimantadine for children older than 1 year of age* and adolescents at high risk who were immunized after circulation of influenza A in the community has begun. Chemoprophylaxis can be beneficial during the interval before a vaccine response (2 weeks after the recommended vaccine schedule of 1 or 2 doses has been completed).

* Use of amantadine and rimantadine in infants (ie, children younger than 1 year of age) has not been evaluated adequately, and neither drug is FDA-approved for use in infants.

- Unimmunized persons providing care to high-risk persons.
- Immunodeficient persons whose antibody response to vaccine is likely to be poor.
- Persons at high risk for whom vaccine is contraindicated, including those with anaphylactic hypersensitivity to egg protein who do not receive desensitization (see Reactions, Adverse Effects, and Contraindications, p 357).
- Any healthy child with age-appropriate development for whom prevention of influenza is considered desirable. These children also should be immunized.

Chemoprophylaxis should not be considered a substitute for immunization. Chemoprophylaxis in immunized persons does not interfere with the immune response to the vaccine and may provide additional protection.

Chemotherapy

Amantadine and rimantadine can reduce the severity and shorten the duration of influenza A illness among healthy adults when administered within 48 hours of illness onset (see Table 3.31, p 354). Among children, rimantadine is approved only for prophylaxis, but many experts believe rimantadine also is appropriate for therapy. Zanamivir is approved for persons 12 years of age and older for treatment of uncomplicated influenza A and B viruses. Zanamivir is inhaled twice a day for 5 days using a special breath-activated plastic inhaler. Oseltamivir is approved for persons 18 years of age and older for treatment of uncomplicated influenza A and B viruses. Safety and efficacy of zanamivir and oseltamivir have not been established for use in preventing influenza.

Information about influenza surveillance is available through the CDC Voice Information System (influenza update, 888-232-3228) or through <http://www.cdc.gov/ncidod/diseases/flu/weekly.htm>

Isosporiasis

(Isospora belli)

CLINICAL MANIFESTATIONS: Protracted, foul-smelling, watery diarrhea is the most common presenting symptom. Manifestations are similar to those caused by *Cryptosporidium* and *Cyclospora* organisms and include abdominal pain, anorexia, and weight loss. Fever, malaise, vomiting, and headache have been reported. Severity of infection ranges from self-limiting in immunocompetent hosts to life-threatening in immunocompromised patients, particularly those with human immunodeficiency virus (HIV) infection.

ETIOLOGY: *Isospora belli* is a coccidian protozoan.

EPIDEMIOLOGY: Humans are the only known host for *I belli.* The frequency of asymptomatic infection with this parasite is unknown. Infection is more common in tropical and subtropical climates and in areas of poor sanitary conditions. Human infection probably occurs by the oral-fecal route and has been linked with contaminated food and water. *Isospora belli* has been reported as a causative agent of traveler's diarrhea in visitors to endemic areas and in institutional outbreaks.

Oocysts are passed unsporulated and require exposure to oxygen and temperatures lower than 37°C (98°F) before becoming infectious. Oocysts are resistant to most disinfectants and may remain viable for months in a cool moist environment.

The **incubation period** is thought to be 8 to 14 days.

DIAGNOSTIC TESTS: Demonstration of oocysts in feces or in duodenal aspirates or finding developmental stages of the parasite in biopsy specimens of the small intestine is diagnostic. Oocysts in stool can be distinguished by their size, which is 5 times larger than *Cryptosporidium* organisms, and by their oval shape. Oocysts can be detected by modified Kinyoun carbolfuchsin and by auramine-rhodamine stains. Concentration techniques may be needed before staining because the organisms often are present in small numbers.

TREATMENT: Trimethoprim-sulfamethoxazole and pyrimethamine-sulfadoxine are effective. In HIV-infected patients who are allergic to sulfonamides, treatment with pyrimethamine (50 to 75 mg/d), followed by daily prophylactic administration of pyrimethamine (25 mg/d), has been effective. Antimicrobial prophylaxis to prevent recurrent disease may be indicated for HIV-infected persons.

ISOLATION OF THE HOSPITALIZED PATIENT: Standard precautions should be used. The risk of nosocomial infection is unknown.

CONTROL MEASURES: None.

Kawasaki Disease

CLINICAL MANIFESTATIONS: Kawasaki disease is a febrile, exanthematous, multisystem illness of importance because of the risk of development of coronary artery abnormalities. Kawasaki disease occurs predominantly in children younger than 5 years of age. Within several days of the onset of fever, other characteristic features of the illness usually appear, including the following: (1) discrete bulbar conjunctival injection without exudate; (2) erythematous mouth and pharynx, strawberry tongue, and red, cracked lips; (3) a polymorphous, generalized, erythematous rash that can be morbilliform, maculopapular, or scarlatiniform or may resemble erythema multiforme; (4) changes in the peripheral extremities consisting of induration of the hands and feet with erythematous palms and soles; and (5) a unilateral cervical lymph node enlarged to at least 1.5 cm in diameter. For the diagnosis of classic Kawasaki disease, patients should have fever for at least 5 days and at least 4 of these 5 features or fever with 3 features and evidence of coronary artery abnormalities. Periungual and groin desquamation often occur during the second to third week of illness. Patients with fever who do not meet these criteria, often infants, can be diagnosed as having atypical Kawasaki disease when coronary artery disease is detected. Irritability, abdominal pain, diarrhea, and vomiting are associated common features. Other findings include urethritis with sterile pyuria (70% of cases), mild hepatic dysfunction (40%), arthritis or arthralgia

(10%–20%), aseptic meningitis (50%), pericardial effusion (20%–40%), gallbladder hydrops (<10%), and myocarditis manifested by congestive heart failure (<5%).

Without aspirin or intravenous immunoglobulin therapy, the mean duration of fever is about 12 days. After the fever resolves, patients can remain anorectic or irritable for 2 to 3 weeks. During this subacute phase, the characteristic desquamation may occur. Recurrence months or years later (ie, second episodes) occurs occasionally (1%–3%).

Routine 2-dimensional echocardiography or angiography demonstrates coronary aneurysm(s) in approximately 20% to 25% of untreated patients. Patients at increased risk for development of coronary aneurysms include males, infants younger than 12 months of age, persons whose fever persists for more than 10 days, those with low serum albumin or hemoglobin concentrations, those who manifest signs or symptoms of cardiac involvement (such as mitral regurgitation or pericardial effusion), and those with thrombocytosis. Coronary aneurysms generally appear 10 days or later after the onset of symptoms. The peak prevalence of coronary aneurysms and coronary dilation occurs 2 to 4 weeks after onset of disease; their appearance later than 6 weeks is uncommon. Giant coronary aneurysms (≥8 mm in diameter) most often are associated with long-term complications. Other medium-sized arterial aneurysms (eg, in iliac, femoral, renal, and axillary vessels) occur uncommonly, virtually always in conjunction with coronary abnormalities. In addition to coronary artery disease, carditis can involve the pericardium, myocardium, or endocardium, and mitral and aortic regurgitation can develop. Carditis generally resolves when fever resolves.

In children with mild coronary dilation or ectasia, coronary artery dimensions often return to baseline within 6 to 8 weeks after onset of disease. Approximately 50% of nongiant coronary aneurysms regress to normal lumen size within 1 to 2 years, although this process may be accompanied by coronary stenosis. In addition, aneurysm regression may result in a poorly compliant, somewhat fibrotic vessel wall.

The current mortality rate in the United States is less than 0.05%. Death results from myocardial infarction resulting from coronary occlusion due to thrombosis or progressive stenosis. Rarely, a large coronary aneurysm may rupture. The majority of fatalities occur within 6 weeks of the onset of symptoms, but myocardial infarction and sudden death can occur months to years after the acute episode. The vasculitis of Kawasaki disease may be a risk factor for premature atherosclerotic disease, but this is uncertain.

ETIOLOGY: The cause is unknown. However, the epidemiologic and clinical features strongly suggest an infectious cause.

EPIDEMIOLOGY: Peak age of occurrence in the United States is between 18 and 24 months. Fifty percent of patients are younger than 2 years of age, and 80% are younger than 5 years of age; children older than 8 years of age rarely develop the disease. The male-female ratio is approximately 1.5:1. The incidence is highest in Asians; 3000 to 3500 cases are estimated to occur annually in the United States. Kawasaki disease was first described in Japan, where a pattern of endemic occurrence with superimposed epidemic outbreaks has emerged. A similar pattern of steady or increasing endemic disease with occasional sharply defined community-wide epidemics has been recognized in diverse locations in North America and Hawaii. Epidemics generally occur during the winter and spring at 2- to 3-year intervals. No evidence indicates person-to-person or common-source spread, although the incidence is somewhat higher in siblings of children with the disease.

The **incubation period** is unknown.

DIAGNOSTIC TESTS: No specific tests are available. The diagnosis is established by fulfillment of the clinical criteria (see Clinical Manifestations, p 360) and exclusion of other possible illnesses, such as measles, streptococcal infection (ie, scarlet fever), viral and rickettsial exanthems, drug reactions (eg, Stevens-Johnson syndrome), staphylococcal scalded skin syndrome, toxic shock syndrome, and juvenile rheumatoid arthritis.* An elevated sedimentation rate and serum C-reactive protein concentration during the first 2 weeks of illness and an elevated platelet count (>450 000/µL [>450 × 10^9/L]) after the 10th day of illness are common laboratory features. These values usually normalize within 6 to 8 weeks.

TREATMENT: Management consists of supportive care, anti-inflammatory therapy, and assessment for possible coronary artery disease. Anti-inflammatory therapy should be initiated when the diagnosis is established or strongly suspected. Specific recommendations are as follows:

Immune Globulin Intravenous. High-dose Immune Globulin Intravenous (IGIV) therapy and aspirin initiated within 10 days of the onset of fever substantially decrease the prevalence of coronary artery dilation and aneurysms detected 2 and 7 weeks later in comparison with treatment with aspirin alone. Significantly more rapid resolution of fever and other indicators of acute inflammation with this therapy also has been demonstrated. Therapy with IGIV should be initiated as soon as possible; its efficacy when initiated later than the 10th day of illness or after aneurysms have been detected has been evaluated incompletely. Therapy with IGIV, however, should be considered for patients diagnosed after day 10 who have manifestations of continuing inflammation (eg, fever and increased sedimentation rate) or of evolving coronary artery disease.

Dose. The optimal therapeutic dose of IGIV is unknown. A dose of 2 g/kg as a single dose, given over 10 to 12 hours, is recommended. Few complications occur from this regimen.

Retreatment. Up to 10% of children with Kawasaki disease treated with IGIV may not respond to the initial dose and may experience persistent (>48 to 72 hours) or recrudescent fever. Other clinical indications of inflammation, such as conjunctival injection and rash, also may persist or recur. If signs and symptoms persist and the diagnosis remains likely, retreatment with a second infusion of 2 g/kg of IGIV, given over 10 to 12 hours, should be considered. Some experts recommend intravenous pulse corticosteroid therapy rather than repeated IGIV dosing, but the safety and efficacy of this remains unclear.

Aspirin. Aspirin usually is given initially in high dosage for its anti-inflammatory effect, and, subsequently, in low dosage to reduce the likelihood of spontaneous

* For further information on the diagnosis of this disease, see the recommendations of the American Heart Association in Dajani AS, Taubert KA, Gerber MA, et al. Diagnosis and therapy of Kawasaki disease in children. *Circulation.* 1993;87:1776–1780

coronary thrombosis through its antiplatelet aggregation action. A dosage of 80 to 100 mg/kg per day in 4 divided doses reduces the duration of fever and clinical signs of inflammation. Monitoring serum salicylate concentrations during high-dose therapy may be helpful in apparent nonresponders because gastrointestinal tract absorption is highly variable in acute Kawasaki disease. The dosage of aspirin in the acute phase of the illness does not seem to affect the subsequent incidence of coronary artery aneurysms. After fever is controlled for at least several days, the aspirin doses should be decreased. A suggested dosage is 3 to 5 mg/kg per day in 1 dose. For patients with no coronary artery abnormalities detected by echocardiography, this regimen should be maintained for 6 to 8 weeks or until the platelet count and erythrocyte sedimentation rate normalize. Low-dose aspirin therapy should be continued indefinitely for persons in whom coronary artery abnormalities are present. Because of the potential risk of Reye syndrome in patients with influenza or varicella receiving salicylates, parents of children receiving aspirin should be instructed to contact their child's physician promptly if the child develops symptoms of or is exposed to either disease.

Cardiac Care.* An echocardiogram should be obtained early in the acute phase of the illness and 6 to 8 weeks after onset. The care of patients with carditis should involve a cardiologist experienced in the management of patients with Kawasaki disease and in assessing echocardiographic studies of coronary arteries in children. Long-term management of patients with Kawasaki disease should be based on the degree of coronary artery involvement. Children should be assessed during the first 2 months to detect evidence of arrhythmias, congestive heart failure, and valvular regurgitation. In addition to prolonged low-dose aspirin therapy to suppress platelet aggregation in patients with persistent coronary artery abnormalities, some experts recommend 4 mg/kg per day of dipyridamole, given in 3 divided doses. Development of giant coronary artery aneurysms (≥8 mm diameter) may require the addition of anticoagulant therapy, such as coumadin, to prevent thrombosis.

Subsequent Immunization. Measles and varicella immunizations should be deferred for 11 months after IGIV administration in children who have received high-dose IGIV for treatment of Kawasaki disease. If the child's risk of exposure to measles is high, the child should be immunized and then reimmunized at or after 11 months following administration of IGIV unless serologic testing indicates successful immunization by the earlier dose (see Measles, p 385, Varicella-Zoster Infections, p 624). The schedule for subsequent administration of other childhood immunizations should not be interrupted. Yearly influenza immunization is indicated for patients 6 months to 18 years of age who require long-term aspirin therapy because of the possible increased risk of development of Reye syndrome (see Influenza, p 351).

ISOLATION OF THE HOSPITALIZED PATIENT: Standard precautions are indicated.

CONTROL MEASURES: None.

* For specific recommendations of the American Heart Association, see Dajani AS, Taubert KA, Takahashi M, et al. Guidelines for long-term management of patients with Kawasaki disease: Report from the Committee on Rheumatic Fever, Endocarditis, and Kawasaki Disease, Council on Cardiovascular Disease in the Young, American Heart Association. *Circulation.* 1994;89:916–922

Legionella pneumophila Infections

CLINICAL MANIFESTATIONS: Legionellosis is associated with 2 clinically and epidemiologically distinct illnesses: legionnaires disease, which varies in severity from a mild to a severe progressive infection characterized by fever, myalgia, cough, and pneumonia, and Pontiac fever, a milder illness without pneumonia. Legionnaires disease may be associated with gastrointestinal tract, central nervous system, and renal manifestations. Respiratory failure and death may occur. Pontiac fever is characterized by an abrupt-onset, self-limited, influenza-like presentation.

ETIOLOGY: *Legionella* species are fastidious aerobic bacilli that stain gram-negative after recovery on artificial media. At least 18 different species have been implicated in human disease, but the majority of *Legionella* infections in the United States are caused by the *Legionella pneumophila* serogroup 1.

EPIDEMIOLOGY: Legionnaires disease is acquired through inhalation of aerosolized water contaminated with *L pneumophila*. Person-to-person transmission has not been demonstrated. More than 80% of cases are sporadic; the sources of infection for these cases may be related to exposure to *L pneumophila*–contaminated water in the patient's home, workplace, or location of medical therapy and to aerosol-producing devices in public places. Outbreaks have been ascribed to common-source exposure to contaminated cooling towers, evaporative condensers, potable water systems, whirlpool spas, humidifiers, and respiratory therapy equipment. Outbreaks have occurred in hospitals, cruise ships, hotels, and other large buildings. The disease occurs most commonly in elderly and immunocompromised persons. Infection in children is uncommon and usually is asymptomatic or mild and unrecognized. Severe disease has occurred in children with malignant neoplasms, severe combined immunodeficiency, chronic granulomatous disease, organ transplantation, or underlying pulmonary disease, children treated with corticosteroids, and neonates.

The **incubation period** for legionnaires disease (pneumonia) is 2 to 10 days; for Pontiac fever, it is 1 to 2 days.

DIAGNOSTIC TESTS: Recovery of *L pneumophila* from respiratory tract secretions, lung tissue, pleural fluid, or other normally sterile fluids by using special culture media provides definitive evidence of infection. The bacterium can be demonstrated in these specimens by direct immunofluorescence and by DNA probes, but these tests are less sensitive and specific than culture. Detection of *L pneumophila* serogroup 1 antigens in urine by commercially available radioimmunoassay or enzyme immunoassay (EIA) is more sensitive and specific than immunofluorescence using respiratory tract secretions and allows rapid diagnosis but only detects infection due to this species and serogroup. For serologic diagnosis, an increase in titer of antibody to *L pneumophila* serogroup 1 to 1:128 or greater, measured by an indirect immunofluorescence antibody assay (IFA), also indicates acute infection. Antibody titers usually increase within 1 to 6 weeks after onset of symptoms, but the increase can be delayed for as long as 12 weeks. The positive predictive value of a single titer of 1:256 or more is low and should not be used for diagnostic purposes. Newer serologic assays, such as EIA or tests using *Legionella* antigens other than serogroup 1, are available commercially but have not been standardized adequately for routine use. Antibodies to *Mycoplasma pneumoniae* and several gram-negative organisms, including *Campylobacter jejuni, Pseudomonas aeruginosa,* and *Bacteroides fragilis,* may cause false-positive IFA test results. Diagnosis of infection by detection of *L pneumophila* DNA by polymerase chain reaction in respiratory tract secretions, serum, or urine holds promise.

TREATMENT: Erythromycin (30 to 50 mg/kg per day; maximum, 4 g/d in 4 divided doses) is the drug of choice. Intravenous high-dose therapy generally is given initially. Once the patient's condition is improving, oral therapy can be substituted. The addition of rifampin (15 mg/kg per day; maximum, 600 mg/d) is recommended for patients with confirmed disease who are severely ill or immunocompromised or in whom the infection does not respond promptly to intravenous erythromycin. Azithromycin also is effective; intravenous azithromycin may be substituted for intravenous erythromycin. Ciprofloxacin, ofloxacin, and levofloxacin are effective but are not approved for persons younger than 18 years of age. Doxycycline and trimethoprim-sulfamethoxazole are alternative drugs. Duration of therapy is 2 weeks for patients with mild disease and 3 weeks for patients who are immunocompromised or have severe disease.

ISOLATION OF THE HOSPITALIZED PATIENT: Standard precautions are recommended.

CONTROL MEASURES: Methods for decontaminating water supplies in common-source outbreaks have included hyperchlorination (or other chemical decontaminants, such as copper-silver ionization) and superheating (to 70°C [158°F]) in conjunction with appropriate mechanical cleaning followed by continuous chlorination or maintenance of a hot water temperature at greater than 50°C (122°F). Insufficient information is available to evaluate the utility of other chemical and physical methods of decontamination.

Leishmaniasis

CLINICAL MANIFESTATIONS: The 3 major clinical syndromes are as follows:

- ***Cutaneous leishmaniasis.*** After inoculation by the bite of an infected sandfly, parasites proliferate locally in mononuclear phagocytes, leading to an erythematous macula or nodule that typically forms a shallow ulcer with raised borders. Lesions commonly are located on exposed areas of the face and extremities and may be accompanied by satellite lesions and regional adenopathy. The clinical manifestations of Old World and New World cutaneous leishmaniasis are similar. Spontaneous resolution of lesions may take from weeks to years and usually results in a flat atrophic scar.
- ***Mucosal leishmaniasis (espundia).*** From the initial cutaneous infection by *Leishmania braziliensis* or related New World species, parasites may disseminate to midline facial structures, including the oral and nasopharyngeal mucosa.

In some patients, granulomatous ulceration follows, leading to facial disfigurement, secondary infection, and mucosal perforation months to years after the cutaneous lesion heals.

- ***Visceral leishmaniasis (kala-azar).*** After cutaneous inoculation of parasites, organisms spread throughout the mononuclear macrophage system and are concentrated in the spleen, liver, and bone marrow. The resulting clinical illness is marked by fever, anorexia, weight loss, splenomegaly, hepatomegaly, lymphadenopathy (in some geographic areas), anemia, leukopenia, thrombocytopenia with hemorrhage, and hypergammaglobulinemia. Secondary pyogenic, gram-negative enteric, and mycobacterial infections are common. Active untreated visceral disease is nearly always fatal. Reactivation of latent visceral leishmaniasis is common in patients with concurrent human immunodeficiency virus (HIV) infection or other immunocompromising conditions.

ETIOLOGY: In the human host, *Leishmania* species are obligate intracellular parasites of mononuclear phagocytes. A single *Leishmania* species can produce different clinical syndromes, and each syndrome can be caused by different species. For example, cutaneous leishmaniasis typically is caused by *Leishmania tropica, Leishmania major, Leishmania aethiopica* (Old World species), and by *Leishmania mexicana, Leishmania amazonensis, L braziliensis, Leishmania panamensis, Leishmania guyanensis, Leishmania peruviana, Leishmania chagasi,* and other New World species. Mucosal leishmaniasis is caused by *L braziliensis* and occasionally other related species. Visceral leishmaniasis is caused by *Leishmania donovani, Leishmania infantum,* and *L chagasi,* as well as *L tropica* and *L amazonensis. Leishmania donovani* and *L infantum* also can cause Old World cutaneous leishmaniasis.

EPIDEMIOLOGY: Leishmaniasis typically is a zoonosis with a variety of mammalian reservoir hosts, including canines and rodents. The vectors are phlebotomine sandflies. The distribution of Old World cutaneous leishmaniasis includes the Middle East, some Asian and African countries, the Indian subcontinent, countries of the former Soviet Union, and, sporadically, southern Europe. New World cutaneous leishmaniasis is found in areas extending from Mexico to northern Argentina, and a few cases have been reported as far north as Texas. Mucosal leishmaniasis occurs primarily in the Amazon basin and the central plains of Brazil but also has been reported in other countries in South and Central America. The distribution of visceral leishmaniasis in the Old World includes southern Europe, the Mediterranean basin, the Middle East, East Africa, China, and the Indian subcontinent. Endemic foci in the New World are found in South and Central America, particularly in Brazil.

The **incubation period** for the different forms of leishmaniasis ranges from several days to months. In cutaneous leishmaniasis, primary skin lesions typically appear several weeks after parasite inoculation. In visceral infection, the incubation period can vary from 6 weeks to 6 months. However, incubation periods from 10 days to 10 years have been reported, and reactivation of previously asymptomatic latent infection can occur in immunosuppressed patients.

DIAGNOSTIC TESTS: Definitive diagnosis is by microscopic identification of intracellular leishmanial organisms on Wright or Giemsa stains of smears or histologic sections of infected tissues. In cutaneous disease, tissue can be obtained by a 3-mm punch biopsy, lesion scrapings, or needle aspiration of the raised nonnecrotic edge (not the center) of the lesion. In visceral leishmaniasis, the organisms can be identified in the spleen and, less commonly, from bone marrow and liver; in East Africa, the organisms also can be identified in the lymph nodes. Blood cultures have been positive in some Indian patients, and in HIV-infected patients, organisms sometimes may be observed in blood smears or buffy-coat preparations. Isolation of parasites by culture of appropriate tissue specimens in specialized media should be attempted when possible. Culture media and further information can be provided by the Centers for Disease Control and Prevention (CDC).

The diagnosis of visceral leishmaniasis and some cases of cutaneous infection can also be aided by serologic or polymerase chain reaction testing, which are available at the CDC. However, a negative serologic test result should never be interpreted as excluding the possibility of a leishmanial infection. In addition, occasional false-positive serologic results may occur in serum samples of patients with other infectious diseases, especially American trypanosomiasis (Chagas disease).

TREATMENT: Because cutaneous lesions may heal without specific therapy, treatment is not always necessary. Treatment is indicated when the ulcers are disabling or disfiguring, when healing is delayed, or when the patient may be infected with *L braziliensis* or other *Leishmania* species associated with mucosal disease. Drug therapy is always indicated when mucosal or visceral infection is present (see Drugs for Parasitic Infections, p 693).

In the United States, the standard drug of choice for leishmaniasis is sodium stibogluconate, a parenteral pentavalent antimonial that usually is given daily for a minimum of 20 days. Stibogluconate is available from the CDC Drug Service (see Appendix I, Directory of Resources, p 743). It generally is well tolerated in young, otherwise healthy patients, but cardiac, pancreatic, and hepatic toxic effects can occur. The related drug, meglumine antimonate (which is not available in the United States) is an alternative agent. Liposomal amphotericin B is approved by the US Food and Drug Administration for treatment of visceral leishmaniasis. For patients with disease refractory to antimonial therapy, amphotericin B, liposomal amphotericin B, or pentamidine should be considered. In selected cases of American cutaneous leishmaniasis, ketoconazole and itraconazole, as well as local heat, have been used successfully. Local therapy is not advisable for infection that could disseminate to cause mucosal leishmaniasis. In selected cases of Old World cutaneous leishmaniasis, various types of local or topical therapy have been used successfully.

ISOLATION OF THE HOSPITALIZED PATIENT: Standard precautions are recommended.

CONTROL MEASURES: Because elimination of infected animal reservoirs and/or sandfly populations is unlikely to occur in most regions that are endemic for leishmaniasis, travelers should be advised to minimize their exposure to sandfly bites by using screened accommodations, fine-mesh bed netting, protective clothing, and insect repellent and by minimizing outdoor exposures from dusk to dawn. Patients infected with *Leishmania* species should not donate blood or be organ donors.

Leprosy

CLINICAL MANIFESTATIONS: Leprosy (Hansen's disease) is a chronic disease mainly involving skin, peripheral nerves, and the mucosa of the upper respiratory tract. The clinical syndromes of leprosy represent a spectrum that reflects the cellular immune response to *Mycobacterium leprae.* Characteristic features are the following:

- ***Tuberculoid:*** one or few well-demarcated, hypopigmented or erythematous, hypoesthetic or anesthetic skin lesions, frequently with raised, active, spreading edges and central clearing. Cell-mediated immune responses are intact.
- ***Lepromatous:*** initial numerous, ill-defined, hypopigmented, or erythematous maculae that progress to papules, nodules, or plaques; and late-occurring hypoesthesia. Dermal infiltration of the face, hands, and feet in a bilateral and symmetric distribution can occur without preceding maculopapular lesions. *Mycobacterium leprae*–specific, cell-mediated immunity is greatly diminished, but serum antibody responses to *M leprae*–derived antigens may occur, or titers of nonspecific antibodies (such as rheumatoid factor or nontreponemal tests for syphilis) may be elevated.
- ***Borderline (dimorphous):*** single or multiple well-defined skin lesions, similar to tuberculoid lesions, but with a raised central area, and delayed development of dysesthesia. Borderline disease often is subdivided into borderline lepromatous, borderline, and borderline tuberculoid.
- ***Indeterminate:*** an early form of leprosy that may develop into any of the other forms; typified by hypopigmented maculae with indistinct edges and no associated dysesthesia.

Serious consequences of leprosy occur from immune reactions and nerve involvement with resulting anesthesia, which can lead to repeated unrecognized trauma, ulcerations, fractures, and bone resorption.

ETIOLOGY: Leprosy is caused by *M leprae.*

EPIDEMIOLOGY: The major mode of transmission is contact with humans who have untreated or drug-resistant multibacillary disease (lepromatous or borderline types). A long duration of exposure, such as to a household contact, is common. However, 70% to 80% of cases in endemic areas do not have a history of household exposure or other contact with a known or suspected case of leprosy, suggesting the possibility of other sources of infection. The major source of infectious material is probably nasal secretions from patients with untreated multibacillary disease, from whom organisms are excreted in large numbers. Little shedding of *M leprae* from involved intact skin occurs. In the United States, 90% of reported cases are imported, occurring in immigrants and refugees from areas endemic for leprosy, particularly Mexico and Southeast Asia. Indigenous cases continue to occur in Texas, California, Louisiana, and Hawaii. The infectivity of lepromatous patients probably ceases soon after treatment is instituted, frequently within a few days or weeks of initiating rifampin therapy or about 3 months after initiating therapy with dapsone or clofazimine.

The **incubation period** ranges from 1 to many years, but usually is 3 to 5 years. The incubation period of tuberculoid cases tends to be shorter than that for lepromatous cases.

DIAGNOSTIC TESTS: Histopathologic examination by an experienced pathologist is the best method for establishing the diagnosis and is the basis for the classification of leprosy. Acid-fast bacilli (AFB) may be found in slit-smears or biopsy specimens of skin lesions but rarely from patients with the tuberculoid and indeterminate forms of disease. Organisms have not been cultured successfully in vitro. Drug resistance is tested by the mouse footpad inoculation test, which is performed only in specialized laboratories, and results require a period of at least 6 months. Clinically, the demonstration of morphologically normal bacilli, ie, organisms with solid staining of the capsule on AFB stains, despite usually effective therapy, suggests possible drug resistance (or poor compliance with therapy), indicating the possible need for a change in therapy.

High titers of predominantly immunoglobulin M serum antibodies against phenolic glycolipid-1 of *M leprae* have been detected in untreated patients with lepromatous or borderline disease. Because elevated antibody titers frequently occur in persons without disease, this test is not diagnostic for leprosy. Titers of these antibodies slowly decrease after years of therapy. This test is experimental and available only in a few reference laboratories.

TREATMENT: Therapy for patients with leprosy should be undertaken in consultation with an expert in leprosy. The Gillis W. Long Hansen's Disease Center, Carville, LA (800-642-2477), provides consultation on clinical and pathologic issues and can provide information about local Hansen's disease clinics and clinicians who have experience with the disease.

Dapsone, one of the primary drugs used in the treatment of leprosy, usually is administered in a dosage of 100 mg/d for adults and 1 mg/kg per day for children. Persons in high-risk groups for glucose-6-phosphate dehydrogenase deficiency should be tested for this disorder before administration. To reduce the risk of drug resistance and possibly shorten the duration of therapy, multidrug therapy is necessary for all patients. Rifampin (600 mg/d for adults or 10 mg/kg per day for children) should be given with dapsone for 1 year for paucibacillary (indeterminate, tuberculoid, and borderline tuberculoid) disease, with close follow-up to detect relapses. Clofazimine (50 mg/d for adults or 1 mg/kg per day for children) should be added for multibacillary (borderline, borderline lepromatous, and lepromatous) disease and continued for at least 2 years. Other drugs, including ofloxacin, sparfloxacin, minocycline, and clarithromycin, have activity against *M leprae* and could be considered for therapy for patients with intolerance to routine drugs or with drug-resistant infections. All clinically compatible patients with demonstrable AFB organisms on skin biopsy specimens or smears should be treated for presumptive multibacillary leprosy.

Corticosteroids are used to treat erythema nodosum leprosum (ENL), which commonly occurs in patients with multibacillary disease after drug therapy is initiated. Occasionally, ENL occurs in untreated patients as well. Short-term, high-dose corticosteroids, followed by maintenance thalidomide, often are useful for managing severe or recurrent ENL reactions. Thalidomide has been approved by the US Food and Drug Administration for ENL. Thalidomide should never be given to a woman of childbearing age unless she is using a reliable means of contraception. Other agents, including clofazimine, also can be used to treat ENL.

The reversal reaction, seen primarily in patients with borderline disease, is characterized by delayed-type hypersensitivity reactions at the site of current or former leprosy lesions and acute neuropathies. These conditions require aggressive treatment with corticosteroids to avoid permanent neurologic sequelae.

Most patients can be treated as outpatients. Rehabilitative measures, including surgery and physical therapy, may be necessary for some patients.

ISOLATION OF THE HOSPITALIZED PATIENT: Standard precautions are indicated.

CONTROL MEASURES: Hand washing is recommended for all persons in contact with a patient with lepromatous leprosy. Disinfection of nasal secretions, handkerchiefs, and other fomites should be considered until treatment is established. Household contacts, particularly those with multibacillary disease, should be examined initially and then annually for at least 5 years. Local public health department regulations for leprosy vary and should be consulted.

A single bacille Calmette-Guérin (BCG) vaccination is reported to be about 50% protective against leprosy, and 1 or 2 repeated doses increases the protection further. Also, the first commercially available leprosy vaccine was approved in India in January 1998. A heat-killed, nonpathogenic *Mycobacterium w,* which has close antigenic similarity to *M leprae,* is given in up to 8 doses to stimulate clearance of bacilli in patients with lepromatous leprosy; improvement is more rapid in such patients than in those receiving multidrug therapy alone. This vaccine is not available in the United States. Neither BCG nor the heat-killed leprosy vaccine are recommended for use for household contacts in the United States, but further evaluation of their role in the control of leprosy is ongoing.

Newly diagnosed cases of leprosy should be reported to local and state public health departments in the United States for reporting to the Centers for Disease Control and Prevention and to the Gillis W. Long Hansen's Disease Center.

Leptospirosis

CLINICAL MANIFESTATIONS: Leptospirosis occurs as 2 clinically recognizable syndromes: anicteric and icteric. The onset of leptospirosis usually is abrupt, with nonspecific, influenza-like, constitutional symptoms of fever, chills, headache, severe myalgia, malaise, and conjunctival suffusion. Gastrointestinal tract symptoms also can occur. Of the infected patients, 90% will present with anicteric illness; however, 10% will present severely ill, with jaundice, renal dysfunction, and central nervous system symptoms (Weil syndrome). This initial "septicemic" phase may be followed by a second, immune-mediated phase, classically known as the biphasic clinical course. Fever and other constitutional symptoms may recur, as may neurologic symptoms. The icteric or severe form of clinical presentation is associated with jaundice, abnormal liver function tests, hepatomegaly, and liver failure; renal involvement includes azotemia, abnormal urine analysis results, and renal failure. Central nervous system involvement occurs most commonly as aseptic meningitis, and complications, such as neuritis and uveitis, occur more commonly in the immune phase.

Conjunctival suffusion, the most characteristic physical finding, occurs in fewer than half the patients. The duration of symptoms varies from less than 1 week to 3 weeks.

ETIOLOGY: All leptospires are spirochetes that are similar in appearance and culture. Historically, they were classified into serovars and serogroups. Members of the genus *Leptospira* are classified by genetic relationships into distinct species (genospecies). The species *borgpetersenii, inadai, interrogans, kirschneri, noguchii, santarosai,* and *weilii* include almost all the pathogenic leptospires.

EPIDEMIOLOGY: The sources for human infection include many species of wild and domestic mammals, particularly dogs, rats, and livestock, that excrete *Leptospira* organisms in urine. Most outbreaks in the United States probably result from recreational exposure to contaminated water. Persons predisposed by occupation include abattoir and sewer workers, veterinarians, farmers, and field workers. Transmission is zoonotic, by direct or indirect contact of mucosal surfaces or abraded or traumatized skin with urine or carcasses of infected animals. Indirect contact occurs from swimming, wading, or splashing in pools, streams, or puddles contaminated by urine from infected animals and, occasionally, causes common-source outbreaks. Asymptomatic human infections occur; however, infection usually is symptomatic. Infected animals can transmit organisms during the 1-month to more than 3-month phase of prolonged leptospiruria. Person-to-person transmission is rare.

The **incubation period** usually is 7 to 13 days, with a range of 2 to 26 days.

DIAGNOSTIC TESTS: Blood and cerebrospinal fluid in the first 7 to 10 days of illness and urine after the first week and during convalescence should be cultured on special media that are not available routinely. Laboratory personnel should be consulted in cases of suspected leptospirosis. The organism also can be recovered by inoculation of body fluids into guinea pigs. Serum antibodies, measured by enzyme immunoassay or agglutination reactions, develop during the second week of illness, but increases in antibody titer can be delayed or absent in some patients. Microscopic agglutination, the confirmatory serologic test, is performed in reference laboratories. Direct darkfield examination of blood or other body fluid specimens has pitfalls that obviate its usefulness, and it is not recommended. Polymerase chain reaction assay for the detection of leptospires has been developed but is not available in commercial laboratories.

TREATMENT: Penicillin is the drug of choice for severely ill patients. Penicillin G (1.5 million U given every 6 hours to adults) administered intravenously for 7 days seems to be effective, even for patients in whom therapy is not started until after the fourth day of the illness. Oral doxycycline therapy for persons with mild illness also seems to shorten the course of illness and reduces the frequency of convalescent leptospiruria. Tetracycline drugs should not be given to children younger than 8 years of age.

ISOLATION OF THE HOSPITALIZED PATIENT: Standard precautions are recommended. These precautions also include urine, which potentially is infectious in persons with leptospirosis.

CONTROL MEASURES:

- Immunization of dogs and livestock prevents disease but not infection (ie, leptospiruria) in animals. The effect of immunization of dogs and livestock on prevention of human disease is unproven, since immunized animals may transmit the organism to humans.
- Protective clothing, boots, and gloves should be worn to reduce risk to persons with occupational exposure.
- Rodent control is indicated.
- Doxycycline, 200 mg, given orally once a week to adults, is effective prophylaxis and should be considered for high-risk occupational groups with short-term exposure. However, indications for doxycycline use for children have not been established.

Listeria monocytogenes Infections

(Listeriosis)

CLINICAL MANIFESTATIONS: *Listeria monocytogenes* infections are relatively uncommon; those affecting children are categorized as maternal, neonatal, or childhood with or without associated predisposing conditions. Maternal infection can be associated with an influenza-like illness, fever, malaise, headache, gastrointestinal tract symptoms, and back pain. Neonatal illness has early-onset and late-onset syndromes similar to those of group B streptococcal infections. Prematurity, pneumonia, and septicemia are common in early-onset disease. Approximately 65% of women experience a symptomatic prodromal illness before diagnosis of listeriosis in their fetus or newborn infant. Amnionitis during labor or asymptomatic infection can occur. Granulomatosis infantisepticum, characterized clinically by an erythematous rash with small pale nodules and histologically by disseminated granulomas, occurs less frequently. Late-onset infection occurs after the first week of life and usually results in meningitis. Infection occurs most commonly in the perinatal period and in patients with decreased cell-mediated immunity resulting from cancer chemotherapy, corticosteroid therapy, immunodeficiency, hepatic or renal disease, or infection with the human immunodeficiency virus. In childhood infections, most patients have meningitis, and almost half have no underlying predisposing condition. *Listeria monocytogenes* rarely causes a diffuse encephalitis. Severe disease in adults associated with contaminated meat products emphasizes that older children and adults can have systemic disease with mortality.

ETIOLOGY: *Listeria monocytogenes* is an aerobic, non–spore-forming, motile, gram-positive bacillus that produces a narrow zone of hemolysis on blood agar medium.

EPIDEMIOLOGY: *Listeria monocytogenes* is distributed widely in the environment, especially in food. Foodborne transmission causes epidemics and sporadic infections. Incriminated foods include unpasteurized milk; soft cheeses and other dairy products; prepared meats, such as hot dogs, deli meat, and pâté; undercooked poultry; and unwashed raw vegetables. Asymptomatic fecal and vaginal carriage in pregnant women can result in sporadic neonatal disease from transplacental or ascending routes of infection or from exposure during delivery. Maternal infection has been associated with abortion, preterm delivery, and other obstetric complications. Late-onset neonatal infection can result from acquisition of the organism during passage through the birth canal or from environmental sources, followed by hematogenous invasion of the organism from intestine. Nosocomial nursery outbreaks also have occurred.

The **incubation period** is variable, ranging from 3 to 10 days; the median incubation period for foodborne transmission is thought to be 3 weeks.

DIAGNOSTIC TESTS: The organism can be recovered on blood agar media from cultures of blood, cerebrospinal fluid (CSF), meconium, gastric washings, placenta, amniotic fluid, and other infected tissues, including joint, pleural, or pericardial fluid. Special techniques (eg, enrichment and selective media) may be needed to recover *L monocytogenes* from sites with mixed flora (eg, vagina and rectum). Gram staining of gastric aspirate material, placental tissue, a biopsy specimen of rash of early-onset infection, or CSF from an infected newborn infant may demonstrate the organism. An isolate of *L monocytogenes* mistakenly can be considered a contaminant or saprophyte because of morphologic similarity to diphtheroids and streptococci. Serologic tests can be useful, particularly in the setting of an epidemiologic investigation.

TREATMENT:

- Initial therapy with intravenous ampicillin and an aminoglycoside, usually gentamicin, is recommended for severe infections. This combination is more effective than ampicillin alone in animal models of *L monocytogenes* infection. After clinical response occurs or for less severe infections in immunocompetent hosts, ampicillin or penicillin alone can be given. The optimal therapeutic regimen, however, has not been established. For the penicillin-allergic patient, the alternative regimen is trimethoprim-sulfamethoxazole. Cephalosporins, including the newer derivatives, are not active against *L monocytogenes.*
- For invasive infections without associated meningitis, 10 to 14 days of treatment usually is satisfactory. For *L monocytogenes* meningitis, most experts recommend 14 to 21 days of treatment.
- The usefulness of culturing the vagina and rectum of the mother of an infected infant and treatment of the mother, if either culture is positive, has not been established.

ISOLATION OF THE HOSPITALIZED PATIENT: Standard precautions are recommended.

CONTROL MEASURES:

- Antimicrobial therapy for infection diagnosed during pregnancy may prevent fetal or perinatal infection and its consequences.
- The incidence of listeriosis has decreased substantially since 1989 when US regulatory agencies began enforcing strict zero-tolerance guidelines for *L monocytogenes* in ready-to-eat foods.
- The general guidelines for preventing listeriosis are similar to those for preventing other foodborne illnesses (thoroughly cook raw food from animal

sources, wash raw vegetables, keep uncooked meats separate from vegetables, avoid unpasteurized dairy products, and wash hands, knives, and cutting boards after exposure to uncooked foods). In addition, persons at high risk for complications from listeriosis (pregnant women and immunocompromised persons) should follow the dietary recommendations in Table 3.33, below.
- Cases of listeriosis should be reported to the regional health department to facilitate early recognition and control of common-source outbreaks.

Table 3.33. **Dietary Recommendations for Persons at High Risk of Listeriosis***

- Avoid soft cheeses (eg, Mexican-style, feta, brie, Camembert, and blue-veined cheese). There is no need to avoid hard cheeses, cream cheese, cottage cheese, or yogurt.
- Leftover foods or ready-to-eat foods (eg, hot dogs) should be reheated until steaming hot before eating.
- Although the risk for listeriosis with foods from delicatessen counters is relatively low, persons at high risk may choose to avoid these foods or to thoroughly reheat cold cuts before eating.

* High-risk patients are those who are immunocompromised by illness, medication, or other therapy and pregnant women.

Lyme Disease

(Borrelia burgdorferi)

CLINICAL MANIFESTATIONS: The clinical manifestations are divided into 3 stages: early localized, early disseminated, and late disease. Early localized disease is characterized by a distinctive rash, termed *erythema migrans,* at the site of a recent tick bite. Erythema migrans begins as a red macula or papule that usually expands over days to weeks to form a large annular erythematous lesion that is 5 cm or more in diameter (median, 15 cm), sometimes with partial central clearing. Localized erythema migrans can vary greatly in size and shape and may have vesicular or necrotic areas in its center. Fever, malaise, headache, mild neck stiffness, myalgia, and arthralgia often accompany the rash. In untreated persons, these associated symptoms may be intermittent and variable over a period of several weeks.

The most common manifestation of early disseminated disease is multiple erythema migrans. This rash usually occurs 3 to 5 weeks after an infective tick bite and consists of secondary annular erythematous lesions similar to, but usually smaller than, the primary lesion. These lesions reflect spirochetemia with dermal dissemination. Other common manifestations of early disseminated illness (which may occur with or without rash) are palsies of the cranial nerves (especially cranial nerve VII), meningitis, and conjunctivitis. Systemic symptoms, such as arthralgia, myalgia, headache, and fatigue, also are common during the early disseminated stage. Carditis, which usually is characterized by various degrees of heart block, occurs rarely.

Late disease is characterized most commonly by recurrent arthritis that usually is pauciarticular and affects the large joints, in particular the knees. Arthritis may occur without a history of earlier stages of illness (including erythema migrans). Central nervous system manifestations also may occur during late disease and include subacute encephalopathy and polyradiculoneuropathy. Late disease is uncommon in children who are treated with antimicrobial agents in the early stage of the disease.

No causal relationship between maternal Lyme disease and abnormalities of pregnancy or congenital disease caused by *Borrelia burgdorferi* has been documented, although transplacental transmission of *B burgdorferi* has been reported. No evidence exists that Lyme disease can be transmitted via human milk.

ETIOLOGY: Infection is caused by the spirochete *B burgdorferi.*

EPIDEMIOLOGY: Lyme disease occurs primarily in 3 distinct geographic regions of the United States. Most cases are reported in the Northeast from Massachusetts to Maryland. The disease also occurs, but with lower frequency, in the upper Midwest, especially in Wisconsin and Minnesota, and, less commonly, on the West Coast, especially northern California. The occurrence of cases in the United States correlates with the distribution and frequency of infected tick vectors (*Ixodes scapularis* [previously known as *Ixodes dammini*] in the East and Midwest and *Ixodes pacificus* in the West). Reported cases in states without known enzootic risks may be imported or, in many cases, may be misdiagnoses resulting from false-positive serologic test results. Endemic Lyme disease also has been reported in Canada, Europe, states of the former Soviet Union, China, and Japan. Most cases occur between April and October. Persons of all ages may be affected.

The **incubation period** from tick bite to appearance of erythema migrans ranges from 3 to 31 days and typically is from 7 to 14 days. Late manifestations occur months to years later.

DIAGNOSTIC TESTS: Diagnosis is made clinically during the early stages of Lyme disease if erythema migrans is present. While cultures of a biopsy specimen of the perimeter of this lesion frequently yield the organism, *Borrelia* cultures (which require special media) are not available commercially. In patients without a rash who manifest signs of a later stage of Lyme disease, diagnosis also should be based on clinical findings, using serologic tests as an adjunct.

The diagnosis of Lyme disease can be difficult, in part because of poor standardization and inappropriate use of serologic diagnostic tests. The immunoglobulin (Ig) M–specific antibody titer usually peaks between weeks 3 and 6 after the onset of infection; specific IgG antibody titers usually rise slowly and generally are highest weeks to months later. Localized erythema migrans typically occurs 1 to 2 weeks after the tick bite; therefore, antibodies against *B burgdorferi* will not be detectable in most patients presenting with erythema migrans. Some patients who are treated early with antimicrobial agents never develop antibodies against *B burgdorferi.* However, most patients with early disseminated disease and virtually all patients with late disease will have antibodies against *B burgdorferi.* As with other infections, once such antibodies develop, they may persist for many years despite cure of the disease. Consequently, tests for antibodies should not be used to assess the success of treatment. Because of the poor sensitivity and specificity of serologic testing for *B burgdorferi* that is available in most commercial laboratories, testing for serum antibodies against *B burgdorferi* should be performed in a reference laboratory when possible. Physicians unfamiliar with the reference laboratories in their area should contact their state health departments for additional information.

The enzyme immunoassay (EIA) is the most commonly used test for detection of antibodies against *B burgdorferi.* This test and the immunofluorescence assay (IFA) may give false-positive results because of cross-reactive antibodies in patients with other spirochetal infections (eg, syphilis, leptospirosis, relapsing fever), certain viral infections (eg, varicella), and certain autoimmune diseases (eg, systemic lupus erythematosus). While antibodies to *B burgdorferi* cross-react with other spirochetes, including *Treponema pallidum,* patients with Lyme disease do not have positive non-treponemal syphilis test results, such as the VDRL or RPR (rapid plasma reagin). In addition, antibodies directed against bacteria in the normal oral flora may cross-react with antigens of *B burgdorferi* and produce a false-positive test result.

Currently, the Western immunoblot test is most useful for corroborating positive or equivocal EIA or IFA results and, as a result, a 2-test approach is recommended for the serologic diagnosis of *B burgdorferi* infection. Serum specimens that give positive or equivocal results by a sensitive EIA or IFA should be tested by a standardized Western immunoblot for the presence of antibodies against proteins specific for *B burgdorferi;* serum specimens that give negative results by a sensitive EIA or IFA do not require immunoblot testing. If a patient with suspected early disease has a negative serologic test result, evidence of infection is best obtained by testing of paired acute- and convalescent-phase serum samples. Persons with early disseminated or late-stage Lyme disease almost always have a robust antibody response to *B burgdorferi* antigens.

Suspected central nervous system involvement with Lyme disease can be confirmed by demonstration of intrathecal production of antibodies against *B burgdorferi.* However, interpretation of antibody tests of cerebrospinal fluid is complex, and physicians should seek the advice of a specialist experienced in the management of patients with Lyme disease to assist them in interpreting results of these tests.

The widespread practice of ordering serologic tests for patients with nonspecific symptoms (such as fatigue or arthralgia) who have a low probability of having Lyme disease is not recommended. Almost all positive serologic test results in these patients are false-positive results. Patients with acute Lyme disease almost always have objective signs of infection (eg, erythema migrans, facial nerve palsy, arthritis). Nonspecific symptoms commonly accompany these specific signs but are almost never the only evidence of Lyme disease.

New, more sensitive and more specific diagnostic tests, such as the polymerase chain reaction, which may be able to identify the presence of even small quantities of spirochetal DNA, are in development. However, physicians should be cautious when interpreting results of these investigational tests until their clinical usefulness has been proven.

Recipients of the recombinant outer surface protein A (rOspA) vaccine have a positive EIA test result because whole-cell *B burgdorferi* is used as the antigen. The Western immunoblot results are not affected by immunization because antibody to specific protein antigens allows identification of non-OspA antibodies and antibody to OspA is not part of the criteria for a positive immunoblot. Therefore, immunoblot testing for non-OspA antibody reactivity is essential for establishing or excluding the diagnosis of Lyme disease in rOspA vaccine recipients.

TREATMENT: See Table 3.34, below.

Early Localized Disease. Doxycycline is the drug of choice for children 8 years of age and older. Precautions to avoid exposure to the sun (eg, the use of sunscreen) should be taken because a rash develops in sun-exposed areas in 20% of persons who take doxycycline. For children younger than 8 years of age, amoxicillin is recommended. For patients allergic to penicillin, alternative drugs are cefuroxime axetil and erythromycin, although erythromycin may be less effective. Most experts treat persons with early Lyme disease for 14 to 21 days, but information is limited about the optimal duration of treatment.

Treatment of erythema migrans almost always prevents development of later stages of Lyme disease. Clinical response to therapy often is slow, and signs and symptoms may persist for several weeks even in successfully treated patients. Erythema migrans usually resolves within several days of initiating treatment.

Early Disseminated and Late Disease. Orally administered antimicrobial agents are recommended for treating multiple erythema migrans and uncomplicated

Table 3.34. **Recommended Treatment of Lyme Disease in Children**

Disease Category	Drug(s) and Dose*
Early localized disease*	
≥8 y	Doxycycline, oral regimen, 100 mg twice a day for 14–21 d
All ages	Amoxicillin, oral regimen, 25–50 mg/kg per day, divided into 2 doses (maximum, 2 g/d) for 14–21 d
Early disseminated and late disease	
Multiple erythema migrans	Same oral regimen as for early disease but for 21 d
Isolated facial palsy	Same oral regimen as for early disease but for 21–28 d†‡
Arthritis	Same oral regimen as for early disease but for 28 d
Persistent or recurrent arthritis§	Ceftriaxone, 75–100 mg/kg, IV or IM, once a day (maximum, 2 g/d) for 14–21 d; or penicillin, 300 000 U/kg per day, IV, given in divided doses every 4 h (maximum, 20 million U/d) for 14–21 d
Carditis	Ceftriaxone or penicillin: see persistent or recurrent arthritis
Meningitis or encephalitis	Ceftriaxone or penicillin: see persistent or recurrent arthritis

* For patients who are allergic to penicillin, cefuroxime axetil and erythromycin are alternative drugs. IV indicates intravenously; IM, intramuscularly.

† Corticosteroids should not be given.

‡ Treatment has no effect on the resolution of the nerve palsy; its purpose is to prevent late disease.

§ Arthritis is not considered persistent or recurrent unless objective evidence of synovitis exists at least 2 months after treatment is initiated. Some experts administer a second course of an oral agent before using an IV-administered antimicrobial agent.

Lyme arthritis. Most experts also recommend oral agents for treatment of nerve palsy, although some experts recommend a lumbar puncture if central nervous system involvement is suspected. If cerebrospinal fluid pleocytosis is found, parenterally administered antimicrobial therapy is indicated. Recurrent or persistent arthritis and central nervous system infection should be treated with parenterally administered antimicrobial agents. Carditis usually is treated with parenteral therapy, although some experts treat mild carditis orally with doxycycline or amoxicillin. The optimal duration of therapy for these different manifestations is not well established, but there is no evidence that children with any manifestation of Lyme disease benefit from prolonged or repeated courses of orally or parenterally administered antimicrobial agents. Accordingly, the maximum duration of a single course of therapy is 4 weeks.

The Jarisch-Herxheimer reaction, characterized by fever, chills, and malaise, can occur transiently when therapy is initiated. Nonsteroidal anti-inflammatory agents may be beneficial, and the antimicrobial agent should be continued.

Pregnancy. Tetracyclines are contraindicated. Otherwise, therapy is the same as recommended for nonpregnant persons.

ISOLATION OF THE HOSPITALIZED PATIENT: Standard precautions are recommended.

CONTROL MEASURES:

Ticks. See Prevention of Tick-borne Infections, p 159.

Chemoprophylaxis. The risk of infection with *B burgdorferi* after a recognized deer tick bite, even in highly endemic areas, is sufficiently low that prophylactic antimicrobial treatment after a tick bite is not indicated routinely. In addition, animal studies indicate that transmission of *B burgdorferi* from infected ticks usually requires a prolonged duration (≥36 hours) of attachment. Analysis of ticks to determine whether they are infected is not indicated because the predictive values of such tests for human disease are unknown.

Blood Donation. Patients with active disease should not donate blood because spirochetemia occurs in early Lyme disease. Patients who have been treated for Lyme disease can be considered for blood donation.

Vaccines.* A Lyme disease vaccine was licensed by the US Food and Drug Administration (FDA) on December 21, 1998, for persons 15 to 70 years of age. This vaccine seems safe and effective, but whether its use is cost-beneficial is not established clearly. Decisions about the use of this vaccine should be based on an assessment of a person's risk as determined by activities and behaviors relating to tick exposure in endemic areas. This vaccine should be considered an adjunct to, not a replacement for, the practice of personal protective measures against tick exposure and the early diagnosis and treatment of Lyme disease. Recommendations for the use of Lyme disease vaccine are as follows:

- The vaccine should be considered for administration to the following persons who are 15 years of age or older:

* American Academy of Pediatrics Committee on Infectious Diseases. Prevention of Lyme disease. *Pediatrics.* 2000;105:142–147

  - Those who reside, work, or recreate in geographic areas of high or moderate risk and whose activities result in frequent or prolonged exposure to vector ticks.
  - Those who visit geographic areas of high risk during the peak Lyme disease transmission season and whose activities result in frequent or prolonged exposure to vector ticks.
- The vaccine may be given to persons who reside, work, or recreate in geographic areas of high or moderate risk and whose activities result in some, but neither frequent nor prolonged, exposure to vector ticks. However, the benefits of vaccine for these persons compared with those of personal protective measures and early treatment of Lyme disease are unclear.
- The vaccine is *not recommended* for the following:
  - Those who reside, work, or recreate in areas of high or moderate risk but who have minimal or no exposure to infected ticks.
  - Persons who reside, work, and recreate in geographic areas of low or no risk.
  - Children younger than 15 years of age until data about the safety and immunogenicity of this vaccine in this age group are available and the FDA has approved the product for use in this age group.
- Persons with a history of Lyme disease
  Immunization should be considered for persons with a history of Lyme disease who are at continued high risk. However, persons with antibiotic treatment–resistant Lyme arthritis should not be immunized because of the association between this condition and immune reactivity to rOspA. Persons with chronic joint or neurologic illness related to Lyme disease, as well as those with second- or third-degree atrioventricular block, were excluded from the phase 3 safety and efficacy trial, and, thus, the safety and efficacy of Lyme disease vaccine for such persons is unknown.
- Simultaneous administration with other vaccines
  The safety and efficacy of the simultaneous administration of rOspA vaccine with other vaccines have not been established. Administration of rOspA vaccine should not interfere with the administration of routinely recommended immunizations. If rOspA vaccine is to be given concurrently with other vaccines, each should be administered in a separate syringe at a separate site.
- Persons with immunodeficiencies
  Data are lacking on the safety and efficacy of rOspA vaccines in persons with immunodeficiencies. General guidelines for administration of inactivated or subunit vaccines should be followed.
- Vaccine use during pregnancy
  Because the safety of rOspA vaccine administered during pregnancy has not been established, immunization of women known to be pregnant is not recommended. A vaccine pregnancy registry has been established by SmithKline Beecham Pharmaceuticals. If a pregnant woman is immunized, health care professionals are encouraged to register this immunization by calling 800-366-8900, extension 5231.

Lymphocytic Choriomeningitis

CLINICAL MANIFESTATIONS: Infection may result in a mild to severe nonspecific illness, which includes fever, malaise, myalgia, retro-orbital headache, photophobia, anorexia, and nausea. Fever usually lasts 1 to 3 weeks, and rash is infrequent. A biphasic febrile course is frequent. Neurologic manifestations varying from aseptic meningitis to severe encephalitis can occur. Arthralgia or arthritis, respiratory tract symptoms, orchitis, and leukopenia occasionally develop. Infection during pregnancy has been associated with abortion and with hydrocephalus, microcephaly, intracranial calcifications, and chorioretinitis in the fetus.

ETIOLOGY: Lymphocytic choriomeningitis (LCM) virus is an arenavirus.

EPIDEMIOLOGY: Lymphocytic choriomeningitis is a chronic infection of the common house mouse. These mice are often asymptomatically infected in nature. In addition, laboratory mice and colonized golden hamsters can be infected and have significant viral shedding. Pet hamsters also have been a source of infection. Humans are infected incidentally by inhalation or ingestion of dust or food contaminated with the virus from the urine, feces, blood, or nasopharyngeal secretions of infected rodents. The disease is most prevalent in young adults. Human-to-human spread of the virus has not been reported.

The **incubation period** is usually 6 to 13 days and occasionally as long as 3 weeks.

DIAGNOSTIC TESTS: The cerebrospinal fluid (CSF) may contain hundreds to thousands of white blood cells, predominantly lymphocytes, and hypoglycorrhachia can occur. The LCM virus can be isolated from blood, CSF, urine, and, rarely, nasopharyngeal secretions. Acute and convalescent serum samples can be tested for increases in antibody titers; demonstration of virus-specific immunoglobulin M antibodies in serum and CSF is useful. Infection of mice trapped in or around houses may be identified by demonstrating serum antibody or viral antigen in liver impression smears.

TREATMENT: Supportive.

ISOLATION OF THE HOSPITALIZED PATIENT: Standard precautions are recommended.

CONTROL MEASURES: Infection can be controlled by preventing rodent infestation in animal and food storage areas. Because the virus is excreted for long periods by rodent hosts, attempts should be made to monitor laboratory and wholesale colonies of mice and hamsters for infection. Pet rodents or wild mice in a patient's home should be considered likely sources of infection. Pregnant women in particular should avoid exposure to rodents and their aerosolized excreta.

Malaria

Clinical Manifestations: The classic symptoms are high fever with chills, rigor, sweats, and headache, which may be paroxysmal. As the infection becomes synchronized, the fever and paroxysms generally occur in a cyclic pattern. Depending on the infecting species, fever appears every other or every third day. Other manifestations can include nausea, vomiting, diarrhea, cough, arthralgia, and abdominal and back pain. Anemia and thrombocytopenia are common, and pallor and jaundice caused by hemolysis may occur. Hepatosplenomegaly may be present.

Infection by *Plasmodium falciparum* is potentially fatal and most commonly manifests as a febrile nonspecific influenza-like illness without localizing signs. With more severe disease, however, *P falciparum* infection may be manifest by one of the following clinical syndromes:

- *Cerebral malaria,* which may have variable neurologic manifestations, including seizures, signs of increased intracranial pressure, confusion, and progression to stupor, coma, and death
- *Severe anemia* due to high parasitemia and consequent hemolysis
- *Hypoglycemia,* sometimes associated with quinine treatment, requiring urgent correction
- *Respiratory failure and metabolic acidosis,* without pulmonary edema
- *Noncardiogenic pulmonary edema,* which is difficult to manage and may be fatal (rare in children)
- *Renal failure* caused by acute tubular necrosis (rare in children younger than 8 years of age)
- *Vascular collapse and shock* associated with hypothermia and adrenal insufficiency
- Children with asplenia are at high risk of death due to malaria.

Syndromes primarily associated with *Plasmodium vivax* and *Plasmodium ovale* are as follows:

- *Hypersplenism* with danger of late splenic rupture
- *Anemia* due to acute parasitemia
- *Relapse*, for as long as 3 to 5 years after the primary infection, due to latent hepatic stages

Syndromes associated with *Plasmodium malariae* infection are as follows:

- *Nephrotic syndrome* from the deposition of immune complexes in the kidney
- *Chronic asymptomatic parasitemia* for as long as several years after the last exposure

Congenital malaria secondary to perinatal transmission may occur rarely. Most congenital cases have been caused by *P vivax* and *P falciparum; P malariae* and *P ovale* account for fewer than 20% of such cases. Manifestations can resemble those of neonatal sepsis, including fever and nonspecific symptoms of poor appetite, irritability, and lethargy.

Etiology: The *Plasmodium* species infecting humans are *P falciparum, P vivax, P ovale,* and *P malariae.*

EPIDEMIOLOGY: Malaria is endemic throughout the tropical areas of the world and is acquired from the bite of the female nocturnal-feeding *Anopheles* mosquitoes. One half of the world's population lives in areas where transmission occurs. Worldwide, there are 300 to 500 million cases annually and 1.5 to 2.7 million deaths. Most deaths occur in young children. Malarial infection poses substantial risks to pregnant women and their fetuses and may result in spontaneous abortion and stillbirth. The risk of malaria is highest for travelers to sub-Saharan Africa, Papua New Guinea, the Solomon Islands, and Vanuatu; the risk is intermediate in Haiti and the Indian subcontinent and is low in most of Southeast Asia and Latin America. Transmission is possible in more temperate climates, including areas in the United States where *Anopheles* mosquitoes are present. Mosquitoes in airplanes flying from tropical climates have been the source of occasional cases in persons working or residing near international airports. However, nearly all of the approximately 1000 annual reported cases in the United States are imported after infection acquired abroad. Other less common modes of malaria transmission are congenital, through transfusions, or through the use of contaminated needles or syringes.

Plasmodium vivax and *P falciparum* are the most common species worldwide. *Plasmodium vivax* malaria is prevalent on the Indian subcontinent and in Central America, and *P falciparum* malaria is prevalent in Africa, Haiti, and Papua New Guinea. Malaria due to *P vivax* and *P falciparum* is common in south Asia, Southeast Asia, Oceania, and South America. *Plasmodium malariae,* although much less common, has a wide distribution. *Plasmodium ovale* malaria occurs most often in West Africa but has been reported in other areas.

Relapses may occur in *P vivax* and *P ovale* malaria because of a persistent hepatic stage of infection. Recrudescence of *P falciparum* and *P malariae* infection occurs when a persistent low-concentration parasitemia causes recurrence of the disease. In hyperendemic areas of Africa and Asia, reinfection in persons with partial immunity often results in a high prevalence of asymptomatic parasitemia.

The spread of chloroquine-resistant *P falciparum* strains throughout the world is of increasing importance. Resistance to other antimalarial drugs is now occurring in many areas where the drugs are used widely. Chloroquine-resistant *P vivax* has been reported in Indonesia, Papua New Guinea, Solomon Islands, and Myanmar.

DIAGNOSTIC TESTS: Definitive diagnosis relies on identification of the parasite on stained blood films. Both thick and thin blood films should be examined. The thick film allows for concentration of the blood to find the parasite that may be present in small numbers, whereas the thin film is most useful for species identification and determination of the level of parasitemia (the percentage of erythrocytes harboring parasites). If the initial blood smears are negative for *Plasmodium* species but malaria remains a possibility, the smear should be repeated every 12 to 24 hours during a 72-hour period. Although rapid screening tests for malarial parasites are being evaluated, blood smears should continue to be performed because data are insufficient to justify using only the quick methods. In hyperendemic areas, the presence of malaria on a blood smear is not conclusive evidence of malaria as a cause of the presenting illness because other infections often are superimposed on low-concentration parasitemia in children with partial immunity. Confirmation and identification of the species of malaria parasites on the blood smear is important in guiding therapy. Serologic testing generally is not helpful, except in epidemiologic surveys. New diagnostic tests in development, including those using polymerase chain reaction, DNA probes, and malarial ribosomal RNA, may provide rapid and accurate diagnosis in the future.

TREATMENT: The choice of malaria chemotherapy is based on the infecting species, possible drug resistance, and the severity of disease (see Drugs for Parasitic Infections, p 693). Severe malaria is defined as a parasitemia greater than 5%, signs of central nervous system or other end-organ involvement, shock, acidosis, and/or hypoglycemia. Patients with severe malaria require intensive care and parenteral treatment until the parasite density falls below 1% and they are able to tolerate oral therapy. Exchange transfusion may be warranted when parasitemia exceeds 10%. Other adjunctive therapies, such as iron chelation, are under investigation but are not yet recommended. For patients with *P falciparum* malaria, sequential blood smears are indicated to monitor treatment. A few new antimalarial drugs are undergoing clinical trials for treatment and chemoprophylaxis of malaria.

ISOLATION OF THE HOSPITALIZED PATIENT: Standard precautions are recommended.

CONTROL MEASURES: Control of the *Anopheles* mosquito population, treatment of infected persons, and chemoprophylaxis of travelers in endemic areas are effective. Measures to prevent contact with mosquitoes, especially from dusk to dawn (because of the nocturnal biting habits of the *Anopheles* mosquito), through the use of bed nets impregnated with insecticide, mosquito repellents, and protective clothing also are beneficial and should be optimized. The most current information on country-specific risks, drug resistance, and resulting recommendations for travelers can be obtained by contacting the 24-hour service of the Centers for Disease Control and Prevention (CDC, see Directory of Resources, p 743).

Chemoprophylaxis for Travelers to Endemic Areas. * The appropriate chemoprophylactic regimen is determined by the traveler's risk of acquiring malaria in the area(s) to be visited and by the risk of exposure to chloroquine-resistant *P falciparum.* Indications for prophylaxis for children are identical to those for adults. Chemoprophylaxis should begin 1 week before arrival in the endemic area (except doxycycline, which should be started 1–2 days before arrival), allowing time for development of adequate blood concentration of the drug and evaluation of any adverse reactions.

Travelers to areas where chloroquine-resistant malaria species have not been reported should take chloroquine, once weekly, starting 1 week before exposure, for the duration of exposure, and for 4 weeks after departure from the endemic area.

Travelers to areas where chloroquine-resistant *P falciparum* exists should take mefloquine, once weekly, starting 1 week before travel, continuing weekly during travel, and for 4 weeks after travel has concluded (see Drugs for Parasitic Infections,

* For further information on prevention of malaria in travelers, see the annual publication of the US Public Health Service, *Health Information for International Travel, 1999–2000.* Atlanta, GA: US Dept of Health and Human Services, Public Health Service, Centers for Disease Control and Prevention, National Center for Infectious Diseases, Division of Quarantine; 1999, or visit the CDC Web site (www.cdc.gov/travel/index.htm).

p 693). Mefloquine is not approved by the US Food and Drug Administration (FDA) for children who weigh less than 15 kg (33 lb), but recent recommendations of the World Health Organization (WHO) and the CDC allow it to be considered for use in children without weight (>5 kg for WHO recommendations) or age restrictions when travel to areas of chloroquine-resistant *P falciparum* cannot be avoided. Mefloquine is contraindicated for use by travelers with a known hypersensitivity to mefloquine or a history of epilepsy or severe psychiatric disorders. Although a warning about concurrent use with ß-blockers is given in the product labeling, a review of available data suggest that mefloquine may be used by persons concurrently receiving ß-blockers if they have no underlying arrhythmia. Mefloquine is not recommended for use by persons with cardiac conduction abnormalities until additional data are available. Caution may be advised for travelers involved in tasks requiring fine motor coordination and spatial discrimination, such as airline pilots. Patients in whom mefloquine prophylaxis fails should be monitored closely if they are treated with quinidine or quinine because either drug may exacerbate the known adverse effects of mefloquine. Because of the frequency of adverse effects, mefloquine should not be used for presumptive self-treatment.

For short-term travelers unable to take mefloquine, doxycycline alone is the preferred alternative regimen (see Drugs for Parasitic Infections, p 693). Travelers taking doxycycline should be advised of the need for strict compliance with daily dosing (in a single dose), the advisability of always taking the drug on a full stomach, and the possible adverse effects, including diarrhea, photosensitivity, and increased risk of monilial vaginitis. Use of doxycycline should be avoided for pregnant women and for children younger than 8 years of age because of the risk of dental staining (see Antimicrobial Agents and Related Therapy, p 646).

Children who cannot take mefloquine or doxycycline can be given chloroquine (with proguanil for travel to sub-Saharan Africa) for prophylaxis, although these drugs are much less effective against chloroquine-resistant malaria. Children should avoid travel to areas with chloroquine-resistant *P falciparum* unless they can take a highly effective drug, such as mefloquine or doxycycline.

Prophylaxis During Pregnancy. Malaria infection in pregnant women may be more severe than in nonpregnant women. Malaria may increase the risk of adverse outcomes in pregnancy, including prematurity, abortion, and stillbirth. For these reasons and because no chemoprophylactic regimen is completely effective, women who are pregnant or likely to become pregnant should avoid travel to areas where they could contract malaria. Women traveling to areas where drug-resistant *P falciparum* has not been reported may take chloroquine prophylaxis. Harmful effects on the fetus have not been demonstrated when chloroquine is given in the recommended doses for malaria prophylaxis. Pregnancy, therefore, is not a contraindication for malaria prophylaxis with chloroquine.

Mefloquine, according to the FDA-approved product labeling, is not recommended for use during pregnancy. However, a review of data from clinical trials and reports of inadvertent use of mefloquine during pregnancy suggests that its use is not associated with adverse fetal or pregnancy outcomes, such as birth defects, stillbirths, and spontaneous abortions, when taken during the second and third trimesters of pregnancy. From the very limited data available so far, mefloquine seems safe during the first trimester of pregnancy. Consequently, mefloquine may be considered for prophylactic use for women who are pregnant or likely to become pregnant when exposure to chloroquine-resistant *P falciparum* is unavoidable.

For other travelers for whom mefloquine is contraindicated and doxycycline is inappropriate (eg, for reasons of age), chloroquine alone or chloroquine plus proguanil have been used as alternatives but are less effective (see Drugs for Parasitic Infections, p 693). In addition, such travelers should carry pyrimethamine-sulfadoxine (Fansidar) for use as presumptive self-treatment if a febrile illness develops while taking chloroquine and professional medical care is not readily available. Resistance to pyrimethamine-sulfadoxine has been reported from Southeast Asia and the Amazon Basin, and, therefore, it should not be used for treatment of malaria acquired in these areas. Travelers should be advised that self-treatment is not considered a replacement for seeking prompt medical help. Pyrimethamine-sulfadoxine should not be taken for routine prophylaxis or by patients with known intolerance to either drug or to other sulfonamide drugs, infants younger than 2 months of age, or pregnant women at term, unless circumstances suggest the potential benefit outweighs the possible risk of hyperbilirubinemia in the infant.

Prevention of Relapses. To prevent relapses of *P vivax* or *P ovale* infection after departure from areas where these species are endemic, use of primaquine phosphate should be considered. Primaquine can cause hemolysis in patients with glucose-6-phosphate dehydrogenase deficiency; thus, all patients should be screened for this condition before primaquine therapy is initiated.

Personal Protective Measures. All travelers to areas where malaria is endemic should be advised to use personal protective measures, including the following: (1) using insecticide-impregnated mosquito nets while sleeping, (2) remaining in well-screened areas, (3) wearing protective clothing, and (4) using mosquito repellents containing DEET.* To be effective, most of these repellents require reapplication frequently. Since adverse reactions, including toxic encephalopathy, seizures, and rashes have been reported with the use of high concentrations of DEET in children, DEET should be used according to the product label. Travelers, particularly children, should be advised against using products containing high concentrations of DEET (>35%) directly on skin. The risk of serious adverse effects is exceedingly low when used according to FDA-approved product label instructions.

Measles

CLINICAL MANIFESTATIONS: Measles is an acute disease characterized by a temperature of 38.3°C or more (≥101°F), cough, coryza, conjunctivitis, an erythematous maculopapular rash, and a pathognomonic enanthem (Koplik spots). Complications, such as otitis media, bronchopneumonia, laryngotracheobronchitis (croup), and diarrhea, occur more commonly in young children. Acute encephalitis, which frequently results in permanent brain damage, occurs in approximately 1 of every 1000 cases. Death, predominantly due to respiratory and neurologic complications, occurs in 1 to 3 of every 1000 cases reported in the United States. Case-fatality rates are increased in children younger than 5 years of age and immunocompromised

* N, N-diethyl-meta-toluamide.

children, including those with leukemia and human immunodeficiency virus (HIV) infection. Sometimes the characteristic rash does not develop in immunocompromised patients.

Subacute sclerosing panencephalitis (SSPE), a rare degenerative central nervous system disease characterized by behavioral and intellectual deterioration and seizures, is a result of a persistent measles virus infection that develops years after the original infection. Widespread measles immunization has led to its virtual disappearance in the United States.

ETIOLOGY: Measles virus is an RNA virus with 1 serotype, classified as a member of the genus Morbillivirus in the Paramyxovirus family.

EPIDEMIOLOGY: The only natural hosts of measles virus are humans and primates. Measles is transmitted by direct contact with infectious droplets or, less commonly, by airborne spread. In temperate areas, the peak incidence of infection usually occurs during the late winter and spring. In the prevaccine era, measles was an epidemic disease with biennial cycles in urban areas. Most cases occurred in preschool- and young school-age children, and few persons remained susceptible by age 20 years. The childhood immunization program in the United States has resulted in a greater than 99% reduction in the reported incidence of measles since measles vaccine was first licensed in 1963.

From 1989 to 1991, the incidence of measles in the United States increased due to low immunization rates in preschool-age children, especially in urban areas. Since 1992, the incidence of measles in the United States has been low (<1000 reported cases per year). Indigenous measles transmission likely was interrupted in 1993, and record low numbers of cases were reported in 1997 and in 1998. Cases of measles continue to occur from importation of the virus from other countries. Cases are considered imported from another country if the rash onset occurs within 18 days after entering the United States and illness cannot be linked to local transmission.

Vaccine failure occurs in as many as 5% of persons who have received a single dose of vaccine at 12 months of age or older. Although possible waning immunity after immunization may be a factor in some cases, most cases of measles in previously immunized children seem to occur in those in whom response to the vaccine was inadequate, ie, primary vaccine failures. Vaccine failure after 2 doses of measles vaccine administered after 12 months of age is uncommon.

Patients are contagious from 1 to 2 days before the onset of symptoms (3 to 5 days before the rash) to 4 days after appearance of the rash. Immunocompromised patients who may have prolonged excretion of the virus in respiratory tract secretions can be contagious for the duration of the illness. Patients with SSPE are not contagious.

The **incubation period** is generally 8 to 12 days from exposure to onset of symptoms. In family studies, the average interval between appearance of rash in the source case and subsequent cases is 14 days, with a range of 7 to 18 days. In SSPE, the mean incubation period of 84 cases reported between 1976 and 1983 was 10.8 years.

DIAGNOSTIC TESTS: Measles virus infection can be diagnosed by a positive serologic test result for measles immunoglobulin (Ig) M antibody, a significant increase in measles IgG antibody level in paired acute (collected within 4 days of rash onset) and convalescent (collected 2 to 4 weeks later) serum specimens by any standard serologic assay, or isolation of measles virus from clinical specimens, such as urine, blood or nasopharyngeal secretions. The state public health laboratory or the Centers for Disease Control and Prevention Measles Laboratory will process these viral specimens free of charge. For more information, contact the state health department. The simplest method to establish the diagnosis is to test for IgM antibody on a single serum specimen collected during the first encounter with a person suspected of having measles. The sensitivity of measles IgM assays varies and may be diminished during the first 72 hours after rash onset. If the result is negative for measles IgM and the patient has a generalized rash lasting more than 72 hours, the measles IgM test should be repeated. Measles IgM is detectable for at least 1 month after rash onset. Persons with febrile rash illness who are seronegative for measles IgM should be tested for rubella using the same specimens. Virus isolation from clinical specimens is useful for tracking the distribution of different measles virus genotypes to determine patterns of importation and transmission. All cases of suspected measles should be reported immediately to the local or state health department, without waiting for the results of diagnostic tests.

TREATMENT: No specific antiviral therapy is available. Measles virus is susceptible in vitro to ribavirin, which has been given by the intravenous and aerosol routes to treat severely affected and immunocompromised children with measles. However, no controlled trials have been conducted, and ribavirin is not approved by the US Food and Drug Administration for treatment of measles.

Vitamin A. The World Health Organization (WHO) and the United Nations International Children's Emergency Fund (UNICEF) recommend administration of vitamin A to all children diagnosed with measles in communities where vitamin A deficiency is a recognized problem and where mortality related to measles is 1% or greater. Vitamin A treatment of children with measles in developing countries has been associated with reduction in morbidity and mortality. Although vitamin A deficiency is not recognized as a major problem in the United States, low serum concentrations of vitamin A have been found in children with severe measles. Hence, vitamin A supplementation should be considered in the following circumstances:

- Patients 6 months to 2 years of age hospitalized with measles and its complications (eg, croup, pneumonia, and diarrhea). Limited data are available about the safety and need for vitamin A supplementation for infants younger than 6 months of age.
- Patients older than 6 months of age with measles who have any of the following risk factors and who are not already receiving vitamin A supplementation: immunodeficiency, clinical evidence of vitamin A deficiency, impaired intestinal absorption, moderate to severe malnutrition, and recent immigration from areas where high mortality rates due to measles have been observed.

Parenteral and oral formulations of vitamin A are available in the United States. The recommended dosage is similar to that recommended by the WHO and UNICEF. The oral form is a capsule.

- Single dose of 200 000 IU, orally, for children 1 year of age and older (100 000 IU for children 6 months to 1 year of age). The higher dose may be associated with vomiting and headache for a few hours.
- The dose should be repeated the next day and at 4 weeks for children with ophthalmologic evidence of vitamin A deficiency.

ISOLATION OF THE HOSPITALIZED PATIENT: In addition to standard precautions, airborne precautions are indicated for 4 days after the onset of the rash in otherwise healthy children and for the duration of illness in immunocompromised patients.

CONTROL MEASURES:

Care of Exposed Persons.

Use of Vaccine. Exposure to measles is not a contraindication to immunization. Available data suggest that live-virus measles vaccine, if given within 72 hours of measles exposure, will provide protection in some cases. If the exposure does not result in infection, the vaccine should induce protection against subsequent measles exposures. Vaccine is the intervention of choice for control of measles outbreaks in schools and child care centers. In addition to vaccine, susceptible household contacts also should receive Immune Globulin (IG) since identification of the index case usually occurs after 72 hours.

Use of IG. Immune Globulin can be given to prevent or modify measles in a susceptible person within 6 days of exposure. The usual recommended dose is 0.25 mL/kg of body weight given intramuscularly; immunocompromised children should receive 0.5 mL/kg (the maximum dose in either instance is 15 mL). Immune Globulin is indicated for susceptible household contacts of patients with measles, particularly contacts younger than 1 year of age, pregnant women, and immunocompromised persons for whom the risk of complications is highest. Infants younger than 5 months of age usually have partial or complete protection as a result of passively acquired measles antibodies. However, infants who are younger than 5 months of age whose mothers develop measles also should receive IG because they are not protected by passive immunity.

Immune Globulin is not indicated for household contacts who have received 1 dose of vaccine at 12 months of age or older unless they are immunocompromised.

Immune Globulin Intravenous (IGIV) preparations generally contain measles antibodies at approximately the same concentration per gram of protein as IG, although the concentration may vary by lot and manufacturer. For patients who regularly receive IGIV, the usual dose of 100 to 400 mg/kg should be more than sufficient for measles prophylaxis after exposures occurring within 3 weeks of receiving IGIV.

HIV Infection.* All children and adolescents with HIV infection and children of unknown infection status born to HIV-infected women who are exposed to wild type measles should receive IGIV (400 mg/kg) or IG prophylaxis (0.5 mL/kg, maximum dose 15 mL), regardless of their immunization status (see HIV Infection,

* American Academy of Pediatrics Committee on Infectious Diseases and Committee on Pediatric AIDS. Measles immunization in HIV-infected children. *Pediatrics.* 1999;103:1057–1060

p 325). An exception is the patient receiving IGIV (400 mg/kg) at regular intervals whose last dose was received within 3 weeks of exposure. Because of the rapid metabolism of IGIV, some experts recommend administration of an additional dose of IGIV if 2 or more weeks have elapsed since IGIV has been administered at the time of measles exposure.

For children who receive IG for modification or prevention of measles after exposure, measles vaccine (if not contraindicated) should be given 5 months (if the dose was 0.25 mL/kg) or 6 months (if the dose was 0.5 mL/kg) after IG administration, provided that the child is at least 12 months old. Longer intervals are required after larger doses of IGIV (see Table 3.35, p 390).

Hospital Personnel. To decrease nosocomial infection, immunization programs should be established to ensure that health care personnel who will be in contact with patients with measles are immune to the disease (see Health Care Personnel, p 74).

Measles Vaccine. The only measles vaccine currently licensed in the United States is a live further-attenuated strain prepared in chick embryo cell culture. Measles vaccines provided through the Expanded Programme on Immunization in developing countries meet the WHO standards and usually are comparable to the vaccine available in the United States. Measles vaccine is available in monovalent (measles only) formulation and in combination formulations, ie, measles-rubella (MR) and measles-mumps-rubella (MMR) vaccines.

The MMR vaccine is the recommended product of choice in most circumstances, especially when administered at 12 months of age or older and including the routinely recommended second dose of measles vaccine, to also provide optimal protection against mumps and rubella. Vaccine (as a combination or monovalent product) in a dose of 0.5 mL is given subcutaneously. Measles and measles-containing vaccines can be given simultaneously with other vaccines (see Simultaneous Administration of Multiple Vaccines, p 26).

Serum measles antibodies develop in approximately 95% of children immunized at 12 months of age and 98% of those immunized at 15 months of age. Protection conferred by a single dose is durable in most persons. However, a very small percentage of immunized persons may lose protection after several years. More than 99% of persons who receive 2 doses separated by at least 1 month (4 weeks) with both doses on or after their first birthday develop serologic evidence of measles immunity. Immunization is not deleterious for persons who already are immune.

Improperly stored vaccine may fail to protect against measles. Since 1979, an improved stabilizer has been added to the vaccine that makes it more resistant to heat inactivation. However, during storage before reconstitution, measles vaccine should be kept at 2°C to 8°C (36°F–46°F) or colder. Freezing is not harmful to the lyophilized vaccine. The vaccine diluent (sterile water) vials may break if frozen and, therefore, should not be frozen. Measles vaccine also must be protected from ultraviolet light (especially after reconstitution), which can inactivate the virus. Vaccine should be shipped at 10°C (50°F) or colder and may be shipped on dry ice. Reconstituted vaccine should be stored in a refrigerator and discarded if not used within 8 hours.

Vaccine Recommendations (see Table 3.36, p 391, for summary).

Table 3.35. **Suggested Intervals Between Immunoglobulin Administration and Measles Immunization (MMR or Monovalent Measles Vaccine)***

Indication for Immunoglobulin	Route	Dose: U or mL	Dose: mg IgG/kg	Interval, mo†
Tetanus (as TIG)	IM	250 U	~10	3
Hepatitis A prophylaxis (as IG)				
Contact prophylaxis	IM	0.02 mL/kg	3.3	3
International travel	IM	0.06 mL/kg	10	3
Hepatitis B prophylaxis (as HBIG)	IM	0.06 mL/kg	10	3
Rabies prophylaxis (as RIG)	IM	20 IU/kg	22	4
Measles prophylaxis (as IG)				
Standard	IM	0.25 mL/kg	40	5
Immunocompromised host	IM	0.50 mL/kg	80	6
Varicella prophylaxis (as VZIG)	IM	125 U/10 kg (maximum, 625 U)	20–39	5
Blood transfusion				
Washed RBCs	IV	10 mL/kg	Negligible	0
RBCs, adenine-saline added	IV	10 mL/kg	10	3
Packed RBCs	IV	10 mL/kg	20–60	5
Whole blood	IV	10 mL/kg	80–100	6
Plasma or platelet products	IV	10 mL/kg	160	7
Replacement (or therapy) of immune deficiencies (as IGIV)	IV	...	300–400	8
ITP (as IGIV)	IV	...	400	8
RSV-IGIV	IV	...	750	9
ITP	IV	...	1000	10
ITP or Kawasaki disease	IV	...	1600–2000	11

* MMR indicates measles-mumps-rubella; IgG, immunoglobulin G; IG, Immune Globulin; TIG, Tetanus IG; IM, intramuscular; HBIG, Hepatitis B IG; RIG, Rabies IG; VZIG, Varicella-Zoster IG; RBC, Red Blood Cell; IV, intravenous; IGIV, IG intravenous; ITP, immune (formerly termed "idiopathic") thrombocytopenic purpura; and RSV-IGIV, Respiratory Syncytial Virus IGIV.

† These intervals should provide sufficient time for decreases in passive antibodies in all children to allow for an adequate response to measles vaccine. Physicians should not assume that children are fully protected against measles during these intervals. Additional doses of IG or measles vaccine may be indicated after exposure to measles (see text).

Age of Routine Immunization. The first dose should be given at 12 to 15 months of age. Delays in administering the first dose contributed to large outbreaks from 1989 to 1991. Initial immunization at 12 months of age is recommended for preschool-age children in high-risk areas, especially large urban areas. The second dose is recommended routinely at school entry (ie, 4 to 6 years of age) but can be given at any earlier age (eg, during an outbreak or before international travel), provided the interval between the first and second doses is at least 1 month (4 weeks). Children who were not reimmunized at school entry should receive the

Table 3.36. **Recommendations for Measles Immunization***

Category	Recommendations
Unimmunized, no history of measles (12–15 mo of age)	A 2-dose schedule (with MMR) is recommended if born after 1956. The first dose is recommended at 12–15 mo of age; the second is recommended at 4–6 y of age
Children 6–11 mo of age in epidemic situations†	Immunize (with monovalent measles vaccine or, if not available, MMR); reimmunization (with MMR) at 12–15 mo of age is necessary, and a third dose is indicated at 4–6 y of age
Children 4–12 y of age who have received 1 dose of measles vaccine at ≥12 mo of age	Reimmunize (1 dose)
Students in college and other post–high school institutions who have received 1 dose of measles vaccine at ≥12 mo of age	Reimmunize (1 dose)
History of immunization before the first birthday	Consider susceptible and immunize (2 doses)
Unknown vaccine, 1963–1967	Consider susceptible and immunize (2 doses)
Further attenuated or unknown vaccine given with IG	Consider susceptible and immunize (2 doses)
Allergy to eggs	Immunize; no reactions likely (see text for details)
Neomycin allergy, nonanaphylactic	Immunize; no reactions likely
Tuberculosis	Immunize; vaccine does not exacerbate infection
Measles exposure	Immunize and/or give IG, depending on circumstances (see text, p 388)
HIV-infected	Immunize (2 doses) unless severely immunocompromised (see text, p 394)
Immunoglobulin or blood	Immunize at the appropriate interval (see Table 3.35, p 390).

* See text for details. MMR indicates measles-mumps-rubella vaccine; IG, Immune Globulin; HIV, human immunodeficiency virus.

† See Outbreak Control (p 395).

second dose by 11 to 12 years of age. If the child receives a dose of measles vaccine before 12 months of age, 2 additional doses are required beginning at 12 to 15 months of age and separated by at least 1 month. By 2001, all school-age children should have received 2 doses of measles-containing vaccine.

High School Students and Older Persons. Because of the continuing occurrence of cases in older children and young adults, emphasis must be placed on identifying and appropriately immunizing potentially susceptible adolescents and young adults in high school, college, and health care settings.

Persons should be considered susceptible unless they have documentation of appropriate immunization, physician-diagnosed measles, laboratory evidence of immunity to measles, or were born before 1957. For children, adolescents, and adults born after 1956, 2 doses of measles vaccine are required for evidence of immunity.

A parental report of immunization is not considered adequate documentation. Physicians should provide an immunization record for patients only if they have administered the vaccine or have seen a record documenting immunization.

Colleges and Other Institutions for Education Beyond High School. Colleges and other institutions should require that all entering students have documentation of physician-diagnosed measles, serologic evidence of immunity, birth before 1957, or receipt of 2 doses of measles-containing vaccines. Students without documentation of any measles immunization or immunity should receive a dose on entry, followed by a repeated dose 1 or more months (4 weeks) later.

Immunization During an Outbreak. During an outbreak, monovalent measles vaccine may be given to infants as young as 6 months of age (see Outbreak Control, p 395). If monovalent vaccine is not available, MMR may be given. However, seroconversion rates after MMR immunization are significantly lower in children immunized before the first birthday than are seroconversion rates in children immunized after the first birthday. Children, therefore, immunized before their first birthday should be immunized with MMR vaccine at 12 to 15 months and again at school entry (4 to 6 years).

International Travel. Persons traveling to foreign countries should be immune to measles. For young children traveling to areas where measles is endemic or epidemic, the age for initial measles immunization may need to be lowered. Infants 6 to 11 months of age should receive a dose of monovalent measles (or MMR) vaccine before departure; then they should receive MMR vaccine at 12 to 15 months of age (at least 1 month [4 weeks] after the initial measles immunization) and again at 4 to 6 years of age. Children 12 to 15 months of age should be given their first dose of MMR vaccine before departure. Children who have received 1 dose and are traveling to areas where measles is endemic or epidemic should receive their second dose before departure, provided the interval between doses is 1 month (4 weeks) or more.

Health Care Facilities. Evidence of having had measles, measles immunity, or receipt of 2 measles immunizations is recommended before beginning employment for all health care professionals born after 1956 (see Health Care Personnel, p 74). For recommendations during an outbreak, see Outbreak Control (p 395).

Adverse Events. A temperature of 39.4°C (103°F) or higher develops in approximately 5% to 15% of susceptible vaccine recipients, usually between 6 and 12 days after MMR immunization; the fever generally lasts 1 to 2 days but may last for as many as 5 days. Most persons with fever are otherwise asymptomatic. Transient rashes have been reported in approximately 5% of vaccine recipients. Transient thrombocytopenia has occurred after administration of measles-containing vaccines, specifically MMR (see Thrombocytopenia, p 394). The reported frequency of central nervous system conditions, including encephalitis and encephalopathy, is less than 1 per million doses administered in the United States. Because the incidence of encephalitis or encephalopathy after measles immunization in the United States is lower than the observed incidence of encephalitis of unknown cause, some or most of the rare reported severe neurologic disorders may be related coincidentally, rather than causally, to measles immunization. After reimmunization, reactions are expected to be clinically similar but much less frequent in occurrence because most of these vaccine recipients already are immune.

High-titer vaccines administered during the mid 1980s in several developing countries were associated with increased mortality in females several months to years after immunization. These high-titer vaccines were never licensed in the United States and are no longer in use in foreign countries.

Seizures. As with any condition that induces fever during the second year of life, children predisposed to febrile seizures can experience seizures after measles immunization. Most are simple febrile seizures and do not increase the risk of subsequent epilepsy or other neurologic disorders. Children with personal histories of seizures or children whose first-degree relatives have histories of seizures may be at a slightly increased risk of a seizure but should be immunized because the benefits greatly outweigh the risks.

Subacute Sclerosing Panencephalitis. Measles vaccine, by protecting against measles, significantly reduces the possibility of developing SSPE.

Measles vaccine is not associated with an increased risk of autism or inflammatory bowel disease.

Precautions and Contraindications (see also Table 3.35 p 390).

Febrile Illnesses. Children with minor illnesses, with or without fever, such as upper respiratory tract infections, may be immunized (see Vaccine Safety and Contraindications, p 30). Fever per se is not a contraindication to immunization. However, if other manifestations suggest a more serious illness, the child should not be immunized until recovery.

Allergic Reactions. Hypersensitivity reactions occur rarely and usually are minor, consisting of wheal and flare reactions or urticaria at the injection site. Reactions have been attributed to trace amounts of neomycin or gelatin, or some other component in the vaccine formulation. Anaphylaxis is rare. Measles vaccine is produced in chick embryo cell culture and does not contain significant amounts of egg white (ovalbumin) cross-reacting proteins. Children with egg allergy are at low risk for anaphylactic reactions to measles-containing vaccines (including MMR), and skin testing of children allergic to eggs is not predictive of reactions to MMR vaccine. Persons with allergies to chickens or feathers are not at increased risk of reaction to the vaccine.

Children who have had a significant hypersensitivity reaction following the first dose of measles vaccine should be (1) tested for measles immunity and, if immune, not receive a second dose or (2) receive evaluation and possible skin testing before receiving a second dose. Children who have had an immediate anaphylactic reaction to prior measles immunization should not be reimmunized but require testing to determine whether they are immune.

Persons who have experienced anaphylactic reactions to topically or systemically administered neomycin should receive measles vaccine only in settings where such reactions could be managed and after consultation with an allergist or immunologist. Most often, however, neomycin allergy manifests as a contact dermatitis, which is not a contraindication to receiving measles vaccine.

Thrombocytopenia. Rarely, MMR vaccine can cause clinically apparent transient and benign thrombocytopenia within 2 months of immunization. In prospective studies, the reported incidence was 1 case per 25 000 to 40 000 immunized children, with a temporal clustering 2 to 3 weeks after immunization. By passive surveillance, the reported rate was approximately 1 per 100 000 doses distributed in Canada and 1 per 2 million doses distributed in the United States. Based on case reports, the risk of vaccine-associated thrombocytopenia may be higher for persons who previously experienced thrombocytopenia, especially when it occurred in temporal association with earlier MMR immunization. The decision to immunize these children should be based on the benefits of protection against measles, mumps, and rubella in comparison with the risks of a recurrence of thrombocytopenia after immunization. No reports of thrombocytopenia associated with receipt of MMR vaccine have resulted in death.

Recent Administration of IG. Immune Globulin preparations interfere with the serologic response to measles vaccine for variable periods depending on the dose administered. Suggested intervals between IG or blood product administration and measles immunization are given in Table 3.35 (p 390). If vaccine is given at less than the indicated intervals, as may be warranted if the risk of exposure to measles is imminent, the child should be reimmunized at or after the appropriate interval for immunization unless serologic testing indicates that measles-specific antibodies were produced.

If IG is to be administered in preparation for international travel, administration of vaccine should precede receipt of IG by at least 2 weeks to preclude interference with replication of the vaccine virus.

Tuberculosis. Tuberculin skin testing is not a prerequisite for measles immunization, and measles vaccine does not exacerbate tuberculosis. If tuberculin skin testing is otherwise indicated, it can be done on the day of immunization. Otherwise, testing should be postponed for 4 to 6 weeks because measles immunization temporarily may suppress tuberculin skin test reactivity.

Altered Immunity. Immunocompromised patients with disorders associated with increased severity of viral infections should not be given live measles virus vaccine while immunodeficient (see Immunocompromised Children, p 56). Their risk of exposure to measles can be reduced by immunizing their close susceptible contacts. Management of immunodeficient and immunosuppressed patients exposed to measles can be facilitated by prior knowledge of their immune status. Susceptible patients with immunodeficiencies should receive IG after measles exposure (see Care of Exposed Persons, p 388).

Corticosteroids. For patients who have received high doses of corticosteroids for 14 days or more and who are not otherwise immunocompromised, the recommended interval before immunization is at least 1 month (see Immunocompromised Children, see p 56).

HIV Infection. Measles immunization (given as MMR vaccine) is recommended at the usual ages for persons with asymptomatic HIV infection and for those with symptomatic infection who are not severely immunocompromised because measles can be severe and often fatal in patients with HIV infection (see HIV Infection, p 325). Severely immunocompromised HIV-infected infants, children, adolescents, and young adults, as defined by low CD4+ T-lymphocyte counts or percentage of total lymphocytes, should not receive measles virus–containing vaccine because vaccine-related pneumonitis has been reported (see HIV Infection, p 325).* All members of the household of an HIV-infected person should receive measles vaccine *unless* they are HIV-infected and severely immunosuppressed, were born before 1957, have had physician-diagnosed measles, have laboratory evidence of measles immunity, have had age-appropriate immunizations, or have a contraindication to measles vaccine.

Regardless of immunization status, symptomatic HIV-infected patients who are exposed to measles should receive IG prophylaxis because immunization may not provide protection (see Care of Exposed Persons, p 388).

Personal or Family History of Seizures. Children with this history should be immunized after advising the parents or guardians that the risk of seizures after measles immunization is increased slightly (see Adverse Events, p 392). Because fever induced by measles vaccine usually occurs between 6 and 12 days after immunization, prevention of vaccine-related febrile seizures is difficult. Parents should be alert to the occurrence of fever after immunization and should treat their children appropriately. Children receiving anticonvulsants should continue such therapy after measles immunization. Prophylactic use of anticonvulsants may not be feasible, because therapeutic concentrations (eg, phenobarbital) are not achieved for some time after initiation of therapy.

Pregnancy. Live-virus measles vaccine, when given as a component of MR or MMR, should not be given to women known to be pregnant or who are considering becoming pregnant within 3 months of immunization. Women who are given monovalent measles vaccine should not become pregnant for at least 30 days. This precaution is based on the theoretical risk of fetal infection, which applies to the administration of any live-virus vaccine to women who might be pregnant or who might become pregnant shortly after immunization. No evidence, however, substantiates this theoretical risk. In the immunization of adolescents and young adults against measles, asking women if they are pregnant, excluding those who are, and explaining the theoretical risks to the others are recommended precautions.

Outbreak Control. Every suspected measles case should be reported immediately to the local health department, and every effort must be made to verify that the illness is measles, especially if this is the first case in the community. Subsequent prevention of the spread of measles depends on prompt immunization of exposed and potentially exposed persons who cannot readily provide documentation of measles immunity, including the date of immunization. Unimmunized persons who have been exempted from measles immunization for medical, religious, or other reasons, if not immunized within 72 hours of exposure, should be excluded from the setting until at least 2 weeks after the onset of rash in the last case of measles.

Schools and Child Care Facilities. During measles outbreaks in child care facilities, schools, and colleges and other institutions of higher education, all students, their siblings, and personnel born after 1956 who cannot provide documentation that they received 2 doses of measles-containing vaccine on or after their first birthday or other evidence of measles immunity should be immunized. Persons receiving

* American Academy of Pediatrics Committee on Infectious Diseases and Committee on Pediatric AIDS. Measles immunization in HIV-infected children. *Pediatrics.* 1999;103:1057–1060

their second dose, as well as unimmunized persons receiving their first dose as part of the outbreak control program, may be readmitted immediately to school.

Health Care Settings. If an outbreak occurs in an area served by a hospital or within a hospital, all employees with direct patient contact who were born after 1956 who cannot provide documentation that they have received 2 doses of measles vaccine on or after their first birthday or other evidence of immunity to measles should receive a dose of measles vaccine. Because some health care personnel who have acquired measles in health care facilities were born before 1957, immunization of older employees who may have occupational exposure to measles also should be considered. Susceptible personnel who have been exposed should be relieved from direct patient contact from the fifth to the 21st day after exposure, regardless of whether they received vaccine or IG after the exposure. Personnel who become ill should be relieved from patient contact for 4 days after rash develops.

Meningococcal Infections

CLINICAL MANIFESTATIONS: Invasive infection usually results in meningococcemia, meningitis, or both. Onset is abrupt in meningococcemia with fever, chills, malaise, prostration, and a rash that initially may be urticarial, maculopapular, or petechial. In fulminant cases, purpura, disseminated intravascular coagulation, shock, coma, and death (Waterhouse-Friderichsen syndrome) can ensue within several hours despite appropriate therapy. The signs of meningococcal meningitis are indistinguishable from those of acute meningitis caused by *Streptococcus pneumoniae* or other meningeal pathogens. Invasive meningococcal infections can be complicated by arthritis, myocarditis, pericarditis, endophthalmitis, and pneumonia. Less common manifestations include pneumonia, occult febrile bacteremia, conjunctivitis, and chronic meningococcemia.

ETIOLOGY: *Neisseria meningitidis* is a gram-negative diplococcus with 13 serogroups (A, B, C, D, 29E, H, I, K, L, W-135, X, Y, and Z). Strains belonging to groups A, B, C, Y, and W-135 are implicated most frequently in systemic disease. The distribution of meningococcal serogroups in the United States has shifted in recent years. Serogroups B, C, and Y each account for approximately 30% of reported cases, but serogroup distribution may vary by location and time. Group A has been associated frequently with epidemics elsewhere in the world, primarily in sub-Saharan Africa.

EPIDEMIOLOGY: Asymptomatic colonization of the upper respiratory tract provides the focus from which the organism is spread. Transmission occurs from person to person through droplets of respiratory tract secretions. Since introduction of *Haemophilus influenzae* type b immunization for infants, *N meningitidis* has become one of the two leading causes of bacterial meningitis in young children and remains an important cause of septicemia. Disease most often occurs in children younger than 5 years of age; the peak attack rate occurs in the 3- to 5-month-old age group. Close contacts of patients with meningococcal disease are at an increased risk for developing infection. Outbreaks have occurred in semiclosed communities, including child care centers, schools, colleges, and military recruit camps. Most cases are sporadic, with fewer than 5% of cases associated with outbreaks. Outbreaks often are heralded by a shift in the age distribution of cases to an older age group. Multilocus enzyme electrophoresis and pulsed-field gel electrophoresis of enzyme-restricted DNA fragments can be used to detect divergence among strains as epidemiologic markers during a suspected outbreak. Patients with deficiency of a terminal complement component (C5-9), properdin deficiencies, or anatomic or functional asplenia are at increased risk for invasive and recurrent meningococcal disease. Patients are considered capable of transmitting the organism for up to 24 hours after initiation of effective treatment.

The **incubation period** is from 1 to 10 days, most commonly less than 4 days.

DIAGNOSTIC TESTS: Cultures of blood and cerebrospinal fluid (CSF) are indicated in all patients with suspected invasive meningococcal disease. Cultures of petechial scraping, synovial fluid, sputum, and other body fluids are positive in some patients. A Gram stain of a petechial scraping, CSF, and buffy coat smear of blood can be helpful on occasion. Since *N meningitidis* can be part of the nasopharyngeal flora, isolation of *N meningitidis* from this site is not helpful. Bacterial antigen detection tests, such as by latex agglutination, may be of value for rapid diagnosis. Detection of meningococcal polysaccharide antigens by a latex agglutination test in urine or serum is not helpful. In contrast, antigen detection in CSF supports the diagnosis of a probable case if the clinical illness is consistent with meningococcal disease. Rapid antigen tests for group B *N meningitidis* may be unreliable. A polymerase chain reaction test has been used in research laboratories to detect *N meningitidis* type B from clinical specimens and currently is used routinely in the United Kingdom.

Case definitions for invasive disease are given in Table 3.37, below.

Table 3.37. Case Definitions for Invasive Meningococcal Disease

Confirmed

- Isolation of *Neisseria meningitidis* from a usually sterile site, eg:
    - Blood
    - Cerebrospinal fluid
    - Synovial fluid
    - Pleural fluid
    - Pericardial fluid
    - Petechial or purpuric lesion

Presumptive

- Gram-negative diplococci in any sterile fluid, such as cerebrospinal fluid, synovial fluid, or aspirate from a petechial or purpuric lesion

Probable

- A positive antigen test for *N meningitidis* in cerebrospinal fluid in the absence of a positive sterile site culture in the setting of a clinical illness consistent with meningococcal disease or clinical purpura fulminans in the absence of a positive blood culture

Susceptibility Testing: Routine susceptibility testing of meningococcal isolates is not indicated. However, *N meningitidis* strains with resistance to penicillin have been identified sporadically from several regions of the United States and have been reported widely from Spain, Italy, and parts of Africa. Selected susceptibility testing of meningococcal isolates should be performed as indicated by the patient's clinical course. Resistant meningococcal strains for which the minimal inhibitory concentration (MIC) to penicillin is more than 1 µg/mL are rare. Most reported isolates are moderately susceptible, with a MIC to penicillin of 0.12 µg/mL or more and less than 1.0 µg/mL. Treatment with high-dose penicillin is effective against moderately susceptible strains. Cefotaxime and ceftriaxone show a high degree of activity against moderately susceptible meningococci. Continued surveillance is necessary to monitor trends in the antimicrobial susceptibility of meningococci in the United States.

Treatment:

- Penicillin G should be administered intravenously in a high dose every 4 to 6 hours for patients with invasive disease. Cefotaxime and ceftriaxone are acceptable alternatives. In a patient with anaphylactoid-type penicillin allergy, chloramphenicol is indicated. Five to 7 days of antimicrobial therapy usually is adequate for most cases of invasive meningococcal disease. For travelers from areas such as Spain, Italy, and parts of Africa, cefotaxime, ceftriaxone, or chloramphenicol is recommended.

Isolation of the Hospitalized Patient: In addition to standard precautions, droplet precautions are recommended until 24 hours after initiation of effective therapy.

Control Measures:

Care of Exposed Persons.

Careful observation. Exposed household, school, or child care contacts must be observed carefully. Exposed persons in whom a febrile illness develops should receive prompt medical evaluation and, if indicated, antimicrobial therapy appropriate for invasive meningococcal infections.

Chemoprophylaxis. The risk of contracting invasive meningococcal disease among contacts of cases is the determining factor in the decision to give chemoprophylaxis (see Table 3.38, p 399). Close contacts of all persons with invasive disease (see Table 3.38), whether sporadic or in an outbreak, are at high risk and should receive prophylaxis within 24 hours of diagnosis of the primary case. Throat and nasopharyngeal cultures are of no value for deciding who should receive prophylaxis.

Household, child care center, and nursery school contacts. Household, child care, and nursery school contacts are at high risk and are considered close contacts. The attack rate for these populations is more than 300 times higher than rates in the general population.

Other contacts. Prophylaxis is warranted for persons who have had contact with the patient's oral secretions through kissing or sharing of toothbrushes or eating utensils, markers of close social contact, during the 7 days before onset of disease

Table 3.38. Disease Risk for Contacts of Index Cases of Invasive Meningococcal Disease*

High risk: chemoprophylaxis recommended (close contact)

- Household contact: especially young children
- Child care or nursery school contact during previous 7 days
- Direct exposure to index patient's secretions through kissing or sharing toothbrushes or eating utensils, markers of close social contact
- Mouth-to-mouth resuscitation, unprotected contact during endotracheal intubation during 7 days before onset of the illness
- Frequently sleeps or eats in same dwelling as index patient

Low risk: chemoprophylaxis not recommended

- Casual contact: no history of direct exposure to index patient's oral secretions, eg, school or work mate
- Indirect contact: only contact is with a high-risk contact, no direct contact with the index patient
- Health care personnel without direct exposure to patient's oral secretions

In outbreak or cluster

- Chemoprophylaxis for persons other than those at high risk should be given only after consultation with the local public health authorities

* Nasopharyngeal aspirate and throat swab cultures are not useful for determining risk.

in the index case. In addition, persons who frequently eat or sleep in the same dwelling within this period should receive chemoprophylaxis. Prophylaxis is not recommended routinely for health care personnel who are considered to be at low risk (Table 3.38) unless they have had intimate exposure, such as occurs with unprotected mouth-to-mouth resuscitation, intubation, or suctioning, before antibiotic therapy was initiated.

Antibiotic regimens (see Table 3.39, p 400). Rifampin, ceftriaxone, and ciprofloxacin are appropriate antibiotics for chemoprophylaxis in adults. The drug of choice in most instances is rifampin. The recommended regimen for rifampin prophylaxis is listed in Table 3.39.

Ceftriaxone given in a single intramuscular dose has been demonstrated to be more effective than oral rifampin in eradicating pharyngeal carriage of group A meningococci. The efficacy of ceftriaxone has been confirmed only for group A strains, but its effect is likely to be similar for other serogroups. Ceftriaxone has the advantages of easier dosage and administration and safety in pregnancy.

Ciprofloxacin given to adults in a single oral dose also is effective in eradicating meningococcal carriage. At present, ciprofloxacin is not recommended for persons younger than 18 years of age or for pregnant women (see Antimicrobial Agents and Related Therapy, p 645).

The index case also should receive chemoprophylaxis before hospital discharge unless the infection was treated with ceftriaxone or cefotaxime.

Table 3.39. **Recommended Chemoprophylaxis Regimens for High-Risk Contacts and Index Cases of Invasive Meningococcal Disease**

Infants, Children, and Adults	Dose	Duration	Percentage of Efficacy	Cautions
Rifampin*				
≤1 mo	5 mg/kg orally every 12 h	2 d		
>1 mo	10 mg/kg (maximum, 600 mg) orally every 12 h	2 d	72–90	May interfere with efficacy of oral contraceptives and some seizure prevention and anticoagulant medications; may stain soft contact lenses
Ceftriaxone				
≤12 y	125 mg intramuscularly	Single dose	97	To decrease pain at injection site, dilute with 1% lidocaine
>12 y	250 mg intramuscularly	Single dose		
Ciprofloxacin*				
≥18 y	500 mg orally	Single dose	90–95	Not recommended for use in persons <18 years of age and pregnant women

*Not recommended for use in pregnant women.

Immunoprophylaxis. Because secondary cases can occur several weeks or more after onset of disease in the index case, meningococcal vaccine is a possible adjunct to chemoprophylaxis when an outbreak is caused by a serogroup contained in the vaccine.

Meningococcal Vaccine. A serogroup-specific quadrivalent meningococcal vaccine against groups A, C, Y, and W-135 *N meningitidis* is approved in the United States for use in children 2 years of age and older. The vaccine consists of 50 µg each of the respective purified bacterial capsular polysaccharides. It is administered subcutaneously as a single 0.5-mL dose and can be given concurrently with other vaccines but at a different site. No vaccine is available for the prevention of group B disease.

A group A meningococcal vaccine is immunogenic in children 3 months of age and older, although a response comparable to that seen in adults is not achieved until 4 or 5 years of age. For children younger than 18 months of age, 2 doses 3 months apart have been given for control of epidemics. When the quadrivalent vaccine is given to infants in a group A outbreak, response to the other meningococcal group polysaccharides usually is poor. The serogroup C polysaccharide does not induce an antibody response before 24 months of age. The groups Y and W135 vaccine polysaccharides have been demonstrated to be immunogenic and safe for children 2 years of age and older.

Indications. Routine immunization of children with meningococcal polysaccharide vaccine is not recommended because the infection rate is low, response is poor in young children, immunity is relatively short-lived, and the response to subsequent vaccine doses may be impaired. However, immunization is recommended for children 2 years of age and older in high-risk groups, including those with functional or anatomic asplenia (see Asplenic Children, p 66), and those with terminal complement component or properdin deficiencies. Immunization of college students is recommended by the American College Health Association. Pediatricians should inform and educate students and parents about the risk of meningococcal disease and the existence of a safe and effective vaccine and immunize students at their request or if educational institutions require it for admission. Immunization may be beneficial for travelers to countries recognized to have hyperendemic or epidemic meningococcal disease caused by a vaccine-preventable serogroup. The vaccine currently is given to all military recruits in the United States.

Reimmunization. Little information is available to determine the need for or timing of reimmunization when the risk of disease continues or recurs. Serum meningococcal antibody in immunized adults seems to persist for as long as 5 years, but in children, especially those initially immunized when younger than 4 years of age, antibody concentrations decline markedly during the first 3 years after immunization. Since reimmunization of young children with quadrivalent vaccine elicits group A but not group C antibodies, only in situations in which there is increased risk of group A disease is reimmunization recommended. Except for outbreak control of group C disease, reimmunization of young children is not recommended. Reimmunization of adults before 5 years after initial immunization does not seem to be necessary even if a new risk of exposure occurs.

Adverse reactions and precautions. Infrequent and mild adverse reactions occur, the most common of which is localized erythema for 1 to 2 days. Studies suggest that altering meningococcal immunization recommendations during pregnancy is unnecessary.

Reporting. All confirmed, presumptive, and probable cases of invasive meningococcal disease must be reported to the regional public health department (see Table 3.37, p 397). Timely reporting can facilitate early recognition of clusters of cases and outbreaks so that appropriate prevention programs can be implemented rapidly.

Counseling and Public Education. When a case of invasive meningococcal disease is detected, the physician needs to provide accurate and timely information about meningococcal disease and the risk of transmission to families and contacts of the index case. Public health questions, such as whether a mass immunization program is needed, should be referred to the local public health department. In appropriate situations, early provision of information in collaboration with the local health department to schools or other groups at increased risk and to the media may help minimize public anxiety and unrealistic or inappropriate demands for intervention.

Microsporidia Infections

(Microsporidiosis)

CLINICAL MANIFESTATIONS: Patients with intestinal infection have watery nonbloody diarrhea. Fever is uncommon. Intestinal infection, often resulting in chronic diarrhea, is most common in immunocompromised persons, especially persons who are infected with the human immunodeficiency virus (HIV). The clinical course is complicated by malnutrition and progressive weight loss. Chronic infection in immunocompetent persons is rare. Other clinical syndromes that can occur in HIV-infected and immunocompetent patients include keratoconjunctivitis, myositis, nephritis, hepatitis, cholangitis, peritonitis, and disseminated disease, but they occur infrequently.

ETIOLOGY: Microsporidia are obligate, intracellular, spore-forming protozoa. The following genera have been implicated in human infection: *Encephalitozoon, Enterocytozoon, Nosema, Pleistophora, Trachipleistophora,* and *Vittaforma,* as have unclassified *"Microsporidium"* species. *Enterocytozoon bieneusi* and *Enterocytozoon (Septata) intestinalis* are important causes of chronic diarrhea in HIV-infected persons.

EPIDEMIOLOGY: Information is limited. In animals such as dogs, pigs, rabbits, and parakeets, transmission occurs by ingestion of Microsporidia spores in food or contact with spores shed into the environment through stools or urine. In humans, fecal-oral contact may have a role in transmission. Spores also have been detected in other body fluids, but their role in transmission is unknown.

The **incubation period** is unknown.

DIAGNOSTIC TESTS: Infection with Microsporidia organisms can be documented by identification of organisms in biopsy specimens from the small intestine. Microsporidia spores also can be detected in formalin-fixed stool specimens or duodenal aspirates stained with a chromotrope-based stain, which is a modification of the trichrome stain, and viewed by light microscopy. Gram, acid-fast, periodic acid–Schiff, and Giemsa stains also can be used to detect organisms in tissue sections. The organisms often are not noticed because they are small, stain poorly, and evoke minimal inflammatory response. Use of one of the stool concentration techniques does not seem to improve the ability to detect *E bieneusi* spores. Identification for classification purposes and diagnostic confirmation of species requires electron microscopy. Reliable serologic tests for the diagnosis of human microsporidiosis are lacking.

TREATMENT: No effective therapy is known. For a limited number of patients, albendazole, metronidazole, and atovaquone have been reported to decrease diarrhea but without eradication of the organism. Albendazole seems to be more effective for cases due to *E intestinalis.* Recurrence of diarrhea is common after therapy is stopped.

ISOLATION OF THE HOSPITALIZED PATIENT: In addition to standard precautions, contact precautions are recommended for diapered and incontinent children for the duration of illness.

CONTROL MEASURES: None have been documented. In HIV-infected persons, reduced exposure may result from attention to hand washing, drinking bottled or boiled water, and thorough cooking of meat.

Molluscum Contagiosum

CLINICAL MANIFESTATIONS: Molluscum contagiosum is a benign, usually asymptomatic viral infection of the skin with no systemic manifestations. It is characterized by relatively few (usually 2 to 20) discrete, flesh-colored to translucent, dome-shaped papules, some with central umbilication. Lesions commonly occur on the trunk, face, and extremities but may be generalized. An eczematous reaction may encircle the lesions in about 10% of patients. Patients with eczema and immunocompromised persons, including persons with human immunodeficiency virus infection, tend to have more intense and widespread eruptions.

ETIOLOGY: The cause is a poxvirus, which is the sole member of the genus Molluscipoxvirus.

EPIDEMIOLOGY: Humans are the only known source of the virus, which is spread by direct contact, including sexual contact, or by fomites, such as towels. Lesions tend to disseminate by autoinoculation. The infectivity generally is low, but occasional outbreaks have been reported. The period of communicability is unknown.

The **incubation period** seems to vary between 2 and 7 weeks but may be as long as 6 months.

DIAGNOSTIC TESTS: The diagnosis usually can be made from the characteristic appearance of the lesions. Wright or Giemsa staining of material expressed from the central core of a lesion reveals characteristic intracytoplasmic inclusions. Electron microscopic examination will identify the typical poxvirus particles.

TREATMENT: Mechanical removal of the central core of each lesion usually results in resolution. EMLA (eutectic mixture of local anesthetics) cream, a topical anesthetic, may be applied 30 minutes to 2 hours before the procedure. Alternatively, topical application of cantharidin (0.7% in collodion), peeling agents such as salicylic and lactic acid preparations, electrocautery, or liquid nitrogen may be successful in removal of lesions. Although lesions can regress spontaneously, treatment may prevent autoinoculation and spread to other persons. Scarring is a rare occurrence.

ISOLATION OF THE HOSPITALIZED PATIENT: Standard precautions are recommended.

CONTROL MEASURES: No control measures are known for isolated cases. For outbreaks, which are common in the tropics, restricting direct body contact and sharing of potentially contaminated fomites (eg, towels and washcloths) may reduce the spread.

Moraxella catarrhalis Infections

CLINICAL MANIFESTATIONS: Common infections include acute otitis media and paranasal sinusitis in children. Bronchopulmonary infection, often occurring in patients with chronic lung disease, can occur. Rare manifestations are bacteremia in immunocompetent or immunocompromised children (sometimes associated with focal infections, such as osteomyelitis, septic arthritis, abscesses, or a rash indistinguishable from that observed in meningococcemia) and conjunctivitis or meningitis in neonates.

ETIOLOGY: *Moraxella catarrhalis* is a gram-negative diplococcus. Almost 100% of strains produce ß-lactamase that mediates resistance to penicillins.

EPIDEMIOLOGY: *Moraxella catarrhalis* is part of the normal flora of the upper respiratory tract of humans. The mode of transmission is presumed to be direct contact with contaminated respiratory tract secretions or droplet spread. Infection is most frequent in infants and young children, but it occurs at all ages. Transmission in families, schools, and child care centers has not been studied. The duration of carriage by infected and colonized children and the period of communicability are unknown.

The **incubation period** is unknown.

DIAGNOSTIC TESTS: The organism can be isolated on blood and chocolate agar culture media after incubation in air or with increased carbon dioxide. Culture of middle ear or sinus aspirates is indicated for patients with unusually severe infection, those in whom the infection fails to respond to treatment, and neonates and other highly susceptible children. Concomitant recovery of *M catarrhalis* with other pathogens (*Streptococcus pneumoniae* or *Haemophilus influenzae*) can occur and indicates a mixed infection.

TREATMENT: Although most strains of *Moraxella* produce ß-lactamase and are resistant to amoxicillin in vitro, this agent remains effective as empiric therapy for otitis media and other respiratory tract infections. When *M catarrhalis* is isolated from appropriately obtained specimens (middle ear fluid, sinus aspirates, or lower respiratory tract secretions), or when initial therapy has been unsuccessful, appropriate antibiotic choices include amoxicillin-clavulanate, cefuroxime, cefprozil, erythromycin, clarithromycin, azithromycin, and trimethoprim-sulfamethoxazole. If parenteral drugs are needed to treat *M catarrhalis* infection, in vitro data indicate that the following drugs are effective: cefuroxime, cefotaxime, ceftriaxone, ceftazidime, and trimethoprim-sulfamethoxazole.

ISOLATION OF THE HOSPITALIZED PATIENT: Standard precautions are recommended.

CONTROL MEASURES: None.

Mumps

CLINICAL MANIFESTATIONS: Mumps is a systemic disease characterized by swelling of one or more of the salivary glands, usually the parotid glands. Approximately one third of infections do not cause clinically apparent salivary gland swelling. More than 50% of persons with mumps have cerebrospinal fluid pleocytosis, but fewer than 10% have clinical evidence of central nervous system infection. Orchitis is a common complication after puberty, but sterility rarely occurs. Other rare complications include arthritis, thyroiditis, mastitis, glomerulonephritis, myocarditis, thrombocytopenia, cerebellar ataxia, transverse myelitis, pancreatitis, and hearing impairment.

ETIOLOGY: Mumps is caused by a paramyxovirus. Other causes of bilateral parotitis include cytomegalovirus and enterovirus, and other causes of unilateral parotitis include tumor, parotid duct obstruction, and bacteria.

EPIDEMIOLOGY: Humans are the only known natural hosts. The virus is spread by direct contact via the respiratory route. Infection can occur throughout childhood. During adulthood, infection is likely to produce more severe disease, including orchitis. Death due to mumps is rare; more than half the fatalities occur in persons older than 19 years of age. Mumps infection during the first trimester of pregnancy can increase the rate of spontaneous abortion. Although mumps virus can cross the placenta, no evidence exists that mumps infection in pregnancy causes congenital malformations. The infection is more common during late winter and spring. The incidence, which has declined markedly since introduction of the mumps vaccine, is now fewer than 1000 cases per year. Most of the reported cases of mumps are in children 5 to 14 years of age. In immunized children, most cases of parotitis are not due to mumps. Outbreaks can occur in highly immunized populations. Like measles vaccine, a single dose of mumps-containing vaccine does not always induce protection. The period of maximum communicability is from 1 to 2 days before the onset of parotid swelling to 5 days after the onset of parotid swelling. Virus has been isolated from saliva up to 7 days before through 9 days after onset of swelling.

The **incubation period** is usually from 16 to 18 days, but cases may occur from 12 to 25 days after exposure.

DIAGNOSTIC TESTS: Children with parotitis lasting 2 days or more without other apparent cause should undergo diagnostic testing to confirm mumps virus as the cause, since mumps is now a rare infection and parotitis may be caused by other agents. Mumps can be confirmed by isolating the virus in cell culture inoculated with throat washings, urine, or spinal fluid; by a significant rise between acute and convalescent titers in serum mumps immunoglobulin (Ig) G antibody titer determined by any standard serologic assay (eg, by complement fixation [CF], neutralization, or hemagglutination inhibition [HAI] test, an enzyme immunoassay [EIA], or a positive mumps IgM antibody test. Past infection is best assessed by

EIA or a neutralization test; CF and HAI tests are unreliable for this purpose. Skin tests also are unreliable and should not be used to test immune status.

TREATMENT: Supportive.

ISOLATION OF THE HOSPITALIZED PATIENT: In addition to standard precautions, droplet precautions are recommended until 9 days after onset of parotid swelling.

CONTROL MEASURES:

School and Child Care. Children should be excluded for 9 days from onset of parotid gland swelling. For control measures during an outbreak, see Outbreak Control, p 408.

Care of Exposed Persons. Mumps vaccine has not been demonstrated to be effective in preventing infection after exposure. However, mumps vaccine can be given after exposure, as immunization will provide protection against subsequent exposures. Immunization during the incubation period has no increased risk. The routine use of mumps vaccine is not advised for persons born after 1956 since most persons are immune. Mumps Immune Globulin is of no value and is no longer manufactured or licensed in the United States.

Mumps Vaccine. Live-virus vaccine is prepared in chick embryo cell cultures. Vaccine is administered by subcutaneous injection of 0.5 mL, either alone as a monovalent vaccine or, preferably, as the combined vaccine containing measles, mumps, and rubella vaccines (MMR). Antibody develops in more than 95% of all susceptible persons after a single dose. Serologic and epidemiologic evidence extending for more than 25 years indicates that vaccine-induced immunity is long-lasting.

Vaccine Recommendations.

- Mumps vaccine should be given as MMR routinely to children at 12 to 15 months of age with a second dose of MMR at 4 to 6 years of age. Reimmunization for mumps can be important because mumps can occur in highly immunized populations, including persons with a history of mumps immunization. Administration of MMR is not harmful if given to a person already immune to one or more of the viruses (from previous infection or immunization).
- Mumps immunization is of particular importance for children approaching puberty, adolescents, and adults who have not had mumps or mumps vaccine. At office visits of prepubertal children and adolescents, the status of immunity to mumps should be assessed. Persons should be considered susceptible unless they have documentation of at least 1 dose of vaccine on or after the first birthday, documentation of physician-diagnosed mumps, or serologic evidence of immunity or were born before 1957.
- Susceptible children, adolescents, and adults born after 1956 should be offered mumps immunization (usually as MMR) before beginning travel since mumps is still endemic throughout most of the world. Because of concern about inadequate seroconversion related to persisting maternal antibodies and because the risk of serious disease from mumps infection is relatively low, persons younger than 12 months of age need not be given mumps vaccine before travel.

- The routine use of mumps vaccine is not advised for persons born before 1957 unless they are considered susceptible, as defined by seronegativity. However, immunization is not contraindicated in these persons if their serologic status is unknown.
- Mumps vaccine can be given simultaneously with other vaccines (see Simultaneous Administration of Multiple Vaccines, p 26).

Adverse Reactions. Adverse reactions attributed to mumps live-virus vaccine are rare. Temporally related reactions, including febrile seizures, nerve deafness, parotitis, meningitis, encephalitis, rash, pruritus, and purpura, may not be related causally. In the United States, the frequency of central nervous system complications after mumps immunization has been lower than the observed incidence in the unimmunized population. Orchitis and parotitis have been reported rarely. Allergic reactions also are rare (see Precautions and Contraindications). Other reactions that occur after immunization with MMR are attributable to the measles and rubella components of the vaccine (see Measles, p 385, and Rubella, p 495).

Reimmunization with mumps vaccine (monovalent or MMR) is not associated with an increased incidence of reactions. Reactions might be expected only among persons not protected by the first dose.

Precautions and Contraindications.

Febrile Illness. Children with minor illnesses with or without fever, such as upper respiratory tract infections, may be immunized (see Vaccine Safety and Contraindications, p 30). Fever per se is not a contraindication to immunization. However, if other manifestations suggest a more serious illness, the child should not be immunized until recovery.

Allergies. The widespread use of the mumps vaccine since 1967 has resulted in only rare isolated reports of allergic reactions. Allergic reactions to components of the vaccine (eg, neomycin) occasionally may occur. Severe allergic reactions, such as anaphylaxis, rarely are reported. Most children with egg hypersensitivity can be safely immunized with MMR. Skin testing before administration of MMR vaccine is not indicated (see Measles, p 385).

Recent Administration of Immune Globulin. Live mumps vaccine should be given at least 2 weeks before or at least 3 months after administration of immune globulin (IG) or blood transfusion because of the theoretical possibility that antibody will neutralize vaccine virus and inhibit a successful immunization. Because high doses of IG (such as those given for the treatment of Kawasaki disease) can inhibit the response to measles vaccine for longer intervals, mumps vaccination, when administered as MMR, should be deferred for a longer period after administration of IG (see Measles, p 385).

Altered Immunity. Patients with immunodeficiency diseases and those receiving immunosuppressive therapy (eg, patients with leukemia, lymphoma, or generalized malignant disease), including high doses of systemically administered corticosteroids, alkylating agents, antimetabolites, or radiation, or who are otherwise immunocompromised should not receive mumps vaccine (see Immunocompromised Children, p 56). The exceptions are patients with human immunodeficiency virus (HIV) infection who are not severely immunocompromised; these patients should be immunized against mumps with MMR (see HIV Infection, p 325). The risk of mumps exposure for patients with altered immunity can be reduced by immunizing their close susceptible contacts. Immunized persons do not transmit mumps vaccine virus.

After cessation of immunosuppressive therapy, mumps vaccine usually should be withheld for an interval of at least 3 months (with the exception of corticosteroid recipients, see the next paragraph). This interval is based on the assumptions that immunologic responsiveness will have been restored in 3 months and the underlying disease for which immunosuppressive therapy was given is in remission or under control. However, because the interval can vary with the intensity and type of immunosuppressive therapy, radiation therapy, underlying disease, and other factors, a definitive recommendation for an interval after cessation of immunosuppressive therapy when mumps vaccine can be administered safely and effectively often is not possible.

Corticosteroids. For patients who have received high doses of corticosteroids for 14 days or more and who are not otherwise immunocompromised, the recommended interval is at least 1 month (see Immunocompromised Children, p 56).

Pregnancy. Susceptible postpubertal females should not be immunized if they are known to be pregnant. If not pregnant, they should be counseled about the potential hazard of fetal infection with vaccine virus before immunization. Live-virus mumps vaccine can infect the placenta, but the virus has not been isolated from fetal tissues of susceptible females who received vaccine and underwent elective abortions. In view of the theoretical risk, however, conception should be avoided for 3 months after mumps immunization with MMR vaccine (see Measles, p 385). Women given monovalent mumps vaccine should not become pregnant for at least 30 days.

Outbreak Control. When determining means to control outbreaks, exclusion of susceptible students from affected schools and schools judged by local public health authorities to be at risk for transmission should be considered. Such exclusion should be an effective means of terminating school outbreaks and rapidly increasing rates of immunization. Excluded students can be readmitted immediately after immunization. Pupils who continue to be exempted from mumps immunization because of medical, religious, or other reasons should be excluded until at least 26 days after the onset of parotitis in the last person with mumps in the affected school. Experience with outbreak control for other vaccine-preventable diseases indicates that this strategy has been highly effective.

Mycoplasma pneumoniae Infections

CLINICAL MANIFESTATIONS: Initial symptoms in patients in whom pneumonia develops, the most prominent manifestation of infection, are nonspecific and include malaise, fever, and, occasionally, headache. Cough, usually associated with widespread rales found on physical examination, develops within a few days and lasts for 3 to 4 weeks. The cough is nonproductive initially but later may become productive, particularly in older children and adolescents. Approximately 10% of children with pneumonia exhibit a rash, most often maculopapular. Roentgenographic abnormalities vary, but bilateral, diffuse infiltrates are common.

The most common clinical syndromes are acute bronchitis and upper respiratory tract infections, including pharyngitis, and, occasionally, otitis media or myringitis, which may be bullous. Coryza, sinusitis, and croup are infrequent.

Unusual manifestations include nervous system disease, such as aseptic meningitis, encephalitis, cerebellar ataxia, transverse myelitis, and peripheral neuropathy, as well as myocarditis, pericarditis, polymorphous mucocutaneous eruptions (including Stevens-Johnson syndrome), hemolytic anemia, and arthritis. In patients with sickle cell disease, Down syndrome, immunodeficiencies, and chronic cardiorespiratory disease, severe pneumonia with pleural effusion can develop.

ETIOLOGY: The mycoplasmas, including *Mycoplasma pneumoniae,* are the smallest free-living microorganisms. These organisms lack a cell wall and are pleomorphic.

EPIDEMIOLOGY: Infected humans are the only known source of infection. *Mycoplasma pneumoniae* is highly transmissible; acquisition is most likely from close contact with a symptomatic person and is presumed to be by droplet spread. Persons of any age can be infected, but specific disease syndromes are age-related. *Mycoplasma pneumoniae* is an uncommon cause of pneumonia in children younger than 5 years of age but is the leading cause of pneumonia in school-age children and young adults. Military and college populations have a high incidence of disease. Infections occur throughout the world, in any season, and in all geographic settings. Community-wide epidemics may occur every 4 to 8 years. Because of the relatively long incubation period, familial spread frequently continues for many months. Cumulative household attack rates approach 100%. Clinical illness within a group, particularly a family, can range from mild upper respiratory tract infection to tracheobronchitis to pneumonia. Asymptomatic carriage after infection can occur for prolonged intervals, commonly for weeks, but has not been associated with transmission of illness. Immunity after infection is not long-lasting.

The **incubation period** is 1 to 4 weeks.

DIAGNOSTIC TESTS: Recovery of *M pneumoniae* in cultures requires special enriched broth or agar media (which is not widely available), is successful in only 40% to 90% of cases, and takes 7 to 21 days. Isolation of *M pneumoniae* in a patient with compatible clinical manifestations suggests causation. Because this organism can be excreted from the respiratory tract for several weeks after an acute infection despite appropriate therapy, isolation of the organism may not indicate acute infection. A polymerase chain reaction test for *M pneumoniae* has been developed but is not available in most clinical microbiologic laboratories.

Serologic diagnosis can be made by demonstrating a 4-fold or greater increase in antibody titer between acute and convalescent serum samples. The antibody titer peaks at about 1 month and persists for 2 to 3 months after infection. The complement fixation (CF) and immunofluorescent (IF) methods are most widely used. Several enzyme immunoassay (EIA) antibody tests and other rapid diagnostic tests for detection of *M pneumoniae* antibodies also are available. The IF test is capable of detecting *Mycoplasma*-specific immunoglobulin (Ig) M and IgG antibodies. Although the presence of IgM antibodies confirms recent *M pneumoniae* infection, they persist in serum for several months and do not necessarily indicate current infection. Since *M pneumoniae* CF and EIA antibodies cross-react with some other antigens, particularly with those of other mycoplasmas, results of these tests should be interpreted cautiously when evaluating febrile illnesses of unknown origin. However, cross-reactivity with other respiratory tract pathogens causing diseases clinically similar to those caused by *M pneumoniae* does not occur. False-negative results occur with both CF and EIA assays.

Serum cold hemagglutinin titers of 1:32 or more are present in more than 50% of patients with pneumonia by the beginning of the second week of illness. Fourfold increases in hemagglutinin titer between acute and convalescent serum samples occur more often in patients with severe *M pneumoniae* than in persons with less severe disease. This test has low specificity for *Mycoplasma* infection, however, and other agents, including adenoviruses, Epstein-Barr virus, and measles, can cause illnesses in infants or children associated with an increase in titer of cold hemagglutinins. A negative test for cold agglutinins does not exclude the diagnosis of mycoplasmal infection. With the wide availability of specific antibody tests, use of this test has been de-emphasized.

Since infections are common and resulting antibodies persist for months or years, measurement of antibody in a single serum sample is of little diagnostic value. However, a CF titer of 1:32 or greater during an acute respiratory tract illness suggests *M pneumoniae* infection.

TREATMENT: Acute bronchitis and upper respiratory tract illness caused by *M pneumoniae* are generally mild and resolve without antibiotic therapy. Erythromycin is the preferred antimicrobial agent for treatment of pneumonia and otitis media in children younger than 8 years of age. Other macrolides, such as clarithromycin and azithromycin, also are effective. Tetracycline is equally effective and may be used for children 8 years of age and older. Most studies with these antimicrobial agents have been conducted in adults, and definitive evidence of their efficacy in children with *M pneumoniae* infection is lacking.

ISOLATION OF THE HOSPITALIZED PATIENT: In addition to standard precautions, droplet precautions are recommended for the duration of illness.

CONTROL MEASURES: Diagnosis of an infected patient should lead to an increased index of suspicion for *Mycoplasma* infection in household members and close contacts. Case finding should be instituted if infection has occurred in many persons in a group. Therapy for each contact should be given if a compatible clinical illness occurs.

Antibiotic prophylaxis for exposed contacts is not recommended routinely. The benefit of chemoprophylaxis has not been assessed adequately, but limited data suggest that prophylaxis may reduce the rate of transmission within families. Persons who are intimately exposed to a person infected with *M pneumoniae* or who live in a house with a person who has an underlying condition that predisposes to severe *Mycoplasma* infection, such as sickle cell disease, should be considered for prophylaxis with erythromycin (or another macrolide) or tetracycline during the acute phase of illness, especially if the illness occurs in a household member.

Nocardiosis

CLINICAL MANIFESTATIONS: A common presentation in immunocompetent children is cutaneous or lymphocutaneous disease after soil contamination at the site of skin injury. Usually the pustular or ulcerative lesions remain localized. Invasive disease occurs most commonly in immunocompromised patients, particularly those with chronic granulomatous disease or human immunodeficiency virus infection or who are receiving long-term corticosteroid therapy. In these children, infection characteristically begins in the lungs, and the illness may be acute, subacute, or chronic. Pulmonary disease often presents as rounded nodular infiltrates that can undergo cavitation. Hematogenous spread may occur from lungs to the brain (single or multiple abscesses), skin (pustules, pyoderma, abscesses, mycetoma), and, occasionally, other organs.

ETIOLOGY: *Nocardia* species are aerobic actinomycetes. Pulmonary or disseminated disease is caused most commonly by the *Nocardia asteroides* complex, which includes *Nocardia farcinica* and *Nocardia nova.* Cutaneous disease is caused most commonly by *Nocardia brasiliensis. Nocardia pseudobrasiliensis* seems to be associated with pulmonary, central nervous system (CNS), and systemic nocardiosis.

EPIDEMIOLOGY: *Nocardia* species are saprophytic soil organisms and are found worldwide. The lungs are the probable portal of entry for pulmonary or disseminated disease. Direct skin inoculation occurs, often as the result of minor trauma with soil contamination. Person-to-person transmission does not occur.

The **incubation period** is unknown.

DIAGNOSTIC TESTS: Stained smears of sputum, body fluids, or pus can demonstrate beaded, branched, weakly gram-positive rods that are variably acid fast. The Brown and Brenn and methenamine silver stains are recommended for demonstrating microorganisms in tissue. Growth of typical colonies occurs on 5% sheep blood, chocolate agar, and most media used for growth of organisms of the *Mycobacteria* genus, including BACTEC 12B broth. *Nocardia* organisms are slow growing; cultures from normally sterile sites should be maintained for 3 weeks in a liquid medium. Serologic tests for *Nocardia* species are hampered by a lack of specificity and sensitivity.

TREATMENT: Trimethoprim-sulfamethoxazole or a sulfonamide alone (eg, sulfisoxazole or sulfamethoxazole) is the drug of choice. Preparations that are less urine soluble, such as sulfadiazine, should be avoided. The infection in immunocompetent patients with lymphocutaneous disease usually responds after 6 to 12 weeks of therapy. Immunocompromised patients and those with invasive disease should be treated for 6 to 12 months and for at least 3 months after apparent cure because of the tendency for relapse. Patients with acquired immunodeficiency syndrome may need even longer therapy. Patients with meningitis or brain abscess should be monitored with serial neuroimaging studies. If response to trimethoprim-sulfamethoxazole does not occur, other agents, such as a tetracycline, amoxicillin-clavulanate, imipenem, or meropenem may be beneficial. Tetracyclines should not be recommended for children younger than 8 years of age who are allergic to sulfonamides. For patients with CNS disease, disseminated disease, or overwhelming infection, amikacin should be included for the first 4 to 12 weeks or until the patient's condition is improved clinically. Drug susceptibility testing, if available, is recommended by some experts for isolates from these patients, as well as for isolates from patients unable to tolerate a sulfonamide. Drainage of abscesses is beneficial, especially for immunocompromised patients.

ISOLATION OF THE HOSPITALIZED PATIENT: Standard precautions are recommended.

CONTROL MEASURES: None.

Onchocerciasis

(River Blindness, Filariasis)

CLINICAL MANIFESTATIONS: The disease involves the skin, subcutaneous tissues, lymphatics, and eyes. Subcutaneous nodules of varying sizes, containing adult worms, develop 6 to 12 months after the initial infection. In patients in Africa, the nodules tend to be found on the lower torso, pelvis, and lower extremities, whereas in patients in Central America, the nodules more often are located on the upper body (the head and trunk) but may occur on the extremities. After the worms mature, microfilariae are produced and migrate in the tissues and may cause a chronic, generalized, pruritic dermatitis. After a period of years, the skin can become lichenified and hypopigmented or hyperpigmented. The presence of microfilariae, living or dead, in the ocular structures, leads to photophobia and inflammation of the cornea, iris, ciliary body, retina, choroid, and optic nerve. Blindness can result if the disease is untreated.

ETIOLOGY: *Onchocerca volvulus* is a filarial nematode.

EPIDEMIOLOGY: Larvae are transmitted by the bites of an infected Simulium black fly that breeds in fast-flowing streams and rivers (hence the colloquial name of the disease, "river blindness"). The disease occurs primarily in equatorial Africa, but small foci are found in southern Mexico, Guatemala, northern South America, and Yemen. Prevalence is greatest among those who live near vector-breeding areas. The adult worms continue to produce microfilariae capable of infecting flies for as long as a decade. The infection is not transmissible by person-to-person contact or blood transfusion.

The **incubation period** from larval inoculation to microfilariae in the skin is approximately 6 to 12 months.

DIAGNOSTIC TESTS: Direct examination of a 1- to 2-mg shave or punch biopsy of the epidermis and upper dermis (taken from scapular or iliac crest area) usually will reveal microfilariae. Adult worms may be demonstrated in excised nodules that have been sectioned and stained. A slit-lamp examination of the anterior chamber of an involved eye may reveal motile microfilariae or corneal lesions typical of onchocerciasis. Microfilariae rarely are found in blood. Eosinophilia is common. Specific serologic tests and polymerase chain reaction techniques for detection of microfilariae in skin are available only at selected research laboratories.

TREATMENT: Ivermectin, a microfilaricidal agent, is the drug of choice for treatment of onchocerciasis. Treatment reduces dermatitis and the risk of developing severe ocular disease, but treatment does not kill the adult worms and, thus, is not curative. One single oral dose of ivermectin (150 µg/kg) should be given annually for 5 to 10 years. Adverse reactions caused by the death of microfilariae include rash, edema, fever, myalgia, and hypotension (which rarely is severe). Contraindications to treatment include pregnancy, central nervous system disorders, and body weight less than 15 kg.

ISOLATION OF THE HOSPITALIZED PATIENT: Standard precautions are recommended.

CONTROL MEASURES: Repellents and protective clothing (long sleeves and pants) can reduce exposure to black fly bites. Treatment of vector breeding sites with larvicides has been effective for controlling black fly populations, particularly in West Africa. A major initiative to distribute ivermectin to all disease-endemic communities to prevent severe morbidity from onchocerciasis has been undertaken.

Papillomaviruses

CLINICAL MANIFESTATIONS: Human papillomaviruses (HPVs) produce epithelial tumors (warts) of the skin and mucous membranes. Cutaneous nongenital warts include common skin warts, plantar warts, flat warts, thread-like (filiform) warts, and epidermodysplasia verruciformis. Those affecting the mucous membranes include anogenital, oral, nasal, and conjunctival warts, as well as respiratory papillomatosis.

Common skin warts are dome-shaped with conical projections that give the surface a rough appearance. They usually are asymptomatic and multiple, occurring on the hands and around or under the nails. When small dermal vessels become thrombosed, black dots appear in the warts. Plantar warts on the foot may be painful and are characterized by marked hyperkeratosis, sometimes with black dots.

Flat warts ("juvenile warts") commonly are found on the face and extremities of children and adolescents. They usually are small, multiple, and flat-topped; they seldom exhibit papillomatosis and rarely cause pain. Filiform warts occur on the face and neck. Cutaneous warts are benign.

The manifestations of anogenital HPV infection range from clinically inapparent infection to condylomata acuminata, which are skin-colored warts with a cauliflower-like surface that vary from a few millimeters to several centimeters in diameter. In males, such warts may be found on the shaft of the penis, the penile meatus, the scrotum, or the perianal area. In females, such warts are seen on the labia and perianal area and less commonly in the vagina and on the cervix. Clinically inapparent infections commonly occur in the vagina, on the cervix, and on the labia and perineum. Most anogenital warts are asymptomatic, but, occasionally, they cause itching, burning, local pain, or bleeding. Some HPV types are associated with genital dysplasia and epithelial cancers of the female and male genital tracts. Specific types of HPV are the causal agents of at least 90% of cervical cancers.

Laryngeal papillomas are rare. They are diagnosed most commonly in children between 2 and 3 years of age and are manifested by a voice change or abnormal cry. When laryngeal papillomas occur in infancy, they have been associated with respiratory tract obstruction. Adult onset also has been described.

Epidermodysplasia verruciformis is a rare, lifelong, severe papillomavirus infection, believed to be a consequence of an inherited deficiency of cell-mediated immunity. The lesions may resemble flat warts but often are similar to tinea versicolor, covering the torso and upper extremities. Most appear during the first decade of life, but malignant transformation, which occurs in approximately one third of affected persons, usually is delayed until adulthood.

ETIOLOGY: Human papillomaviruses are members of the Papovaviridae family and are DNA viruses. More than 70 types have been identified, but a small number of HPV types account for most warts. Those causing nongenital warts generally are distinct from those causing anogenital infections. Of the latter, only a small number have a strong association with malignant neoplasms.

EPIDEMIOLOGY: Papillomaviruses are widely distributed among mammals but are species-specific. Cutaneous warts occur frequently among school-age children; prevalence rates are as high as 50%. Human papillomavirus infections are thought to be transmitted from person to person by close contact. Nongenital warts are acquired through minor trauma to the skin. An increase in the incidence of plantar warts has been associated with swimming in public pools. The intense and often widespread appearance of warts in patients with compromised cellular immunity (particularly patients who have undergone transplantation and persons with human immunodeficiency virus infection) suggests that alterations in immunity predispose to reactivation of latent intraepithelial infection.

Anogenital warts primarily are transmitted by sexual contact but may be acquired at the time of delivery or by transmission from nongenital sites. When they are found in a prepubertal child beyond infancy, sexual abuse must be considered. Evidence of genital HPV infection has been detected in as many as 38% of sexually active adolescent females. Anogenital HPV infection is the most common viral sexually transmitted disease in the United States.

Laryngeal papillomas are believed to be transmitted through aspiration of infectious secretions during passage through the infected birth canal.

The **incubation period** is unknown but is estimated to range from 3 months to several years. Papillomavirus acquired by a neonate at the time of delivery may not cause clinical manifestations for several years.

DIAGNOSTIC TESTS: Most cutaneous and anogenital warts are diagnosed by clinical inspection. Detection of cervical HPV infection may be enhanced by use of colposcopy with application of 3% to 5% acetic acid (vinegar), which causes the lesion to turn white. This characteristic, however, is not specific for HPV infection, and false-positive test results are common. When the diagnosis is questionable, histologic examination of a biopsy specimen can be diagnostic.

Human papillomavirus cannot be cultured. Tests for the detection of HPV nucleic acids in cervical cells are available commercially. Clinical indications for HPV testing are unclear.

TREATMENT: Most nongenital warts eventually regress spontaneously but may persist for months or years. The optimal treatment for warts that do not resolve spontaneously has not been identified. Most methods of treatment rely on chemical or physical destruction of the infected epithelium, such as application of salicylic acid products or cryotherapy with liquid nitrogen. Daily treatment with tretinoin has been useful for widespread flat warts in children. Care must be taken to avoid a deleterious cosmetic result with therapy. Oral cimetidine at moderately high doses (25–40 mg/kg per day for 2–3 months) has been used for treatment of refractory warts; however, the efficacy of cimetidine has not been established in controlled clinical trials.

The optimal treatment for anogenital (exophytic) warts has not been identified. Spontaneous regression is possible within months in a minority of cases. The application of podophyllum resin or patient-applied podofilox (the major cytotoxic ingredient of podophyllum resin) often is the initial therapy of choice. Neither agent has been tested for safety and efficacy in children, and their use is contraindicated in pregnancy. Other treatment modalities are cryotherapy, trichloroacetic acid, imiquimod (patient-applied), electrocautery, laser surgery, and surgical excision (see Table 4.3, p 663). Although most forms of therapy are successful for the initial removal of warts, treatment does not eradicate HPV infection from the surrounding normal tissue. Therefore, recurrences are common and probably due to reactivation rather than reinfection. Many unproven compounds are being used to treat HPV. Agents associated with local tissue damage can be harmful.

Human papillomavirus infection of the cervix in adolescents is common and can be associated with epithelial dysplasia. Hence, the care of adolescents with cervical dysplasia requires a physician who is knowledgeable in the diagnosis and treatment of HPV infection.

Laryngeal papillomas are difficult to treat. Local recurrence is common, and repeated surgical procedures for removal usually are necessary. Extension or dissemination of laryngeal papillomas into the trachea, bronchi, or lung parenchyma is a rare complication that can result in increased morbidity and mortality. Interferon has been used as an investigational treatment and may be of benefit for patients with frequent recurrences.

Oral warts can be removed through cryotherapy, electrocautery, or surgical excision.

ISOLATION OF THE HOSPITALIZED PATIENT: Standard precautions are recommended.

CONTROL MEASURES: Suspected child abuse should be reported to the appropriate local agency if anogenital warts are found in a prepubertal child beyond infancy. Although data are limited, sexual transmission of anogenital warts probably can be decreased by using condoms or refraining from intercourse until therapy is completed and lesions have healed. Although HPV infection may persist for life, the degree and duration of contagiousness in patients with a history of genital infection is unknown.

Examination of sex partners is unnecessary for management of anogenital warts because the role of reinfection probably is minimal and treatment to reduce transmission is not realistic since therapy may not be curative. However, sex partners may benefit from examination to assess presence of anogenital warts or other sexually transmitted diseases. Female sex partners of patients with genital warts should be informed that cytologic screening for cervical cancer is recommended for all sexually active women.

Although laryngeal papillomatosis is believed to be acquired in most cases during passage through the birth canal, this condition has occurred in infants delivered by cesarean section. Because the preventive value of cesarean delivery is unknown, it should not be performed to prevent transmission of HPV to the newborn.

For a report of an expert panel on prevention of genital HPV infection and sequelae, see www.cdc.gov/nchstp/dstd/Report_Publications/99HPVReport.htm/

Paracoccidioidomycosis

(South American Blastomycosis)

CLINICAL MANIFESTATIONS: Disease occurs primarily in adults and is rare in children. The site of primary infection is the lungs. Clinical patterns of disease include acute pneumonia, chronic pneumonia, and dissemination. Dissemination to skin, mucous membranes, lymph nodes, liver, spleen, bone, central nervous system, gastrointestinal tract, and adrenals is common in children. Chronic granulomatous lesions of the mucous membranes, especially of the mouth and palate, are typical but infrequent findings. Infection may be latent for years before causing illness.

ETIOLOGY: *Paracoccidioides brasiliensis* is a dimorphic fungus with a yeast and a mycelial phase.

EPIDEMIOLOGY: The infection occurs primarily in South America, where it is endemic. Cases also have been reported in Central America and Mexico. The natural reservoir is unknown, although soil is suspected. The mode of transmission is unknown; person-to-person transmission does not occur.

The **incubation period** is highly variable, ranging from 1 month to many years.

DIAGNOSTIC TESTS: Round, multiple-budding cells may be seen in 10% potassium hydroxide preparations of sputum specimens, bronchoalveolar lavage specimens, scrapings from ulcers, and material from lesions or in tissue biopsy specimens. The organism can be cultured easily on most enriched media, including blood agar at 37°C (98°F) and Sabouraud dextrose agar (with cycloheximide) at 24°C (75°F). Complement fixation, enzyme immunoassay, and immunodiffusion methods are useful for detecting specific antibodies. Skin testing is not reliable for diagnosis because nonreactivity is common and false-positive tests can occur. However, skin test positivity developing during therapy portends a good prognosis.

TREATMENT: Amphotericin B is the drug of choice for persons with severe paracoccidioidomycosis, but amphotericin B is not curative in itself (see Drugs for Invasive and Other Serious Fungal Infections, p 672). Itraconazole is the treatment for less severe or localized infection. For adults, itraconazole seems to be superior to ketoconazole and to cause fewer adverse effects. However, the safety and efficacy of itraconazole for treatment for children have not been established. Children also should receive maintenance therapy with itraconazole (4-10 mg/kg daily; maximum 200 mg twice daily) or a sulfonamide (trimethoprim-sulfamethoxazole, 8-10 mg/kg of trimethoprim daily). Prolonged therapy for at least 6 months is necessary to minimize the relapse rate.

ISOLATION OF THE HOSPITALIZED PATIENT: Standard precautions are recommended.

CONTROL MEASURES: None.

Paragonimiasis

CLINICAL MANIFESTATIONS: The disease has an insidious onset and a chronic course. The 2 major forms of paragonimiasis described are (1) classical paragonimiasis, which involves the lungs, and (2) nonclassical paragonimiasis, which results in a larval migrans syndrome. In classical infections, pulmonary disease is associated with chronic cough and dyspnea, but most infections probably are inapparent or result in mild symptoms. Heavy infections cause paroxysms of coughing that often produces blood-tinged sputum, which is brown because of the presence of *Paragonimus* eggs. Hemoptysis can be severe. Pleural effusion, pneumothorax, bronchiectasis, and pulmonary fibrosis with clubbing can develop. Extrapulmonary manifestations also may involve the abdominal cavity, skin, and, uncommonly, the central nervous system with meningoencephalitis and seizures due to invasion of the brain by adult flukes. Symptoms tend to subside after approximately 5 years but can persist for as many as 20 years.

Nonclassical paragonimiasis is associated with migratory subcutaneous nodules containing juvenile worms, but hemoptysis does not occur. Pleural effusion is common, as is invasion of the brain.

ETIOLOGY: Classical paragonimiasis is caused by *Paragonimus westermani* and *Paragonimus heterotremus* adult flukes and their eggs. The adult flukes of *P westermani* are up to 12 mm long and 7 mm wide and occur throughout the Far East. A triploid pathogenic form of *P westermani,* which is larger, produces more eggs, and elicits greater disease, has been described in Japan, Korea, Taiwan, and parts of eastern China. *Paragonimus heterotremus* occurs in southeast Asia and adjacent parts of China. Nonclassical paragonimiasis is caused by larval stages of *Paragonimus skrjabini* and *Paragonimus miyazakii.* The worms rarely mature. *Paragonimus skrjabini* occurs in China and *P miyazakii* in Japan. African forms include *Paragonimus africanus* (Nigeria, Cameroon) and *Paragonimus uterobilateralis* (Liberia, Guinea,

Nigeria, Gabon). *Paragonimus mexicanus* occurs in Mexico, Costa Rica, Ecuador, and Peru. *Paragonimus kellicoti,* a lung fluke of mink and opossums in the United States, also can cause a zoonotic infection in humans.

EPIDEMIOLOGY: Transmission occurs when raw or undercooked freshwater crabs or crayfish containing larvae (metacercariae) are ingested. The metacercariae exist in the small intestine and penetrate the abdominal cavity, where they remain for a few days before migrating to the lungs. *Paragonimus westermani* and *P heterotremus* mature within the lungs over 6 to 10 weeks when they begin egg production. Eggs escape from pulmonary capsules into the bronchi and exit from the human host in sputum or feces. Eggs hatch in freshwater within 3 weeks, giving rise to miracidia. Miracidia penetrate freshwater snails and emerge several weeks later as cercariae, which encyst within the muscles and viscera of freshwater crustaceans before maturing into infective metacercariae. Transmission also occurs when humans ingest raw pork, usually from wild pigs, containing the juvenile stages of *Paragonimus* species (described in Japan).

Humans are accidental ("dead-end") hosts for *P skrjabini* and *P miyazakii.* These flukes cannot mature in humans and, hence, do not produce eggs.

Paragonimus species also infect a variety of other mammals such as canids, mustelids, felids, and rodents, which can serve as animal reservoir hosts.

The **incubation period** is not known, although egg production can begin about 1 month after ingestion of *P westermani* metacercariae.

DIAGNOSTIC TESTS: Microscopic examination of stools, sputum, pleural effusion, cerebrospinal fluid, and other tissue aspirates may reveal eggs. A Western blot serologic antibody test, available at the Centers for Disease Control and Prevention, is sensitive and specific but does not distinguish active from past infection. Charcot-Leyden crystals and eosinophils in sputum are useful diagnostic elements. Chest radiographs may be normal or resemble those from patients with tuberculosis. Misdiagnosis is possible unless paragonimiasis is suspected.

TREATMENT: Praziquantel in a 2-day course is the drug of choice and is associated with high cure rates as demonstrated by the disappearance of egg production and chest radiographic lesions in the lungs. The drug also is effective for some extrapulmonary manifestations. Bithionol is an alternative drug.

ISOLATION OF THE HOSPITALIZED PATIENT: Standard precautions are recommended.

CONTROL MEASURES: Cooking of crabs for several minutes until the meat has congealed and turned opaque kills the metacercariae. Similarly, meat from wild pigs should be well cooked before eating. Control of the animal reservoirs is not possible.

Parainfluenza Viral Infections

CLINICAL MANIFESTATIONS: Parainfluenza viruses are the major cause of laryngotracheobronchitis (croup), but they also frequently cause upper respiratory tract infection, pneumonia, or bronchiolitis. Infections can be particularly severe and persistent in immunodeficient children.

ETIOLOGY: Parainfluenza viruses are enveloped RNA viruses classified as paramyxoviruses. Four antigenically distinct types—1, 2, 3, and 4 (with 2 subtypes, 4A and 4B)—have been identified.

EPIDEMIOLOGY: Parainfluenza viruses are believed to be transmitted from person to person by direct contact and exposure to contaminated nasopharyngeal secretions through respiratory tract droplets and fomites. Parainfluenza viral infections are ubiquitous and epidemic as well as sporadic. Type 1 viruses tend to produce outbreaks of respiratory tract illness, usually croup, in the autumn of every other year. A major increase in the number of cases of croup in the autumn indicates a parainfluenza type 1 outbreak. Type 2 virus also can cause outbreaks of respiratory tract illness in the autumn, often in conjunction with type 1 outbreaks, but type 2 outbreaks tend to be less severe, irregular, and less frequent. Parainfluenza type 3 virus usually is most prominent during the spring and summer in temperate climates but frequently continues into the autumn, especially in years when autumn outbreaks of parainfluenza types 1 or 2 are absent. Infections with types 4A and 4B are recognized less commonly, sporadic, and generally mild clinically.

Illness from primary infection with types 1 and 2 occurs predominantly in 2- to 6-year-old children. Infection with type 3 virus usually is acquired initially during the first 2 years of life and is a major cause of lower respiratory tract disease in infants. Reinfections can occur at any age, but they usually are milder, primarily causing upper respiratory tract illness. Severe lower respiratory tract disease, with prolonged shedding of the virus, can develop in immunodeficient persons. In these patients, infection may spread beyond the respiratory tract to the liver and lymph nodes.

Immunocompetent children with primary parainfluenza infection shed the virus from 3 to 6 days before the onset of clinical symptoms until about 10 days after the symptoms have disappeared. Children with type 1 infection shed the virus for an average of 4 to 7 days, but shedding can last as long as 2 weeks. The average period of shedding for type 3 infections is 8 to 9 days but can last as long as 3 weeks or more.

The **incubation period** is from 2 to 6 days.

DIAGNOSTIC TESTS: Virus may be isolated from nasopharyngeal secretions usually within 4 to 7 days of culture inoculation or earlier by using centrifugation of a specimen onto a monolayer of susceptible cells with subsequent staining for viral antigen (shell viral assay). Confirmation is by rapid antigen detection, usually immunofluorescence. Rapid antigen identification techniques, including immunofluorescent assays, enzyme immunoassays, radioimmunoassays, and fluoroimmunoassays, can be used to detect the virus in nasopharyngeal secretions, but the sensitivity of the tests can vary. Serologic diagnosis, made retrospectively by a significant rise in antibody titer between serum samples obtained during acute infection and convalescence, may be confusing because increases in heterotypic antibody levels due to infections caused by other serotypes of parainfluenza and mumps viruses are common. Furthermore, infection may not always be accompanied by a significant homotypic antibody response.

TREATMENT: Specific antiviral therapy is not available. Racemic epinephrine aerosol is given frequently to severely affected, hospitalized patients with laryngotracheobronchitis to reduce airway obstruction. Parenteral dexamethasone in high doses (greater than 0.3 mg/kg), oral dexamethasone (0.15 to 0.6 mg/kg), and nebulized corticosteroids have been demonstrated to lessen the severity and duration of symptoms and hospitalization in patients with moderate to severe laryngotracheobronchitis. Oral dexamethasone doses of 0.15 mg/kg also are effective for outpatients with less severe croup. Management is otherwise supportive.

ISOLATION OF THE HOSPITALIZED PATIENT: In addition to standard precautions, contact precautions are recommended for hospitalized infants and young children for the duration of illness. Strict adherence to infection control procedures, including prevention of environmental contamination by respiratory secretions and careful hand washing, should control nosocomial spread.

CONTROL MEASURES: Efforts should be aimed at reducing nosocomial infection. Hand washing should be emphasized.

Parasitic Diseases

Many parasitic diseases traditionally have been considered exotic and, therefore, frequently are not included in differential diagnoses of patients in the United States, Canada, and Europe. Nevertheless, these organisms are among the most common causes of morbidity and mortality in various and diverse geographic locations worldwide. Tourists returning to their own countries, immigrants from endemic areas, and immunocompromised persons are at risk for acquiring parasitic infections in nonendemic areas. Physicians and clinical laboratory personnel need to be aware of where these infections may be acquired, clinical presentations, and methods of diagnosis so that tourists can be warned appropriately before travel and evaluated on return to the United States.

Table 3.40 (p 421) gives details on some infrequently encountered parasitic diseases.

Consultation and assistance in diagnosis and management of parasitic diseases are available from government agencies (eg, Centers for Disease Control and Prevention [CDC] and state health departments) and university departments or divisions of geographic medicine, tropical medicine, pediatric infectious disease, international health, and public health.

The CDC distributes a number of drugs that are not available commercially in the United States for treatment of parasitic diseases. These drugs are indicated by footnotes in the table entitled Drugs for Parasitic Infections (p 693). To request these drugs, a physician must contact the CDC Drug Service (see Directory of Resources, p 743), and provide the following information: (1) the physician's name,

Table 3.40. **Additional Parasitic Diseases***

Diseases and/or Agent	Where Infection May Be Acquired	Definitive Host	Intermediate Host	Modes of Human Infection	Directly Communicable (Person to Person)	Diagnostic Laboratory Tests in Humans	Causative Form of Parasite	Manifestations in Humans
Angiostrongylus cantonensis	Pacific islands, Eastern Asia, Puerto Rico, Cuba, Africa, and Louisiana	Rats	Snails and slugs	Eating uncooked infected mollusks	No	Eosinophils in CSF; identification of larvae in CSF or at autopsy	Larval worms	Meningo-encephalitis
Angiostrongylus costaricensis	Central and South America	Rodents	Snails and slugs	Eating uncooked infected mollusks	No	Gel diffusion	Larval worms	Abdominal pain
Anisakiasis	Cosmopolitan, mainly Japan	Marine mammals	Certain salt-water fish, squid, and octopus	Eating uncooked infected fish	No	Identification of recovered larvae in granulomas or vomitus	Larval worms	Acute gastro-intestinal disease
Clonorchis sinensis	Far East	Humans, cats, dogs, other animals	Certain fresh-water snails	Eating uncooked infected freshwater fish	No	Eggs in stool or duodenal fluid	Larvae and mature flukes	Abdominal pain; hepatobiliary disease
Dracunculiasis *(Dracunculus medinensis)*	Foci in Africa	Humans	Crustacea copepods	Drinking infected water	No	Adult worm in skin, subcutaneous tissues	Adult female worm	Inflammatory response; systemic and local in skin and subcutaneous tissue

Table 3.40. **Additional Parasitic Diseases,* continued**

Diseases and/or Agent	Where Infection May Be Acquired	Definitive Host	Intermediate Host	Modes of Human Infection	Directly Communicable (Person to Person)	Diagnostic Laboratory Tests in Humans	Causative Form of Parasite	Manifestations in Humans
Fascioliasis (*Fasciola hepatica*)	Foci throughout tropics and temperate areas	Humans and many animals	Certain freshwater snails and vegetation	Eating uncooked infected plants, such as watercress	No	Eggs in feces, duodenal fluid, or bile	Larvae and mature worms	Disease of liver and biliary tree; acute gastrointestinal disease
Fasciolopsiasis (*Fasciolopsis buski*)	Far East	Humans, pigs, dogs	Certain freshwater snails, plants	Eating uncooked infected plants	No	Eggs or worm in feces or duodenal fluid	Larvae and mature worms	Diarrhea, constipation vomiting, anorexia, edema of face and legs, ascites
Intestinal capillariasis (*Capillaria philippinensis*)	Philippines, Thailand	Humans	Fish	Ingestion of uncooked infected fish	Uncertain	Eggs and parasite in feces	Larvae and mature worms	Protein-losing enteropathy, ascites, emaciation

* For recommended drug treatment, see Drugs for Parasitic Infections (p 693). CSF indicates cerebrospinal fluid.

address, and telephone number; (2) the type of infection to be treated and the method by which the infection was diagnosed; and (3) the patient's name, age, weight, sex, and, if the patient is female, whether she is pregnant. Consultation with a medical officer from the CDC may be required before a drug is distributed.

Important human parasitic infections are discussed in individual chapters in Section 3; the diseases are arranged alphabetically, and the discussions include recommendations for drug treatment. Tables 4.13, 4.14, and 4.15, reproduced from *The Medical Letter* (see Drugs for Parasitic Infections, p 693), provide dosage recommendations and other relevant information for specific antiparasitic drugs. Although the recommendations for administration of these drugs given in the disease-specific chapters are similar, they may not be identical in all instances because of differences of opinion among experts. Both sources should be consulted.

Parvovirus B19

(Erythema Infectiosum, Fifth Disease)

Clinical Manifestations: Infection with parvovirus B19 is recognized most often as erythema infectiosum (EI), which is characterized by mild systemic symptoms, fever in 15% to 30% of patients, and, frequently, a distinctive rash. Before onset of these manifestations, a brief, mild, nonspecific illness consisting of fever, malaise, myalgias, and headache, followed approximately 7 to 10 days later by the characteristic exanthema, may occur in some patients. The facial rash is intensely red with a "slapped cheek" appearance and often accompanied by circumoral pallor. A symmetric, maculopapular, lace-like, and often pruritic rash also occurs on the trunk, moving peripherally to involve the arms, buttocks, and thighs. The rash can fluctuate in intensity and recur with environmental changes, such as temperature and exposure to sunlight, for weeks or months. Arthralgia and arthritis occur infrequently among infected children but commonly among adults, especially women.

Infection with the causative agent of EI, human parvovirus B19, also can cause asymptomatic infection, a mild respiratory tract illness with no rash, a rash atypical for EI that may be rubelliform or petechial, arthritis in adults (in the absence of manifestations of EI), chronic bone marrow failure in immunodeficient patients, and transient aplastic crisis lasting 7 to 10 days in patients with hemolytic anemias (eg, sickle cell disease, and autoimmune hemolytic anemia) and other conditions associated with low hemoglobin levels, including hemorrhage, severe anemia, and thalassemia. Chronic parvovirus B19 infection has been detected in some human immunodeficiency virus (HIV)-infected patients with severe anemia, at rates up to 17% in those with hematocrit values of 24% (0.24) or less and in 31% of those with hematocrit values of 20% (0.20) or less. In addition, parvovirus B19 infection has been associated with thrombocytopenia and neutropenia. Patients with aplastic crisis may have a prodromal illness with fever, malaise, and myalgia, but rash usually is absent. The red blood cell aplasia is related to lytic infection in erythrocyte precursors.

Parvovirus B19 infection occurring during pregnancy can cause fetal hydrops and death but is not a proven cause of congenital anomalies. The risk of fetal death is probably between 2% and 6%, with the greatest risk when infection occurs during the first half of pregnancy.

ETIOLOGY: Human parvovirus B19 is a DNA-containing virus.

EPIDEMIOLOGY: Parvovirus B19 is distributed worldwide and is a common cause of infection in humans, who are the only known hosts. Modes of transmission include contact with respiratory tract secretions, percutaneous exposure to blood or blood products, and vertical transmission between a mother and her fetus. Parvovirus B19 infections are ubiquitous, and cases of EI can occur sporadically or as part of community outbreaks, which often occur in elementary or junior high schools during the late winter and early spring. Secondary spread among susceptible household members is common and occurs in approximately 50% of susceptible contacts. The transmission rate in schools is less, but infection can be an occupational risk for school and child care personnel, with approximately 20% of susceptible persons becoming infected. However, 50% of children are seropositive by 15 years of age, and more than 90% of elderly persons are seropositive. In young children, antibody seroprevalence is generally 5% to 10%. The annual seroconversion rate in women of childbearing age has been reported as 1.5%. The timing of the presence of parvovirus B19 DNA in serum and respiratory tract secretions indicates that persons with EI are most infectious before illness onset and are unlikely to be infectious after onset of the rash and other associated symptoms. In contrast, patients with aplastic crises are contagious from before the onset of symptoms and through the week after onset or even longer. Transmission from patients with aplastic crisis to hospital personnel can occur.

The **incubation period** from acquisition of infection to onset of initial symptoms is usually between 4 and 14 days but can be as long as 21 days. Rash and joint symptoms occur 2 to 3 weeks after acquisition of infection.

DIAGNOSTIC TESTS: The most feasible methods of diagnosis are direct detection of parvovirus B19 antigen or DNA in clinical specimens and serologic tests. In the healthy host, detection of serum parvovirus B19–specific immunoglobulin (Ig) M antibody is preferred, and detection indicates infection probably occurred within the previous 2 to 4 months. By using a radioimmunoassay or enzyme immunoassay, antibody may be detected in 90% or more of patients at the time of the EI rash and by the third day of illness in patients with transient aplastic crisis. Serum IgG antibody indicates previous infection and immunity. These assays are available through commercial laboratories and through some state health and research laboratories. However, their sensitivity and specificity may vary, particularly for IgM antibody. The optimal method for detecting chronic infection in the immunocompromised patient is demonstration of virus by nucleic acid hybridization or polymerase chain reaction (PCR) assay, because parvovirus B19 antibody is variably present in persistent infection. Since parvovirus B19 DNA can be detected by PCR in serum after the acute viremic phase for up to 9 months in some patients, PCR detection of parvovirus B19 DNA does not necessarily indicate acute infection. The less sensitive nucleic acid hybridization assays usually are positive for only 2 to 4 days after onset of illness. For HIV-infected patients with severe anemia, dot blot hybridization of serum may be a more appropriate assay. Parvovirus B19 has not been grown in standard cell culture, but the virus has been cultivated in experimental cell culture.

TREATMENT: For most patients, only supportive care is indicated. Patients with aplastic crises may require transfusion. For the treatment of chronic infection in immunodeficient patients, intravenous immunoglobulin therapy seems to be effective and should be considered. Some cases of B19 infected hydrops fetalis have been treated successfully with intrauterine blood transfusions.

ISOLATION OF THE HOSPITALIZED PATIENT: In addition to standard precautions, droplet precautions are recommended for those caring for hospitalized children with aplastic crises or immunosuppressed patients with chronic infection and anemia for the duration of hospitalization. For patients with transient aplastic or erythrocyte crisis, these precautions should be maintained for 7 days.

Pregnant health care personnel should be informed of the potential risks to the fetus from parvovirus B19 infections and about preventive measures that may reduce these risks, eg, attention to strict infection control procedures and not caring for immunocompromised patients with chronic parvovirus infection or patients with parvovirus B19–associated aplastic crises, as both groups of patients have highly contagious disease.

CONTROL MEASURES:

- Women who are exposed to children at home or at work (eg, teachers or child care workers) are at increased risk of infection with parvovirus B19. However, because of widespread inapparent infection in adults and children, all women are at some degree of risk of exposure, particularly those with school-age children. In view of the high prevalence of parvovirus B19, the low incidence of ill effects on the fetus, and the fact that avoidance of child care or classroom teaching can reduce but not eliminate the risk of exposure, routine exclusion of pregnant women from the workplace where EI is occurring is not recommended. Women of childbearing age who are concerned can undergo serologic testing for IgG antibody to parvovirus B19 to determine their susceptibility to infection.
- Pregnant women who find that they have been in contact with children who were in the incubation period of EI or with children who were in aplastic crisis should have the relatively low potential risk explained to them, and the option of serologic testing should be offered. Fetal ultrasonography may prove useful in these situations.
- Children with EI may attend child care or school, because they are no longer contagious.
- Transmission of parvovirus B19 is likely to be reduced through use of routine infection control practices, including hand washing and disposal of used facial tissues.
- Pediatricians, as child care advocates, should act as consultants in providing greater access to testing facilities, assistance in interpreting test results, and reassurance to pregnant women.

Pasteurella multocida Infections

CLINICAL MANIFESTATIONS: The most common manifestation in children is cellulitis at the site of a scratch or bite of a cat, dog, or other animal. This finding usually occurs within 24 hours after the bite or scratch and includes swelling, erythema, tenderness, and serous or sanguinopurulent discharge. Regional lymphadenopathy, chills, and fever can occur. Local complications, such as septic arthritis, osteomyelitis, and tenosynovitis, are common. Less common complications include septicemia, meningitis, respiratory tract infections (eg, pneumonia, pulmonary abscesses, and empyema), appendicitis, hepatic abscess, peritonitis, urinary tract infection, and ocular infections, including conjunctivitis, corneal ulcer, and endophthalmitis.

ETIOLOGY: *Pasteurella multocida* is a facultatively anaerobic, bipolar staining, gram-negative coccobacillus that is a primary pathogen in animals.

EPIDEMIOLOGY: The organism is found in the oral flora of 70% to 90% of cats, 25% to 50% of dogs, and the mouths of many other animals. Transmission occurs from the bite or scratch of a cat or dog or, less commonly, from another animal. Respiratory spread from animals to humans also occurs. Human-to-human spread has not been documented.

The **incubation period** usually is less than 24 hours.

DIAGNOSTIC TESTS: *Pasteurella multocida* can be isolated from skin lesion drainage or other sites of infection (eg, joint fluid, cerebrospinal fluid, sputum, pleural fluid, or suppurative lymph nodes). Although *P multocida* resembles several other organisms morphologically (such as *Haemophilus influenzae, Neisseria* species, and fastidious gram-negative rods, particularly *Actinobacillus*) and grows on many culture media at 37°C (98°F), laboratory differentiation is not difficult.

TREATMENT: The drug of choice is penicillin. Other effective agents include ampicillin, amoxicillin-clavulanate, cefuroxime, cefpodoxime, trimethoprim-sulfamethoxazole, and tetracycline. For patients allergic to ß-lactam agents, tetracycline is effective but should not be given to children younger than 8 years of age. For polymicrobial infection, which frequently occurs with *Staphylococcus aureus,* oral amoxicillin-clavulanate or intravenous ampicillin-sulbactam or ticarcillin-clavulanate (for severe infection) can be given. Parenterally administered, broad-spectrum cephalosporins, such as cefotaxime or cefoxitin, are active against *P multocida* in vitro, but the therapeutic experience with these drugs for *P multocida* infections is limited. The duration of therapy usually is 7 to 10 days for local infections and 10 to 14 days for more severe infections. Wound drainage or débridement may be necessary.

ISOLATION OF THE HOSPITALIZED PATIENT: Standard precautions are recommended. For culture-proven pneumonia, contact precautions are indicated in addition to standard precautions.

CONTROL MEASURES: Limiting contact with wild and domestic animals can prevent *P multocida* infections. Animal bites and scratches should be irrigated, cleansed, and débrided promptly. Minimal data exist about advisability of surgical closure of the wounds. Antimicrobial prophylaxis with penicillin or amoxicillin-clavulanate may be given, but data supporting efficacy are limited (see Table 2.18 in Bite Wounds, p 156).

Pediculosis Capitis

(Head Lice)

CLINICAL MANIFESTATIONS: Itching is the most common symptom of head lice infestation, but many children are asymptomatic. Adult lice or eggs (nits) are found in the hair, usually behind the ears and near the nape of the neck. Excoriations and crusting caused by secondary bacterial infection may occur and often are associated with regional lymphadenopathy. In temperate climates, head lice deposit their eggs on a hair shaft 3 to 4 mm from the scalp. Because hair grows at a rate of about 1 cm per month, the duration of infestation can be estimated by the distance of the nit from the scalp.

ETIOLOGY: *Pediculus humanus capitis* is the head louse. Both nymphs and adult lice feed on human blood.

EPIDEMIOLOGY: Head lice infestation in children attending child care and in school-age children is common in the United States. Head lice are not a sign of poor hygiene, and all socioeconomic groups are affected. Infestations are less common in African American children than in children of other races. Head lice infestation is not influenced by hair length or frequency of shampooing or brushing. Head lice are not a health hazard because they are not responsible for spread of any disease. Transmission occurs by direct contact with hair of infested persons and, less commonly, by contact with their personal belongings, such as combs, hair brushes, and hats. Head lice can survive only 1 to 2 days away from the scalp, and their eggs cannot hatch at a lower ambient temperature than that close to the scalp.

The **incubation period** from laying of the eggs to hatching of the first nymph is 6 to 10 days. Mature adult lice capable of reproducing do not appear until 2 to 3 weeks later.

DIAGNOSTIC TESTS: Identification of eggs, nymphs, and lice with the naked eye is possible; the diagnosis can be confirmed by using a hand lens or microscope. Adult lice seldom are seen because they move rapidly and conceal themselves effectively.

TREATMENT: The following agents are effective for treating pediculosis of the scalp (see Drugs for Parasitic Infections, p 693). Safety is a major concern with pediculicides because the infestation itself does not present a risk to the host. Pediculicides should be used only as directed and with care.

- ***Permethrin (1%).*** Permethrin is available without a prescription in a 1% cream rinse that is applied to the scalp and hair for 10 minutes. Permethrin has several advantages over the other pediculicides: a low potential for toxic effects, a high cure rate, and high ovicidal activity. Although activity continues for 2 weeks or more after application, most experts advise a second treatment 7 to 10 days after the first. Widespread resistance to permethrin has been reported in other countries. Although resistance to permethrin has been documented in the United States, the prevalence of this resistance is not known.
- ***Pyrethrin-based products.*** These 10-minute shampoos are available without prescription. Ovicidal activity is low, there is no residual activity, and repeated application 7 to 10 days later is necessary to kill newly hatched lice. Resistance to these compounds has not been documented in the United States but has been reported in other countries. These products are contraindicated in persons allergic to chrysanthemums.
- ***Lindane (1%).*** This 4-minute shampoo requires a prescription in the United States and is indicated primarily for persons who have not responded to or are intolerant of other approved therapies. Ovicidal activity is low, and repeated application 7 to 10 days later often is recommended. Lindane resistance has been reported from a number of countries. Lindane is contraindicated for use in premature infants, persons with known seizure disorders, and persons with hypersensitivity to the product; lindane should be used with caution in patients with inflamed or traumatized skin, in children younger than 2 years of age, and in pregnant or nursing women. Although lindane has the highest potential for toxic effects of all pediculicides, serious adverse effects rarely have been reported when used according to product instructions. Toxic effects with lindane usually have been associated with misuse, such as ingestion, excessive doses, or prolonged or repeated administration.
- ***Malathion (0.5%).*** This pesticide is highly effective for treatment of head lice and is safe when used as directed. The only preparation currently available in the United States is a 0.5% lotion, recommended for use in an 8- to 12-hour application that is to be repeated in 7 to 9 days if lice are still present at that time. Malathion lotion is flammable and, if ingested, can cause severe respiratory distress.

Because pediculicides kill lice shortly after application, the detection of living lice on scalp inspection 24 hours or more after treatment suggests incorrect use of the pediculicide, a very heavy infestation, reinfestation, or resistance to therapy. In such situations, after excluding incorrect use, immediate retreatment with a different pediculicide followed by a second application 7 days later is recommended.

Itching or mild burning of the scalp caused by inflammation of the skin in response to topical therapeutic agents can persist for many days after lice are killed and is not a reason for retreatment. Topical corticosteroids and oral antihistamines may be beneficial for relieving these signs and symptoms.

Removal of nits after treatment with a pediculicide is not necessary to prevent spread. If removal of nits is attempted for aesthetic reasons or to decrease diagnostic confusion, loosening the glue by which the nits are attached to hair may be facilitated by combing with a fine-toothed nit comb following pretreatment with a commercial formic acid rinse designated for this purpose, or soaking the hair with white vinegar (3% to 5% acetic acid) and then applying a damp towel soaked in the same solution for 30 to 60 minutes. Data are needed to determine whether suffocation of lice by application of occlusive agents, such as petroleum jelly, olive oil, or mayonnaise, is effective as a method of treatment.

ISOLATION OF THE HOSPITALIZED PATIENT: In addition to standard precautions, contact precautions are recommended until the patient has been treated with an appropriate pediculicide.

CONTROL MEASURES: Household and other close contacts should be examined and treated if infested. Differentiation of nits from benign hair casts (a layer of follicular cells that easily slides off the hair shaft), plugs of desquamated epithelial cells, and external debris can be difficult. Bedmates should be treated prophylactically. Children should not be excluded or sent home early from school because of head lice. Parents of affected children should be notified and informed that their child must be properly treated before returning to school the next day. After proper application of an appropriate pediculicide, reinfestation of children from an untreated infested contact is more common than treatment failure.

"No-nit" policies requiring that children be free of nits before they return to child care or school have not been effective in controlling head lice transmission and are not recommended. Lice incubating in egg cases (nits) are so close to the scalp that they are difficult to remove with nit combs. Egg cases further from the scalp are easier to remove but are empty and, thus, are of no consequence. To keep children from missing school or child care, it is recommended that settings with no-nit policies assist families with the removal of any nits on the day after treatment.

Most children can be treated effectively without extra efforts to treat their clothing or bedding. Although fomites do not have a major role in transmission of head lice, some parents may wish to disinfest headgear, pillow cases, and towels by washing them in hot water and machine drying (using a hot cycle). Combs and hair brushes can be washed with a pediculicide shampoo or soaked in hot water. Temperatures exceeding 53.5°C (128.3°F) for 5 minutes are lethal to lice and eggs. Although rarely necessary, dry cleaning clothing or simply storing contaminated items in well-sealed plastic bags for 10 days also is effective. Disinfesting furniture, such as chairs and sofas, is not necessary. Environmental insecticide sprays increase chemical exposure of household members and have not been helpful in the control of head lice. Vacuuming is a safe and effective alternative to spraying. Treatment of dogs, cats, or other pets is not indicated.

Pediculosis Corporis

CLINICAL MANIFESTATIONS: Intense itching, particularly at night, is common with body lice infestations. Body lice and their eggs live in the seams of clothing. Infrequently, a louse can be seen feeding on the skin. Secondary bacterial infection of the skin caused by scratching is common.

ETIOLOGY: *Pediculus humanus corporis* (or *humanus*) is the body louse. Both nymphs and adult lice feed on human blood.

EPIDEMIOLOGY: Body lice generally are found on persons with poor hygiene. Fomites have a role in transmission. Body lice cannot survive away from a blood source for longer than 10 days. In contrast with head lice, body lice are well-recognized vectors of disease (eg, epidemic typhus, trench fever, and relapsing fever).

The **incubation period** from laying of the eggs to hatching of the first nymph is 6 to 10 days. Mature adult lice capable of reproducing do not appear until 2 to 3 weeks later.

DIAGNOSTIC TESTS: Identification of eggs, nymphs, and lice with the naked eye is possible; the diagnosis can be confirmed by using a hand lens or microscope. Adult lice seldom are seen because they move rapidly and conceal themselves effectively.

TREATMENT: Treatment consists of improving hygiene and cleaning clothes. Infested clothing can be washed and dried at hot temperatures to kill the lice. Pediculicides are not necessary.

ISOLATION OF THE HOSPITALIZED PATIENT: In addition to standard precautions, contact precautions are recommended until the patient has been treated.

CONTROL MEASURES: The most important factor in the control of body lice infestation is the ability to change and wash clothing. Close contacts should be examined and treated appropriately.

Pediculosis Pubis

CLINICAL MANIFESTATIONS: Pruritus of the anogenital area is a common symptom in pubic lice infestations ("crabs"). Many hairy areas of the body can be infested, including the eyelashes, eyebrows, beard, axilla, perianal area, and, rarely, the scalp. A characteristic sign of heavy pubic lice infestation is the presence of bluish or slate-colored maculae on the chest, abdomen, or thighs, known as maculae ceruleae.

ETIOLOGY: *Phthirus pubis* is the pubic or crab louse. Both nymphs and adult lice feed on human blood.

EPIDEMIOLOGY: Pubic lice infestations are common in adolescents and young adults and usually are transmitted through sexual contact. The pubic louse also can be transferred by contaminated items, such as towels. Pubic lice can be found on the eyelashes of younger children and, while other modes of transmission are possible, may be evidence of sexual abuse. Infested persons should be examined for other sexually transmitted diseases, including syphilis and infection with *Neisseria gonorrhoeae, Chlamydia trachomatis,* hepatitis B, and human immunodeficiency virus.

The **incubation period** from laying of the eggs to hatching of the first nymph is 6 to 10 days. Mature adult lice capable of reproducing do not appear until 2 to 3 weeks later.

DIAGNOSTIC TESTS: Identification of eggs, nymphs, and lice with the naked eye is possible; the diagnosis can be confirmed by using a hand lens or microscope. Adult lice seldom are seen because they move rapidly and conceal themselves effectively.

TREATMENT: The pediculicides used to treat pediculosis capitis are effective for the treatment of pubic lice. Retreatment is recommended 7 to 10 days later. For infestation of eyelashes by pubic lice, petrolatum ointment applied 3 to 4 times daily for 8 to 10 days is effective. Nits should be removed by hand from the eyelashes.

ISOLATION OF THE HOSPITALIZED PATIENT: In addition to standard precautions, contact precautions are recommended until the patient has been treated with an appropriate pediculicide.

CONTROL MEASURES: All sexual contacts should be treated.

Pelvic Inflammatory Disease

CLINICAL MANIFESTATIONS: Pelvic inflammatory disease (PID) denotes a spectrum of inflammatory disorders of the female upper genital tract, including endometritis, parametritis, salpingitis, oophoritis, tubo-ovarian abscess, and pelvic peritonitis. Pelvic inflammatory disease typically presents with dull, continuous, bilateral lower abdominal or pelvic pain that may range from indolent to severe. Additional symptoms can include fever, vomiting, an abnormal vaginal discharge, and irregular vaginal bleeding (signaling endometritis). Some patients have sharp right upper abdominal quadrant pain as a result of perihepatitis. Symptoms often begin within a week after the onset of menses.

Common examination findings include fever, lower abdominal tenderness, tenderness on lateral motion of the cervix, adnexal tenderness that is generally but not always bilateral, and adnexal fullness. Leukocytosis, an erythrocyte sedimentation rate more than 15 mm/h, and an adnexal mass demonstrated by abdominal or transvaginal ultrasonography are common findings.

No single symptom, sign, or laboratory finding is sensitive and specific for the diagnosis of acute PID. Many patients are afebrile and have only mild pain and tenderness, no abnormal vaginal discharge, and no leukocytosis. Pelvic inflammatory disease may be asymptomatic (silent PID). Combinations of findings that improve sensitivity (ie, correctly detect more women who have PID) do so only while reducing specificity (ie, incorrectly including more women who do not have PID). The diagnostic criteria currently recommended by the Centers for Disease Control and Prevention are presented in Table 3.41, p 432.

Many episodes of PID go unrecognized, some because patients are asymptomatic (silent PID) and others because the symptoms are mild and nonspecific, so the diagnosis is not considered.

Complications of PID may include perihepatitis (Fitz-Hugh–Curtis syndrome) and tubo-ovarian abscess. Important long-term sequelae are recurrent infection, chronic pelvic pain, a 6-fold increase in the incidence of ectopic pregnancy, and

Table 3.41. Criteria for Clinical Diagnosis of Pelvic Inflammatory Disease (PID)*

Minimum Criteria

Empiric treatment of PID should be instituted on the basis of the presence of all of the following minimum clinical criteria for pelvic inflammation and in the absence of an established cause other than PID:

- Lower abdominal tenderness,
- Adnexal tenderness, and
- Cervical motion tenderness

Additional Criteria

Because incorrect diagnosis and management may cause unnecessary morbidity, more detailed diagnostic evaluation is warranted for women with severe clinical signs to increase the specificity of the diagnosis.

The following are the additional criteria for diagnosing PID:

- Oral temperature >38.3°C (101°F),
- Abnormal cervical or vaginal discharge,
- Elevated erythrocyte sedimentation rate,
- Elevated C-reactive protein level, and
- Laboratory documentation of cervical infection with *Neisseria gonorrhoeae* or *Chlamydia trachomatis*

The following are the definitive criteria for diagnosing PID:

- Histopathologic evidence of endometritis on endometrial biopsy
- Transvaginal or abdominal ultrasonography showing tubo-ovarian abscess or consistent fallopian tube abnormalities
- Laparoscopic abnormalities consistent with PID

* Adapted from the Centers for Disease Control and Prevention. 1998 Guidelines for treatment of sexually transmitted diseases. *MMWR Morb Mortal Wkly Rep.* 1998;47(RR-1):1–116. No single symptom, sign, or laboratory finding is sensitive and specific for the diagnosis of pelvic inflammatory disease. Combinations of findings that improve sensitivity do so only at the expense of reduced specificity, and vice versa.

infertility resulting from tubal occlusion. The risk of tubal infertility is estimated to be 10% after a single episode of PID and more than 50% after 3 or more episodes. Factors that may increase the likelihood of infertility are older age at the time of infection, chlamydial disease, PID determined to be severe laparoscopically, and delayed antibiotic treatment.

ETIOLOGY: Sexually transmitted organisms, especially *Neisseria gonorrhoeae* and *Chlamydia trachomatis,* are implicated in most cases of PID. However, other organisms, such as anaerobes, including *Bacteroides* and *Peptostreptococcus* species; facultative anaerobes, including *Gardnerella vaginalis, Streptococcus* species, and coliform bacteria; and genital tract mycoplasmas, including *Mycoplasma hominis* and *Ureaplasma urealyticum,* also are associated with PID.

EPIDEMIOLOGY: As is true for other sexually transmitted diseases (STDs), the incidence of PID is highest among adolescents and young adults. Other risk factors for PID include numerous sexual partners, use of an intrauterine device, douching, and previous episodes of PID. Barrier methods of contraception reduce the incidence of all STDs. Oral contraceptive pills reduce the likelihood of PID in the face of gonococcal or chlamydial cervicitis. Ascending pelvic infection is a rare complication of gonococcal vaginitis in prepubertal girls.

An **incubation period** for PID is undefined. In women with gonococcal cervicitis, symptoms of PID generally appear during the first half of the menstrual cycle.

DIAGNOSTIC TESTS: The diagnosis of PID usually is based on clinical findings (see Table 3.41, p 432) and is supported by the findings of a preponderance of leukocytes in cervical secretions, leukocytosis, an elevated C-reactive protein level or erythrocyte sedimentation rate, the identification of *N gonorrhoeae* in an endocervical culture, and the presence of *C trachomatis* in a rapid detection test of endocervical secretions (see *Chlamydia trachomatis,* p 208 and *Neisseria gonorrhoeae,* p 254). An endocervical culture for *N gonorrhoeae* and an endocervical test for *C trachomatis* should be obtained before treatment is begun. Ultrasonography and laparoscopy are most useful when appendicitis, ruptured ovarian cyst, or ectopic pregnancy is a leading alternative to the diagnosis of PID. Laparoscopy also permits bacteriologic samples to be obtained directly from tubal exudate or the cul-de-sac. However, laparoscopy cannot detect endometritis and is not indicated in most cases. Because an adolescent's recollection of her menstrual history is not always reliable, and because PID and ectopic pregnancy can both produce abdominal pain and irregular bleeding, a pregnancy test is indicated in the diagnostic evaluation of the adolescent with suspected PID.

TREATMENT: Since the clinical diagnosis of PID, even in the most experienced hands, is imprecise, and because the consequences of untreated infection are substantial, most experts provide antimicrobial therapy to patients who fulfill the minimum criteria rather than limiting therapy to patients who fulfill the additional criteria for the diagnosis of PID (Table 3.41, p 432). To minimize the risks of progressive infection and subsequent infertility, treatment should not await culture results but should be instituted as soon as the clinical diagnosis is made.

Observation and treatment in the hospital are suggested for the following reasons: (1) a surgical emergency, such as ectopic pregnancy or appendicitis, cannot be excluded, (2) compliance with or tolerance of an outpatient treatment regimen and follow-up within 72 hours cannot be assured, (3) the patient's illness is severe (eg, pelvic or tubo-ovarian abscess, overt peritonitis), (4) the patient is immunodeficient (human immunodeficiency virus [HIV] infection with low CD4 lymphocyte count, immunosuppression therapy), (5) the patient is pregnant, or (6) the patient has failed to respond to outpatient therapy. Although, in the past, many experts have recommended hospitalization for all adolescent patients with PID, data to support this recommendation are lacking.

The choice of an antibiotic regimen for PID is empiric, broad spectrum, and directed against the most common causative agents. Antimicrobial regimens consistent with those recommended by the Centers for Disease Control and Prevention

Table 3.42. Recommended Treatment of Pelvic Inflammatory Disease (PID)*

Inpatient: Regimen A[†]

Cefoxitin, 2 g IV every 6 h

OR

Cefotetan,[||] 2 g every 12 h

PLUS

Doxycycline, 100 mg IV or orally every 12 h

OR

Inpatient: Regimen B[¶]

Clindamycin, 900 mg IV every 8 h

PLUS

Gentamicin: loading dose, 2.0 mg/kg IV or IM, followed by maintenance, 1.5 mg/kg IV every 8 h. Single daily dosing may be substituted.

NOTE

Regimens A and B are continued for 24 to 48 h after significant clinical improvement is demonstrated and are followed by doxycycline, 100 mg orally twice a day (regimen A[#]), or clindamycin, 600 mg orally 3 times a day (regimen B[#]), to complete a 14-d total course.

Ambulatory: Regimen A[‡]

Ofloxacin,[§] 400 mg orally twice a day for 14 d

PLUS

Metronidazole, 500 mg orally twice a day for 14 d

OR

Ambulatory: Regimen B

Cefoxitin, 2 g IM, with concurrent probenecid, 1 g orally once

Ceftriaxone, 250 mg IM once

OR

Equivalent parenteral cephalosporin[||]

PLUS

Doxycycline, 100 mg orally twice a day for 14 d

* IV indicates intravenous; IM, intramuscular. For further alternative treatment regimens, see Centers for Disease Control and Prevention. 1998 guidelines for treatment of sexually transmitted diseases. *MMWR Morb Mortal Wkly Rep.* 1998;47(RR-1):1–116

† Many experts recommend hospitalization for all patients with PID, particularly adolescents.

‡ Patients with inadequate response to outpatient therapy after 72 hours should be reevaluated for possible misdiagnosis and should receive parenteral therapy.

§ Fluoroquinolones are contraindicated for patients younger than 18 years of age, for pregnant women, and during lactation (see Antimicrobials and Related Therapy, p 645).

|| Data to indicate whether expanded spectrum cephalosporins (ceftizoxime, cefotaxime, ceftriaxone) can replace cefoxitin or cefotetan are limited. Many authorities believe they also are effective therapy for PID, but they are less active against anaerobes.

¶ Alternative parenteral regimens include ofloxacin plus metronidazole, ampicillin-sulbactam plus doxycycline, and ciprofloxacin plus doxycycline plus metronidazole.

\# For continued oral therapy for tubo-ovarian abscess, recurrent PID, and postsurgical PID, many clinicians use clindamycin (or metronidazole), as well as doxycycline, to provide more effective anaerobic coverage.

(1998) are summarized in Table 3.42 (above). Clinical outcome data are lacking about the use of other cephalosporin antibiotics, such as ceftizoxime, cefotaxime, and ceftriaxone. Some experts believe that these agents can be used to replace cefoxitin or cefotetan for PID treatment; however, cefoxitin and cefotetan are more active against anaerobes. Fluoroquinolones are not recommended for use in patients younger than 18 years of age when other effective alternatives are available. Consideration should be given to selecting an antibiotic that provides broad anaerobic coverage (clindamycin or metronidazole) for patients with tubo-ovarian abscess, recurrent PID, or recent pelvic surgery. If the patient has an intrauterine device in place, the device should be removed immediately. In patients treated orally or parenterally, clinical improvement can be expected within 72 hours after initiation of treatment. Accordingly, outpatients should be reevaluated routinely on the third or fourth day of treatment.

Isolation of the Hospitalized Patient: Standard precautions are recommended.

Control Measures:

- Male sexual partners of patients with PID should receive diagnostic evaluation for gonococcal and chlamydial urethritis and then should be treated presumptively for both infections if they had sexual contact with the patient during the 60 days preceding onset of symptoms in the patient. A large proportion of these males will be asymptomatic.
- The patient should abstain from intercourse until she and her partner(s) have completed treatment.
- The patient and her partner(s) should be encouraged to use condoms consistently.
- The patient should be tested for syphilis and HIV infection, and a Papanicolaou smear should be obtained.
- Unimmunized or incompletely immunized patients should begin or complete hepatitis B immunization (see Recommended Childhood Immunization Schedule, p 22).
- Because of the high risk of reinfection, some experts recommend that patients with PID whose initial test for *N gonorrhoeae* and *C trachomatis* was positive be retested 4 to 6 weeks after completing treatment.
- The diagnosis of PID provides an opportune time to educate the adolescent about prevention of STDs, including abstinence, consistent use of barrier methods of protection, and the importance of receiving periodic screening for STDs.

Pertussis

Clinical Manifestations: Pertussis begins with mild upper respiratory tract symptoms (catarrhal stage) and can progress to severe paroxysms of cough (paroxysmal stage), often with a characteristic respiratory whoop, followed by vomiting. Fever is absent or minimal. Symptoms wane gradually (convalescent stage). Disease in infants younger than 6 months of age may be atypical; apnea is a common manifestation and whoop often is absent. Similarly, older children and adults can have atypical manifestations, with persistent cough and no whoop. The duration of classic pertussis is 6 to 10 weeks; however, more than half of the primary cases last less than 6 weeks, and a quarter of the patients have cough for 3 weeks or less. Complications include seizures, pneumonia, encephalopathy, and death. Pertussis is most severe when it occurs during the first year of life (particularly for preterm infants). According to data from the Centers for Disease Control and Prevention based on cases reported to local and state health departments from 1980 to 1989, pneumonia, seizures, and encephalopathy occurred in 22%, 3%, and 1%, respectively, of infants with pertussis. The case-fatality rate was 1.3% in infants younger than 1 month of age and 0.3% in infants 2 to 11 months of age. However, because more than 40% of these reported cases were hospitalized, these complication rates are likely to be representative of more severe illness. In a recent study of unimmunized outpatients in Germany, the complication rates were appreciably lower. Infection in immunized children and older persons often is mild. Pertussis does not seem to cause permanent pulmonary sequelae.

ETIOLOGY: *Bordetella pertussis* is a fastidious, gram-negative, pleomorphic bacillus. A whooping cough syndrome also may be caused by *Bordetella parapertussis, Mycoplasma pneumoniae, Chlamydia trachomatis, Chlamydia pneumoniae, Bordetella bronchiseptica,* and certain adenoviruses. *Bordetella parapertussis* may cause an appreciable portion of the clinical cases of pertussis, especially milder cases, and has been reported as the single agent or as a dual infection with *B pertussis* in up to 40% of laboratory-confirmed cases.

EPIDEMIOLOGY: Humans are the only known hosts of *B pertussis.* Transmission occurs by close contact via respiratory tract secretions of patients with disease. Asymptomatic infection has been demonstrated but is unlikely to be a factor in transmission. Pertussis occurs endemically with 3- to 5-year cycles of increased disease. As many as 90% of nonimmune household contacts acquire the disease. Adolescents and adults are an important source of pertussis, accounting in 1997 for as many as 46% of reported cases. Infants and young children frequently are infected by older siblings or adults who often have mild or atypical illness. While pertussis can occur at any age, in 1997, approximately 24% of reported cases in the United States occurred in infants younger than 6 months of age, including 18% in infants younger than 3 months of age, and approximately 43% of reported cases occurred in children younger than 5 years of age. Widespread immunization with pertussis vaccine since the 1940s is primarily responsible for the current low morbidity and mortality rates of pertussis in the United States. Patients are most contagious during the catarrhal stage before the onset of paroxysms; communicability then diminishes rapidly but may persist for 3 weeks or more after onset of cough. Erythromycin therapy decreases infectivity and may limit spread. Nasopharyngeal cultures usually become negative for *B pertussis* within 5 days after initiating therapy.

The **incubation period** is 6 to 20 days, usually 7 to 10 days.

DIAGNOSTIC TESTS: Culture of *B pertussis* requires inoculation of nasopharyngeal mucus, obtained by aspiration or with a Dacron (polyethylene terephthalate) or calcium alginate swab, on special media (such as Regan-Lowe or fresh Bordet-Gengou), with incubation for 10 to 14 days. Because these media may not be available routinely, laboratory personnel should be informed when *B pertussis* is suspected. Although for optimal results specimens should be inoculated at the bedside or taken promptly to the laboratory in special transport media, reasonable rates of positive culture have been obtained by preincubation in Regan-Lowe transport medium for submission to the laboratory. The organism is recovered most frequently in the catarrhal or early paroxysmal stage and rarely is found after the fourth week of illness. A positive culture is diagnostic. Negative cultures are common, particularly late in the course of the disease, from patients who have been immunized previously or from patients receiving antibiotics. The direct immunofluorescent assay (DFA) of nasopharyngeal secretions has variable sensitivity and low specificity, requires experienced personnel for interpretation, and is not a reliable criterion for laboratory confirmation of the diagnosis. Since false-positive and false-negative DFA results occur, culture confirmation of all suspected pertussis cases should be attempted. Rapid progress in the investigational application of nucleic acid amplification methods, such as polymerase chain reaction on nasopharyngeal specimens and on cultures, suggests that these tests may offer a more sensitive and rapid means for the diagnosis of infection with *B pertussis* and *B parapertussis* in the future.

No single serologic test is diagnostic of pertussis. *Bordetella pertussis* infections stimulate a heterogeneous antibody response that differs among individuals, depending on age and previous exposure to the organism or to its antigens by immunization. In research laboratories, the serologic diagnosis of pertussis has excellent sensitivity and specificity when an acute serum specimen is collected early in the illness and paired acute- and convalescent-phase serum specimens are tested. Measurement of agglutinating antibodies has long been the standard for serologic testing for pertussis. During the past decade, however, the enzyme immunoassays for immunoglobulin (Ig) G and IgA antibody to *Bordetella* antigens increasingly have become the methods of choice, but these assays are not available widely or standardized.

Although an increased white blood cell count with an absolute lymphocytosis often is present in patients with classic *B pertussis* but not *B parapertussis* infection, it is a nonspecific finding, especially in infants, who often develop lymphocytosis from other infections. The degree of elevation of the white blood cell count and lymphocytosis usually parallels the severity of the patient's cough.

Because laboratory confirmation of pertussis can be difficult, clinicians often need to make the diagnosis on the basis of characteristic manifestations of prolonged paroxysmal coughing with supportive associated findings, such as inspiratory whoop, posttussive emesis, and lymphocytosis.

TREATMENT:

- Infants younger than 6 months of age and other patients with potentially severe disease often require hospitalization for supportive care to manage coughing paroxysms, apnea, cyanosis, feeding difficulties, and other complications. Intensive care facilities may be required for severe cases.
- Antimicrobial agents given during the catarrhal stage may ameliorate the disease. After paroxysms are established, however, antimicrobial agents usually have no discernible effect on the course of illness but are recommended to limit the spread of the organisms to others. The drug of choice is erythromycin (40 to 50 mg/kg per day orally in 4 divided doses; maximum, 2 g/d); some experts prefer the estolate preparation. The recommended duration of therapy to prevent bacteriologic relapse is 14 days. Studies suggest that the newer macrolides, azithromycin (10–12 mg/kg per day orally in 1 dose) or clarithromycin (15–20 mg/kg per day orally in 2 divided doses; maximum,

1 g/d), may be effective in shorter courses of 5 to 7 days; however, their efficacy is unproven. Erythromycin resistance of *B pertussis* has been reported, but rarely.

An association between orally administered erythromycin and infantile hypertrophic pyloric stenosis (IHPS) has been reported in infants younger than 6 weeks of age. The risk of IHPS after treatment with other macrolides (eg, azithromycin and clarithromycin) is unknown. Since confirmation of erythromycin as a contributor to cases of IHPS will require additional investigation, and since alternative therapies are not as well studied, the AAP continues to recommend use of erythromycin for prophylaxis and treatment of disease caused by *B pertussis.* Physicians who prescribe erythromycin to newborn infants should inform parents about the potential risks of developing IHPS and signs of IHPS. Cases of pyloric stenosis following use of oral erythromycin should be reported to MEDWATCH (see MEDWATCH, p 726).

- Trimethoprim-sulfamethoxazole is another possible alternative, but its efficacy is unproven.
- Corticosteroids, albuterol (a β_2-adrenergic stimulant), and pertussis-specific immunoglobulin each may be effective in reducing paroxysms of coughing, but further evaluation is required before they can be recommended. Pertussis-specific immunoglobulin currently is an investigational product.

ISOLATION OF THE HOSPITALIZED PATIENT: In addition to standard precautions, droplet precautions are recommended for 5 days after initiation of effective therapy or until 3 weeks after the onset of paroxysms if appropriate antimicrobial therapy is not given.

CONTROL MEASURES:

Care of Exposed Persons.

Household and Other Close Contacts.

Immunization. Close contacts younger than 7 years of age who are unimmunized or who have received fewer than 4 doses of pertussis vaccine (diphtheria and tetanus toxoids and acellular pertussis [DTaP] or diphtheria and tetanus toxoids and pertussis [DTP]) should have pertussis immunization initiated or continued, according to the recommended schedule. Children who received their third dose 6 months or more before exposure should be given a fourth dose at this time. Children who have had 4 doses of pertussis vaccine should receive a booster dose of DTaP unless a dose has been given within the last 3 years or they are 7 years of age or older.

Chemoprophylaxis. Erythromycin (40–50 mg/kg per day orally in 4 divided doses; maximum, 2 g/d) for 14 days, as tolerated, is recommended for all household contacts and other close contacts, such as those in child care, irrespective of age and immunization status. A recent study indicates that a 10-day course of erythromycin is equally effective. Some experts recommend the estolate preparation. For erythromycin use in infants younger than 4 weeks of age, see Treatment, p 437. The newer macrolides, clarithromycin and azithromycin, are potential, but not proven, alternatives for patients who cannot tolerate erythromycin (see Treatment, p 437). Prompt use of chemoprophylaxis in household contacts effectively limits secondary transmission. The rationale for administering chemoprophylaxis to all household and other close contacts irrespective of age or immunization status is that pertussis immunity is not absolute and may not prevent infection. Persons with mild illness that may not be recognized as pertussis can transmit the infection.

Persons who have been in contact with an infected person should be monitored closely for respiratory tract symptoms for 20 days after last contact with the infected person.

Child Care. Exposed children, especially incompletely immunized children, should be observed for respiratory tract symptoms for 20 days after contact has been terminated. Pertussis immunization and chemoprophylaxis should be given as recommended for household and other close contacts. Symptomatic children with cough should be excluded from child care, pending physician evaluation. Children with pertussis, if their medical condition allows, may return to or enter a child care facility 5 days after initiation of erythromycin or other recommended drug therapy. Chemoprophylaxis should be considered for adult staff with close or extensive contact. Staff members should be monitored for respiratory tract symptoms, undergo culture for pertussis if symptoms develop, and be given antimicrobial therapy if cough develops within 20 days of exposure (see Treatment, p 437).

Schools. Students and staff with pertussis should be excluded from school; if their medical condition allows, they may return 5 days after initiation of erythromycin therapy (or other recommended drug therapy). Persons who do not receive appropriate antimicrobial therapy should be excluded from school for 21 days after onset of symptoms. Other public health recommendations to control pertussis transmission have not been established. School-wide or classroom chemoprophylaxis generally has not been recommended, usually because of the delay in recognition of outbreaks and difficulties of implementation. The immunization status of children younger than 7 years of age should be reviewed and vaccine given, if indicated, as for household and other close contacts. Pertussis should be considered in the differential diagnosis of persons with cough illness who may have been exposed. Parents and employees should be notified about possible exposures to pertussis. Exclusion of exposed persons with cough illness, pending physician evaluation, should be considered. The local health department should be consulted about the possible implementation of this and other control measures.

Immunization. Universal immunization with pertussis vaccine of children younger than 7 years of age is critical for the control of pertussis. The pertussis vaccines recommended for use in the United States are acellular vaccines in combination with diphtheria and tetanus toxoids (DTaP) and, for acellular and whole cell products, in combination with *Haemophilus influenzae* type b conjugate vaccine. Recommendations for use of DTaP are similar to recommendations for use of DTP, which continues to be given to infants and children in many countries in the world. Acellular vaccines are adsorbed onto an aluminum salt and, thus, are administered intramuscularly. Acellular vaccines contain one or more immunogens derived from *B pertussis* organisms. These antigens include detoxified pertussis toxin (ie, pertussis toxoid [PT], also termed lymphocytosis-promoting factor), filamentous hemagglutinin, fimbrial proteins (agglutinogens), and pertactin (an outer membrane 69-kd protein). As of January 2000, 5 acellular pertussis–containing vaccines (DTaP) are licensed in the United States, and 4 have been approved by the US Food and Drug

Administration (FDA) for use in infants and for primary immunization (see Table 3.43, p 441). Licensure of additional products is anticipated. Although licensed vaccines differ in their formulation of pertussis antigens, their efficacy seems similar. All DTaP vaccines currently contain PT. Detailed information on acellular pertussis vaccines, including efficacy, adverse events, and vaccine composition, is summarized in an American Academy of Pediatrics statement on DTaP.* Vaccine recommendations are updated and published each January in *Pediatrics.*

Efficacy of acellular pertussis vaccines originally was demonstrated in Japan in children 2 years of age and older. Trials of several acellular vaccines in Europe and Africa have documented efficacy comparable to that of whole-cell pertussis vaccine given to infants as the primary 3-dose series. The immunogenicity of the antigens in the acellular vaccines is similar to that of whole-cell DTP vaccine. However, antibody responses do not correlate with protection against disease and, thus, cannot be used to predict efficacy. Duration of protection after immunization with acellular pertussis vaccine has not been established; studies of this question, however, are in progress.

The rates of local reactions (erythema and induration at the injection site), fever, and other common systemic symptoms (drowsiness, fretfulness, and anorexia) are substantially lower with acellular pertussis vaccines than with whole-cell pertussis vaccines. Whether the rare, more serious adverse events associated with DTP will occur less frequently after acellular pertussis vaccine is not known (see Adverse Events After Pertussis Immunization, p 443).

Dose and Route. Each dose of DTaP is 0.5 mL, given intramuscularly. The use of reduced volume of individual doses of pertussis vaccines or multiple doses of reduced volume (fractional doses) is not recommended, including for premature or low-birth-weight infants. The effect of such practices on the frequency of serious adverse events and on protection against disease has not been determined.

Interchangeability of Acellular Pertussis Vaccines. When feasible, the same DTaP vaccine product should be used for the first 3 doses of the pertussis immunization series. No data exist on the safety, immunogenicity, or efficacy of different DTaP vaccines when administered interchangeably in the primary series. However, in circumstances in which the type of DTaP product(s) received previously is not known or the previously administered product(s) is not readily available, any of the DTaP vaccines licensed for use in the primary series may be used. For the fourth and fifth dose, any licensed product is acceptable, irrespective of prior vaccines received. These recommendations may change as data become available about the response to different DTaP vaccines administered interchangeably in a primary series or as the fourth or fifth doses.

Antipyretic Prophylaxis. Administration of acetaminophen or other appropriate antipyretic at the time of immunization with DTaP and at 4 and 8 hours after immunization decreases the subsequent incidence of febrile and local reactions.

Recommendations for Routine Childhood Immunization. A total of 5 doses of pertussis vaccine is recommended by the time of school entry, unless contraindicated (see Contraindications to Pertussis Immunization, p 445, and Precautions for Pertussis Immunization, p 446). If the fourth dose of pertussis vaccine is given

* See American Academy of Pediatrics Committee on Infectious Diseases. Acellular pertussis vaccine: recommendations for use as the initial series in infants and children. *Pediatrics.* 1997;99:282–288

Table 3.43. **Licensed DTaP-Containing Vaccines***

	Tripedia (DTaP)	ACEL-IMUNE (DTaP)	Infanrix (DTaP)	Certiva (DTaP)	TriHIBit† (DTaP-Hib)
Pharmaceutical Co.	Aventis Pasteur, Swiftwater, Pa	Lederle Laboratories, Pearl River, NY (distributed by Wyeth-Lederle Vaccines, Wyeth-Ayerst Laboratories, Philadelphia, Pa	SmithKline Beecham, Philadelphia, Pa	North American Vaccine, Inc, Beltsville, Md	Aventis Pasteur
Antigens	PT, FHA	PT, FHA, fimbria 2, pertactin	PT, FHA, pertactin	PT	PT, FHA
Recommended use	**First 4 doses,** children 6 wk to 6 y; can be used for the fifth dose for a child who has received one or more doses of whole-cell DTP	**All 5 doses,** children 6 wk to 6 y	**First 4 doses,** children 6 wk to 6 y; can be used for the fifth dose for a child who has received one or more doses of whole-cell DTP	**First 4 doses,** children 6 wk to 6 y; can be used for the fifth dose for a child who has received one or more doses of whole-cell DTP	**Only fourth dose;** TriHIBit can be used for the fourth dose after 3 doses of DTaP or whole-cell DTP and a primary series of any Hib vaccine

* DTaP recommended schedule is 2, 4, 6, and 15 to 18 months and 4 to 6 years. The fourth dose can be given as early as 12 months, provided 6 months have elapsed since the third dose was given. The fifth dose is not necessary if the fourth dose was given on or after the fourth birthday. DTaP indicates diphtheria and tetanus toxoids and acellular pertussis vaccine; Hib, *Haemophilus influenzae* type b vaccine; PT, pertussis toxoid; FHA, filamentous hemagglutinin; and DTP, diphtheria and tetanus toxoids and pertussis vaccine. Refer to manufacturers' package inserts for comprehensive product information regarding indications and use of the vaccines listed.

† TriHIBit is ActHib reconstituted with Tripedia.

after the fourth birthday because of delays in completing the immunization schedule, the fifth dose is not indicated. The first dose is given at 2 months of age, followed by 2 additional doses at intervals of approximately 2 months. The fourth dose is recommended at 15 to 18 months of age. The fifth dose is given before school entry (kindergarten or elementary school) at 4 to 6 years of age to protect these children from pertussis in ensuing years and to decrease transmission of the disease to younger children.

In the United States, DTaP is preferred for all doses because of the decreased likelihood of vaccine-associated adverse events, such as fever and local reactions. Combination products containing pertussis vaccine may be given, provided they are approved by the FDA for the child's current age and administration of the other components of the vaccine also is justified.

Other recommendations are as follows:

- For the fourth dose, DTaP may be given as early as 12 months of age if the interval between the third and fourth doses is at least 6 months and the child is considered unlikely to return for a visit at the recommended age of 15 to 18 months for this dose.
- Simultaneous administration of DTaP and other recommended vaccines is acceptable. Vaccines should not be mixed in the same syringe unless the specific combination is approved by the FDA (see Simultaneous Administration of Multiple Vaccines, p 26, and *Haemophilus influenzae* Infections, p 262).
- If pertussis is prevalent in the community, immunization can be started as early as 6 weeks of age, and doses in the primary series can be given as frequently as 4 weeks apart.
- Pertussis immunization is not recommended for persons 7 years of age or older.
- For children who have begun their primary immunization schedule with DTP, an FDA-approved DTaP vaccine should be used to complete the pertussis immunization schedule.
- Children who have a contraindication to pertussis immunization should receive no further doses of pertussis-containing vaccine (see Contraindications to Pertussis Immunization, p 445, and Precautions for Pertussis Immunization, p 446).

Recommendations for Scheduling Pertussis Vaccine in Special Circumstances.

- For the child whose pertussis immunization schedule is resumed after deferral or interruption of the recommended schedule, the next dose in the sequence should be given, irrespective of the interval since the last dose, ie, the schedule is not reinitiated (see Lapsed Immunizations, p 27).
- For children who have received fewer than the recommended number of doses of pertussis vaccine but who have received the recommended number of DT doses for their age (ie, those started on DT, then given DTaP or DTP), dose(s) of DTaP should be given to complete the recommended pertussis immunization schedule. However, the total number of doses of diphtheria and tetanus

toxoids (as DT, DTaP, or DTP) should not exceed 6 before the fourth birthday. A monovalent pertussis vaccine preparation* may be used instead.

- Children who have had well-documented pertussis should complete the immunization series with at least DT; some experts recommend including the pertussis component as well, ie, administration of DTaP. Although well-documented pertussis disease (ie, positive culture for *B pertussis* or epidemiologic linkage to a culture-positive case) is likely to confer immunity against pertussis, the duration of such immunity is unknown.
- During pertussis outbreaks, such as in a hospital, pertussis immunization usually is not recommended for adult contacts. Evaluation of acellular pertussis vaccines for use in adolescents and adults is in progress, and these vaccines should be used only under appropriate research protocols until they are licensed for use in this population.

Medical Records. Charts of children for whom pertussis immunization has been deferred should be flagged, and the immunization status of these children should be assessed periodically to ensure that they are immunized appropriately.

Adverse Events After Pertussis Immunization.

- ***Local and febrile reactions.*** Reactions to DTaP vaccine most commonly include redness, edema, induration, and tenderness at the injection site; drowsiness; fretfulness; anorexia; vomiting; crying; and slight to moderate fever. These local and systemic manifestations following pertussis immunization occur within several hours of immunization and subside spontaneously without sequelae. They are significantly less common with DTaP than with DTP. Children with such reactions should receive subsequent doses of pertussis vaccine as scheduled.

  Bacterial or sterile abscesses at the site of the injection are rare. Bacterial abscesses indicate contamination of the product or nonsterile technique and should be reported (see Reporting of Adverse Events, p 31). The causes of sterile abscesses are unknown. Their occurrence usually does not contraindicate further doses of DTaP.
- ***Allergic reactions.*** The rate of anaphylaxis to DTP is estimated to be approximately 2 cases per 100 000 injections; the incidence of allergic reactions following immunization with DTaP is unknown. Severe anaphylactic reactions and resulting deaths, if any, are rare following pertussis immunization. The transient urticarial rashes that occasionally occur after pertussis immunization, unless appearing immediately (ie, within minutes), are unlikely to be anaphylactic (IgE-mediated) in origin. These rashes probably represent a serum sickness–type reaction caused by circulating antigen-antibody complexes due to one of the antigens in pertussis vaccine and corresponding antibody acquired from an earlier dose or transplacentally. Because formation of such complexes depends on a precise balance between concentrations of circulating antigen and antibody, such reactions are unlikely to recur after a subsequent dose and are not contraindications to further doses.

* Available from Bio Port Corporation, Lansing, Mich.

- ***Seizures.*** The incidence of seizures occurring within 48 hours of administration of whole-cell pertussis (ie, DTP) vaccine has been estimated to be 1 case per 1750 doses administered. In field trials in Europe of DTaP vaccine and postlicensure surveillance of adverse events associated with DTaP in the United States, the incidence of seizures has been substantially less than that associated with DTP.

  Most seizures occurring after immunization with DTP are brief, self-limited, and generalized. They usually occur in febrile children after the third or fourth dose of the vaccine series. These characteristics suggest that seizures associated with pertussis vaccine usually are febrile seizures. These seizures have not been demonstrated to result in the subsequent development of recurrent afebrile seizures (ie, epilepsy) or other neurologic sequelae. Predisposing factors to seizures occurring within 48 hours include underlying convulsive disorder, personal history of seizures, and family history of seizures (see Infants and Children With Underlying Neurologic Disorders, p 446, and Children With a Personal or Family History of Seizures, p 68).
- ***Hypotonic-hyporesponsive episodes.*** These episodes (also termed *collapse* or *shock-like state*) have been reported to occur at a frequency of 1 per 1750 doses of DTP vaccine administered. However, rates seem to vary widely, ranging from 3.5 to 291 cases per 100 000 immunizations in other observations. The rate following immunization with DTaP is currently unknown; however, in a large Italian trial, these episodes occurred significantly less often following immunization with DTaP than with DTP. A follow-up study of a group of children who experienced hypotonic-hyporesponsive episode (HHE) following immunization with DTP demonstrated no evidence of subsequent serious neurologic damage or intellectual impairment.
- ***Temperature of 40.5°C (104.8°F) or greater.*** Following administration of DTP vaccine, approximately 0.3% of recipients have been reported to develop temperature of 40.5°C (104.8°F) or greater within 48 hours. The rate following DTaP is significantly less.
- ***Prolonged crying.*** Persistent, severe, inconsolable screaming or crying for 3 or more hours sometimes is observed within 48 hours of immunization with DTP (1 of 100 doses administered). The frequency of inconsolable crying for 3 or more hours is significantly less following immunization with DTaP. Distinguishing between these features and crying from pain can be difficult and requires close questioning of the patient's caregiver. The significance of persistent crying is unknown. It has been noted after receipt of immunizations other than pertussis vaccine and is not known to be associated with sequelae.

Frequency of Adverse Events Following Immunization With DTaP. Moderate to severe systemic events, including temperature of 40.5°C (104.8°F) or higher, persistent inconsolable crying lasting 3 hours or more, and collapse (HHE) rarely have been reported after immunization with DTaP, but each of these events occurs less frequently than after immunization with DTP. When these events occur after the administration of DTP, they seem to be without sequelae; the limited experience with DTaP suggests a similar outcome. Because DTaP causes high fever less frequently than DTP, seizures are anticipated to be much less likely after receipt of DTaP than after DTP.

Alleged Reactions to Pertussis Immunization. The temporal relation of DTP immunization and severe adverse events, such as death, encephalopathy, onset of a seizure disorder, developmental delay, or learning or behavioral problems, does not establish causation by immunization. Many of the manifestations of alleged vaccine reactions have other causes, such as viral encephalitis, concurrent infections, preexisting neurologic disorders, and metabolic and other congenital abnormalities. For example, whereas infantile spasms frequently have their onset during the first 6 months of life and, in some cases, have been related temporally to the administration of pertussis vaccine, epidemiologic data demonstrate that the vaccine does not cause infantile spasms. Sudden infant death syndrome (SIDS) has occurred after DTP immunization, but several studies provide evidence that DTP immunization is not associated causally with SIDS. A large case-control study of SIDS in the United States demonstrated that SIDS victims were no more likely to have recently received DTP immunization than control children who did not have SIDS. Because SIDS occurs most commonly at the age when DTP immunization is recommended, coincidental, temporal associations between the death and immunization by chance alone are expected.

Evaluation of Adverse Events Temporally Associated With Pertussis Immunization. Appropriate diagnostic studies should be undertaken to establish the cause of serious adverse events occurring temporally with immunization rather than assuming that they are caused by the vaccine. However, the cause of events temporally related to immunization cannot always be established even after diagnostic studies.

Severe Acute Neurologic Illness and Permanent Brain Damage. Permanent neurologic disability (brain damage) and even death previously have been considered uncommon sequelae of rare, severe, adverse neurologic events temporally related to whole-cell pertussis vaccine (DTP). Because no specific clinical syndromes or neuropathologic findings have been recognized in these cases, determination of whether pertussis vaccine is the cause of a specific child's deficit is not possible. Such adverse events can occur in immunized and unimmunized children, particularly during the first year of life. Hence, epidemiologic studies have been necessary to determine the risk of severe sequelae after acute events temporally related to pertussis immunization.

The only case-control study that addressed the issue of whether acute neurologic illness associated with DTP immunization results in permanent brain damage is the National Childhood Encephalopathy Study in England, conducted from 1976 to 1979.

The results of this study and the 10-year follow-up do not establish a causal relationship between whole-cell pertussis immunization and chronic neurologic disorders. Other studies also have not provided evidence to support a causal relationship between DTP immunization and serious acute neurologic illness resulting in permanent neurologic injury. Limited experience with acellular pertussis vaccine does not allow conclusions about the frequency of rare, serious, adverse effects temporally associated with its administration.

Contraindications to Pertussis Immunization. Adverse events after pertussis immunization that contraindicate further administration of DTaP are as follows:

- ***An immediate anaphylactic reaction.*** Further immunization with any of the 3 vaccine components in DTaP or DTP should be deferred because of the uncertainty about which antigen may be responsible. Persons who experience anaphylactic reaction may be referred to an allergist for evaluation and desensitization to tetanus toxoid if a specific allergy can be demonstrated.
- ***Encephalopathy within 7 days,*** defined as severe, acute, central nervous system disorder unexplained by another cause, which may be manifested by major alterations of consciousness or by generalized or focal seizures that persist for more than a few hours without recovery within 24 hours. Studies indicate that such events associated with DTP are evident within 72 hours of immunization; prudence, however, usually justifies considering such an illness occurring within 7 days of DTP as a possible contraindication to further doses of pertussis vaccine, and DT should be substituted for each of the recommended subsequent doses of diphtheria and tetanus toxoid.

Precautions for Pertussis Immunization. If the following adverse events occur in temporal relation to immunization with DTaP, the decision to administer additional doses of pertussis vaccine should be considered carefully. Although these events once were regarded as contraindications, they now are considered precautions because they have not been proven to cause permanent sequelae:

- A seizure, with or without fever, occurring within 3 days of immunization with DTP or DTaP
- Persistent, severe, inconsolable screaming or crying for 3 or more hours within 48 hours
- Collapse or shock-like state (HHE) within 48 hours
- Temperature of 40.5°C (104.8°F) or higher, unexplained by another cause, within 48 hours

Before administration of each dose of pertussis vaccine, the child's parent or guardian should be asked about possible adverse events after the previous dose.

Although the risks of giving subsequent doses of pertussis vaccine to a child who has had one of these events are unknown, the possibility of another reaction of similar or greater severity may justify discontinuing pertussis immunization. However, in circumstances of increased risk, such as during a community outbreak of pertussis, the potential benefit of pertussis immunization may outweigh the risk of another reaction. The decision to give or withhold immunization should be based on the clinical assessment of the earlier reaction, the likelihood of pertussis exposure in the child's community, and the potential benefits and risks of pertussis vaccine.

Infants and Children With Underlying Neurologic Disorders. The decision to give pertussis vaccine to infants and children with underlying neurologic disorders can be difficult and must be made on an individual basis after careful and continuing consideration of the risks and benefits (see also Children With a Personal or Family History of Seizures, p 68). In some cases, these disorders may constitute a cause for deferring pertussis immunization and, based on the medical history of the child, subsequent administration of pertussis vaccine. Because outbreaks of pertussis continue to occur in the United States, the decision to defer immunization should be reassessed at each subsequent medical visit, and the decision to give pertussis vaccine should be based on the adjudged risks and consequences of a seizure after DTaP immunization in comparison with the risk of pertussis and its complications. Children with associated neurologic deficits may be at increased risk of complications if pertussis develops. Children traveling to or residing in areas of endemic or epidemic pertussis are at increased risk of developing pertussis. Efforts should be undertaken to ensure pertussis immunization of children attending child care centers, special clinics, or residential care institutions.

The different categories of neurologic disorders and the relevant recommendations are as follows:

- ***A progressive neurologic disorder characterized by developmental delay or neurologic findings.*** These conditions are reason for deferral of pertussis immunization, often permanently. Administration of DTaP may coincide with or hasten the recognition of inevitable manifestations of the disorder, with resulting confusion about causation. Examples include infantile spasms and other epilepsies beginning in infancy. Such disorders should be differentiated from those that are nonprogressive with symptoms that may change as the child matures.
- ***Infants and children with a personal history of seizures.*** Children with a personal history of seizures have an increased risk of seizures after receipt of DTP. No evidence indicates that these vaccine-associated seizures induce permanent brain damage, cause epilepsy, aggravate neurologic disorders, or affect the prognosis for children with underlying disorders. However, because the risk of a postimmunization seizure is increased, pertussis immunization of children with recent seizures should be deferred until a progressive neurologic disorder is excluded. Infants and children with well-controlled seizures or those in whom a seizure is unlikely to recur may be immunized with DTaP. Administration of acetaminophen or other appropriate antipyretic also should be considered at the time of immunization and every 4 hours for the ensuing 24 hours.
- ***Infants and children known to have, or suspected of having, neurologic conditions that predispose to seizures or neurologic deterioration.*** Such conditions include tuberous sclerosis and certain inherited metabolic or degenerative diseases. Deferral of pertussis immunization should be considered for these patients. Seizures or encephalopathy can occur in the normal course of these disorders and, thus, may occur after any immunization. Immunization with DTaP may be associated with the occurrence of overt manifestations of the disorders with resulting confusion about causation. Hence, children with unstable or evolving neurologic disorders that may predispose to seizures or neurologic deterioration should be observed before immunization to ascertain the diagnosis and prognosis of the primary neurologic disorder. Pertussis immunization with DTaP should be reconsidered at each visit. Children whose condition is resolved, corrected, or controlled can be immunized. No evidence indicates that prematurity in the absence of other factors increases the risk of seizures after immunization, and prematurity is not a reason to defer immunization (see Preterm Infants, p 54). Similarly, stable neurologic conditions, such as developmental delay or cerebral palsy, are not contraindications to pertussis immunization.

- ***Temporary deferment of pertussis immunization.*** Children in the first year of life with neurologic disorders that necessitate temporary deferment of pertussis immunization should not receive either DTaP or DT because, in the United States, the risk of acquiring diphtheria or tetanus by children younger than 1 year of age is remote. At or before the first birthday, the decision to give pertussis vaccine as DTaP or DT should be made to ensure that the child is at least immunized against diphtheria and tetanus; as children become ambulatory, their risk of tetanus-prone wounds increases.

  Children with neurologic disorders that are recognized after the first birthday frequently will have received one or more doses of pertussis-containing vaccine. The physician may temporarily defer additional doses of DTaP in anticipation of stabilization of the child's neurologic status. If the physician determines that the child probably should not receive further pertussis immunizations, DT immunization should be completed according to the recommended schedule (see Diphtheria, p 230, and/or Tetanus, p 563).

Children With a Family History of Seizures (see also Children With a Personal or Family History of Seizures, p 68). A history of seizure disorders or adverse events after receipt of a pertussis-containing vaccine in a family member is not a contraindication to pertussis immunization. Although the risk of seizures after immunization with DTP in children with a family history of seizures is increased, these seizures usually are febrile in origin and generally have a benign outcome. In addition, the risk of fever is less with DTaP immunization, and any risk of resulting febrile seizure is considerably outweighed by the continuing risk of pertussis in the United States. Because of the substantial number of children with a family history of seizures who, if not immunized, would remain susceptible to pertussis, DTaP is recommended for these children.

Advice to Parents of Children at Increased Risk of Seizures. Parents of children who may be at increased risk of a seizure, such as from personal or family history of seizures, after pertussis immunization should be informed of the risks and benefits of pertussis immunization in these circumstances. Advice should be provided about fever and fever control (see Antipyretic Prophylaxis, p 440) and appropriate medical care in the unlikely event of a seizure.

Pinworm Infection

(Enterobius vermicularis)

CLINICAL MANIFESTATIONS: Pinworm infection (enterobiasis) causes pruritus ani and, rarely, pruritus vulvae. Although pinworms have been found in the lumen of the appendix, most evidence indicates that they are not related causally to acute appendicitis. Many clinical findings, such as grinding of the teeth at night, weight loss, and enuresis, have been attributed to pinworm infections, but proof of a causal relationship has not been established. Urethritis, vaginitis, salpingitis, or pelvic peritonitis may occur from aberrant migration of the adult worm from the perineum.

ETIOLOGY: *Enterobius vermicularis* is a nematode, or roundworm.

EPIDEMIOLOGY: Enterobiasis occurs worldwide and commonly clusters within families. In the past, 5% to 15% of the population in the United States was estimated to be infected, but the incidence seems to have declined. Prevalence rates are higher in preschool-age and school-age children, in primary caretakers of infected children, and in institutionalized persons, of whom up to 50% of the population may be infected.

Transmission occurs by multiple routes, with fecal-oral being the most important. Worm eggs are transmitted directly by fingers and hands or fomites, such as via shared toys, bedding, clothing, toilet seats, and baths. Because female pinworms usually die after depositing eggs on the perianal skin, reinfection by autoinfection or infection acquired from others is necessary to maintain enterobiasis in a person. The period of communicability is as long as the female nematodes are discharging eggs on perianal skin. The eggs remain infective in an indoor environment, usually 2 to 3 weeks. Humans are the only known natural hosts; dogs and cats do not harbor *E vermicularis.*

The **incubation period** from ingestion of an egg until an adult gravid female migrates to the perianal region is 1 to 2 months or longer.

DIAGNOSTIC TESTS: Diagnosis usually is made when adult worms are visualized in the perianal region, which is best examined 2 to 3 hours after the child is asleep, or in the stool. Alternatively, transparent (not translucent) adhesive tape can be applied to the perianal skin to collect any eggs that may be present; the tape is then applied to a glass slide and examined under a low-power microscopic lens. Three consecutive specimens should be obtained when the patient first awakens in the morning and before washing.

TREATMENT: The drugs of choice are mebendazole, pyrantel pamoate, and albendazole, given in a single dose and repeated in 2 weeks. For children younger than 2 years of age, in whom experience with these drugs is limited, the risks and benefits should be considered before drug administration. Other alternatives include piperazine and pyrvinium pamoate, but they are less effective and more cumbersome to use. Reinfection with pinworms occurs easily; prevention should be discussed concurrently with treatment. Infected persons should bathe in the morning; bathing removes a large proportion of the eggs. Frequently changing the infected person's underclothes, bedclothes, and bed sheets may reduce the egg contamination of the local environment and the risk of reinfection. Specific personal hygiene measures (eg, washing hands before eating or preparing food, keeping finger nails short, avoiding scratching of the perianal region, and avoiding nail biting) may reduce the risk of autoinfection and of continued transmission. Measures such as cleaning or vacuuming the entire house or washing bedclothes and bed sheets daily are not necessary. Repeated infections should be treated the same as the first one. Families may need to be treated as a group. Vaginitis is self-limited and does not require separate treatment.

ISOLATION OF THE HOSPITALIZED PATIENT: Standard precautions are indicated.

CONTROL MEASURES: Control is difficult in child care centers and schools because the rate of reinfection is high. In institutions, mass and simultaneous treatment, repeated in 2 weeks, can be effective.

Plague

CLINICAL MANIFESTATIONS: Plague most commonly presents as the bubonic form, with acute onset of fever and painful swollen regional lymph nodes (buboes). Buboes develop most commonly in the inguinal region but also occur in axillary or cervical areas. Less commonly, plague presents in the septicemic form (hypotension, acute respiratory distress, intravascular coagulopathy) or as pneumonic plague (cough, fever, dyspnea, and hemoptysis) and, rarely, as meningeal plague. Fever, chills, headache, and rapidly progressive weakness are characteristic in all cases. Occasionally, patients present with mild lymphadenitis or with prominent gastrointestinal tract symptoms, which may obscure the correct diagnosis.

ETIOLOGY: Plague is caused by *Yersinia pestis,* a pleomorphic, bipolar staining, gram-negative coccobacillus.

EPIDEMIOLOGY: Plague is a zoonotic infection of rodents and their fleas that occurs in many areas of the world. Plague has been reported throughout the western United States, but most human cases occur in New Mexico, Arizona, California, and Colorado and arise as isolated cases or in small clusters. In the United States, human plague is a rural disease, usually associated with epizootic infections in ground squirrels, prairie dogs, and other wild rodents. Bubonic plague usually is transmitted by the bites of infected rodent fleas and uncommonly by direct contact with tissues and fluids of infected rodents or carnivores, including domestic cats. Septicemic plague occurs most often as a complication of bubonic plague but may result from direct contact with infectious materials or from a flea bite. Primary pneumonic plague is acquired by inhalation of respiratory droplets from a human or animal with respiratory plague or from exposure to aerosols in the laboratory. Secondary pneumonic plague arises from hematogenous seeding of the lungs with *Y pestis* in patients with bubonic or septicemic plague. Epidemics of human plague occur usually as a consequence of epizootics in domestic rodents or after exposures to pneumonic plague.

The **incubation period** usually is 2 to 6 days for bubonic plague and 2 to 4 days for primary pneumonic plague.

DIAGNOSTIC TESTS: Plague is characterized by massive growth of *Y pestis* in affected tissues, especially lymph nodes, spleen, and liver. The organism has a bipolar (safety-pin) appearance when stained with Wayson or Gram stain. The microbiology laboratory should be informed when plague organisms are suspected in submitted specimens to minimize risks of transmission to laboratory personnel. A positive fluorescent antibody test for the presence of *Y pestis* in direct smears or cultures of a bubo aspirate, sputum, cerebrospinal fluid, or blood provides presumptive evidence of *Y pestis* infection. A single positive serologic test result by passive hemagglutination assay or enzyme immunoassay in an unimmunized patient who has not previously had plague also provides presumptive evidence of infection. Seroconversion and/or a 4-fold difference in antibody titer between 2 serum specimens obtained 4 weeks to 3 months apart provides serologic confirmation. The diagnosis of plague usually is confirmed by culture of *Y pestis* from blood, bubo aspirate, or other clinical specimen. Polymerase chain reaction for rapid diagnosis of *Y pestis* is not available in commercial laboratories. Isolates suspected as *Y pestis* should be reported immediately to the state health department and submitted to the Division of Vector-Borne Infectious Diseases of the Centers for Disease Control and Prevention.

TREATMENT: For children, streptomycin (30 mg/kg per day in 2 or 3 divided doses, given intramuscularly) is the treatment of choice in most cases. Gentamicin in standard doses for age given intramuscularly or intravenously is an equally effective alternative to streptomycin. Tetracycline (25 to 50 mg/kg per day in 4 divided doses) or chloramphenicol (initial dose, 25 mg/kg; subsequently, 50 mg/kg per day in 4 divided doses) also is effective. Tetracycline should not be given to children younger than 8 years of age unless the benefits of its use outweigh the risks of dental staining (see Antimicrobial Agents and Related Therapy, p 646). Chloramphenicol is the treatment of choice for plague meningitis. The usual duration of antimicrobial treatment is 7 to 10 days or several days after lysis of fever.

Drainage of abscessed buboes may be necessary; drainage material is infectious until effective antimicrobial therapy has been given.

ISOLATION OF THE HOSPITALIZED PATIENT: For patients with bubonic plague, standard precautions are recommended. Droplet precautions also are indicated for all patients until pneumonia is excluded and appropriate therapy has been initiated. In patients with pneumonic plague, droplet precautions should be continued for 48 hours after initiation of appropriate treatment.

CONTROL MEASURES:

Care of Exposed Persons. Household members and other persons with intimate exposure to a patient with plague should report any fever or other illness to their physician. Persons with close exposure (within about 2 meters) to a patient with pneumonic plague should receive antimicrobial prophylaxis; for exposed children younger than 8 years of age, prophylactic trimethoprim-sulfamethoxazole is recommended, whereas for adults and children 8 years of age and older, doxycycline is recommended. Prophylaxis is given for 7 days.

Other Measures. State public health authorities should be notified immediately of any suspected cases of human plague. The public should be educated about risk factors for plague, measures to prevent the disease, and the signs and symptoms of infection. Persons living in plague-endemic areas should be informed about the role of dogs and cats in bringing plague-infected rodents and their fleas into the peridomestic environment, the need for control of fleas and confinement of pets, and the importance of avoiding contact with sick and dead animals. Other preventive measures include surveillance of rodent populations and the use of insecticides and rodent control measures by health authorities when surveillance indicates the occurrence of plague epizootics.

Vaccine.* An inactivated whole-cell *Y pestis* vaccine is recommended only for persons whose occupation regularly places them at high risk for exposure to *Y pestis* or plague-infected rodents (eg, some field biologists and laboratory workers). Primary immunization consists of 3 intramuscular doses; the second and third doses are given 1 to 3 months and 5 to 6 months, respectively, after the first dose. Booster doses can be given 3 times at 6-month intervals when vaccine recipients have continuing high risk of exposure and a serum passive hemagglutination *Y pestis* antibody titer of less than 1:128. Additional booster doses can be administered at 1- to 2-year intervals. Since safety and immunogenicity have been evaluated only in persons 18 years of age and older, recommendations for immunization of children have not been established.

Immunized persons should take the same preventive measures as unimmunized persons.

Pneumococcal Infections†

CLINICAL MANIFESTATIONS: The pneumococcus is the most common cause of acute otitis media and of invasive bacterial infections in children. Many children with bacteremia have no identifiable primary focus of infection. Pneumococci also are a frequent cause of sinusitis and of community-acquired pneumonia. Since introduction of *Haemophilus influenzae* type b conjugate immunization, pneumococci and meningococci have become the two most common causes of bacterial meningitis in infants and young children.

ETIOLOGY: *Streptococcus pneumoniae* (pneumococci) are lancet-shaped, gram-positive diplococci. Ninety pneumococcal serotypes have been identified. Serotypes 4, 6B, 9V, 14, 18C, 19F, and 23F (Danish serotyping system) cause most invasive childhood pneumococcal infections in the United States. Serotypes 6B, 9V, 14, 19A, 19F, and 23F are the most frequent isolates associated with resistance to penicillin.

EPIDEMIOLOGY: Pneumococci are ubiquitous; many persons are colonized in the upper respiratory tract. Transmission is from person to person, presumably by respiratory droplet contact. Among young children who acquire a new pneumococcal serotype in the nasopharynx, illness (usually otitis media) occurs in 15%, generally within 1 month of acquiring the new serotype. Viral upper respiratory tract infections, including influenza, may predispose to pneumococcal infections. Pneumococcal

---

* Available from Greer Laboratories, Inc, Lenoir, NC, 286445-0800; telephone 800-438-0088 or 704-754-5327.

† On February 17, 2000, the Food and Drug Administration approved a license application for pneumococcal 7-valent conjugate for active immunization of infants and toddlers against invasive disease caused by *Streptococcus pneumoniae* due to capsular serotypes included in the vaccine, beginning at 2 months of age. Information about recommendations for use of this vaccine will be published in *Pediatrics* and is available at: http://www.aap.org.

infections are most common in infants, young children, and the elderly and are more common in African Americans and some Native American populations than in other racial and ethnic groups. Also, these infections are increased in incidence and severity in persons with congenital or acquired humoral immunodeficiency (eg, agammaglobulinemia), including human immunodeficiency virus (HIV) infection, absent or deficient splenic function (eg, sickle cell disease, congenital or surgical asplenia), nephrotic syndrome, chronic renal failure, organ transplantation, diabetes mellitus, chronic pulmonary disease, or congestive heart failure. Patients with cerebrospinal fluid (CSF) leaks from a congenital malformation or complicating skull fracture or neurosurgical procedures, can have recurrent pneumococcal meningitis. Mortality from pneumococcal disease is highest in patients who have meningitis. Pneumococcal infections are most prevalent during the winter months. The period of communicability is unknown but may be as long as the organism is present in respiratory tract secretions and probably is less than 24 hours after effective antimicrobial therapy is begun.

The **incubation period** varies by type of infection and can be as short as 1 to 3 days.

DIAGNOSTIC TESTS: Material obtained from a suppurative focus should be Gram stained and cultured by appropriate microbiologic techniques. Blood cultures should be obtained from all patients with suspected invasive pneumococcal disease; cultures of CSF and other body fluids (eg, pleural fluid) also may be indicated. The white blood cell (WBC) count may be of assistance in suspected bacteremia caused by *S pneumoniae;* young children with high temperatures and leukocytosis (particularly a WBC count of >15 000 cells per microliter [$>15.0 \times 10^9$/L]) have an increased likelihood of bacteremia. Although the predictive value of an elevated WBC count for pneumococcal bacteremia is not high, a normal WBC count is highly predictive of the absence of bacteremia. Recovery of pneumococci from an upper respiratory tract culture is not useful in patients with otitis media, pneumonia, or sinusitis. Rapid methods to detect pneumococcal capsular antigen in CSF, pleural and joint fluid, and concentrated urine usually are of limited value.

Susceptibility Testing.* All *S pneumoniae* isolates from normally sterile body fluids (ie, CSF, blood, middle ear, pleural or joint fluid) should be tested for in vitro antimicrobial susceptibility to determine the minimum inhibitory concentration (MIC) to penicillin and to cefotaxime or ceftriaxone. *Nonsusceptible* is defined to include both *intermediate resistance* and *highly resistant* isolates. Accordingly, current definitions of in vitro susceptibility and nonsusceptibility are as follows:

		Nonsusceptible, µg/mL	
Drug	Susceptible, µg/mL	Intermediate	Resistant
Penicillin	≤0.06	0.1–1.0	≥2.0
Cefotaxime	≤0.5	1.0	≥2.0
Ceftriaxone	≤0.5	1.0	≥2.0

* For further information, see American Academy of Pediatrics Committee on Infectious Diseases. Therapy for children with invasive pneumococcal infection. *Pediatrics.* 1997;99:289–299

For patients with meningitis whose organism is *nonsusceptible* to penicillin, cefotaxime, and ceftriaxone, additional susceptibility testing to vancomycin, rifampin, and, possibly, meropenem should be performed. If the patient has a nonmeningeal infection caused by a *nonsusceptible* isolate to penicillin, cefotaxime, and ceftriaxone, susceptibility testing to clindamycin, erythromycin, rifampin, trimethoprim-sulfamethoxazole, meropenem, and vancomycin should be considered, depending on the patient's response to antimicrobial therapy.

When quantitative testing methods are not available, the qualitative screening test using a 1-µg oxacillin disk on an agar plate reliably identifies all penicillin-*susceptible* pneumococci based on the criterion of a disk zone diameter of 20 mm or greater. Organisms with an oxacillin disk zone size of less than 20 mm are potentially *nonsusceptible* and require quantitative susceptibility testing. The oxacillin disk test is used as a screening test for resistance to ß-lactam drugs (ie, penicillins and cephalosporins).

TREATMENT: *Streptococcus pneumoniae* strains that are nonsusceptible to penicillin G, cefotaxime, ceftriaxone, and other antimicrobial agents have been identified in many regions of the United States and worldwide in increasing frequency in recent years. Nonsusceptible strains most often have intermediate resistance to penicillin (ie, in vitro MIC of 0.1 to 1 µg/mL); however, resistant strains (ie, MIC of ≥2 µg/mL) are becoming more common. In children in the United States, more than 40% of isolates from sterile body sites in some geographic areas are nonsusceptible to penicillin G, and as many as 50% of these isolates are resistant. Approximately 50% of penicillin-nonsusceptible strains also are nonsusceptible to cefotaxime or ceftriaxone. The prevalence of nonsusceptible strains varies geographically, but these organisms have appeared unexpectedly in communities that previously had only susceptible *S pneumoniae.*

Vancomycin resistance has not been reported. If a strain with an in vitro MIC greater than 1.0 µg/mL to vancomycin is isolated, the state health department should be notified promptly and arrangements made for confirmatory testing.

Recommendations for treatment of pneumococcal infections are as follows.

***Bacterial Meningitis Possibly or Proven To Be Caused by* S pneumoniae.** Combination therapy with vancomycin and cefotaxime or ceftriaxone should be administered initially to all children 1 month of age or older with definite or probable bacterial meningitis because of the increased prevalence of penicillin-, cefotaxime-, and ceftriaxone-resistant *S pneumoniae.* Some experts, however, recommend that vancomycin need not be used if compelling evidence indicates that the cause is an organism other than *S pneumoniae* (eg, gram-negative diplococci on a CSF smear during an outbreak of meningococcal disease).

For children with severe hypersensitivity to the ß-lactam antibiotics (ie, penicillins and cephalosporins), the combination of vancomycin and rifampin should be considered. Vancomycin should not be given alone because bactericidal concentrations in the CSF are difficult to sustain, and clinical experience to support its use as monotherapy is minimal. Rifampin also should not be given as monotherapy because resistance may develop during therapy. Other possible antimicrobial agents for the treatment of pneumococcal meningitis include meropenem or chloramphenicol (which only should be used for pneumococcal meningitis if the in vitro minimal bactericidal concentration is ≤4 µg/mL).

Table 3.44. **Antimicrobial Therapy for Infants and Children With Bacterial Meningitis Caused By *Streptococcus pneumoniae* Based on Susceptibility Test Results**

Susceptibility Test Results*	Antibiotic Management†
Susceptible to penicillin	Discontinue vancomycin **AND** Begin penicillin **OR** Continue cefotaxime or ceftriaxone alone‡
Nonsusceptible to penicillin *(intermediate or resistant)* **AND** *Susceptible* to cefotaxime and ceftriaxone	**Discontinue vancomycin** and Continue cefotaxime or ceftriaxone
Nonsusceptible to penicillin *(intermediate or resistant)* **AND** *Nonsusceptible* to cefotaxime and ceftriaxone *(intermediate or resistant)* **AND** *Susceptible* to rifampin	Continue vancomycin and cefotaxime or ceftriaxone. Rifampin may be added to vancomycin in selected circumstances (see text).

* Based on susceptibility studies.

† See Table 3.45, p 456, for dosage. Some experts recommend the maximum dosages.

‡ Some physicians may choose this alternative for convenience and cost savings.

A lumbar puncture should be considered after 24 to 48 hours of therapy for the following reasons: (1) the organism is penicillin-*nonsusceptible* by oxacillin disk or quantitative (MIC) testing, results from cefotaxime and ceftriaxone quantitative susceptibility testing are not yet available, and the patient's condition has not improved or has worsened; or (2) the child has received dexamethasone, which might interfere with the ability to interpret clinical response, such as resolution of fever.

Based on available results of susceptibility testing of the pneumococcal isolate, therapy should be modified according to the guidelines in Table 3.44, above. If the organism is susceptible to penicillin or cefotaxime or ceftriaxone, **vancomycin should be discontinued,** and penicillin or cefotaxime or ceftriaxone should be continued. Vancomycin should be continued only if the organism is nonsusceptible to penicillin and to cefotaxime or ceftriaxone.

Addition of rifampin to vancomycin after 24 to 48 hours of therapy should be considered if the organism is susceptible to rifampin and (1) after 24 to 48 hours, despite therapy with vancomycin and cefotaxime or ceftriaxone, the clinical condition has worsened; (2) the subsequent gram-stained smear or culture of CSF indicates failure to eradicate or to reduce substantially the number of organisms; or (3) the organism has an unusually high cefotaxime or ceftriaxone MIC (≥4 µg/mL). Consultation with an infectious disease specialist should be considered in such circumstances.

Table 3.45. **Dosages of Intravenous Antimicrobial Agents for Invasive Pneumococcal Infections in Infants and Children***

Antimicrobial	Meningitis		Nonmeningeal Infections	
	Dosage, kg/d	Dose Interval	Dosage, kg/d	Dose Interval
Penicillin G	250 000–400 000 U[†]	4–6 h	Same	Same
Cefotaxime	225–300 mg	8 h	75–100 mg	Same
Ceftriaxone	100 mg	12–24 h	50–75 mg	Same
Vancomycin	60 mg	6 h	40–45 mg	Same
Rifampin[‡]	20 mg	12 h	Not indicated	...
Chloramphenicol[§]	75–100 mg	6 h	Same	Same
Clindamycin[§]	Not indicated	...	25–40 mg	6–8 h
Meropenem[‖]	120 mg	8 h	60 mg	8 h
Imipenem-cilastatin[¶]	...	...	60 mg	6 h

* Doses are for children 1 month of age or older.
† Because 1 U = 0.6 µg/mL, this range is equal to 150 to 240 mg/kg per day.
‡ Indications for use are not completely defined.
§ Drug should be considered only for patients with life-threatening allergic response following administration of ß-lactam antibiotics.
‖ Drug is approved for pediatric patients 3 months of age and older.
¶ Drug is not approved for use in patients younger than 12 years of age and is not recommended for patients with meningitis because of its potential epileptogenic properties.

Dexamethasone. For infants and children 6 weeks of age and older, adjunctive therapy with dexamethasone should be considered after weighing the potential benefits and possible risks. The CSF concentrations of vancomycin, ceftriaxone, cefotaxime, and rifampin, when given in the recommended dosages for patients with meningitis (see Table 3.45, above) in children treated with dexamethasone are adequate to treat meningitis caused by most nonsusceptible strains of *S pneumoniae.* Dexamethasone can lead to decreased fever and a misleading impression of clinical improvement, even though CSF sterilization may not have been achieved.

Children With Probable Aseptic Meningitis. During the summer and autumn, many young children will be hospitalized for severe headaches, vomiting, fever, stiff neck, and CSF pleocytosis caused by enteroviruses. Although antibiotics are not usually indicated, some physicians choose to give antimicrobial therapy until the CSF and blood cultures are negative. Vancomycin should *not* be used in these circumstances unless the child has a toxic appearance and/or is hypotensive and pneumococcal infection is suspected.

Nonmeningeal Invasive Pneumococcal Infections Requiring Hospitalization. For nonmeningeal invasive infections in previously well children who are not critically ill, antimicrobial agents currently in use to treat *S pneumoniae* and other potential pathogens should be initiated at the usually recommended dosages (see Table 3.45, above).

For critically ill infants and children with invasive infections potentially due to *S pneumoniae,* additional initial antimicrobial therapy for possible penicillin-, cefotaxime-, or ceftriaxone-nonsusceptible strains may be considered. Such patients include those with myopericarditis or severe multilobar pneumonia with hypoxia or hypotension. If vancomycin is administered, it should be discontinued as soon as antimicrobial susceptibility test results demonstrate effective alternative agents.

If the organism is highly resistant to penicillin, cefotaxime, and ceftriaxone, therapy should be modified based on the clinical response, susceptibility to other antimicrobial agents, and results of follow-up cultures of blood and other body fluids. Consultation with an infectious disease specialist should be considered.

For children with severe hypersensitivity to the ß-lactam antibiotics (ie, penicillins and cephalosporins), initial management for a potential pneumococcal infection should include clindamycin or vancomycin, in addition to antimicrobial drugs for other potential pathogens as indicated. Vancomycin should not be continued if the organism is susceptible to other appropriate non–ß-lactam antibiotics. Consultation with an infectious disease specialist should be considered.

Nonmeningeal Invasive Pneumococcal Infections in the Immunocompromised Host. The preceding recommendations for management of possible pneumococcal infections requiring hospitalization also apply to immunocompromised children, provided they are not critically ill. However, for critically ill patients, consideration should be given to initiating therapy with vancomycin and cefotaxime or ceftriaxone. Vancomycin should be discontinued as soon as antimicrobial susceptibility test results indicate that effective alternative antimicrobial agents are available.

Dosages. The recommended dosages of intravenous antimicrobial agents for treatment of invasive pneumococcal infections are given in Table 3.45 (p 456).

Otitis Media. Most experts recommend empiric initial treatment of acute otitis media with high-dose oral amoxicillin (80–90 mg/kg per day). Standard duration of therapy is 10 days, but uncomplicated cases among children older than 2 years of age can be treated for 5 days. Based on concentrations in middle ear fluid and in vitro activity, no currently available oral antibiotic has better activity than amoxicillin against resistant *S pneumoniae.*

For patients with clinically defined treatment failures when assessed after 3 to 5 days of initial therapy, suitable alternative agents should be active against penicillin-nonsusceptible pneumococci as well as ß-lactamase–producing *H influenzae* and *Moraxella catarrhalis.* Such agents include oral cefuroxime axetil, intramuscular ceftriaxone, and high-dose oral amoxicillin-clavulanate. Amoxicillin-clavulanate should be given at 80 to 90 mg/kg per day of the amoxicillin component (eg, the 7:1 formulation) to reduce the incidence of diarrhea. Erythromycin-sulfisoxazole, clarithromycin, and azithromycin are appropriate alternatives for penicillin-allergic patients.

Myringotomy should be considered for recurrent treatment failures or severe cases in order to obtain cultures to guide therapy. For multiply drug-resistant strains of *S pneumoniae,* the use of clindamycin, rifampin, or other agents in consultation with an expert in infectious diseases should be considered.

Sinusitis. Antimicrobial agents effective for the treatment of acute otitis media also are likely to be effective for acute sinusitis and are recommended.

ISOLATION OF THE HOSPITALIZED PATIENT: Standard precautions are recommended, including for patients with infections caused by drug-resistant *S pneumoniae.*

Control Measures:

Child Care, Household, and School. No isolation precautions are necessary for children in child care or school who have pneumococcal disease. The need for or benefit of prophylactic antibiotic treatment of contacts of a person with pneumococcal disease has not been demonstrated, and chemoprophylaxis is not recommended.

Active Immunization. The 23-valent pneumococcal vaccine is composed of purified capsular polysaccharide antigens of 23 pneumococcal serotypes. This vaccine is given intramuscularly. Each vaccine dose (0.5 mL) contains 25 µg of each polysaccharide antigen. These capsular antigens are those of serotypes causing 88% of cases of bacteremia and meningitis in adults, almost 100% of cases of bacteremia and meningitis in children, and 85% of cases of acute otitis media. Like other polysaccharide antigens, many of the pneumococcal serotypes in the vaccine have limited immunogenicity in children younger than 2 to 3 years of age. The effectiveness of pneumococcal vaccines in preventing pneumonia has been demonstrated in healthy young adults and older children who have an increased incidence of invasive pneumococcal disease. Immunized children with sickle cell disease or children who have undergone splenectomy have experienced significantly less bacteremic pneumococcal infections than unimmunized patients.

Multivalent protein conjugate pneumococcal vaccines that are immunogenic in infants and children younger than 2 years of age have been developed. Preliminary results suggest these vaccines are efficacious in preventing meningitis, bacteremia, pneumonia, and otitis media caused by serotypes of *S pneumoniae* contained in the vaccine. Licensure of a 7-valent protein conjugate pneumococcal vaccine for use in infants beginning at 2 months of age is anticipated. Once this vaccine is approved by the US Food and Drug Administration, the American Academy of Pediatrics (AAP) recommendations for use can be found at http://www.aap.org/ and will be published in *Pediatrics.*

Adverse Reactions. Mild side effects, such as erythema and pain at the injection site, are common with the 23-valent polysaccharide vaccine. Fever, myalgia, and severe local reactions are uncommon. Severe systemic reactions, such as anaphylaxis, have been reported rarely. No data are available to allow estimates of adverse reaction rates among persons who received more than 2 doses of pneumococcal polysaccharide vaccine.

Recommendations for Immunization.

- Children 2 years of age and older at increased risk of acquiring invasive pneumococcal infections or of serious disease if they become infected should be immunized. Indications are the following: (1) sickle cell disease; (2) functional or anatomic asplenia; (3) nephrotic syndrome or chronic renal failure; (4) conditions associated with immunosuppression, such as organ or bone marrow transplantation, drug therapy or cytoreduction therapy (including long-term systemic corticosteroid therapy); (5) HIV infection (see HIV Infection, p 325); and (6) CSF leaks.
- Other indications for pneumococcal immunization that are recommended by the Advisory Committee on Immunization Practices (ACIP) of the Centers for Disease Control and Prevention include persons 2 years of age and older

with chronic cardiovascular disease (eg, congestive heart failure or cardiomyopathy), chronic pulmonary disease (eg, cystic fibrosis, but not asthma), diabetes mellitus, or chronic liver disease (eg, cirrhosis).

- Pneumococcal immunization of persons 2 years of age and older living in special environments or social settings in which the risk of invasive pneumococcal disease or its complications is high (eg, Alaskan Native and certain American Indian populations) is recommended by the ACIP and the AAP.* Additional booster doses are not recommended.
- Parents and other caregivers of immunized children with functional or anatomic asplenia should be informed that immunization does not guarantee protection from fulminant pneumococcal disease and death. The patients, if old enough to be responsible for their health care (eg, adolescents) also should be informed. Asplenic patients with unexplained fever or manifestations of sepsis should receive prompt medical attention, including treatment for suspected bacteremia, the initial signs and symptoms of which may be subtle. Antimicrobial agents selected for initial empiric treatment should be effective against *Neisseria meningitidis,* as well as *S pneumoniae.*
- When elective splenectomy is to be performed, pneumococcal polysaccharide vaccine should be given approximately 2 weeks or more before the operation, if possible, to increase the likelihood of eliciting a protective antibody response. Similarly, in planning cancer chemotherapy or immunosuppressive therapy for patients with Hodgkin disease or persons who are to undergo bone marrow or solid-organ transplantation, immunization should precede initiation of chemotherapy or immunosuppression by approximately 2 weeks or more, if possible. Immunization during chemotherapy or radiation therapy often results in poor serum antibody responses and is not likely to be effective in preventing pneumococcal infection. Patients who received vaccine during chemotherapy or radiation therapy should be reimmunized 3 months after discontinuation of the therapy.
- Immunization with the pneumococcal vaccine is not recommended for preventing otitis media or any other pneumococcal infection during the first 2 years of life.
- Reimmunization is recommended for children 2 to 10 years of age who are at high risk of severe pneumococcal infection. These children include those who (1) have sickle cell disease; (2) are functionally or anatomically asplenic; (3) have conditions associated with a rapid antibody decline after initial immunization, such as from nephrotic syndrome, renal failure, or transplantation; or (4) are at increased risk because of HIV infection or other conditions associated with immunosuppression, including malignant neoplasm (eg, leukemia, lymphoma, and Hodgkin disease). If the child is younger than 10 years of age, reimmunization is recommended 3 to 5 years after a previous dose of pneumococcal polysaccharide vaccine. Reimmunization also is indicated for high-risk older children and adults 5 or more years after being immunized with pneumococcal polysaccharide vaccine. Reimmunization once only is recommended.

---

* American Academy of Pediatrics Committee on Native American Child Health and Committee on Infectious Diseases. Immunizations for Native American children. *Pediatrics.* 1999;104:564–567

- Pneumococcal vaccines may be given concurrently with other vaccines (see Simultaneous Administration of Multiple Vaccines, p 26). No data indicate that administration of pneumococcal vaccine with MMR (measles, mumps, rubella), DTaP (diphtheria and tetanus toxoids and acellular pertussis), poliovirus, *H influenzae* type b, hepatitis B virus, influenza, or other vaccines increases the severity of reactions or diminishes antibody responses.

Contraindications and Precautions. Immunization generally should be deferred during pregnancy because the effect of the vaccine on the fetus is unknown. However, the risk of severe pneumococcal disease during pregnancy must be weighed against the potential hazards of the vaccine, and in high-risk persons immunization is justified.

Passive Immunization. Immune Globulin Intravenous administration is recommended for preventing pneumococcal infection in patients with congenital or acquired immunodeficiency diseases, including persons with HIV infection who have recurrent pneumococcal infections (see HIV Infection, p 325).

Chemoprophylaxis. Daily antimicrobial prophylaxis is recommended for children with functional or anatomic asplenia, irrespective of their immunization status, for prevention of pneumococcal disease (see Asplenic Children, p 66). Oral penicillin V (125 mg twice a day for children younger than 5 years of age; 250 mg twice a day for children 5 years of age and older) is recommended.

The results of a multicenter study demonstrated that oral penicillin V (125 mg twice a day) given to infants and young children with sickle cell anemia reduced the incidence of pneumococcal bacteremia by 84% compared with the placebo control group. Based on this study, daily penicillin prophylaxis for children with sickle cell anemia beginning before 2 months of age is recommended.

The number of cases of penicillin-resistant invasive pneumococcal infections and the prevalence of nasopharyngeal carriage of penicillin-resistant strains in patients with sickle cell disease have increased in recent years. Parents, thus, should be informed that penicillin prophylaxis no longer may be as effective at preventing invasive pneumococcal infections as in the past.

The age at which prophylaxis is discontinued often is an empiric decision. Children with sickle cell anemia who had received penicillin prophylaxis for prolonged periods, who are receiving regular medical attention, and who have not had a prior severe pneumococcal infection or a surgical splenectomy may safely discontinue prophylactic penicillin at 5 years of age. However, they must be counseled to seek medical attention for all febrile events. The duration of prophylaxis for children with asplenia due to other causes is unknown; however, some experts continue prophylaxis throughout childhood.

Pneumocystis carinii Infections

CLINICAL MANIFESTATIONS: In infants and children, a subacute diffuse pneumonitis with dyspnea at rest, tachypnea, oxygen desaturation, nonproductive cough, and fever develop characteristically. However, the magnitude of these signs and symptoms may vary, and in some immunocompromised children and adults, the onset can be acute and fulminant. The chest radiograph often shows bilateral diffuse interstitial or alveolar disease; rarely, lobar, miliary, and nodular lesions occur as well. Occasionally, the chest radiograph at the time of diagnosis appears normal. Mortality in immunocompromised patients is high, ranging from 5% to 40% if treated, and almost 100% if untreated.

Etiology: *Pneumocystis carinii* seems to be an unusual or primitive fungus, based on DNA sequence homologies. It, however, retains several morphologic and biologic similarities to the protozoa, most notably susceptibility to a number of antiprotozoal agents but resistance to most antifungal agents.

Epidemiology: *Pneumocystis carinii* is ubiquitous in mammals worldwide, particularly rodents. This organism has a tropism for growth on respiratory tract surfaces of mammals. Whether *P carinii* in animals is infectious for humans has not been determined. *Pneumocystis carinii* isolates recovered from mice, rats, and ferrets are diverse genetically from each other and from human *P carinii* and do not seem to cross-infect other animals. Asymptomatic infection occurs early in life, with more than 75% of healthy persons acquiring antibody by 4 years of age. In developing countries and in times of famine in industrialized countries, *P carinii* pneumonia (PCP) has occurred in epidemics, primarily affecting malnourished infants and children. Epidemics also have occurred in premature infants. In industrialized countries today, PCP occurs almost entirely in immunocompromised persons with deficient cell-mediated immunity, particularly persons with human immunodeficiency virus (HIV) infection, recipients of immunosuppressive therapy after organ transplantation or treatment for malignant neoplasm, and children with congenital immunodeficiency syndromes. *Pneumocystis carinii* pneumonia is the most common serious opportunistic infection in infants and young children with perinatally acquired HIV infection and is one of the most common pediatric acquired immunodeficiency syndrome (AIDS)-defining illnesses. Although onset of disease can occur at any age, including rare instances during the first month of life, PCP most frequently occurs in HIV-infected children between 3 and 6 months of age. The incidence of PCP is decreasing as chemoprophylaxis is more widely implemented. The mode of transmission is unknown. Proposed hypotheses are as follows: (1) person-to-person transmission by the respiratory route (airborne transmission has been demonstrated in experimental animals), and (2) acquisition from the environment. Circumstantial evidence suggests that person-to-person transmission can occur, but identifying any contact with an infected person before onset is rare. Primary infection probably accounts for disease during infancy. While reactivation of latent infection with immunosuppression has been proposed as an explanation for disease after the first 2 years of life, animal models of PCP do not support the existence of latency. Recurrences in immunocompromised patients, especially those with AIDS, are common. In patients with lymphoma or leukemia, the disease can occur during remission or relapse. The period of communicability is unknown.

The **incubation period** is unknown.

Diagnostic Tests: A definitive diagnosis of PCP is made by demonstration of organisms in lung tissue or respiratory tract secretions. The most sensitive and specific diagnostic procedures have been open lung biopsy and transbronchial biopsy. However, bronchoscopy with bronchoalveolar lavage, induction of sputum in older children and adolescents, and intubation with deep endotracheal aspiration are less invasive and often diagnostic and have been sufficiently sensitive in patients with HIV infection who have an increased number of organisms compared with non–HIV-infected patients with PCP. Methenamine silver, toluidine blue O, calcofluor white, and fluorescein-conjugated monoclonal antibody are the most useful stains for identifying the thick-walled cysts of *P carinii*. Extracystic trophozoite forms are identified with Giemsa stain, modified Wright-Giemsa stain, and fluorescein-conjugated monoclonal antibody. Serologic tests and polymerase chain reaction assays for detecting *P carinii* infection are experimental and are not recommended for diagnosis. Many children and adults with HIV infection and PCP have elevated serum concentrations of lactate dehydrogenase, but this abnormality is not specific for PCP.

TREATMENT: The drug of choice is trimethoprim-sulfamethoxazole (15 to 20 mg/kg per day of trimethoprim; 75 to 100 mg/kg of sulfamethoxazole daily in divided doses every 6 hours), usually given intravenously. Oral therapy should be reserved for patients with mild disease who do not have malabsorption or diarrhea. The rate of adverse reactions is higher in HIV-infected patients than in patients without HIV infection; the incidence in HIV-infected children treated with trimethoprim-sulfamethoxazole is approximately 15% but may be as high as 60% in adults with HIV infection. If the adverse reaction is not severe, continuation of therapy is recommended, because 50% of patients with adverse reactions subsequently have been treated successfully with trimethoprim-sulfamethoxazole.

Parenterally administered pentamidine (4 mg/kg per day of salt given once a day) is an alternative drug for children and adults who cannot tolerate trimethoprim-sulfamethoxazole or who have severe disease and who have not responded to trimethoprim-sulfamethoxazole after 5 to 7 days of therapy. The therapeutic efficacy of parenteral pentamidine in adults with PCP has been similar to that of trimethoprim-sulfamethoxazole. However, pentamidine is associated with a high incidence of adverse reactions, including pancreatitis, renal dysfunction, hypoglycemia, hyperglycemia, hypotension, fever, and neutropenia. Pentamidine should not be used concomitantly with didanosine, since both drugs can cause pancreatitis. If a recipient of didanosine develops PCP and requires pentamidine, didanosine should be discontinued until 1 week after the pentamidine therapy has been discontinued.

Atovaquone is approved for the oral treatment of mild to moderate PCP in adults who are intolerant of trimethoprim-sulfamethoxazole. Experience with the use of atovaquone in children is limited.

Other potentially useful drugs identified by in vitro studies, animal models, and clinical trials in adults include dapsone with trimethoprim, trimetrexate with leucovorin, and clindamycin with primaquine. Experience with the use of these combinations in children is limited.

A minimum duration of 2 weeks of therapy is recommended; many experts advise 3 weeks of therapy for patients with AIDS. In patients with AIDS, continuous lifelong prophylaxis should be initiated at the end of therapy for acute infection.

Corticosteroids seem to be beneficial in the treatment of HIV-infected adults with moderate to severe PCP (as defined by an arterial oxygen pressure [PaO_2] of less than 70 mm Hg or an arterial-alveolar gradient of more than 35 mm Hg). For adolescents older than 13 years of age and adults, 80 mg/d of oral prednisone in 2 divided doses for the first 5 days of therapy, 40 mg once a day on days 6 through 10, and 20 mg once a day on days 11 through 21 is recommended. Although no controlled studies of the use of corticosteroids in young children have been performed, most experts would include corticosteroids as part of therapy for children with moderate to severe PCP. The optimal dose and duration of corticosteroid therapy for children have not been determined, but most experts suggest 2 mg/kg per day of prednisone or its equivalent for 7 to 10 days, followed by a tapering dose during the next 10 to 14 days.

Chemoprophylaxis. Prophylaxis against a first episode of PCP is indicated for many patients with significant immunocompromise, including persons with HIV infection and those with primary or acquired immunodeficiency, such as from chemotherapy or other immunosuppressive therapy (see HIV Infection, p 325).

Because half of all cases of PCP in children with perinatally acquired HIV occur in infants 3 to 6 months of age, identification as early as possible of infants who have been exposed perinatally to HIV is essential so that prophylaxis can be initiated before they are at risk. The most effective means to implement this recommendation is by diagnosing maternal HIV infection before or during pregnancy (see HIV Infection, p 325). Prophylaxis for PCP is recommended for all infants born to HIV-infected women beginning at 4 to 6 weeks of age (see Table 3.46, p 464). Prophylaxis for PCP should be discontinued for children in whom HIV infection has been excluded. Children whose HIV infection status is not determined should continue prophylaxis throughout the first year of life.

For HIV-infected infants and children, PCP prophylaxis should be continued or administered in the following situations: (1) any CD4+ T-lymphocyte count indicates severe immunosuppression for age (see Table 3.46, p 464), (2) a rapidly declining CD4+ T-lymphocyte count occurs, or (3) severely symptomatic HIV disease (Category C) is present (see HIV Infection, p 325, and Table 3.46, p 464). Criteria are the same for older children and adolescents except for different age-specific definitions of low absolute CD4+ cell counts. For adolescents or adults, PCP prophylaxis is indicated if the patient has unexplained fever for 2 or more weeks or a history of oropharyngeal candidiasis.

Human immunodeficiency virus–infected children older than 1 year of age, not previously receiving PCP prophylaxis (eg, those children not previously identified or whose PCP prophylaxis was discontinued), should begin prophylaxis if at any time their CD4+ T-lymphocyte cell counts indicate severe immunosuppression (see Table 3.46, p 464).

The recommended drug regimen for prophylaxis in all immunocompromised patients (whether from HIV infection, malignant neoplasm, or other causes) is trimethoprim-sulfamethoxazole administered for 3 consecutive days each week (see Table 3.47, p 465, for dosage). For patients who cannot tolerate the drug, aerosolized pentamidine administered by the Respirgard II nebulizer for persons 5 years of age or older is an alternative; daily oral dapsone is another alternative drug for prophylaxis in children, especially children younger than 5 years of age (see Table 3.47, p 465). Intravenous pentamidine also has been used, but it seems to be less effective and potentially more toxic than other prophylactic regimens.

Table 3.46. Recommendations for *Pneumocystis carinii* Pneumonia (PCP) Prophylaxis for Human Immunodeficiency Virus (HIV)-Exposed Infants and Children, by Age and HIV-Infection Status*

Age and HIV Infection Status	PCP Prophylaxis†
Birth to 4–6 wk, HIV-exposed	No prophylaxis
4–6 wk to 4 mo, HIV-exposed	Prophylaxis
4–12 mo	
HIV-infected or indeterminate	Prophylaxis
HIV-infection excluded‡	No prophylaxis
1–5 y, HIV-infected	Prophylaxis if: CD4+ T-lymphocyte count is <500/µL or percentage is <15%§‖
≥5 y, HIV-infected	Prophylaxis if: CD4+ T-lymphocyte count is <200/µL or percentage is <15%‖

*Modified from Centers for Disease Control and Prevention. 1999 USPHS/IDSA guidelines for the prevention of opportunistic infections in persons infected with human immunodeficiency virus. *MMWR Morb Mortal Wkly Rep.* 1999;48(RR-10):1–59, 61–66

† Children who have had PCP should receive lifelong PCP prophylaxis.

‡ HIV infection can be excluded reasonably among children who have had 2 or more negative results of HIV diagnostic tests (ie, HIV culture or polymerase chain reaction), both of which are performed at ≥1 month of age and 1 of which is performed at ≥4 months of age; or 2 or more negative results of HIV immunoglobulin G antibody tests performed at ≥6 months of age among children who have no clinical evidence of HIV disease (see HIV Infection, p 325).

§ Children 1 to 2 years of age who were receiving PCP prophylaxis and had a CD4+ T-lymphocyte count of less than 750/µL or percentage of <15% at younger than 12 months of age should continue prophylaxis.

‖ Prophylaxis should be considered on a case-by-case basis for children who might otherwise be at risk for PCP, such as children with rapidly declining CD4+ counts or percentages or children with Category C status of HIV infection.

Other drugs with potential for prophylaxis include pyrimethamine plus dapsone plus leucovorin, pyrimethamine-sulfadoxine, and oral atovaquone. Experience with these drugs in adults and children is limited. These agents should be considered only in unusual situations in which the recommended regimens are not tolerated or cannot be used. The safety of discontinuing any prophylaxis in HIV-infected children receiving highly active antiretroviral therapy has not been studied.

Although prophylaxis substantially reduces the risk of PCP, pulmonary and extrapulmonary *P carinii* infections have occurred in HIV-infected adults and children receiving prophylaxis.

Isolation of the Hospitalized Patient: Standard precautions are recommended. In addition, some experts recommend that patients with PCP not share a room with immunocompromised patients, although data are insufficient to support this recommendation as standard practice.

Control Measures: Appropriate therapy for infected patients and prophylaxis in immunocompromised patients are the only available means of control. Detailed guidelines have been issued recently by the Centers for Disease Control and Preven-

Table 3.47. Drug Regimens for *Pneumocystis carinii* Pneumonia Prophylaxis for Children 4 Weeks of Age or Older*

Recommended regimen:

Trimethoprim-sulfamethoxazole, 150 mg/m^2 per day of trimethroprim with 750 mg/m^2 per day of sulfamethoxazole administered orally in divided doses twice a day 3 times per week on consecutive days (eg, Monday-Tuesday-Wednesday)

Acceptable alternative trimethoprim-sulfamethoxazole dosage schedules:

- 150 mg/m^2 per day of trimethoprim with 750 mg/m^2 per day of sulfamethoxazole administered orally **as a single daily dose** 3 times per week on consecutive days (eg, Monday-Tuesday-Wednesday).
- 150 mg/m^2 per day of trimethoprim with 750 mg/m^2 per day of sulfamethoxazole administered orally in divided doses twice a day and **administered 7 days per week.**
- 150 mg/m^2 per day of trimethoprim with 750 mg/m^2 per day of sulfamethoxazole administered orally in divided doses twice a day and administered 3 times per week on alternate days (eg, Monday-Wednesday-Friday).

Alternative regimens if trimethoprim-sulfamethoxazole is not tolerated†:

- **Dapsone (children ≥1 mo of age)**
  2 mg/kg (maximum 100 mg) administered orally once a day or 4 mg/kg (maximum 200 mg) orally every week
- **Aerosolized pentamidine (children ≥5 y old)**
  300 mg administered via Respirgard II inhaler monthly
- **Atovaquone (children 1–3 mo of age and >24 mo of age)**
  30 mg/kg orally once a day
  (children 4–24 mo of age)
  45 mg/kg orally once a day

* Modified from Centers for Disease Control and Prevention. 1999 USPHS/IDSA guidelines for the prevention of opportunistic infections in persons infected with human immunodeficiency virus. *MMWR Morb Mortal Wkly Rep.* 1999;48(RR-10):1–59, 61–66

† If dapsone, aerosolized pentamidine, and atovaquone are not tolerated, some clinicians use intravenous pentamidine (4 mg/kg) administered every 2 to 4 weeks.

tion and the Infectious Diseases Society of America and endorsed by the American Academy of Pediatrics.*

Poliovirus Infections

CLINICAL MANIFESTATIONS: Approximately 95% of poliovirus infections are asymptomatic. Nonspecific illness with low-grade fever and sore throat (minor illness) occurs in 4% to 8% of people who become infected. Aseptic meningitis, sometimes with paresthesias, occurs in 1% to 5% of patients a few days after the

* Centers for Disease Control and Prevention. 1999 USPHS/IDSA guidelines for the prevention of opportunistic infections in persons infected with human immunodeficiency virus. *MMWR Morb Mortal Wkly Rep.* 1999;48(RR-10):1–59, 61–66

minor illness has resolved. Rapid onset of asymmetric acute flaccid paralysis with areflexia of the involved limb occurs in 0.1% to 2% of infections, and residual paralytic disease involving the motor neurons (paralytic poliomyelitis) occurs in approximately 1 per 250 infections. Cranial nerve involvement and paralysis of respiratory muscles can occur. Findings in the cerebrospinal fluid (CSF) are characteristic of viral meningitis with mild pleocytosis and lymphocytic predominance.

Adults who contracted paralytic poliomyelitis during childhood may develop the postpolio syndrome 30 to 40 years later. Postpolio syndrome is characterized by muscle pain and exacerbation of weakness.

ETIOLOGY: Polioviruses are enteroviruses and consist of 3 serotypes: 1, 2, and 3.

EPIDEMIOLOGY: Poliovirus infections occur only in humans. Spread is by the fecal-oral and oral-oral (respiratory) routes. Infection is more common in infants and young children and occurs at an earlier age among children living in poor hygienic conditions. The risk of paralytic disease after infection increases with age. In temperate climates, poliovirus infections are most common during the summer and autumn; in the tropics, the seasonal pattern is variable with a less pronounced peak of activity.

The last reported case of poliomyelitis due to indigenously acquired, wild-type poliovirus in the United States occurred in 1979. The only identified imported case of paralytic poliomyelitis since 1986 occurred in 1993 in a child transported to United States for medical care. Since 1979, all other cases have been vaccine-associated paralytic poliomyelitis (VAPP) that are attributable to oral poliovirus (OPV) vaccine. An average of 8 cases of VAPP have been reported annually in the United States from 1980 to 1996. The circulation of wild-type polioviruses has ceased in the United States, and the risk of contact with imported wild-type polioviruses is decreasing rapidly because of the successful eradication of poliomyelitis from the western hemisphere in 1991 and the ongoing global eradication program of the World Health Organization. All suspected cases of paralytic poliomyelitis are reviewed by a panel of expert consultants before final classification occurs. Confirmed cases then are further classified based on epidemiologic and laboratory criteria.

Communicability of poliovirus is greatest shortly before and after onset of clinical illness when the virus is present in the throat and excreted in high concentration in feces. The virus persists in the throat for about 1 week after onset of illness and is excreted in feces for several weeks and rarely for months. Patients potentially are contagious as long as fecal excretion persists. In recipients of OPV vaccine, the virus persists in the throat for 1 to 2 weeks and is excreted in feces for several weeks, although in rare cases, excretion for more than 2 months can occur. Immunodeficient patients can excrete virus for prolonged periods of more than 6 months.

The **incubation period** of abortive poliomyelitis is 3 to 6 days. For the onset of paralysis in paralytic poliomyelitis, the incubation period usually is 7 to 21 days, but occasionally it is as short as 4 days.

DIAGNOSTIC TESTS: Poliovirus can be recovered from the pharynx, feces, urine, and, rarely, CSF by isolation in cell culture. Two or more stool and throat swab specimens for enterovirus isolation should be obtained at least 24 hours apart from patients with suspected paralytic poliomyelitis as early in the course of the illness as possible, ideally within 14 days of onset of symptoms. Fecal material is most likely to yield virus.

If a poliovirus is isolated from a patient with paralysis, the isolate should be sent to the Centers for Disease Control and Prevention through the state health department for testing to distinguish a wild-type virus from a vaccine strain. Since infants and children who are immunized with OPV can excrete vaccine virus in feces for several weeks, the incidental isolation of poliovirus from enteric sites in healthy young infants should be assumed to be the result of administration of or exposure to OPV, unless an epidemiologic or clinical reason to suspect otherwise exists. Serologic testing of acute and convalescent serum samples should be performed when paralytic poliomyelitis is suspected, but interpretation of serologic test results can be difficult. Hence, the diagnostic test of choice for confirming poliovirus disease is viral culture of stool specimens and throat swabs obtained as early in the course of illness as possible (see preceding paragraph).

TREATMENT: Supportive.

ISOLATION OF THE HOSPITALIZED PATIENT: Standard precautions are recommended.

CONTROL MEASURES:

Immunization of Infants and Children.

Vaccines. The 2 types of poliovirus vaccines are inactivated vaccine given parenterally (subcutaneously or intramuscularly) and live-virus vaccine given orally. Inactivated poliovirus (IPV) vaccine contains the 3 types of poliovirus grown in monkey kidney cells and inactivated with formaldehyde. The IPV vaccine in use in the United States since 1987 has higher potency than earlier formulations. Trace amounts of streptomycin, neomycin, and polymyxin B are present in IPV vaccine. The OPV vaccine contains attenuated poliovirus types 1, 2, and 3, produced in monkey kidney cell cultures.

Immunogenicity and Efficacy. Both IPV and OPV vaccines in their recommended schedules are highly immunogenic and effective in preventing poliomyelitis.

Administration of IPV vaccine results in seroconversion in 95% or more of vaccine recipients to each of the 3 serotypes after 2 doses and in 99% to 100% of recipients after 3 doses. Immunity is prolonged, perhaps lifelong. Mucosal immunity is induced by enhanced-potency IPV vaccine but to a lesser extent than that with OPV vaccine; on reinfection, IPV-immunized children excrete polioviruses from stool but not from the oropharynx. A 3-dose series of OPV vaccine in the United States results in sustained, probably lifelong immunity. Immunization with 2 or more doses of OPV vaccine induces excellent serum antibody responses and a high degree of intestinal immunity against poliovirus reinfection, which explains its effectiveness in controlling wild-virus circulation.

Administration With Other Vaccines. Either IPV or OPV vaccine may be given concurrently with other routinely recommended childhood vaccines (see Simultaneous Administration of Multiple Vaccines, p 26).

Adverse Reactions. No serious adverse events have been associated with use of the currently available IPV vaccine. Since IPV vaccine contains trace amounts of streptomycin, neomycin, and polymyxin B, allergic reactions are possible in recipients with hypersensitivity to one or more of these antibiotics.

The OPV vaccine can cause VAPP. Before the expanded use of IPV vaccine in the United States, which began in 1997, the overall risk of VAPP was approximately 1 case per 2.4 million doses of OPV vaccine distributed. The rate after the first dose was approximately 1 case per 750 000 doses, including vaccine recipient and contact cases.

Schedule. The American Academy of Pediatrics recommends a 4-dose all-IPV vaccine schedule for routine immunization of all infants and children in the United States. The first 2 doses should be given at 2-month intervals beginning at 2 months of age (minimum age of 6 weeks), and a third dose is recommended at 6 to 18 months of age. Doses may be given at 4-week intervals when accelerated protection is indicated. Administration of the third dose at 6 months of age has the potential advantage of enhancing the likelihood of completion of the primary series and does not compromise seroconversion. A supplemental dose of IPV vaccine should be given before the child enters school, ie, at 4 to 6 years of age. A fourth dose is not necessary if the third dose was given on or after the child's fourth birthday.

The OPV vaccine should be used only for the following special circumstances, unless otherwise contraindicated:

- Mass vaccination campaigns to control outbreaks of paralytic poliomyelitis.
- Unimmunized children who will be traveling in fewer than 4 weeks to areas where polio is endemic or epidemic, ie, those for whom the time before departure is insufficient for administration of 2 doses of IPV vaccine.
- Children of parents who do not accept the recommended number of vaccine injections to fulfill the current childhood immunization schedule. However, OPV vaccine , if available, should be given only for the third or fourth dose or both.

Whenever OPV vaccine is administered, the risk of VAPP in recipients and contacts should be discussed with parents or caregivers. The availability of OPV vaccine in the United States is expected to be limited beginning in 2000.*

The OPV vaccine is the vaccine of choice for global eradication. It is recommended in the following areas: (1) locations with continued or recent circulation of wild-type poliovirus; (2) most developing countries where the higher cost of IPV vaccine prohibits its use; and (3) where inadequate sanitation necessitates an optimal mucosal barrier to wild-type virus circulation.

Issues in Scheduling IPV Vaccine Administration. Until appropriate combination vaccines are available, administration of IPV vaccine necessitates additional injections. In scheduling IPV vaccine administration, the following options should be considered to decrease the number of injections at the 2- and 4-month visits:

- Hepatitis B vaccine administration at birth and ages 1 and 6 months.
- Additional visits, assuming that the child is likely to return.
- Use of available combination vaccines.

---

* For recommendations for the use of remaining supplies of OPV vaccine during the transition to the all-IPV vaccine schedule, see American Academy of Pediatrics Committee on Infectious Diseases. Prevention of poliomyelitis: recommendations for the use of only inactivated poliovirus vaccine for routine immunization. *Pediatrics.* 1999;104:1404–1406

Vaccine Interchangeability. Until the recommended all-IPV vaccine schedule becomes fully implemented, 4 doses of any combination of IPV or OPV vaccine by 4 to 6 years of age should be considered equivalent to a complete poliovirus immunization series when administered according to the recommendations for minimum ages and intervals between doses.

Children Incompletely Immunized. Children who have not received the recommended doses of poliovirus vaccines on schedule should receive sufficient doses of IPV vaccine to complete the immunization series for their age (see Lapsed Immunizations, p 27).

Vaccine Recommendations for Adults. Most adults residing in the United States are immune as the result of immunization received during childhood and have a small risk of exposure to wild-type poliovirus in the United States. Immunization is recommended for certain adults who are at a greater risk of exposure to wild-type polioviruses than the general population, including the following:

- Travelers to areas or countries where poliomyelitis is or may be epidemic or endemic
- Members of communities or specific population groups with disease caused by wild-type polioviruses
- Laboratory workers handling specimens that may contain wild-type polioviruses
- Health care personnel in close contact with patients who may be excreting wild-type polioviruses

For unimmunized adults, primary immunization with IPV vaccine is recommended. Two doses of IPV vaccine should be given at intervals of 1 to 2 months (4 to 8 weeks); a third dose is given 6 to 12 months after the second unless the risk of exposure is increased, such as when traveling to areas where wild-type poliovirus is known to be circulating. If time does not allow 3 doses of IPV vaccine to be given according to the recommended schedule before protection is required, the following alternatives are recommended:

- If protection is not needed until 8 weeks or more, 3 doses of IPV vaccine should be given at least 4 weeks apart.
- If protection is not needed for 4 to 8 weeks, 2 doses of IPV vaccine should be given at least 4 weeks apart.
- If protection is needed in fewer than 4 weeks, a single dose of either IPV vaccine or OPV vaccine (if available) should be given.

The remaining doses of vaccine to complete the primary immunization schedule should be given subsequently at the recommended intervals if the person remains at an increased risk.

Recommendations in other circumstances are as follows:

- ***Incompletely immunized adults.*** Those who previously received less than a full primary course of OPV or IPV vaccine should be given the remaining required doses of IPV vaccine regardless of the interval since the last dose and the type of vaccine that was received previously.
- ***Adults who are at an increased risk of exposure to wild-type poliovirus and who previously completed primary immunization with OPV or IPV vaccine.*** These adults should receive a single dose of IPV vaccine.

Precautions and Contraindications to Immunization.

Immunodeficiency Disorders. Patients with immunodeficiency disorders, including human immunodeficiency virus (HIV) infection, combined immunodeficiency, abnormalities of immunoglobulin synthesis (ie, antibody deficiency syndromes), leukemia, lymphoma, or generalized malignant neoplasm, or those being given immunosuppressive therapy with pharmacologic agents (see Immunocompromised Children, p 56) or radiation therapy should receive IPV vaccine. A protective immune response to IPV vaccine in an immunodeficient patient cannot be ensured.

Household Contacts of Persons With Immunodeficiency Disease, Altered Immune States, Immunosuppression Due to Therapy for Other Disease, or Known HIV Infection. The IPV vaccine is recommended for these persons, and OPV vaccine should not be used. If OPV vaccine is administered inadvertently to a household contact of an immunodeficient or HIV-infected person, close contact between the patient and the OPV vaccine recipient should be minimized for approximately 4 to 6 weeks after immunization. Household members should be counseled on practices that will minimize exposure of the immunodeficient or HIV-infected person to excreted polio vaccine virus. These practices include hand washing after contact with the child and avoidance of diaper changing.

Pregnancy. Immunization during pregnancy generally should be avoided for reasons of theoretical risk, although no convincing evidence indicates that the rates of adverse events to IPV vaccine are increased in pregnant women or their developing fetuses. If immediate protection against poliomyelitis is needed, IPV is recommended (see Vaccine Recommendations for Adults, p 469).

Hypersensitivity or Anaphylactic Reactions Following IPV Vaccine, OPV Vaccine, or the Antibiotics Contained in These Vaccines. The IPV vaccine is contraindicated for persons who have experienced an anaphylactic reaction following a previous dose of IPV vaccine or to one of the following antibiotics: streptomycin, polymyxin B, and neomycin.

Breastfeeding and mild diarrhea are not contraindications to IPV or OPV vaccine administration.

Reporting of Adverse Events Following Vaccination. All cases of VAPP and other serious adverse events associated temporally with poliomyelitis vaccine should be reported (see Reporting of Adverse Events, p 31).

Case Reporting and Investigation. A suspected case of poliomyelitis should be reported promptly to the state health department and result in an immediate epidemiologic investigation. Poliomyelitis should be considered in the differential diagnosis of all cases of acute flaccid paralysis, including Guillain-Barré syndrome and transverse myelitis. If the course is clinically compatible with poliomyelitis, specimens should be obtained for viral studies (see Diagnostic Tests, p 466). If the evidence implicates wild-type poliovirus infection, an intensive investigation will be conducted, and a public health decision will be made about the need for supplementary immunizations, choice of vaccine, and other action.

PRION DISEASES

Transmissible Spongiform Encephalopathies*

CLINICAL MANIFESTATIONS: Transmissible spongiform encephalopathies (TSEs or prion diseases) comprise a group of rare, rapidly progressive, universally fatal neurodegenerative syndromes of humans and animals that are characterized by neuronal degeneration, spongiform change, gliosis, and accumulation of an abnormal protease-resistant amyloid protein, (protease-resistant prion protein [PrP^{res}] or scrapie prion protein [PrP^{sc}]) distributed diffusely throughout the brain and sometimes also in discrete plaques. Although other human organ systems have not been shown to be symptomatically or pathologically involved, accumulation of PrP^{res} in certain animal TSEs has been reported.

The human TSEs include Creutzfeldt-Jakob disease (CJD); Gerstmann-Sträussler-Scheinker disease; fatal familial insomnia, a fatal sporadic insomnia; and kuru. Classic CJD can be sporadic (approximately 85% of cases), familial (approximately 15%), or iatrogenic (<1%). Iatrogenic CJD has been acquired through injection of cadaveric pituitary hormones (growth hormone and human gonadotropin), dura mater allografts, corneal transplantation, and instrumentation of the brain at neurosurgery or depth-electrode electroencephalographic recording. In 1996, an outbreak of variant CJD (vCJD) emerged in the United Kingdom and France and has been linked to exposure to tissues from bovine spongiform encephalopathy–infected cattle.

Creutzfeldt-Jakob disease commences as a dementing syndrome in approximately two thirds of affected persons, occurring with progressive defects in memory, personality, and other higher cortical functions; approximately one third of patients present with a cerebellar syndrome of ataxia and dysarthria. Iatrogenic CJD may present with dementia (as in dural allograft transplants) or with cerebellar signs (as observed in virtually all peripherally inoculated disease). Myoclonus develops in at least 80% of affected persons at some point in the course of disease. Death usually supervenes in weeks to months; survival exceeding a year is observed in only approximately 10% of patients with sporadic CJD.

The vCJD is distinguished from classic CJD by young age of onset, "psychiatric" presentation, and other features, such as painful sensory symptoms, delayed onset of overt neurologic signs, absence of the diagnostic electroencephalographic changes, and a more prolonged duration of illness. In vCJD, "florid" or "daisy" plaques and marked accumulation of PrP^{res} in the central nervous system and in lymphoid tissues are found.

ETIOLOGY: The infectious particle or prion responsible for the human and animal prion diseases is widely thought to be protein-based, without a nucleic acid component, although some experts remain skeptical of the prion hypothesis. Proponents of the hypothesis postulate that sporadic CJD arises from a rare spontaneous misfolding of the normal protease-sensitive host protein (PrP^{sen}) or control PrP (PrP^{c}) to yield

* Whitley RJ, MacDonald N, Asher D. Transmissible spongiform encephalopathies (TSE): a review for pediatricians. *Pediatrics.* In press

the abnormal protease-resistant form associated with infectivity. Prion protein conformational changes are propagated by a "recruitment reaction" (the nature of which is unknown) in which abnormal PrP serves as a template or lattice for the conformational conversion of neighboring PrP^{sen} molecules.

The protein coding sequence of the PrP gene also influences susceptibility to iatrogenic and sporadic CJD through an amino acid polymorphism at codon 129, encoding methionine or valine in humans. A large majority of patients in whom sporadic or iatrogenic CJD develops are homozygous for methionine or valine at this site (approximately 80% methionine) in contrast with 40% to 50% of an unselected population; to date all patients with vCJD who have been tested have been homozygous for methionine.

EPIDEMIOLOGY: Classic CJD is rare, occurring at approximately 1 case per million total population per year. The onset of disease peaks in the 60- to 69-year-old age group. Familial CJD occurs at about one tenth the frequency of sporadic CJD, with onset of disease approximately 10 years earlier than sporadic CJD.

Case control studies of CJD found a family history of CJD to be the only consistently recognized risk factor. No statistically significant increased risk was observed for treatment with blood, blood components, or plasma derivatives, although all studies to date have lacked sufficient statistical power to detect small risks exceeding that of the control population.

As of December 1, 1999, vCJD was reported in 45 persons in the United Kingdom and 1 in France. Most patients with vCJD were younger than 40 years of age, and several were adolescents. The eventual number of vCJD cases is not predictable yet.

The **incubation period** for iatrogenic CJD varies by route of exposure and can range from 1.5 to 30 years or possibly more.

DIAGNOSTIC TESTS: The diagnosis of human prion diseases can be obtained with certainty only by neuropathologic examination of affected brain tissue. A progressive neurologic syndrome in a person bearing a pathogenic mutation of the prion gene may be presumed a prion disease. The failure to identify a unique prion nucleic acid component precludes detection of the infective particle by genome amplification. To date, there is no validated sensitive and specific noninvasive diagnostic test of human prion disease, but extensive research is ongoing in this area.

TREATMENT: No treatment slows or stops the progressive neurodegenerative syndromes of the prion diseases. Supportive therapy is targeted to management of the fulminant dementia, spasticity, rigidity, and seizures that can arise in the course of the illness. Psychological support may help families of affected persons. Genetic counseling is indicated in familial disease.

ISOLATION OF THE HOSPITALIZED PATIENT: Standard precautions are recommended. The available evidence indicates that even prolonged intimate contact with CJD-infected persons has not resulted in transmission of disease. Tissues associated with high levels of infectivity (eg, brain, eyes, and spinal cord of affected persons) and instruments in contact with those tissues are considered biohazards; incineration, prolonged autoclaving at elevated temperature and pressure, and exposure to a solution of sodium hydroxide of 1N or greater or a solution of sodium hypochlorite of 5.25% or greater (undiluted household chlorine bleach) for 1 hour has been reported to markedly reduce infectivity. Cerebrospinal fluid should be regarded as infectious. Person-to-person transmission of CJD by blood, milk, saliva, urine, or feces has not been reported. These body fluids can be handled using standard infection control procedures.

CONTROL MEASURES: Immunization against the prion diseases is not available, and no immune response to infection has been demonstrated. Iatrogenic transmission of CJD through cadaveric pituitary hormones has been obviated by use of recombinant products. Recognition that CJD can be spread by transplantation of infected dura and corneas has led to more stringent donor-selection criteria and improved collection protocols. The effect of vCJD on health care is unclear at present (see Blood Safety, p 88). Regimens for postexposure prophylaxis have been proposed but not validated. A suspected or confirmed diagnosis of CJD in a child or adolescent should be reported to the CJD Surveillance Unit, Division of Viral and Rickettsial Diseases, Centers for Disease Control and Prevention, Atlanta, GA 30333; telephone, 404-639-3311). Current precautionary policies of the US Food and Drug Administration about risk of CJD and human blood or blood products are accessible on the Internet at http://www.fda.gov/cber/whatsnew.html.

Q Fever

CLINICAL MANIFESTATIONS: Acute Q fever usually is characterized by abrupt onset of fever, chills, weakness, headache, and anorexia, as well as other nonspecific systemic symptoms. Cough and chest pains can signify pneumonia, which occurs in about half the patients. Weight loss and weakness can be pronounced. Hepatosplenomegaly frequently is noted, and rash is unusual. The illness lasts 1 to 4 weeks and then resolves gradually. Chronic Q fever is infrequent; endocarditis and hepatitis are the major manifestations. Although acute Q fever is rarely fatal, mortality among patients with endocarditis is 30% to 60%.

ETIOLOGY: *Coxiella burnetii,* the cause of Q fever, is unique among rickettsiae because it undergoes a host-dependent phase variation, and it is highly resistant to heat, desiccation, and chemicals. While considered a rickettsia, *C burnetii* has been reclassified in the γ subgroup of Proteobacteria.

EPIDEMIOLOGY: Animal infection is widespread, usually asymptomatic, and primarily involves a large variety of domestic farm animals (especially sheep, goats, and cows), but also cats, dogs, rodents, marsupials, other mammalian species, and some wild and domestic bird species. Tick vectors may be important for maintaining animal reservoirs. Infectious organisms can persist in the environment for many years. Human disease is uncommon but may be asymptomatic or unrecognized. The disease occurs endemically throughout the world, typically in areas where cattle are raised and sheep and goats are herded. The disease has been transmitted to humans by inhalation of aerosols spontaneously generated from infected material, such as placental tissue from infected cats or farm animals, and by exposure to infected animals or tissues on farms or ranches or in research facilities. Consumption of raw milk is a risk factor for infection. Persons who work with animals, including farmers, ranchers, and research laboratory workers, as well as persons in other occupations or with avocational interests resulting in close contact with infected animals or tissues, are at increased risk. Q fever has occurred among flocks of sheep used as experimental subjects in medical research facilities, and transmission to research investigators and technical personnel has been documented. The handling of animal fetuses and products of conception is a major means of infection. Although seasonal trends are not obvious, in some areas, the disease coincides with the lambing season in the early spring. Because the birth of farm animals, such as sheep, goats, and cows, is a somewhat controllable event, the disease can occur throughout the year in areas where planned animal births are permitted. Evidence for human intrauterine infection has been reported. The risk of chronic infection is increased by immunodeficiency and by underlying cardiovascular disease.

The **incubation period** varies from 9 to 39 days but usually is between 14 and 22 days.

DIAGNOSTIC TESTS: Isolation of *C burnetii* from blood usually is not attempted because of the hazard to laboratory workers. Specific antiphase I and antiphase II immunofluorescent, enzyme immunoassay, complement fixation, and immune adherence hemagglutination antibody tests using paired serum specimens are used diagnostically. Specific immunoglobulin (Ig) M, IgG, and IgA tests using immunofluorescence or enzyme immunoassay methods are available in reference and research laboratories. In research laboratories, immunoblotting techniques have been used to diagnose chronic Q fever; polymerase chain reaction can detect small numbers of organisms in tissue and has been used to detect *C burnetti* DNA in environmental specimens. DNA hybridization in conjunction with polymerase chain reaction can detect small numbers of organisms in blood, urine, and tissue, and restriction in length polymorphism can be used to differentiate isolates obtained from animals and humans. *Coxiella burnetii* infection does not cause a positive serum Weil-Felix test.

TREATMENT: Tetracycline or doxycycline is the drug of choice, and chloramphenicol is an alternative. Tetracyclines should not be given to children younger than 8 years of age unless the benefit is greater than the risk of dental staining (see Antimicrobial Agents and Related Therapy, p 646). Therapy should be initiated promptly and continued until the patient has been afebrile for 2 to 3 days. In chronic Q fever, relapses can occur necessitating repeated courses of antimicrobial therapy. The organism can remain latent in tissues for years; treatment of chronic disease is extremely difficult. Treatment of chronic endocarditis is prolonged and appears to be more effective when tetracycline or doxycycline is combined with rifampin, trimethoprim-sulfamethoxazole, or a fluoroquinolone. In patients younger than 18 years of age, fluoroquinolones usually are contraindicated (see Antimicrobial Agents and Related Therapy, p 645). Relapses can occur after discontinuation of treatment.

ISOLATION OF THE HOSPITALIZED PATIENT: Standard precautions are recommended.

CONTROL MEASURES: Experimental vaccines for domestic animals and laboratory workers are promising but not available in the United States. Recommendations have been made to reduce the risk of infection in research facilities involving sheep.* Special safety practices are recommended for nonpropagative laboratory procedures involving *C burnetii* and for all propagative procedures, necropsies of infected animals, and manipulation of infected human and animal tissues. Otherwise, no specific management is recommended for persons who have been exposed. Flash pasteurization of milk at 71.6°C (160.8°F) for 15 seconds or 62.9°C (145.1°F) for 30 minutes destroys the organism, but the epidemiologic role of milk in transmission is uncertain.

Rabies†

CLINICAL MANIFESTATIONS: Infection with rabies virus characteristically produces an acute illness with rapidly progressive central nervous system manifestations, including anxiety, dysphagia, and seizures. Illness almost invariably progresses to death. Some patients may present with paralysis. The differential diagnosis of all acute encephalitic illnesses of unknown cause with atypical focal neurologic signs or with paralysis should include rabies.

ETIOLOGY: Rabies virus is an RNA virus classified in the Rhabdovirus family.

EPIDEMIOLOGY: In the United States, the number of cases of human rabies has declined steadily since the 1950s, reflecting widespread rabies immunization of dogs and the availability of effective immunoprophylaxis after exposure to a rabid animal. Between 1980 and 1997, 12 (33%) of 36 rabies cases diagnosed in the United States were related to rabid animals outside the United States. In contrast, 21 (58%) were bat variants. Despite the large focus of rabies in raccoons in the eastern United States, no human deaths have been attributed to the raccoon rabies virus variant. Rarely, airborne transmission has been reported in the laboratory and in caves serving as habitats for bats. Transmission also has occurred by transplantation of corneas from patients dying of undiagnosed rabies. Person-to-person transmission by bite has not been documented, although the virus has been isolated from the saliva of patients. The epidemiology of rabies is aided by strain identification using monoclonal antibodies and nucleotide sequencing.

Wildlife rabies exists throughout the United States except for Hawaii, which remains rabies free. Wildlife, including raccoons, skunks, foxes, coyotes, bats, and other species, is the most important potential source of infection for humans and

* Bernard KW, Parham GL, Winkler WG, Helmick CG. Q fever control measures: recommendations for research facilities using sheep. *Infect Control.* 1982;3:461–465; and Harrison RJ, Vugia DJ, Ascher MS. Occupational health guidelines for control of Q fever in sheep research. *Ann N Y Acad Sci.* 1990;590:283–290

† For further information, see Centers for Disease Control and Prevention. Human rabies prevention: United States, 1999: recommendations of the Advisory Committee on Immunization Practices [published correction appears in *MMWR Morb Mortal Wkly Rep.* 1999;48:16]. *MMWR Morb Mortal Wkly Rep.* 1999;48(RR-1):1–21

domestic animals in the United States. Rabies in small rodents (squirrels, hamsters, guinea pigs, gerbils, chipmunks, rats, and mice) and lagomorphs (rabbits and hares) is rare, but rabies may occur in woodchucks or other large rodents in areas where raccoon rabies is common. The virus is present in saliva and is transmitted by bites or, rarely, by contamination of mucosa or skin lesions by infectious material. Worldwide, most rabies cases in humans result from dog bites in areas where canine rabies is enzootic. Most dogs, cats, and ferrets become ill within 4 or 5 days of viral shedding, and no case of human rabies in the United States has been attributed to a dog, cat, or ferret that has remained healthy throughout the standard 10-day period of confinement.

The **incubation period** in humans averages 4 to 6 weeks but ranges from 5 days to more than 1 year. Incubation periods of up to 6 years have been confirmed by antigenic typing and nucleotide sequencing of strains.

DIAGNOSTIC TESTS: Infection in animals can be diagnosed by demonstration of virus-specific fluorescent antigen in brain tissue. Suspected rabid animals should be euthanized in a manner that preserves brain tissue for appropriate examination. Virus can be isolated from saliva, brain, and other tissues in suckling mice or in tissue culture. The diagnosis in suspected human cases can be made postmortem and sometimes antemortem by fluorescent microscopy of skin biopsy specimens from the nape of the neck, by isolation of the virus from saliva, by detection of antibody in the cerebrospinal fluid (CSF) or serum in unimmunized persons, and by detection of viral nucleic acid in infected tissues. Laboratory personnel should be consulted before submission of specimens so that appropriate collection and transport of materials can be arranged.

TREATMENT: Once symptoms have developed, no drug or vaccine improves the prognosis. Only a few patients with human rabies have survived with intensive supportive care; all other patients have died despite treatment.

ISOLATION OF THE HOSPITALIZED PATIENT: Standard precautions are recommended for the duration of illness. If the patient has bitten another person or the patient's saliva has contaminated an open wound or mucous membrane, the involved area should be washed thoroughly and postexposure prophylaxis should be administered (see Care of Exposed Persons, p 478).

CONTROL MEASURES:

Education of children by parents, teachers, and health care personnel to avoid contact with stray or wild animals is of primary importance. Children should be cautioned against provoking or attempting to capture stray or wild animals and against touching carcasses. Inadvertent contact of family members and pets with potentially rabid animals, such as raccoons, foxes, coyotes, and skunks, may be diminished by securing garbage and refuse to decrease attraction of domestic and wild animals. Similarly, chimneys and other potential portals of entry for wild animals, including bats, should be identified and covered. International travelers to areas of endemic canine rabies should be warned to avoid exposure to stray dogs, and, if travelling to an area where immediate access to medical care and biologics is limited, preexposure prophylaxis is indicated.

Table 3.48. **Rabies Postexposure Prophylaxis Guide**

Animal Type	Evaluation and Disposition of Animal	Postexposure Prophylaxis Recommendations
Dogs, cats, and ferrets	Healthy and available for 10 days of observation	Prophylaxis only if animal develops signs of rabies*
	Rabid or suspected of being rabid†	Immediate immunization‡ and RIG
	Unknown (escaped)	Consult public health officials for advice
Bats, skunks, raccoons, foxes, and most other carnivores; woodchucks	Regarded as rabid unless geographic area is known to be free of rabies or until animal proven negative by laboratory tests†	Immediate immunization‡ and RIG
Livestock, rodents, and lagomorphs (rabbits and hares)	Consider individually	Consult public health officials. Bites of squirrels, hamsters, guinea pigs, gerbils, chipmunks, rats, mice, other rodents, rabbits, and hares almost never require antirabies treatment.

*During the 10-day holding period, at the first sign of rabies in the biting dog, cat, or ferret, treatment with Rabies Immune Globulin (human) (RIG) and vaccine should be initiated. The suspect animal should be euthanized immediately and tested.

† The animal should be euthanized and tested as soon as possible. Holding for observation is not recommended. Immunization is discontinued if immunofluorescent test of the animal is negative.

‡ See text.

Exposure Risk and Decisions to Give Immunoprophylaxis. Exposure to rabies results from a break in the skin caused by the teeth of a rabid animal or by contamination of scratches, abrasions, or mucous membranes with saliva from a rabid animal. The decision to immunize an exposed person ordinarily should be made in consultation with the local health department, which can provide information on the risk of rabies in a particular area for each species of animal, and in accordance with the guidelines in Table 3.48 above. In the United States, raccoons, skunks, foxes, and bats are more likely to be infected than other animals, but coyotes, cattle, dogs, cats, ferrets, and other species occasionally are infected. Bites of rodents (such as squirrels and rats) or lagomorphs (rabbits and hares) rarely require specific antirabies prophylaxis. Additional factors must be considered when deciding whether immunoprophylaxis is indicated. An unprovoked attack is more suggestive of a rabid animal than a bite that occurs during attempts to feed or handle an animal. Properly immunized dogs, cats, and ferrets have only a minimal chance of developing rabies. However, in rare instances, rabies has developed in properly immunized animals.

Postexposure prophylaxis for rabies is recommended for all persons bitten by wild mammalian carnivores or bats or by domestic animals that may be infected. Exposures other than bites rarely have resulted in infection, but seemingly insignificant physical contact with bats may result in viral transmission even without a clear history of a bite. Postexposure prophylaxis is recommended for persons who report an open wound, scratch, or mucous membrane that has been contaminated with saliva or other potentially infectious material (eg, brain tissue) from a rabid animal. Because the injury inflicted by a bat bite or scratch may be small and not evident or the circumstances of contact may preclude accurate recall (eg, a bat in a room of a sleeping person, previously unattended child, mentally disabled person, or intoxicated person), prophylaxis is indicated for situations in which a bat is physically present if a bite or mucous membrane exposure cannot be reliably excluded, unless prompt testing of the bat has excluded rabies virus infection. Prophylaxis always should be initiated as soon as possible after bites by known or suspected rabid animals.

Postexposure prophylaxis also is recommended for persons who report a possibly infectious exposure (eg, bite, scratch, or open wound or mucous membrane contaminated with saliva or other infectious material) to a human with rabies. However, exposure to a human with rabies has not been documented as a means of rabies transmission except after corneal transplantation from donors who died of unsuspected rabies encephalitis. Casual contact with an infected person (eg, by touching a patient) or contact with noninfectious fluids or tissues (eg, urine or feces) alone does not constitute an exposure and is not an indication for prophylaxis (see Care of Hospital Contacts, below).

Handling of Suspect Animals. A suspect dog, cat, or ferret that has bitten a human should be captured, confined, and observed by a veterinarian for 10 days. Any illness in the animal should be reported immediately to the local health department. If signs of rabies develop, the animal should be euthanized and its head removed and shipped under refrigeration (iced, not frozen) to a qualified laboratory for examination.

Other biting animals that may have exposed a person to rabies should be reported immediately to the local health department. Management of animals depends on the species, the circumstances of the bite, and the epidemiology of rabies in the area. Prior immunization of an animal may not preclude the necessity for euthanasia and testing if the period of viral shedding is unknown for that species. Because clinical manifestations of rabies in a wild animal cannot be interpreted reliably, a suspect wild mammal should be euthanized at once and its brain examined for evidence of rabies. The exposed person need not be treated if results of rapid examination of the brain by fluorescent antibody procedures are negative for rabies.

Care of Hospital Contacts. Immunization of hospital contacts of a patient with rabies should be reserved for persons who were bitten or whose mucous membranes or open wounds have come in contact with saliva, CSF, or brain tissue of a patient with rabies (see Care of Exposed Persons). Other hospital contacts of a patient with rabies do not require immunization.

Care of Exposed Persons.

Local Wound Care. The immediate objective of postexposure prophylaxis is to prevent virus from entering neural tissue. Prompt and thorough local treatment of all lesions is essential, because virus may remain localized to the area of the bite for a variable time. All wounds should be flushed thoroughly and cleaned with soap and water. Quaternary ammonium compounds (such as Zephiran), which were recommended in the past, are no longer considered superior to soap. The need for tetanus

Table 3.49. **US Food and Drug Administration–Approved Rabies Vaccines and Rabies Immune Globulin**

Category	Product	Manufacturer	Method of Administration*
Human rabies vaccine	Human diploid cell vaccine (HDCV) (Imovax)†	Pasteur-Merieux Connaught	IM or ID
	Rabies vaccine adsorbed (RVA)	Bio Port‡	IM
	Purified chick embryo cell (PCEC) (RabAvert)	Chiron Corporation	IM
Rabies Immune Globulin	Imogam Rabies-HT	Pasteur-Merieux Connaught	Infiltrate around wound§
	BayRab	Bayer	Infiltrate around wound§

* IM indicates intramuscular; ID, intradermal.
† Products are Imovax Rabies and Imovax Rabies I.D.
‡ Distributed by SmithKline Beecham Pharmaceuticals.
§ Any remaining volume should be administered IM.

prophylaxis and measures to control bacterial infection also should be considered. The wound, if possible, should not be sutured.

Immunoprophylaxis. After wound care is completed, concurrent use of passive *and* active immunoprophylaxis is required for optimal therapy (see Table 3.48, p 477). Prophylaxis should begin as soon as possible after exposure, ideally within 24 hours. However, a delay of several days or more may not compromise effectiveness, and prophylaxis should be initiated if otherwise indicated, regardless of the interval between exposure and initiation of therapy. In the United States only the human product, rabies immune globulin (RIG), which is preferable to equine serum that was used previously, is available for passive immunization. Licensed tissue culture rabies vaccine should be used for active immunization. Physicians can obtain expert counsel from their local or state health departments.

Active Immunization (Postexposure). Four formulations of 3 rabies vaccines are available commercially for preexposure and postexposure prophylaxis in the United States (see Table 3.49, above). A 1.0-mL dose of any of the 3 vaccines is given intramuscularly in the deltoid area or anterolateral aspect of the thigh on the first day of postexposure prophylaxis, and repeated doses are given on days 3, 7, 14, and 28 after the first dose. An immunization series should be initiated and completed with 1 vaccine product; clinical studies evaluating efficacy or frequency of adverse reactions when the series is completed with a second product have not been conducted. The volume of the dose is not reduced for children. Serologic testing to document seroconversion after administration of any of the 3 rabies vaccine series is unnecessary but has been advised occasionally for recipients who may be immunocompromised.

Care should be taken to ensure that the vaccine is administered intramuscularly. Intradermal vaccine is not advised for postexposure prophylaxis in the United States, although for reasons of cost and availability, intradermal regimens are used in some countries. Because antibody responses in adults who received vaccine in the gluteal area sometimes have been less than in those who were injected in the deltoid muscle, the latter site always should be used, except in infants and young children in whom the anterolateral thigh is the appropriate site.

- ***Adverse reactions and precautions with human diploid cell vaccine, rabies vaccine adsorbed, and purified chick embryo cell.*** Reactions, primarily reported in adults, after immunization with these rabies vaccines are less common than with previously available vaccines. Reactions are uncommon in children. In adults, local reactions, such as pain, erythema, and swelling or itching at the injection site, are reported in 15% to 25%, and mild systemic reactions, such as headache, nausea, abdominal pain, muscle aches, and dizziness, are reported in 10% to 20%. Several cases of neurologic illness resembling Guillain-Barré syndrome that resolved without sequelae in 12 weeks and an acute, generalized, transient neurologic syndrome temporally associated with human diploid cell vaccine (HDCV) have been reported but are not thought to be related causally.

  Immune complex–like reactions in persons receiving booster doses of HDCV have been observed possibly due to interaction between the stabilizer (propiolactone) and human albumin. The reaction, characterized by onset 2 to 21 days after inoculation, presents with a generalized urticaria and can include arthralgia, arthritis, angioedema, nausea, vomiting, fever, and malaise, is not life-threatening, and occurs in as many as 6% of adults receiving booster doses as part of a preexposure immunization regimen. It is rare in persons receiving primary immunization with HDCV. Similar allergic reactions with primary or booster doses are not reported with purified chick embryo cell (PCEC) or rabies vaccine adsorbed (RVA).

  If the patient has a serious allergic reaction to HDCV, the RVA or the PCEC vaccine may be given according to the same schedule as HDCV. All suspected serious, systemic, neuroparalytic or anaphylactic reactions to the rabies vaccine should be reported immediately (see Reporting of Adverse Events, p 31).

  Although the safety of the use of rabies vaccine during pregnancy has not been studied specifically in the United States, pregnancy should not be considered a contraindication to the use of vaccine after exposure.
- ***Nerve tissue vaccines.*** Inactivated nerve tissue vaccines are not licensed in the United States but are available in many areas of the world. These preparations induce neuroparalytic reactions in between 1:2000 and 1:8000 recipients, perhaps as a result of sensitization to myelin. Immunization with nerve tissue vaccine should be discontinued if meningeal or neuroparalytic reactions develop. Corticosteroids can be used for treatment of complications, but they should be used only for life-threatening reactions because they definitely increase the risk of rabies in experimentally inoculated animals.

Passive Immunization. Human RIG should be used concomitantly with the first dose of vaccine for postexposure prophylaxis to bridge the time between initiation of medical attention and active antibody production by the vaccine recipient (see Table 3.49, p 479). If vaccine is not available immediately, RIG should be given alone and immunization started later. If RIG is not available immediately, vaccine should be given followed by RIG when obtained in the first 7 days after beginning treatment. If administration of vaccine and RIG is delayed, both should be used regardless of the interval between exposure and treatment.

The recommended dose of RIG is 20 IU/kg of body weight. As much of the dose as possible should be used to infiltrate the wound(s). The remainder is given intramuscularly using a separate syringe and needle. In cases of multiple severe wounds in which RIG is insufficient for infiltration, dilution in saline to an adequate volume (2-fold or 3-fold) has been recommended to ensure that all wound areas receive infiltrate. For children with a small muscle mass, it may be necessary to administer RIG at multiple sites. Human RIG is supplied in 2-mL (300 IU) and 10-mL (1500 IU) vials. Passive antibody can inhibit the response to rabies vaccines; therefore, the recommended dose should not be exceeded. Vaccine never should be administered in the same parts of the body or with the same syringe used to give RIG. Hypersensitivity reactions to RIG rarely, if ever, occur.

Purified equine RIG or antisera containing rabies antibodies is available outside the United States and generally is accompanied by a low rate of serum sickness (<1%). It is administered at a dose of 40 IU/kg, and desensitization is required.

Administration of RIG is not recommended for the following exposed persons: (1) those who previously received postexposure prophylaxis with HDCV, RVA, or PCEC; (2) those who received a 3-dose, intramuscular, preexposure regimen of HDCV, RVA, or PCEC; (3) those who received a 3-dose, intradermal, preexposure regimen of HDCV with the product used in the United States; and (4) those who have a documented adequate rabies titer after previous immunization with any other rabies vaccine. These persons should receive two 1.0-mL doses of HDCV, RVA, or PCEC; doses are given on the day of exposure and on day 3.

Preexposure Control Measures, Including Immunization. The relatively low frequency of reactions to HDCV, RVA, and PCEC has made the provision of preexposure immunization practical for persons in high-risk groups, such as veterinarians, animal handlers, certain laboratory workers, and persons traveling to live in areas where canine rabies is common. Others, such as spelunkers, whose vocational or avocational pursuits may result in frequent exposures to wildlife also should be considered for preexposure prophylaxis.

The RVA and PCEC vaccines are licensed for intramuscular administration only. Intramuscular (1.0 mL) and intradermal (0.1 mL) dosage formulations of HDCV are available for preexposure use. The preferred site of administration for intradermal vaccine is the skin in the deltoid area. The preexposure immunization schedule is the same for both routes of administration: 1-mL injection each given on days 0, 7, and 21 **or** 28. This series of immunizations has resulted in the development of antibodies in all persons properly immunized. For this reason, routine serologic testing for rabies antibody is not indicated.

Persons who are taking chloroquine or related antimicrobial drugs, such as mefloquine, should receive rabies vaccine by the intramuscular but not the intradermal route to minimize the potential for vaccine failure. Serum antibodies usually will still be present in most American vaccine recipients 2 years after the primary series given intramuscularly but may be less persistent in vaccine recipients in other circumstances, especially if antimalarial compounds are used. Preexposure booster immunization with HDCV (1.0 mL intramuscularly or 0.1 mL intradermally) or with RVA or PCEC intramuscularly will produce an effective anamnestic response.

An immune complex–like reaction occurred among 6% of persons who received booster doses of HDCV 2 to 21 days after administration of the booster dose. Rabies serum antibody titers should be determined at 6-month intervals for those at continuous risk (rabies research laboratory workers, rabies biologics production workers) and at intervals up to 2 years for those with risk of frequent exposure (rabies diagnostic laboratory workers, spelunkers, veterinarians and staff, and animal-control and wildlife workers in rabies-enzootic areas). Booster doses of vaccine should be administered only as appropriate to maintain serum antibody concentrations. The Centers for Disease Control and Prevention currently specifies complete viral neutralization at a 1:5 or greater titer by the rapid fluorescent-focus inhibition test as acceptable; the World Health Organization specifies 0.5 IU/mL or more as acceptable.

Public Health. A variety of approved public health measures, including immunization of dogs, cats, and ferrets and elimination of stray dogs and selected wildlife, are used to control rabies in animals. In regions where oral immunization of wildlife with recombinant rabies vaccine is undertaken, the incidence of rabies among foxes and raccoons may be reduced. Unimmunized dogs, cats, ferrets, or other pets bitten by a known rabid animal should be euthanized immediately. If the owner is unwilling to allow the animal to be euthanized, the animal should be placed in strict isolation for 6 months and immunized 1 month before release. If the animal has been immunized within 1 to 3 years, depending on the vaccine administered and local regulations, the animal should be reimmunized and observed for 45 days.

Case Reporting. All patients who are suspected of having rabies should be reported promptly to public health authorities.

Rat-Bite Fever

CLINICAL MANIFESTATIONS: Rat-bite fever is caused by either of two organisms and is characterized by fever of abrupt onset, chills, a maculopapular or petechial rash predominantly on the extremities, muscle pain, and headache. Specific clinical manifestations depend on the infecting organism. With *Streptobacillus moniliformis* infection (streptobacillary or Haverhill fever), the bite usually heals promptly, exhibits no or minimal inflammation, and is followed by nonsuppurative migratory polyarthritis or arthralgia in approximately 50% of patients. Complications include soft tissue and solid-organ abscesses, arthritis, pneumonia, endocarditis, myocarditis, pericarditis, and meningitis. With *Spirillum minus* infection, a period of initial apparent healing at the site of the bite usually is followed by ulceration, regional lymphangitis and lymphadenopathy, a distinctive rash of red or purple plaques, and, rarely, arthritic symptoms.

ETIOLOGY: The causes are *S moniliformis,* a microaerophilic, gram-negative, pleomorphic bacillus, and *S minus,* a small, gram-negative, spiral organism with bipolar flagellar tufts.

EPIDEMIOLOGY: Rat-bite fever is a zoonotic illness. *Streptobacillus moniliformis* and *S minus* are found in upper respiratory tract secretions of infected animals.

Streptobacillus moniliformis is transmitted by the bite of rats, squirrels, mice, cats, and weasels; by ingestion of contaminated food or milk products; and by contact with an infected animal. *Haverhill fever* refers to infection after ingestion of milk or water contaminated with *S moniliformis. Spirillum minus* is transmitted by the bites of rats and mice. On rare occasions, *S moniliformis* and *S minus* have been reported to be transmitted from person to person by a blood transfusion. *Streptobacillus moniliformis* infection accounts for most cases of rat-bite fever in the United States; *S minus* infections occur primarily in Asia. Both diseases are rare.

The **incubation period** for *S moniliformis* usually is 3 to 10 days but can be as long as 3 weeks; for *S minus* it is 7 to 21 days.

DIAGNOSTIC TESTS: *Streptobacillus moniliformis* can be isolated from blood, synovial fluid, aspirates from abscesses, or material from the bite lesion by inoculation into bacteriologic media enriched with blood, serum, or ascitic fluid. Because it is a fastidious organism, laboratory personnel should be notified that rat-bite fever is suspected. *Spirillum minus* has not been recovered on artificial media. Organisms can be visualized by the use of darkfield microscopy in wet mounts of blood, exudate of the initial lesion, and lymph nodes. Blood specimens also should be stained with Giemsa or Wright stain. *Spirillum minus* can be recovered from blood, lymph nodes, or local lesions by intraperitoneal inoculation of mice or guinea pigs.

TREATMENT: Procaine penicillin should be administered intramuscularly for 7 to 10 days for rat-bite fever caused by either agent. Initial intravenous penicillin G therapy for 5 days followed by oral penicillin V also has been successful. Tetracycline, chloramphenicol, or streptomycin may be substituted when a patient is allergic to penicillin. Tetracycline should not be given to children younger than 8 years of age unless the benefits of therapy are greater than the risks (see Antimicrobials and Related Therapy, p 646). Patients with endocarditis should receive intravenous high-dose penicillin G for at least 4 weeks. The addition of streptomycin initially may be useful.

ISOLATION OF THE HOSPITALIZED PATIENT: Standard precautions are recommended.

CONTROL MEASURES: Exposed persons should be observed for symptoms. Because the attack rate of rat-bite fever due to *S moniliformis* after a rat bite is 10%, some experts recommend postexposure administration of penicillin. Rat control is important in the control of disease.

Respiratory Syncytial Virus

CLINICAL MANIFESTATIONS: Respiratory syncytial virus (RSV) causes acute respiratory tract illness in patients of all ages. In infants and young children, RSV is the most important cause of bronchiolitis and pneumonia. During the first few weeks of life, particularly among preterm infants, infection with RSV may produce minimal respiratory tract signs. Lethargy, irritability, and poor feeding, sometimes accompanied by apneic episodes, may be the major manifestations. Most previously healthy infants infected with RSV do not require hospitalization, and many who are hospitalized improve within a few days with supportive care and are discharged in fewer than 5 days. Conditions that increase the risk of severe or fatal RSV infection are cyanotic or complicated congenital heart disease, especially conditions causing pulmonary hypertension; underlying pulmonary disease, especially bronchopulmonary dysplasia; prematurity; and immunodeficiency disease or therapy causing immunosuppression at any age. Long-term sequelae of RSV infection among infants are difficult to assess. Some evidence suggests that in subpopulations of infected children, long-term abnormalities in pulmonary function develop that may manifest as recurrent wheezing. This, however, may reflect an underlying predisposition to reactive airway disease, rather than RSV being the sole cause.

Infection with RSV in older children and adults usually manifests as an upper respiratory tract illness, occasionally with bronchitis. Exacerbation of asthma or other chronic lung conditions also is common.

ETIOLOGY: Respiratory syncytial virus is an enveloped RNA paramyxovirus that lacks neuraminidase and a hemagglutinin. Two major subtypes (A and B) have been identified and often circulate concurrently. The clinical and epidemiologic significance of strain variation has not been determined, but evidence suggests that antigenic differences may affect susceptibility to infection, and some strains may be more virulent than other strains.

EPIDEMIOLOGY: Humans are the only source of infection. Transmission usually is by direct or close contact with contaminated secretions, which may involve droplets or fomites. The RSV can persist on environmental surfaces for many hours and for half an hour or more on hands. Infection among hospital personnel can occur by self-inoculation with contaminated secretions. Hospital-acquired infections are frequent among hospital personnel and infants and have a significant effect on morbidity, mortality, and duration of hospitalization. Nosocomial spread of RSV on wards housing organ recipients or patients with other immunocompromised conditions has been associated with severe and fatal disease in children and adults.

Initial RSV infection usually occurs during the first 2 years of life and is the most common viral agent causing lower respiratory tract illness in infancy. Reinfection throughout life is common.

Respiratory syncytial virus usually occurs in annual epidemics during the winter and early spring in temperate climates and infects almost all children during the first 3 years of life. Spread among household and child care contacts, including adults, is common. The period of viral shedding usually is 3 to 8 days, but it may last longer, especially in young infants in whom shedding may continue for as long as 3 to 4 weeks.

The **incubation period** ranges from 2 to 8 days; 4 to 6 days is most common.

DIAGNOSTIC TESTS: Rapid diagnostic procedures, including immunofluorescent and enzyme immunoassay techniques for detection of viral antigen in clinical specimens, are available commercially and generally are reliable during RSV outbreaks. The sensitivity of these assays in comparison with culture varies between 53% and 96%, with most in the 80% to 90% range. Viral isolation from nasopharyngeal secretions in cell cultures requires 3 to 5 days, but results and sensitivity vary among laboratories because methods of isolation are exacting and RSV is a relatively labile virus with infectivity that decreases rapidly at room temperature and after freeze-thawing. An experienced viral laboratory should be consulted for optimal methods of collection and transport of specimens. Serologic testing of acute and convalescent serum samples can be used to confirm infection; however, the sensitivity of serologic diagnosis of infection is low among young infants. Polymerase chain reaction technology has been applied to detection of RSV but is not available commercially.

TREATMENT: Primary treatment is supportive and should include hydration, treatment of hypoxia with supplemental oxygen, and, if necessary, mechanical ventilation. Ribavirin has in vitro antiviral activity against RSV, but ribavirin aerosol treatment for RSV infection is controversial. The high cost, aerosol route of administration, concern about potential toxic effects among exposed health care personnel, and conflicting results of efficacy trials all contribute to this controversy.* Decisions about ribavirin administration should be based on the particular clinical circumstances and physicians' experience.

Corticosteroids. In previously healthy infants with RSV bronchiolitis, corticosteroids are not effective and are not indicated.

Antibiotics. Antibiotics rarely are indicated since bacterial lung infection and bacteremia are uncommon in infants hospitalized with RSV bronchiolitis or pneumonitis.

Prevention of RSV Infections. Two products are available to prevent RSV infection: Respiratory Syncytial Virus Immune Globulin Intravenous (RSV-IGIV),† prepared from donors selected for high serum titers of RSV neutralizing antibody, and palivizumab,‡ a humanized mouse monoclonal antibody that is given intramuscularly. Both have been approved for prevention of RSV disease in children younger than 24 months of age with bronchopulmonary dysplasia or with a history of premature birth (<35 weeks' gestation). Neither RSV-IGIV nor palivizumab has been approved for treatment of RSV infection. RSV-IGIV is given once per month just before and monthly throughout the RSV season at a dose of 15 mL/kg (750 mg/kg). Palivizumab is administered intramuscularly in a dose of 15 mg/kg once a month during the RSV season.

Recommendations by the American Academy of Pediatrics for the use of palivizumab and RSV-IGIV are as follows:

- Palivizumab or RSV-IGIV prophylaxis should be considered for infants and children younger than 2 years of age with chronic lung disease (CLD) who have required medical therapy for CLD within 6 months before the anticipated RSV season. Palivizumab is preferred for most high-risk children because of its ease of administration, safety, and effectiveness. Patients with more severe CLD may benefit from prophylaxis for 2 RSV seasons, especially those who require medical therapy. Decisions about individual patients may need addi-

* American Academy of Pediatrics Committee on Infectious Diseases. Reassessment of indications for ribavirin therapy in respiratory syncytial virus infections. *Pediatrics*. 1996;97:137–140

† RespiGam, Medimmune Inc, Gaithersburg, Md.

‡ For additional information, see American Academy of Pediatrics Committee on Infectious Diseases and Committee on Fetus and Newborn. Prevention of respiratory syncytial virus infections: indications for the use of palivizumab and update on the use of RSV-IGIV. *Pediatrics*. 1998;102:1211–1216

tional consultation from neonatologists, intensivists, or pulmonologists. There are limited data on the efficacy of palivizumab during the second year of age; risk of severe RSV disease exists for children with CLD who require medical therapy. Although children with less severe underlying disease may receive some benefit for the second season, immunoprophylaxis may not be necessary.

- Infants born at 32 weeks of gestation or earlier without CLD or who do not meet the aforementioned criteria also may benefit from RSV prophylaxis. For these infants, major risk factors to consider are gestational age and chronologic age at the start of the RSV season. Infants born at 28 weeks of gestation or earlier may benefit from prophylaxis up to 12 months of age. Infants born at 29 to 32 weeks of gestation may benefit most from prophylaxis up to 6 months of age. Decisions about duration of prophylaxis should be individualized according to the duration of the RSV season. Pediatricians may wish to use RSV rehospitalization data from their own region to assist in the decision-making process.
- Given the large number of patients born between 32 and 35 weeks of gestation and the cost of the drug, the use of palivizumab and RSV IGIV in this population should be reserved for infants with additional risk factors until more data are available.
- Palivizumab and RSV-IGIV are not licensed by the US Food and Drug Administration for patients with congenital heart disease (CHD). Available data indicate that RSV-IGIV is contraindicated in patients with cyanotic CHD. However, patients with CLD, who were born prematurely, or both, who meet the criteria in the first and second recommendations and who also have asymptomatic acyanotic CHD (eg, patent ductus arteriosus or ventricular septal defect) may benefit from prophylaxis.
- Palivizumab or RSV-IGIV prophylaxis has not been evaluated in randomized trials in immunocompromised children. Although specific recommendations for immunocompromised patients cannot be made, children with severe immunodeficiencies (eg, severe combined immunodeficiency or severe acquired immunodeficiency syndrome) may benefit from prophylaxis. If these infants and children are receiving standard IGIV monthly, physicians may consider substituting RSV-IGIV during the RSV season.
- Prophylaxis for RSV should be initiated at the onset of the RSV season and terminated at the end of the RSV season. In most areas of the United States, the usual time for the beginning of RSV outbreaks is October to December, and termination is March to May, but regional differences occur. Physicians should consult with health departments or diagnostic virology laboratories in their area or the Centers for Disease Control and Prevention if such information is not available locally.
- The RSV is known to be transmitted in the hospital setting and to cause serious disease in high-risk infants. In high-risk hospitalized infants, the major means to prevent RSV disease is strict observance of infection control practices, including the use of rapid means to identify and segregate RSV-infected

infants. If an RSV outbreak is documented in a high-risk unit (eg, pediatric intensive care unit), primary emphasis should be placed on proper infection control practices. The need for and efficacy of prophylaxis in these situations has not been evaluated.

- Palivizumab does not interfere with the response to vaccines.
  - In contrast, in infants and children receiving RSV-IGIV prophylaxis, immunization with measles-mumps-rubella and varicella vaccines should be deferred for 9 months after the last dose. The use of RSV-IGIV should not alter the primary immunization schedule for other routinely recommended vaccines. The manufacturer of RSV-IGIV has suggested that an additional dose of vaccine may be needed to assure an adequate immune response to DTaP (diphtheria and tetanus toxoids and acellular pertussis), *Haemophilus influenzae* b conjugate, and oral poliovirus vaccine, but more information is needed before recommendations can be made. The available data at this time do not support the need for supplemental doses of any of these routinely administered vaccines.

ISOLATION OF THE HOSPITALIZED PATIENT: In addition to standard precautions, contact precautions are recommended for the duration of RSV-associated illness among infants and young children, including patients treated with ribavirin. The effectiveness of these precautions depends on compliance and necessitates scrupulous adherence to good hand-washing practices and use of gloves and gown when entering the patient's room. Patients with laboratory-documented RSV infection can be cared for in the same room.

CONTROL MEASURES: The control of nosocomial RSV is complicated by the continuing chance for introduction through infected patients, staff, and visitors. During the peak of RSV season, many infants and children hospitalized with respiratory tract symptoms will be infected with RSV and should be managed with contact precautions (see Isolation of the Hospitalized Patient,). Early identification of RSV-infected patients (see Diagnostic Tests, p 484) is important so that appropriate precautions can be instituted promptly. During large outbreaks, a variety of measures have been demonstrated to be effective, including the following: (1) laboratory screening of patients for RSV infection, (2) segregating infected patients and staff, (3) excluding visitors with respiratory tract infections, and (4) excluding staff with respiratory tract illness or RSV infection from caring for susceptible infants. These additional measures may be most important for preventing transmission to patients with compromised cardiac, pulmonary, or immune systems.

A critical aspect of RSV prevention among high-risk infants is education of parents and other caregivers about the importance of reducing exposure to and transmission of RSV. Preventive measures include limiting, where feasible, exposure to contagious settings (eg, child care centers) and emphasis on hand washing in all settings including the home, especially during periods when the contacts of high-risk children have respiratory infections.

Rhinovirus Infections

CLINICAL MANIFESTATIONS: Rhinoviruses are the most frequent causes of the common cold or rhinosinusitis. Rhinoviruses also can be associated with pharyngitis and otitis media and with exacerbations of bronchitis and reactive airway disease. Nasal discharge usually is watery and clear at the onset but often becomes mucopurulent and viscus after a few days and may persist for 10 to 14 days. Malaise, headache, myalgias, and low-grade fever also may occur.

ETIOLOGY: Rhinoviruses are RNA viruses classified as picornaviruses. At least 100 antigenic serotypes have been identified by neutralizing antibodies. Infection with one type confers some type-specific immunity, but immunity is of variable degree and brief duration and offers little protection against other types.

EPIDEMIOLOGY: Only humans and chimpanzees are infected with human rhinoviruses. Transmission occurs predominantly by person-to-person contact through self-inoculation by contaminated secretions on hands, but in some circumstances, transmission may occur by aerosol. Infections occur throughout the year, but peak activity is most frequent in the autumn and spring. Several serotypes usually circulate simultaneously, but the prevalent serotypes circulating in a given population tend to change over time. By adulthood, antibodies to many serotypes have developed. Household spread is common. The period of communicability is variable but generally correlates with viral shedding in nasopharyngeal secretions, which is most abundant during the first 2 to 3 days of infection and usually ceases by 7 to 10 days, although shedding may continue for up to 3 weeks.

The **incubation period** is usually 2 to 3 days but occasionally up to 7 days.

DIAGNOSTIC TESTS: Inoculation of nasal secretions in appropriate cell cultures for viral isolation is the best means of establishing a specific diagnosis. The large number of antigenic types make serologic testing to diagnose infection impractical.

TREATMENT: Only symptomatic treatment is given. Placebo-controlled studies have indicated that over-the-counter antihistamine-decongestant cold medications are no more effective than placebo in children younger than 5 years of age. In contrast, controlled studies in adults have shown significant shortening of symptoms with early treatment with antihistamines. Antibiotics do not prevent secondary bacterial infection but may complicate later therapy by encouraging the emergence of resistant bacteria (see Judicious Use of Antimicrobial Agents, p 647).

ISOLATION OF THE HOSPITALIZED PATIENT: In addition to standard precautions, contact precautions are recommended for hospitalized infants and children for the duration of illness.

CONTROL MEASURES: Frequent hand washing and hygienic measures in schools, households, and other settings where transmission is common may help reduce the spread of rhinoviruses. Use of disinfectant sprays in the environment is of no proven benefit.

Rickettsial Diseases

The rickettsiae are pleomorphic bacteria, most of which have arthropod vectors. Humans are incidental hosts, except for epidemic (louse-borne) typhus, when humans are the principal reservoir and the human body louse is the vector. Rickettsiae are obligate intracellular parasites and cannot be grown in cell-free media. They have typical bacterial cell walls and cytoplasmic membranes and divide by binary fission. Their natural life cycles typically involve mammalian reservoirs, and animal-to-human or vector-to-human transmission occurs as a result of environmental or occupational exposure.

Ticks are the vector for many rickettsial diseases. Thus, control measures involve prevention of tick transmission of rickettsial agents to humans (see Prevention of Tick-borne Infections, p 159).

Rickettsial infections have many features in common, including the following:

- Multiplication of the organism in an arthropod host.
- Intracellular replication.
- Limited geographic and seasonal occurrence related to arthropod life cycles, activity, and distribution.
- Zoonotic diseases.
- Humans are incidental hosts (except for louse-borne typhus).
- Local primary lesions occur with some rickettsial diseases.
- Fever, rash (especially in spotted fever and typhus group rickettsiae), headache, myalgias, and respiratory tract symptoms are prominent features.
- Systemic capillary and small-vessel endothelial damage is the primary pathologic feature of spotted fever and typhus group rickettsial infections.
- With the exception of Q fever, rickettsialpox, and ehrlichiosis, nonspecific serum *Proteus vulgaris* agglutinins (Weil-Felix test) develop during infection. However, their presence frequently is unreliable for diagnosis. Specific serologic assays for rickettsial illnesses are available and should replace the nonspecific Weil-Felix test.
- Group-specific antibodies are detectable in the serum of most patients within 7 to 14 days after onset of illness.
- Various serologic tests exist for detecting these antibodies. The indirect fluorescent antibody assay is recommended in most cases because of its relative simplicity, sensitivity, and specificity.
- The polymerase chain reaction (PCR) to detect rickettsiae in blood or tissue is promising for early diagnosis of many rickettsial diseases.
- In experienced laboratories, immunohistologic or PCR testing of skin biopsy specimens of patients with rash can be used to diagnose rickettsial infections.
- Treatment early in the course of illness can blunt or delay serologic responses.
- Rickettsial diseases can be severe and fatal, so prompt and specific therapy is important for successful patient outcome. Appropriate antimicrobial treatment is most effective for patients who are treated during the first week of illness. If the disease remains untreated in the second week, even optimal therapy is less effective at preventing complications of the illness.

- Immunity against reinfection by the same agent after natural infection usually is of long duration, except in the case of scrub typhus caused by *Rickettsia tsutsugamushi.* Among the 4 groups of rickettsial diseases, partial or complete cross-immunity usually is conferred by infections within groups but not among groups. Reinfection with *Ehrlichia* organisms has been reported.
- Many rickettsial diseases, including Rocky Mountain spotted fever, ehrlichiosis, and Q fever, may be reportable to state and local health departments.

For details, including treatment, the following chapters on rickettsial diseases should be consulted:

- Ehrlichiosis (Human)
- Q Fever
- Rickettsialpox
- Rocky Mountain Spotted Fever
- Endemic Typhus (Flea-borne Typhus or Murine Typhus)
- Epidemic Typhus (Louse-borne Typhus)

A number of other epidemiologically distinct but clinically similar tick-borne spotted fever infections caused by rickettsiae have been recognized. The causative agents of some of these infections share the same group antigen as *Rickettsia rickettsii;* these include *Rickettsia conorii,* the causative agent of boutonneuse fever (also known as Kenya tick-bite fever, African tick typhus, Mediterranean spotted fever, India tick typhus, and Marseilles fever) that is endemic in southern Europe, Africa, and the Middle East; *Rickettsia sibirica,* the causative agent of Siberian tick typhus, endemic in central Asia; *Rickettsia australis,* the causative agent of North Queensland tick typhus, endemic in eastern Australia; and *Rickettsia japonica,* the causative agent of a spotted fever rickettsiosis, endemic in Japan. All of these infections have clinical, pathologic, and epidemiologic features similar to those of Rocky Mountain spotted fever and are treated similarly. The specific diagnosis is confirmed serologically. These conditions are of importance among persons traveling to endemic areas.

Rickettsialpox

CLINICAL MANIFESTATIONS: Rickettsialpox is characterized by generalized erythematous papulovesicular eruptions on the trunk, face, extremities (including palms and soles), and mucous membranes after the appearance of a primary lesion at the site of the bite of the mouse mite vector. An eschar develops at the site about the time of fever onset. Regional lymph nodes in the area of the primary eschar typically become enlarged. Systemic disease lasts about 1 week; manifestations can include chills, fever, headache, drenching sweats, myalgias, anorexia, and photophobia. The disease is self-limited and rarely associated with complications.

ETIOLOGY: Rickettsialpox is caused by *Rickettsia akari,* which is classified with the spotted-fever–group rickettsiae and related antigenically to *Rickettsia rickettsii.*

EPIDEMIOLOGY: The natural host for *R akari* in the United States is *Mus musculus,* the common house mouse. The disease is transmitted by a mouse mite *(Liponyssoides sanguineus).* Disease risk is heightened in areas infested with mice. The disease is found in large urban settings and has been recognized in the northeastern United States, Ohio, Utah, Croatia, Ukraine, Russia, Korea, and South Africa. All age groups can be affected. No seasonal pattern of disease occurs. The disease is not communicable and currently is rare in the United States.

The **incubation period** is 9 to 14 days.

DIAGNOSTIC TESTS: *Rickettsia akari* can be isolated from blood during the acute stage of disease, but culture is not attempted routinely and is available only in specialized laboratories. An indirect fluorescent antibody assay (IFA) or complement fixation test for *R rickettsii* (the cause of Rocky Mountain spotted fever) will demonstrate a 4-fold change in antibody titers between acute and convalescent serum samples, because antibodies to *R akari* have extensive cross-reactivity with those against *R rickettsii.* Absorption of serum samples before IFA testing can distinguish between antibody responses to *R rickettsii* and *R akari.* The Weil-Felix test for all *Proteus vulgaris* OX agglutinins is negative. Direct fluorescent antibody testing of paraffin-embedded eschars and histopathologic examination of papulovesicles for distinctive features are useful diagnostic techniques.

TREATMENT: Doxycycline or chloramphenicol will shorten the course of the disease; symptoms resolve within 48 hours after initiation of therapy. Tetracyclines should not be given to children younger than 8 years of age unless the benefits of therapy are greater than the risks (see Antimicrobials and Related Therapy, p 646). Treatment is effective when given for 3 to 5 days; relapse is rare.

ISOLATION OF THE HOSPITALIZED PATIENT: Standard precautions are recommended.

CONTROL MEASURES: Disinfestation with residual insecticides and rodent control measures limit or eliminate the vector. No specific management of exposed persons is necessary.

Rocky Mountain Spotted Fever

CLINICAL MANIFESTATIONS: Rocky Mountain spotted fever (RMSF) is a systemic, small vessel vasculitis with a characteristic rash that usually occurs before the sixth day of illness. Fever, severe headache, myalgia, confusion, photophobia, nausea, vomiting, and anorexia are major clinical features. Abdominal pain and diarrhea are noted less frequently. The rash initially is erythematous and macular and later can become maculopapular and, frequently, petechial. Rash first appears on the wrists and ankles, spreading within hours proximally to the trunk. The palms and soles typically are involved. Although early development of a rash is a useful diagnostic sign, in up to 20% of cases, the rash fails to develop. Thrombocytopenia of varying severity develops in most cases, and anemia has been noted in approximately 30% of patients. Leukopenia is noted less frequently. The illness can last as long as 3 weeks and can be severe, with prominent central nervous system, cardiac, pulmonary, gastrointestinal tract, and renal involvement, disseminated intravascular coagulation, and shock leading to death. Significant long-term neurologic (paraparesis; hearing loss; peripheral neuropathy; bladder and bowel incontinence; and cerebellar, vestibular, and motor dysfunction) and nonneurologic (disability from limb amputation) sequelae are common in patients with severe RMSF.

ETIOLOGY: *Rickettsia rickettsii* is an obligate intracellular pathogen and a member of the spotted fever group of rickettsiae.

EPIDEMIOLOGY: The disease is transmitted to humans by the bite of a tick. Many small wild animals and dogs have antibodies to *R rickettsii,* but their role as natural hosts is not clear since ticks are reservoirs and vectors of *R rickettsii.* In ticks, the agent is transmitted transovarially and between stages. Persons with occupational or recreational exposure to the tick vector (eg, pet owners, animal handlers, and outdoor persons) are at an increased risk of acquiring the organism. Persons of all ages, races, and socioeconomic status and both sexes can be infected, but most cases occur in persons younger than 15 years of age. April through October are the months of highest prevalence. Laboratory-acquired infection has resulted from accidental inoculation and aerosol contamination. Transmission has occurred on rare occasions by blood transfusion. Mortality is highest in males, persons older than 30 years of age, and persons with no known tick bite or attachment. Delay in disease recognition and the resulting late initiation of appropriate antimicrobial therapy increase the risk of death. Factors contributing to delayed diagnosis include absence of rash, initial presentation before the fourth day of illness, and presentation during months other than May through August.

The disease is widespread in the United States. Most cases are reported in the south Atlantic, southeastern, and south central states. Focal sites in an affected area can account for much of the morbidity in an area. The dog tick *(Dermacentor variabilis)* primarily is responsible for transmission in these geographic areas and some areas of western United States. Summer is the season of highest prevalence. In the western United States, the northern Rocky Mountain states have the highest incidence; the vector usually is the wood tick *(Dermacentor andersoni).* The Lone Star tick *(Amblyomma americanum)* is a vector of *R rickettsii* in the south central United States. Transmission parallels the tick season in a given geographic area. The disease also occurs in Canada, Mexico, and Central and South America.

The **incubation period** usually is about 1 week but ranges from 2 to 14 days. It seems to be related to the size of the rickettsial inoculum.

DIAGNOSTIC TESTS: The diagnosis can be established by one of the multiple rickettsial group-specific serologic tests. A 4-fold or greater change in titer between acute- and convalescent-phase serum specimens is diagnostic when determined by indirect immunofluorescence antibody (IFA), enzyme immunoassay (EIA), complement fixation (CF), latex agglutination (LA), indirect hemagglutination (IHA), or microagglutination (MA) tests. The IFA, EIA, and IHA are the most sensitive and specific tests. Antibodies are detected by IFA 7 to 10 days after onset of illness. A probable diagnosis can be established by a single convalescent serum titer of 1:64 or greater by IFA, 1:16 or greater by CF, or 1:128 or greater by LA, IHA, or MA. The nonspecific and insensitive Weil-Felix serologic test (*Proteus vulgaris* OX-19 and OX-2 agglutinins) is not recommended.

Culture of *R rickettsii* usually is not attempted because of the danger of transmission to laboratory personnel; only the laboratories with adequate biohazard containment equipment should attempt isolation of rickettsiae. *Rickettsia rickettsii* have been identified by immunofluorescent staining of skin biopsy specimens obtained from the site of the rash. With adequate specimens, this method can be 70% sensitive and 100% specific, but it is not widely available. Polymerase chain reaction (PCR) for detection of *R rickettsii* in blood and biopsy specimens during the acute phase of the illness confirms the diagnosis, but this test is available only in reference laboratories. The PCR is specific but not sensitive.

TREATMENT: Treatment is based on clinical features and epidemiologic considerations. Treatment before day 5 of illness in children with compatible clinical manifestations affords the highest likelihood of good outcome. Treatment need not be initiated if another cause is determined. Doxycycline is the drug of choice. While tetracyclines generally should not be given routinely to children younger than 8 years of age (see Antimicrobial Agents and Related Therapy, p 646), most experts consider doxycycline to be the drug of choice for children of any age. Reasons for this preference include the following: (1) tetracycline staining of teeth is dose-related, (2) doxycycline is less likely to stain developing teeth than other tetracyclines, and (3) doxycycline is effective against RMSF and ehrlichiosis, while chloramphenicol may not be (see Ehrlichiosis [Human], p 234). Also, a retrospective study indicated that chloramphenicol may be less effective than tetracyclines for the treatment of RMSF. Therapy is continued until the patient has been afebrile for at least 2 or 3 days; the usual duration of therapy is 7 to 10 days.

ISOLATION OF THE HOSPITALIZED PATIENT: Standard precautions are recommended.

CONTROL MEASURES: Control of ticks in their natural habitat is not practical. Avoidance of tick-infested areas is the best preventive measure. If a tick-infested area is entered, persons should wear protective clothing and apply tick or insect repellents to clothes and exposed body parts for added protection. They should be taught to thoroughly inspect themselves, their children (bodies and clothing), and pets for ticks after spending time outdoors during the tick season and to remove ticks promptly (see Prevention of Tick-borne Infections, p 159).

There is no role for antimicrobial agents in preventing RMSF. No licensed *R rickettsii* vaccine is available in the United States.

Rotavirus Infections

CLINICAL MANIFESTATIONS: Infection can result in diarrhea, usually preceded or accompanied by emesis and fever. In severe cases, dehydration, electrolyte abnormalities, and acidosis may occur. In immunocompromised children, including those with human immunodeficiency virus infection, persistent infection can develop.

ETIOLOGY: Rotaviruses (Rv) are RNA viruses belonging to the family Reoviridae, with at least 7 distinct antigenic groups (A to G). Group A viruses are the major causes of Rv diarrhea worldwide. Group B and C viruses also have been identified as causes of gastroenteritis in humans. Serotyping is based on the VP7 glycoprotein (G) and VP4 protease-cleaved hemagglutinin (P); G types 1 to 4 and 9 and P types 1A and 1B most commonly are associated with disease.

EPIDEMIOLOGY: Most human infections result from contact with infected persons. Infections due to Rv occur in many animal species, but transmission from animals to humans has not been documented. However, reassortment among Rvs, whether human or animal, can occur and generate new strains. Rotavirus is present in high titer in stools of patients with diarrhea, which is the only body specimen consistently positive for the virus. Rotavirus is present in stool before the onset of diarrhea and can persist for 10 to 12 days after the onset of symptoms in normal hosts. Transmission is presumed to be by the fecal-oral route. Rotavirus can be found on toys and hard surfaces in child care centers, indicating that fomites may serve as a mechanism of transmission. Respiratory transmission also may have a role in disease transmission. Spread within families and institutions is common. Rotavirus is the most common cause of nosocomially acquired diarrhea in children and is an important cause of acute gastroenteritis in children attending child care. Common-source outbreaks have been reported.

Human Rv infections occur worldwide and may occur earlier in life and may be more frequent in lower socioeconomic areas. Worldwide, Rvs are the single most common agent of severe diarrhea in children younger than 2 years of age and, in developing countries, are a major cause of dehydration and death.

In North America, the annual epidemic peak characteristically starts in the autumn in Mexico and the southwest United States, moving sequentially to reach the northeast United States and maritime Canada by spring. Specific seasonal patterns in tropical climates are less pronounced.

Virtually all children are infected by 3 years of age. The rate of hospitalization from Rv diarrhea in infected children can be as high as 2.5%. Although clinically apparent cases of gastroenteritis most commonly occur in infants and children between 4 and 24 months of age, serologic assays have demonstrated infection in other age groups. Reinfections are common and tend to be milder than first infections. From 30% to 50% of adult contacts of infected infants have reinfections, although only a minority manifest symptoms. Infections in neonates often are asymptomatic. Breastfeeding has not been proven to prevent infection but may be associated with milder disease and should be encouraged.

Following exposure to Rv, the **incubation period** usually is from 1 to 3 days.

DIAGNOSTIC TESTS: Enzyme immunoassay (EIA) and latex agglutination assays for group A Rv antigen detection in stool are available commercially. However, EIAs are more sensitive for the detection of antigen late in the course of illness. Both assays have high specificity, but false-positive and nonspecific reactions can occur in neonates and in persons with underlying intestinal disease. These nonspecific reactions can be distinguished from true positive ones by the performance of confirmatory assays. Virus also can be identified in stool by electron microscopy and by specific nucleic acid amplification techniques.

TREATMENT: No specific antiviral therapy is available. Oral or parenteral fluids are given to prevent and correct dehydration.* Orally administered human immunoglobulins given as an investigational therapy in immunocompromised patients with prolonged infections have reduced viral shedding and shortened the duration of diarrhea.

ISOLATION OF THE HOSPITALIZED PATIENT: In addition to standard precautions, contact precautions are indicated for the duration of the illness. In view of the prolonged fecal shedding of low concentration of virus after recovery, continuation of contact precautions for the duration of hospitalization can be justified, particularly if transmission can occur to immunocompromised and premature infants.

CONTROL MEASURES:

Child Care. General measures for interrupting enteric transmission in child care centers are recommended (see Children in Out-of-Home Child Care, p 105). Children with Rv diarrhea in whom stool cannot be contained by diapers or toilet use should be excluded from child care centers until diarrhea ceases. Surfaces should be washed with soap and water. A 70% ethanol solution will inactivate Rv and may help prevent disease transmission resulting from contact with environmental surfaces.

Vaccines. A vaccine to prevent Rv infection and disease is not available. The rhesus rotavirus tetravalent vaccine (Rotashield) approved by the US Food and Drug Administration in August 1998 and incorporated into the 1999 routine immunization schedule is no longer recommended for use because of the association of this vaccine and intussusception. This product was withdrawn voluntarily from the market in October 1999. Children who received Rv vaccine during the period of approval are not at increased risk for development of intussusception in the future.

Rubella

CLINICAL MANIFESTATIONS:

Congenital Rubella. The most commonly described anomalies associated with the congenital rubella syndrome are ophthalmologic (cataracts, retinopathy, and congenital glaucoma), cardiac (patent ductus arteriosus, peripheral pulmonary artery stenosis), auditory (sensorineural deafness), and neurologic (behavioral disorders, meningoencephalitis, and mental retardation). In addition, infants with congenital rubella frequently are growth-retarded and may have radiolucent bone disease, hepatosplenomegaly, thrombocytopenia, and purpuric skin lesions (giving a "blueberry muffin" appearance). Mild forms of the disease can be associated with few or no obvious clinical manifestations at birth. The occurrence of congenital defects is 50% or greater if infection occurs during the first month of gestation, 20% to 30% if during the second month, and 5% if during the third or fourth month.

* American Academy of Pediatrics Provisional Committee on Quality Improvement, Subcommittee on Gastroenteritis. Practice parameter: the management of acute gastroenteritis in young children. *Pediatrics.* 1996;97:424–435

Postnatal Rubella. Rubella usually is a mild disease characterized by a generalized erythematous maculopapular rash, generalized lymphadenopathy (commonly suboccipital, postauricular, and cervical), and slight fever. Transient polyarthralgia and polyarthritis rarely occur in children and are common in adolescents and adults, especially females. Encephalitis and thrombocytopenia are rare complications.

ETIOLOGY: Rubella virus is an RNA virus classified as a Rubivirus in the Togaviridae family.

EPIDEMIOLOGY: Humans are the only source of infection. Postnatal rubella is transmitted primarily through direct or droplet contact from nasopharyngeal secretions. The peak incidence of infection is in the late winter and early spring. Approximately 25% to 50% of infections are asymptomatic. Immunity from wild-type or vaccine virus usually is prolonged, but reinfection on rare occasions has been demonstrated and rarely has resulted in congenital rubella. The period of maximal communicability seems to be the few days before and 5 to 7 days after the onset of the rash. Volunteer studies have demonstrated the presence of rubella virus in nasopharyngeal secretions from 7 days before to 14 days after the onset of the rash. A small number of infants with congenital rubella continue to shed virus in nasopharyngeal secretions and urine for 1 year or more and can transmit infection to susceptible contacts. In approximately 10% to 20% of these patients, virus can be isolated from the nasopharynx when the infant is 6 months old.

Before widespread use of rubella vaccine, rubella was an epidemic disease, occurring in 6- to 9-year cycles, with most cases occurring in children. The incidence of rubella in the United States has declined by approximately 99% from the prevaccine era. The risk of acquiring rubella has declined in all age groups, including adolescents and young adults. In the vaccine era, most cases have occurred in young unimmunized adults in outbreaks in colleges and occupational settings. Although the number of susceptible persons has decreased since introduction and widespread use of rubella vaccine, recent serologic surveys have indicated that approximately 10% of young adults are susceptible to rubella.

The **incubation period** for postnatally acquired rubella ranges from 14 to 23 days, usually 16 to 18 days.

DIAGNOSTIC TESTS: Rubella virus most consistently can be isolated from nasal specimens by inoculation of appropriate cell culture. Laboratory personnel should be notified that rubella is suspected since additional testing is required to detect the virus. Throat swabs, blood, urine, and cerebrospinal fluid also can yield virus, particularly in congenitally infected infants. A 4-fold or greater rise in antibody titer or seroconversion between acute and convalescent serum titers indicates infection. Detection of rubella-specific immunoglobulin (Ig) M antibody usually indicates recent postnatal infection or congenital infection in a newborn infant, but false-positive results occur. Congenital infection also can be confirmed by stable or increasing serum concentrations of rubella-specific IgG over several months. Every effort should be made to establish a laboratory diagnosis when rubella infection is suspected in pregnant women or newborn infants. The diagnosis of congenital rubella infection in children older than 1 year of age is difficult; serologic testing usually is not diagnostic, and viral isolation, while confirmatory, is possible in only a small proportion of congenitally infected children of this age. The hemagglutination inhibition (HAI) rubella antibody test, which previously was the most frequently used method of serologic screening, generally has been supplanted by a number of equally or more sensitive assays for determining rubella immunity, including latex agglutination, fluorescence immunoassay, passive hemagglutination, hemolysis-in-gel, and enzyme immunoassay tests. Some persons in whom antibody has been absent by HAI testing have been found to be immune when their serum specimen was tested by more sensitive assays.

TREATMENT: Supportive.

ISOLATION OF THE HOSPITALIZED PATIENT: In addition to standard precautions, for postnatal rubella, droplet precautions are recommended for 7 days after the onset of the rash. Contact isolation is indicated for children with proven or suspected congenital rubella until they are at least 1 year old, unless nasopharyngeal and urine cultures after 3 months of age are repeatedly negative for rubella virus.

CONTROL MEASURES:

School and Child Care. Children with postnatal rubella should be excluded from school or child care for 7 days after the onset of the rash. Patients with congenital rubella in child care should be considered contagious until they are at least 1 year old, unless nasopharyngeal and urine cultures are repeatedly negative for rubella virus. Mothers of these infants should be made aware of the potential hazard of their infants to susceptible pregnant contacts.

Care of Exposed Persons. When a pregnant woman is exposed to rubella, a blood specimen should be obtained as soon as possible and tested for rubella antibody. An aliquot of frozen serum should be stored for possible repeated testing at a later time. The presence of rubella-specific IgG antibody in a properly performed test at the time of exposure indicates that the person most likely is immune. If antibody is not detectable, a second blood specimen should be obtained 2 to 3 weeks later and tested concurrently with the first specimen. If the second test result is negative, another blood specimen should be obtained 6 weeks after the exposure and also tested concurrently with the first specimen; a negative test result in both specimens indicates that infection has not occurred, and a positive test in the second but not the first (seroconversion) indicates recent infection.

Immune Globulin. The routine use of immune globulin (IG) for postexposure prophylaxis of rubella in early pregnancy is not recommended. Administration of IG should be considered only if termination of the pregnancy is not an option. Limited data indicate that intramuscular IG in a dose of 0.55 mL/kg may decrease clinically apparent infection in an exposed susceptible person from 87% to 18% compared with placebo. However, the absence of clinical signs in a woman who has received intramuscular IG does not guarantee that fetal infection has been prevented. Infants with congenital rubella have been born to mothers who were given IG shortly after exposure.

Vaccine. Live-virus rubella vaccine given after exposure has not been demonstrated to prevent illness but theoretically can prevent illness if administered within 3 days of exposure. Immunization of exposed nonpregnant persons may be indicated because if the exposure did not result in infection, immunization will protect the person in the future. Immunization of a person who is incubating natural rubella or who already is immune is not associated with increased risk of adverse effects.

Rubella Vaccine. The live-virus rubella vaccine distributed in the United States is the RA 27/3 strain grown in human diploid cell cultures. Vaccine is administered by subcutaneous injection of 0.5 mL, alone or, preferably, as the combined vaccine containing measles and mumps vaccines (MMR). Vaccine can be given simultaneously with other vaccines (see Simultaneous Administration of Multiple Vaccines, p 26). Serum antibody to rubella is induced in 95% or more of the recipients after a single dose at 12 months of age or older. Clinical efficacy and challenge studies have demonstrated that 1 dose confers long-term, probably lifelong, immunity against clinical and asymptomatic infection in more than 90% of immunized persons. Asymptomatic reinfection has occurred.

Because of the 2-dose recommendation for measles vaccine as MMR, 2 doses of rubella vaccine now are given routinely. This provides an added safeguard against primary vaccine failures.

Vaccine Recommendations. Rubella vaccine is recommended to be administered in combination with measles and mumps vaccine (MMR) when a child is 12 to 15 months of age and at school entry at 4 to 6 years, according to recommendations for routine measles immunization; those who have not received this dose at school entry should receive their second dose as soon as possible but no later than 11 to 12 years of age (see Measles, p 385).

Special emphasis must continue to be placed on the immunization of at-risk postpubertal males and females, especially college students, military recruits, and health care personnel. Those who have not received at least 1 dose of vaccine or who have no serologic evidence of immunity to rubella are considered susceptible and should be immunized with MMR vaccine. Birth before 1957 is not acceptable evidence of rubella immunity for women who could become pregnant because it provides only presumptive evidence, not proof, of rubella immunity. Clinical diagnosis of infection usually is unreliable and should not be accepted as evidence of immunity. Women should be informed of the theoretical risk to the fetus if they are pregnant or become pregnant within 3 months of immunization (see Precautions and Contraindications, p 499, for further discussion). Specific recommendations are as follows:

- Postpubertal females without documentation of presumptive evidence of rubella immunity should be immunized, unless they are known to be pregnant. Postpubertal females should be advised not to become pregnant for 3 months after receiving rubella vaccine.
- During annual health care examinations, premarital and family planning visits, and visits to sexually transmitted disease clinics, postpubertal females should be assessed for rubella susceptibility and, if deemed susceptible, should be immunized with MMR vaccine. Serologic prescreening is indicated only if aggressive follow-up and immunization are implemented.
- Routine prenatal screening for rubella immunity should be undertaken, and rubella vaccine, given as MMR vaccine, should be administered to susceptible women during the immediate postpartum period before discharge. Physicians can help ensure immunization of susceptible women by inquiring

about the immune status of the mothers of their patients during medical visits for well-child care of newborn infants.

- Previous or simultaneous administration of IG (human) or blood products may require reimmunization (see Precautions and Contraindications, below).
- Breastfeeding is not a contraindication to postpartum immunization (for additional information, see Human Milk, p 98). Although the vaccine virus has been transmitted to breastfed infants, the infants remained asymptomatic.
- Special efforts should be made to be certain that all persons are protected who plan to attend or work in educational institutions, child care centers, or other places where they are likely to be exposed to, or spread, rubella.
- All susceptible health care personnel who may be exposed to patients with rubella should be immunized for the prevention or transmission of rubella to pregnant patients, as well as for their own health.

Adverse Reactions.

- Of susceptible children who receive MMR vaccine, fever develops in 5% to 15% from 5 to 12 days after immunization. Rash occurs in approximately 5% of immunized persons. Mild lymphadenopathy occurs commonly.
- Joint pain, usually in small peripheral joints, has been reported in approximately 0.5% of young children. Arthralgia and transient arthritis tend to be more frequent in susceptible postpubertal females, occurring in approximately 25% and 10%, respectively, of vaccine recipients. Joint involvement usually begins 7 to 21 days after vaccination and generally is transient. Persistent or recurrent joint symptoms have been reported in adult women by 1 group of investigators from Canada, but subsequent studies in the United States have not supported this relationship.
- The incidence of joint manifestations after immunization is lower than that after natural infection at the corresponding age. In addition, in persons who are reimmunized, the likelihood of these manifestations can be expected to be considerably less than that in previously immunized persons, most of whom already are immune.
- Transient peripheral neuritic complaints, such as paresthesia and pain in the arms and legs, also have been reported, although rarely.
- Central nervous system manifestations have been reported, but no causal relationship with rubella vaccine has been established.
- Thrombocytopenia can occur after rubella immunization with MMR (see Measles, p 385).

Precautions and Contraindications.

- ***Pregnancy.*** Rubella vaccine should not be given to pregnant women. If vaccine is given inadvertently or if pregnancy occurs within 3 months of immunization, the patient should be counseled on the theoretical risks to the fetus, estimated to be 1.6%, based on data accumulated by the Centers for Disease Control and Prevention (CDC) from 226 susceptible women who received rubella vaccine (the RA27/3 strain) during the first trimester. Of the offspring, 2% had asymptomatic infection, but none had congenital defects. In view of these observations, receipt of rubella vaccine during pregnancy is not an indication for interruption of pregnancy.

Routine serologic testing of postpubertal women before immunization is unnecessary. Serologic testing is a potential impediment to protection of these women against rubella because it requires two visits, one to identify susceptible persons and one to administer vaccine. However, a sample of blood may be obtained before immunization and stored for at least 3 months. If a woman becomes pregnant or has become pregnant after immunization, the preimmunization specimen can be tested. Demonstration of rubella antibody in the prevaccine specimen indicates immunity and eliminates anxiety about fetal injury from rubella vaccine virus. Immunizing susceptible children whose mothers or other household contacts are pregnant does not cause a risk. Most immunized persons intermittently shed small amounts of virus from the pharynx 7 to 28 days after immunization, but no evidence of transmission of the vaccine virus from immunized children has been found in studies of more than 1200 susceptible household contacts.

- ***Febrile illness.*** Children with minor illnesses with or without fever, such as upper respiratory tract infection, may be immunized (see Vaccine Safety and Contraindications, p 30). Fever per se is not a contraindication to immunization. However, if other manifestations suggest a more serious illness, the child should not be immunized until recovery has occurred.
- ***Recent administration of IG.*** Immunoglobulin preparations may interfere with the serologic response to rubella vaccine. Since rubella vaccine usually is given as MMR and because high doses of IG (such as those given for the treatment of Kawasaki disease) can inhibit the response to the measles vaccine for longer intervals, rubella immunization as part of the MMR vaccine necessitates deferral for longer periods in such circumstances (see Section 1, p 1). Rubella vaccine may be given to postpartum women at the same time as anti-Rh_0 (D) IG (Rhogam) or after blood products are given, but these women should be tested 8 or more weeks later to determine if they have developed an active antibody response.
- ***Altered immunity.*** Immunocompromised patients with disorders associated with increased severity of viral infections should not receive live-virus rubella vaccine while immunodeficient (see Immunocompromised Children, p 56). The exceptions are patients with symptomatic human immunodeficiency virus (HIV) infection who are not severely immunocompromised; these patients may be immunized against rubella with MMR (see HIV Infection, p 325). The risk of rubella exposure for patients with altered immunity can be reduced by immunizing their close susceptible contacts.

Corticosteroids. For patients who have received high doses of corticosteroids for 14 days or more and who are not otherwise immunocompromised, the recommended interval before immunization is at least 1 month (see Immunocompromised Children, p 56).

Surveillance for Congenital Infections. Accurate diagnosis and reporting of the congenital rubella syndrome are extremely important in assessing the control of rubella. All birth defects in which rubella infection is etiologically suspected should be investigated thoroughly and reported to the CDC through local or state health departments.

Salmonella Infections

CLINICAL MANIFESTATIONS: Nontyphoidal *Salmonella* organisms cause asymptomatic carriage, gastroenteritis, bacteremia, and focal infections (such as meningitis and osteomyelitis). These disease categories are not mutually exclusive but represent a spectrum of illness caused by *Salmonella* organisms. The most common illness associated with nontyphoidal *Salmonella* organisms is gastroenteritis, in which diarrhea, abdominal cramps and tenderness, and fever are frequent manifestations. The site of infection usually is the small intestine, but colitis can occur.

Salmonella typhi and several other *Salmonella* serotypes cause protracted bacteremic illness referred to as enteric or typhoid fever. The onset of illness typically is gradual, with manifestations such as fever, constitutional symptoms (eg, headache, malaise, anorexia, and lethargy), abdominal pain and tenderness, hepatomegaly, splenomegaly, rose spots, and changes in mental status. Constipation may be an early feature. Diarrhea occurs more commonly in children than in adults. Enteric fever may present as a mild nondescript febrile illness in young children. Sustained or intermittent bacteremia can occur in enteric fever and nontyphoidal *Salmonella* bacteremia. Recognizable focal infections may occur in as many as 10% of patients with *Salmonella* bacteremia. Recurrent *Salmonella* bacteremia is an acquired immunodeficiency syndrome (AIDS)-defining condition for adolescents and adults infected with the human immunodeficiency virus (HIV).

ETIOLOGY: *Salmonella* organisms are gram-negative bacilli that belong to the Enterobacteriaceae family. Most serotypes that cause human disease are in serogroups A through E. *Salmonella typhi* is classified in serogroup D. In 1997, the most frequently reported human isolates in the United States were *Salmonella typhimurium* (serogroup B), *Salmonella heidelberg* (B), *Salmonella enteritidis* (D), *Salmonella newport* (C2), *Salmonella infantis* (C1), *Salmonella agona* (B), *Salmonella thompson* (C1), and *Salmonella montevideo* (C1).

EPIDEMIOLOGY: The principal reservoirs for nontyphoidal *Salmonella* organisms are animals, including poultry, livestock, reptiles, and pets. The major vehicles of transmission are foods of animal origin, including poultry, red meat, eggs, unpasteurized milk, and other dairy products. Many other foods, such as fruits, vegetables, alfalfa sprouts, and rice, have been implicated. These foods usually are contaminated by contact with animal products or an infected human. Other modes of transmission include ingestion of contaminated water (primary route); contact with infected reptiles (eg, pet turtles, iguanas, and others); and contact with contaminated medications, dyes, and medical instruments. Ingestion of raw or improperly cooked eggs or unpasteurized milk can produce severe disease. Unlike nontyphoidal *Salmonella* serotypes, *S typhi* is found only in humans. Cases of typhoid fever in the United States usually are acquired during foreign travel to countries that lack safe drinking water and food or by consumption of food contaminated by a chronic carrier. Approximately 400 cases per year of typhoid fever are reported in the United States.

Age-specific attack rates for *Salmonella* infection are highest in persons younger than 5 years and older than 70 years of age and peak early during the first year of life. Invasive infections and mortality are more frequent in infants, elderly persons, and persons with an underlying disease, particularly hemoglobinopathies (including sickle cell disease), malignant neoplasm, AIDS, and other immunosuppressive conditions. Most reported cases are sporadic, but outbreaks in institutions are common. Nosocomial epidemics have been reported. In 1996 through 1998, *Salmonella* organisms were second to *Campylobacter* organisms as the cause of laboratory-confirmed cases of enteric pathogens as reported by the Foodborne Diseases Active Surveillance Network (FoodNet). Typhoid fever, while uncommon in the United States, is endemic in many developing areas of the world.

The risk of transmission exists throughout the duration of fecal excretion, which occurs for a variable period. Twelve weeks after infection, 45% of children younger than 5 years of age excrete *Salmonella* organisms compared with 5% of older children and adults; antimicrobial therapy can prolong excretion. Approximately 1% of patients continue to excrete *Salmonella* organisms for more than 1 year.

The **incubation period** for gastroenteritis is 6 to 72 hours. For enteric fever, the incubation period is 3 to 60 days but typically is 7 to 14 days.

DIAGNOSTIC TESTS: Isolation of *Salmonella* organisms from cultures of stool, blood, urine, and material from foci of infection, as indicated by the suspected *Salmonella* syndrome is diagnostic. Serologic tests for *Salmonella* agglutinins ("febrile agglutinins," the Widal test) may suggest the diagnosis of *S typhi* infection, but because of false-positive and false-negative results, these tests are not recommended. DNA probes and monoclonal antibodies against protein antigens of *S typhi* are being evaluated.

TREATMENT:

- Antimicrobial therapy usually is not indicated for patients with uncomplicated (noninvasive) gastroenteritis caused by nontyphoidal *Salmonella* species because therapy does not shorten the duration of disease. Although of unproven benefit, antimicrobial therapy is recommended for *Salmonella* gastroenteritis occurring in patients with an increased risk of invasive disease, including infants younger than 3 months of age and persons with malignant neoplasms, hemoglobinopathies, HIV infection or other immunosuppressive illnesses or therapy, chronic gastrointestinal tract disease, or severe colitis.
- Ampicillin, amoxicillin, trimethoprim-sulfamethoxazole (TMP-SMX), cefotaxime, or ceftriaxone is recommended for susceptible strains in patients for whom therapy is indicated. Strains acquired in developing countries often exhibit resistance to many antimicrobial agents but usually are susceptible to ceftriaxone or cefotaxime and to fluoroquinolones (eg, ciprofloxacin or ofloxacin). However, the fluoroquinolones are not recommended for use in patients younger than 18 years of age unless the benefits of therapy outweigh the potential risks for use of the drug (see Antimicrobial Agents and Related Therapy, p 645). Domestically acquired *S typhimurium* infections are increasingly drug-resistant. Approximately one third of all *S typhimurium* isolates are resistant to ampicillin, chloramphenicol, streptomycin, sulfonamides, and tetracycline.

- In invasive *Salmonella* disease (such as typhoid, non–*S typhi* bacteremia, or osteomyelitis), appropriate drugs are ampicillin, amoxicillin, cefotaxime, ceftriaxone, chloramphenicol, TMP-SMX, or a fluoroquinolone (see Antimicrobial Agents and Related Therapy, p 645). Drug of choice, route of administration, and duration of therapy are based on susceptibility of the organism, site of infection, host, and clinical response. For susceptible *S typhi,* administration of a 14-day course of ampicillin, chloramphenicol, or TMP-SMX is adequate. For severely ill patients, parenteral therapy is indicated. For typhoid fever due to multiply antimicrobial-resistant (ampicillin, chloramphenicol, TMP-SMX) strains, such as are acquired routinely in India, Pakistan, and Egypt, therapeutic options include a 7- to 10-day course of ceftriaxone or a 5- to 7-day course of ofloxacin or ciprofloxacin. Some patients require more prolonged courses of treatment. Relapse is common after completion of therapy; retreatment is indicated. Strain susceptibility should be interpreted with caution; clinical failure has been reported in patients with typhoid fever treated with cephalexin, aminoglycosides, furazolidone, and second-generation cephalosporins despite in vitro susceptibility. For invasive infections caused by nontyphoidal *Salmonella* in immunocompetent hosts without localization, such as bacteremia or enteric fever, patients also should be treated for 14 days; those with localized infection, such as osteomyelitis or abscess, and patients with bacteremia and HIV infection should receive 4 to 6 weeks of therapy to prevent relapse. For *Salmonella* meningitis, ceftriaxone or cefotaxime is recommended, often for 4 weeks or longer.
- Chronic (1 year or more) *S typhi* carriage may be eradicated in some children by high-dose parenteral ampicillin or high-dose oral amoxicillin combined with probenecid (see Antimicrobial Agents and Related Therapy, p 645), or cholecystectomy. Ciprofloxacin is the drug of choice for chronic adult carriers of *S typhi.*
- Corticosteroids may be beneficial to patients with severe enteric fever, which is characterized by delirium, obtundation, stupor, coma, or shock. These drugs, however, should be reserved for critically ill patients in whom relief of the manifestations of toxemia may be life saving. The usual regimen is high-dose dexamethasone given intravenously at an initial dose of 3 mg/kg, followed by 1 mg/kg every 6 hours for a total course of 48 hours.

Isolation of the Hospitalized Patient: In addition to standard precautions, contact precautions should be used for diapered and incontinent children for the duration of illness. In children with typhoid fever, precautions should be continued until cultures of 3 consecutive stool specimens obtained at least 48 hours after cessation of antimicrobial therapy are negative for *S typhi.*

Control Measures: Important measures include proper sanitation methods for food processing and preparation, sanitary water supplies, proper hand washing, sanitary sewage disposal, exclusion of infected persons from handling food, prohibiting the sale of reptiles for pets, reporting cases to appropriate health authorities, and investigating outbreaks. Eggs and other foods of animal origin should be cooked thoroughly. Raw eggs and food containing raw eggs should not be eaten. Notification of public health authorities and determination of serotype are of primary importance in detection and investigation of outbreaks.

Child Care. Outbreaks of *Salmonella* infection are unusual in child care programs, and specific strategies for controlling infection in out-of-home child care have not been evaluated. General measures for interrupting enteric transmission in child care centers are recommended (see Children in Out-of-Home Child Care, p 105).

When *S typhi* disease is identified in a symptomatic child care attendee or staff member, stool specimens from other attendees and staff members should be cultured, and all infected persons should be excluded until 3 consecutive stool cultures are negative for *S typhi.*

When species other than *S typhi* are identified in a symptomatic child care attendee or staff member with enterocolitis, older children and staff do not need to be excluded unless they are symptomatic. Stool cultures are not required from asymptomatic contacts. Antimicrobial therapy is not recommended for persons with asymptomatic infection or uncomplicated diarrhea or who have been exposed to an infected person.

Typhoid Vaccine. Resistance to infection with *S typhi* is enhanced by typhoid immunization, but the degree of protection with currently available vaccines is limited and can be overcome by ingestion of a large bacterial inoculum. Three typhoid vaccines are available for civilian use in the United States (see Table 3.50, p 505); a fourth, an acetone-inactivated parenterally administered vaccine, is available only to the military in the United States.

The demonstrated efficacy of the 3 licensed vaccines ranges from 17% to 66%. Selection of vaccine is based on the age of the child, need for booster doses, possible contraindications (see Contraindications and Precautions, p 506), and reactions (see Adverse Events, p 505). Either oral Ty21a or intramuscular Vi CPS is the vaccine of choice, unless contraindicated.

Indications. In the United States, immunization is recommended only for the following:

- ***Travelers to areas where a risk of exposure to* S typhi *is recognized.*** Risk is greatest for travelers to developing countries, especially Latin America, Asia, and Africa, who have prolonged exposure to contaminated food and drink. Such travelers need to be cautioned that typhoid vaccine is not a substitute for careful selection of food and drink.
- ***Persons with intimate exposure to a documented typhoid fever carrier,*** such as occurs with continued household contact.
- ***Laboratory workers with frequent contact with* S typhi *and persons living in typhoid-endemic areas outside the United States.***

Dosages. For primary immunization, the following dosage is recommended for each vaccine:

- ***Oral Ty21a vaccine.*** Children (6 years of age and older) and adults should take 1 enteric-coated capsule every 2 days for a total of 4 capsules. Each capsule should be taken with cool liquid, no warmer than 37°C (98°F), approximately 1 hour before meals. The capsules must be kept refrigerated, and all 4 doses must be taken to achieve maximal efficacy.

Table 3.50. **Commercially Available Typhoid Vaccines Available in the United States**

Typhoid Vaccine	Type	Route	Minimum Age of Receipt, y	No. of Doses*	Booster Frequency, y	Adverse Effects (Incidence, %)
Ty21a	Live-attenuated	Oral	6	4	5	<5
Vi CPS	Polysaccharide	Intra-muscular	2	1	2	<7
Heat-phenol–inactivated	Killed whole-cell	Subcu-taneous	0.5	2	3	<35

*Primary immunization. For further information on dosage, schedules, and adverse events, see text.

- ***Vi capsular polysaccharide vaccine.*** Primary immunization of persons 2 years of age and older with Vi CPS consists of one 0.5 mL (25 µg) dose administered intramuscularly.
- ***Parenteral inactivated vaccine.*** This vaccine is indicated for use only in children younger than 2 years of age who are at high risk of exposure. Many experts avoid use of this vaccine because of the high rate of adverse events. Immunization consists of 2 doses (0.25 mL each) given subcutaneously at a minimum interval of 4 weeks.

Booster Doses. In circumstances of continued or repeated exposure to *S typhi,* booster doses are recommended to maintain immunity after primary immunization.

The optimal booster schedule for persons who have received the oral Ty21a vaccine has not been determined. Continued efficacy for 5 years after immunization has been demonstrated; however, the manufacturer of Ty21a vaccine recommends reimmunization with the entire 4-dose series every 5 years if continued or renewed exposure to *S typhi* is expected.

The manufacturer of Vi CPS recommends a booster dose every 2 years after the primary dose if continued or renewed exposure is expected.

If the parenteral inactivated vaccine is used initially, booster doses should be administered every 3 years if continued or renewed exposure is expected. A single booster dose of parenteral inactivated vaccine is sufficient, even if more than 3 years have elapsed since the prior immunization.

No data have been reported concerning the use of one vaccine as a booster after primary immunization with a different vaccine. However, using the primary series of 4 doses of the oral Ty21a vaccine or 1 dose of Vi CPS as a booster for persons previously immunized with heat-phenol–inactivated vaccine is a reasonable alternative to administration of a booster dose of heat-phenol–inactivated vaccine.

Adverse Events. Ty21a produces minimal, if any, adverse reactions. Reported adverse effects have included abdominal discomfort, nausea, vomiting, fever, headache, and rash or urticaria.

Reported adverse events from Vi CPS also are minimal and include fever (0% to 1%), headache (1.5% to 3%), and local reaction of erythema or induration of 1 cm or greater (7%).

Parenteral inactivated vaccines can produce several systemic and local adverse reactions, including fever (7% to 24%), headache (9% to 10%), and severe local pain and swelling (3% to 35%). More severe reactions have been reported sporadically, including hypotension, chest pain, and shock.

Contraindications and Precautions. The only contraindication to administration of one of the parenteral typhoid immunizations is a history of severe local or systemic reactions after a previous dose. No data have been reported for any of the 3 typhoid vaccines in pregnant women. Since the oral vaccine is a live-attenuated vaccine, it should not be administered to immunocompromised persons, including those known to be infected with HIV. Because the antimalarial drug mefloquine can inhibit the growth of the live Ty21a strain in vitro, immunization with Ty21a vaccine should be delayed for at least 24 hours before or after a dose of this drug. The vaccine manufacturer advises that Ty21a vaccine should not be administered to persons receiving antimicrobial agents until 24 hours or more after a dose. No data exist on the immunogenicity of Ty21a vaccine when administered concurrently or within 4 weeks of other vaccines. In the absence of such data, if typhoid immunization is warranted, it should not be delayed because of the administration of other vaccines.

Scabies

CLINICAL MANIFESTATIONS: Scabies is characterized by an intensely pruritic, erythematous, papular eruption caused by burrowing of adult female mites in the upper layers of the epidermis, where they create serpiginous burrows. Itching is most intense at night. In older children and adults, the sites of predilection are the interdigital folds, flexor aspects of the wrists, extensor surfaces of the elbows, anterior axillary folds, belt line, thighs, navel, genitalia, areolae, abdomen, intergluteal cleft, and buttocks. In children younger than 2 years of age, the eruption generally is vesicular and often occurs in areas usually spared in older children and adults such as the head, neck, palms, and soles. The eruption is caused by a hypersensitivity reaction to the proteins of the parasite.

The characteristic scabies burrow appears as a gray or white, tortuous, thread-like line. Excoriations are common, and most burrows are obliterated by scratching before a patient is seen by a physician. Occasionally, 2- to 5-mm red-brown nodules are present, particularly on covered parts of the body such as the genitalia, groin, and axilla. These scabies nodules are a granulomatous response to the dead mite antigens and feces; the nodules can persist for weeks and even months after effective treatment. Cutaneous secondary bacterial infection can occur and usually is caused by *Streptococcus pyogenes* or *Staphylococcus aureus.*

Norwegian scabies is an uncommon form of infestation characterized by a large number of mites and widespread, crusted, hyperkeratotic lesions. Norwegian scabies usually occurs in debilitated, developmentally disabled, or immunologically compromised persons.

ETIOLOGY: The mite, *Sarcoptes scabiei* subsp *hominis,* is the cause of scabies. *Sarcoptes scabiei* subsp *canis,* acquired from dogs, can cause a self-limited and mild infestation, usually involving the area in direct contact with the infested animal.

EPIDEMIOLOGY: Humans are the source of infestation. Transmission usually occurs through prolonged, close, personal contact. Because of the large number of mites in exfoliating scales, even minimal contact with a patient with crusted (Norwegian) scabies may result in transmission. Infestation acquired from dogs and other animals is uncommon. Scabies can be transmitted as long as the patient remains infested and untreated, including the interval before symptoms develop. Scabies is endemic in many countries and occurs worldwide in cycles thought to be 15 to 30 years long. Scabies affects persons from all socioeconomic levels without regard to age, sex, or standards of personal hygiene.

The **incubation period** in persons without previous exposure usually is 4 to 6 weeks. Persons who previously were infested are sensitized already and develop symptoms 1 to 4 days after repeated exposure to the mite; however, these reinfestations usually are milder than the original episode.

DIAGNOSTIC TESTS: Diagnosis is confirmed by identification of the mite or mite eggs, or scybala (feces) from scrapings of papules or intact burrows, preferably from the terminal portion where the mite generally is found. Mineral oil, microscope immersion oil, or water applied to the skin facilitates the collection of scrapings. A number 15 scalpel is used to scrape the burrow. The scrapings and oil then are placed on a slide under a glass coverslip and examined microscopically under low power. Adult female mites average 330 to 450 µm in length.

TREATMENT: Infested children and adults should apply lotion or cream containing a scabicide over their entire body below the head. Because scabies can affect the head, scalp, and neck in infants and young children, treatment of the entire head, neck, and body in this age group is required. The drug of choice, particularly for infants, young children, and pregnant or nursing women, is 5% permethrin, a synthetic pyrethroid (Elimite). Alternative drugs are lindane (Kwell) and 10% crotamiton (Eurax). Permethrin should be removed by bathing after 8 to 14 hours, and lindane after 8 to 12 hours. Crotamiton is applied once a day for 2 days followed by a cleansing bath 48 hours after the last application, but crotamiton is associated with frequent treatment failures. Ivermectin in a single dose administered orally is effective for the treatment of severe or crusted (Norwegian) scabies and should be considered for patients whose infestation is refractory to topical therapy. This drug is not approved for this indication by the US Food and Drug Administration.

Lindane is contraindicated for premature infants, persons with known seizure disorders, and persons with hypersensitivity to the product. Lindane should be used cautiously in young infants, women who are pregnant or breastfeeding, and patients with inflamed or traumatized skin. The frequency of lindane applications should not exceed that recommended by the manufacturer to avoid the possibility of neurologic toxic effects from absorption through skin.

Because scabietic lesions are the result of a hypersensitivity reaction to the mite, itching may not subside for several weeks despite successful treatment. The use of oral antihistamines and topical corticosteroids can help relieve this itching.

Topical or systemic antibiotic therapy is indicated for secondary bacterial infections of the excoriated lesions.

Isolation of the Hospitalized Patient: In addition to standard precautions, contact precautions are recommended until the patient has been treated with an appropriate scabicide.

Control Measures:

- Prophylactic therapy is recommended for household members. Manifestations of scabies infestation can appear as late as 2 months after exposure, during which time patients can transmit scabies. All members of the household should be treated at the same time to prevent reinfestation. Bedding and clothing worn next to the skin during the 4 days before initiation of therapy should be laundered in a washer with hot water and dried using a hot cycle. The mites do not survive more than 3 to 4 days without skin contact. Clothing that cannot be laundered should be removed from the patient and stored for several days to a week to avoid reinfestation.
- Children should be allowed to return to child care or school after treatment has been completed.
- Epidemics and localized outbreaks may require stringent and consistent measures to treat contacts. Caregivers who have had prolonged skin-to-skin contact with infested patients may benefit from prophylactic treatment.
- Environmental disinfestation is unnecessary and unwarranted. Thorough vacuuming of environmental surfaces is recommended following use of a room by a patient with crusted (Norwegian) scabies.
- Persons with crusted (Norwegian) scabies and their close contacts must be treated promptly and aggressively to avoid outbreaks.

Schistosomiasis

Clinical Manifestations: Initial entry of the infecting larvae (cercariae) through the skin frequently is accompanied by a transient, pruritic, papular rash (cercarial dermatitis). After penetration, the organism enters the bloodstream and migrates through the lungs. Each of the 3 major human schistosome parasites lives in some part of the venous plexus that drains the intestines or the bladder, depending on the *Schistosoma* species. Four to 8 weeks after exposure, an acute illness can develop, manifested by fever, malaise, cough, rash, abdominal pain, diarrhea, nausea, lymphadenopathy, and eosinophilia (Katayama fever). In acute infections with heavy infection due to *Schistosoma mansoni* or *Schistosoma japonicum,* a mucoid bloody diarrhea accompanied by tender hepatomegaly occurs. The severity of symptoms associated with chronic disease is related to the worm burden. Persons with low to moderate worm burdens can be asymptomatic; heavily infected persons can have a range of symptoms caused primarily by inflammation and fibrosis triggered by eggs produced by adult worms. Portal hypertension can develop and cause hepatosplenomegaly, ascites, and esophageal varices. Long-term involvement of the colon produces abdominal pain and bloody diarrhea. Other organ systems can be involved from eggs embolized, eg, to the lungs causing pulmonary hypertension or to the central nervous system, notably the spinal cord in *S mansoni* or *Schistosoma haema-*

tobium infections. In *S haematobium* infections, the bladder becomes inflamed and fibrotic. Symptoms and signs include dysuria, urgency, terminal microscopic and gross hematuria, secondary urinary tract infections, and nonspecific pelvic pain.

Swimmer's itch (cercarial dermatitis) is caused by the larvae of other avian and mammalian schistosome species that penetrate human skin but do not complete the life cycle and do not cause chronic fibrotic disease. Manifestations include mild to moderate pruritus at the penetration site a few hours after exposure, followed in 5 to 14 days by an intermittent pruritic, sometimes papular, eruption. In previously sensitized persons, more intense papular eruptions may occur for 7 to 10 days after exposure.

ETIOLOGY: The trematodes (flukes) *S mansoni, S japonicum, S haematobium,* and, rarely, *Schistosoma mekongi* and *Schistosoma intercalatum* cause disease. All species have similar life cycles. Swimmer's itch is caused by multiple avian and mammalian species of *Schistosoma.*

EPIDEMIOLOGY: Humans are the principal hosts for the major species. Persistence of schistosomiasis depends on the presence of an appropriate snail as an intermediate host. Eggs excreted in stool *(S mansoni and S japonicum)* or urine *(S haematobium)* into fresh water hatch into motile miracidia, which infect snails. After development in the snails, cercariae emerge and penetrate the skin of humans encountered in the water. Children frequently are infected after infancy when they begin to explore the environment.

Schistosoma mansoni occurs throughout tropical Africa, in several Caribbean islands including Puerto Rico, and in Venezuela, Brazil, Suriname, and the Arabian peninsula. *Schistosoma japonicum* is found in China, the Philippines, and Indonesia. *Schistosoma haematobium* occurs in Africa and the eastern Mediterranean region. *Schistosoma mekongi* is limited to a small area of the Mekong delta in Southeast Asia (Kampuchea and Laos). *Schistosoma intercalatum* is found in Central Africa. Children frequently are involved in transmission because of habits of uncontrolled defecation, urination, and frequent wading in infected waters. Communicability lasts as long as live eggs are excreted in the urine and feces. Adult worms of the *S mansoni* species have been documented to live as long as 26 years in the human host. Thus, schistosomiasis can be diagnosed in patients many years after they have left the endemic areas.

Swimmer's itch occurs in all regions of the world after exposure to fresh, brackish, or salt water containing larvae that do not complete their life cycle in humans.

The **incubation period** is variable but is approximately 8 weeks for *S haematobium* and 4 weeks for *S mansoni* and *S japonicum.*

DIAGNOSTIC TESTS: Infection with *S mansoni* and other species (except *S haematobium)* is determined by microscopic examination of concentrated stool specimens to detect characteristic eggs. In light infections, several specimens may have to be examined before eggs are found, and a biopsy of the rectal mucosa may be necessary. The fresh tissue obtained should be compressed between 2 glass slides and examined under low power (unstained) for eggs. *Schistosoma haematobium* is diagnosed by examining filtered urine for eggs. Egg excretion often peaks between noon and 3 PM.

Biopsy of the bladder mucosa may be necessary. Serologic tests, available through the Centers for Disease Control and Prevention and some commercial laboratories, may be particularly helpful for detecting light infections or before eggs appear in the stool or urine.

Swimmer's itch can be difficult to differentiate from other causes of dermatitis. A skin biopsy may demonstrate larvae, but their absence does not exclude the diagnosis.

TREATMENT: The drug of choice for schistosomiasis caused by any species is praziquantel; the alternative drug for *S mansoni* is oxamniquine. No satisfactory alternative drug for *S japonicum* is available. Swimmer's itch is a self-limited disease that requires only symptomatic treatment of the urticarial rash.

ISOLATION OF THE HOSPITALIZED PATIENT: Standard precautions are recommended.

CONTROL MEASURES: Elimination of the intermediate snail host is difficult to achieve in most areas. Thus, treatment of infected populations, sanitary disposal of human waste, and education about the source of infection are the key elements of current control measures. Travelers to endemic areas should be advised to avoid contact with freshwater streams and lakes.

Shigella Infections

CLINICAL MANIFESTATIONS: In mild infections, manifestations consist of watery or loose stools, with minimal or no constitutional symptoms, of several days duration. Abrupt onset of fever, systemic toxic effects, headache, and profuse watery diarrhea occur in patients with small-bowel infection. Seizures can occur. Abdominal cramps, tenderness, tenesmus, and mucoid stools with or without blood characterize large-bowel disease (bacillary dysentery). Rare complications include bacteremia, Reiter syndrome (after *Shigella flexneri* infection), hemolytic-uremic syndrome (from *Shigella dysenteriae* type 1 infection), colonic perforation, and toxic encephalopathy (ekiri syndrome), which can be lethal within 4 to 48 hours of onset.

ETIOLOGY: *Shigella* are gram-negative bacilli in the family Enterobacteriaceae. Four species (of more than 40 serotypes) have been identified. *Shigella sonnei* currently accounts for almost three quarters of the cases in the United States, and *S flexneri* accounts for a large percentage of the remainder. *Shigella dysenteriae* type 1 (the Shiga bacillus) is rare in the United States but widespread in rural Africa and the Indian subcontinent. *Shigella boydii* is uncommon in the United States.

EPIDEMIOLOGY: Feces of infected humans are the source of infection. No animal reservoir is known. Predisposing factors include crowded living conditions, poor hygiene, closed population groups with substandard environmental sanitation (eg, residential homes for retarded children), and travel to countries with substandard food and water sanitation. Because transmission of *Shigella* organisms can occur after ingestion of a small bacterial inoculum, fecal-oral transmission from person-to-person contact is the common route by which children are infected. Other modes of transmission include ingestion of contaminated food or water, contact with a contaminated inanimate object, and anal intercourse. Houseflies also are vectors through physical transport of infected feces. Infection, particularly with *S sonnei,* is most common in children 1 to 4 years of age and is an important problem in child care centers in the United States. *Shigella flexneri* and the other species are more frequent in older children and adults and often are associated with sources outside the United States. Communicability exists until the organism no longer is present in feces. Even without antimicrobial therapy, the convalescent carrier state usually ceases within 4 weeks of the onset of illness. A chronic carrier state (>1 year) is rare.

The **incubation period** varies from 1 to 7 days but typically is 2 to 4 days.

DIAGNOSTIC TESTS: Cultures of feces or rectal swab specimens containing feces should be performed. Blood should be cultured only in severely ill, immunocompromised, or malnourished patients because bacteremia is rare. A stool smear stained with methylene blue may disclose polymorphonuclear leukocytes or erythrocytes, a finding indicative of enterocolitis, which is consistent with but not specific for *Shigella* infection.

TREATMENT:

- Antimicrobial therapy is effective for shortening the duration of diarrhea and eradicating organisms from feces and is recommended for all patients with dysentery due to *Shigella* species. Small-bowel disease often is self-limited (48 to 72 hours) but may progress to dysentery. In mild illness, the primary indication for treatment is to prevent spread of the organism.
- Antimicrobial susceptibility testing of clinical isolates is indicated because resistance to antimicrobial agents is common. Plasmid-mediated, multiple antimicrobial resistance has been identified in all *Shigella* species.
- For susceptible strains, ampicillin and trimethoprim-sulfamethoxazole are effective; amoxicillin is less effective. The oral route of therapy is acceptable except for seriously ill patients. For cases in which susceptibility is unknown or an ampicillin- and trimethoprim-sulfamethoxazole–resistant strain is isolated, either parenteral ceftriaxone or a fluoroquinolone should be given. Experts disagree about the benefit of therapy with oral third-generation cephalosporins, such as cefixime. For resistant strains, ciprofloxacin or ofloxacin should be considered. The latter two agents are not recommended for use for persons younger than 18 years of age except in exceptional circumstances (see Antimicrobial Agents and Related Therapy, p 645).
- Antimicrobial therapy should be administered for 5 days.
- Antidiarrheal compounds that inhibit intestinal peristalsis are contraindicated because they may prolong the clinical and bacteriologic course of disease.

ISOLATION OF THE HOSPITALIZED PATIENT: In addition to standard precautions, contact precautions are indicated for the duration of illness.

CONTROL MEASURES:

Child Care. General measures for interrupting enteric transmission in child care centers are recommended (see Children in Out-of-Home Child Care, p 105). Hand washing is the single most important measure to decrease transmission rates.

When *Shigella* infection is identified in a child care attendee or staff member, stool specimens from other symptomatic attendees and staff members should be cultured. Stool specimens from household contacts who have diarrhea also should be cultured. All symptomatic persons in whom *Shigella* organisms are isolated from stool should receive antimicrobial therapy (see Treatment, p 511) and should not be permitted to reenter the program until the diarrhea has ceased and stool cultures are negative for *Shigella*. If several persons are infected, a cohort system should be considered until stool cultures no longer yield *Shigella* organisms.

General Control Measures. Strict attention to hand washing is essential to limit spread. Other important control measures include sanitary water supply, food processing, and sewage disposal; exclusion of infected persons as food handlers; prevention of contamination of food by flies; and case reporting to appropriate health authorities (eg, hospital infection control personnel and public health department).

Vaccination. No vaccine is available commercially.

Sporotrichosis

CLINICAL MANIFESTATIONS: Sporotrichosis manifests most commonly as cutaneous infection, although pulmonary and disseminated forms occur. Inoculation occurs at a site of minor trauma, causing an ulcerative subcutaneous nodule that is firm and slightly tender but often painless. Secondary lesions may spread along lymphatic channels to form multiple nodules that ulcerate and suppurate. The extremities and face are the most common sites of infection in children.

Extracutaneous sporotrichosis commonly affects bones and joints, particularly those of the hands, elbows, ankles, or knees, but any organ can be affected. Disseminated disease generally occurs after hematogenous spread from primary skin or lung infection. Disseminated sporotrichosis may involve multiple foci (eg, eyes, genitourinary system, or central nervous system) and occurs predominantly in immunocompromised patients. Pulmonary sporotrichosis clinically resembles tuberculosis and occurs after inhalation or aspiration of aerosolized spores. Pulmonary and disseminated sporotrichosis are uncommon in children.

ETIOLOGY: *Sporothrix schenckii* is a dimorphic fungus that grows as an oval or cigar-shaped yeast at 37°C (98°F).

EPIDEMIOLOGY: *Sporothrix schenckii* is a ubiquitous organism that is most common in tropical and subtropical regions of Central and South America. In the United States, it is found predominantly in the Midwest. The fungus is isolated from soil and plants, including hay, straw, thorny plants (especially roses), and sphagnum moss. Cutaneous disease occurs from inoculation of debris containing the organism into a wound. Persons engaging in gardening or farming are at risk for infection. Inhalation of spores can lead to pulmonary disease. Rarely, transmission from infected cats has led to cutaneous disease.

The **incubation period** is 7 to 30 days after cutaneous inoculation but may be as long as 6 months.

DIAGNOSTIC TESTS: A culture positive for *S schenkii* from tissue, wound drainage, or sputum is diagnostic of infection. A positive blood culture result suggests the multifocal form of sporotrichosis associated with immunodeficiency. Histopathologic examination of tissue can be helpful, but the organism is difficult to detect in biopsy samples. No standardized serologic test is available.

TREATMENT: The time-honored treatment for sporotrichosis has been a saturated solution of potassium iodide (SSKI) given orally until several weeks after all lesions were healed. Treatment with SSKI may be limited by side effects, including gastrointestinal tract symptoms, rhinorrhea, and rash. Itraconazole is the drug of choice for cutaneous and extracutaneous disease in adults; however, no controlled studies to document the efficacy of itraconazole have been reported, and the safety of this drug for use in children has not been established. Amphotericin B or itraconazole is the treatment of choice for systemic or multifocal infection. Osteoarticular, pulmonary, or disseminated infection responds less well than cutaneous infection to amphotericin B or itraconazole, despite prolonged therapy. Surgical débridement or excision may be necessary to achieve resolution of skeletal and cavitary pulmonary disease.

ISOLATION OF HOSPITALIZED PATIENTS: Standard precautions are indicated.

CONTROL MEASURES: Eliminating exposure to the organism through the use of protective gloves and clothing in occupational and avocational activities associated with infection can reduce risk of disease.

Staphylococcal Food Poisoning

CLINICAL MANIFESTATIONS: Staphylococcal food poisoning is characterized by the abrupt and sometimes violent onset of severe nausea, abdominal cramps, vomiting, and prostration, often accompanied by diarrhea. Low-grade fever or subnormal temperature may occur. The duration of illness typically is 1 to 2 days, but the intensity of symptoms may require hospitalization. The short incubation period, brevity of illness, and usual lack of fever help distinguish staphylococcal from other types of food poisoning, except that caused by *Bacillus cereus*. Chemical food poisoning usually has an even shorter incubation period. *Clostridium perfringens* food poisoning usually has a longer incubation period and infrequently is accompanied by vomiting. Patients with foodborne *Salmonella* or *Shigella* infection usually have fever and a longer incubation period (see Appendix V, Clinical Syndromes Associated With Foodborne Diseases, p 767).

ETIOLOGY: Enterotoxins produced by strains of *Staphylococcus aureus* and, rarely, *Staphylococcus epidermidis*, elicit the symptoms of staphylococcal food poisoning.

Of the 8 immunologically distinct heat-stable enterotoxins (A, B, C1-3, D, E, and F), enterotoxins A and D are the most common in the United States. Enterotoxin F, which is identical to the toxin associated with toxic shock syndrome, has not been implicated in outbreaks of food poisoning.

EPIDEMIOLOGY: Illness is caused by ingestion of food containing a staphylococcal enterotoxin. Foods usually involved are those that come in contact with food handlers' hands, either without subsequent cooking or with inadequate heating or refrigeration, such as pastries, custards, salad dressing, sandwiches, poultry, sliced meat, and meat products. When these foods remain at room temperature for several hours before being eaten, toxin-producing staphylococci multiply and elaborate heat-stable toxin. The organisms may be of human origin from purulent discharges of an infected finger or eye, abscesses, acneiform facial eruptions, nasopharyngeal secretions, or apparently normal skin, or, less commonly, of bovine origin, such as contaminated milk or milk products, especially cheese.

The **incubation period** is from 30 minutes to 8 hours, usually 2 to 4 hours.

DIAGNOSTIC TESTS: Recovery of large numbers of staphylococci from stool or vomitus supports the diagnosis. In an outbreak setting, demonstration of enterotoxin or a large number of staphylococci ($>10^5$ colony-forming units per gram of specimen) in epidemiologically implicated food confirms the diagnosis. Identification (by pulsed-field gel electrophoresis) of the same types of *S aureus* from stool or vomitus of 2 or more ill persons or from the stool or vomitus of an ill person and an implicated food or a person who handled the food also confirms the diagnosis. Local health authorities should be notified to help determine the source of the outbreak.

TREATMENT: Antimicrobial agents are not indicated.

ISOLATION OF THE HOSPITALIZED PATIENT: Standard precautions are recommended.

CONTROL MEASURES: Reducing the time from initial food preparation to service and holding cooked food no more than 4 hours at room temperature will help to prevent the disease. Cooked foods should be refrigerated at temperatures less than 5°C (41°F). People with boils, abscesses, and other purulent lesions of the hands, face, or nose should be excluded temporarily from handling food.

Staphylococcal Infections

CLINICAL MANIFESTATIONS: *Staphylococcus aureus* causes a wide variety of localized or invasive suppurative infections and 3 toxin-mediated syndromes: toxic shock syndrome (see Toxic Shock Syndrome, p 576), scalded skin syndrome, and food poisoning (see Staphylococcal Food Poisoning, p 513). Localized infections include furuncles, carbuncles, impetigo (bullous and nonbullous), paronychia, ecthyma, cellulitis, lymphadenitis, and wound infections. Infections of implanted prosthetic materials, as well as localized infections, may be associated with bacteremia. Bacteremia can be complicated by septicemia, endocarditis, pericarditis, pneumonia, muscle or visceral abscesses, arthritis, osteomyelitis, septic thrombophlebitis of large vessels and other foci of infection. Meningitis is rare. *Staphylococcus aureus* infections can be fulminant, frequently are associated with metastatic foci, and require prolonged therapy to achieve cure. Risk factors for severe staphylococcal infections include neutropenia; chronic diseases including diabetes mellitus, cirrhosis, and nutritional disorders; transplantation; and disorders of neutrophil function. *Staphylococcus aureus* also causes foreign body infections, including those associated with intravascular catheters or grafts, pacemakers, peritoneal catheters, cerebrospinal fluid shunts, and prosthetic joints.

Coagulase-negative Staphylococcus: Most coagulase-negative staphylococcus represent contamination of culture material (see Diagnostic Tests, p 518). Of the isolates that do not represent contamination, most come from infections that are nosocomial, and most patients with coagulase-negative staphylococcal infections have obvious disruptions of host defense caused by surgery, catheter or prosthesis insertion, or immunosuppression. Coagulase-negative staphylococci are the single most frequent cause of late-onset septicemia among premature infants, especially infants weighing less than 1500 g at birth, and of episodes of nosocomial bacteremia in all age groups. Coagulase-negative staphylococci are responsible for bacteremia in children undergoing treatment for leukemia, lymphoma, or solid tumors, as well as in bone marrow transplant recipients. Infections often are associated with intravascular catheters, cerebrospinal fluid shunts, peritoneal or urinary catheters, vascular grafts or intracardiac patches, prosthetic cardiac valves, pacemaker wires, and prosthetic joints. Mediastinitis following open-heart surgery, endophthalmitis following intraocular trauma, and omphalitis and scalp abscesses in neonates have been described. Coagulase-negative staphylococci also may enter the bloodstream from the respiratory tracts of mechanically ventilated premature infants or from the gastrointestinal tracts of infants with necrotizing enterocolitis. Some species of coagulase-negative staphylococci are associated with urinary tract infection, including *Staphylococcus saprophyticus* in adolescent girls or young adult women, often following sexual intercourse, and *Staphylococcus epidermidis* and *Staphylococcus haemolyticus* in hospitalized patients with urinary catheters. In general, coagulase-negative staphylococcal infections have an indolent clinical presentation.

ETIOLOGY: Staphylococci are gram-positive cocci that appear microscopically as grape-like clusters. There are 32 species that are related closely on the basis of DNA base composition, but only 14 species are indigenous to humans. *Staphylococcus aureus* is the only species that produces coagulase. Of the other 13 coagulase-negative species, *S epidermidis, S haemolyticus, S saprophyticus,* and *Staphylococcus lugdunensis* most often are associated with infections. Staphylococci are ubiquitous and can survive extreme conditions of drying, heat, low oxygen, and high salt environments. *Staphylococcus aureus* has many surface receptors that allow it to bind to tissues and foreign bodies coated with fibronectin, fibrinogen, and collagen, allowing a low inoculum of organisms to adhere to sutures, catheters, prosthetic valves, and other devices. Coagulase-negative staphylococci produce an exopolysaccharide slime biofilm that makes these organisms, as they bind to medical devices (eg, catheters), relatively inaccessible to host defenses and to antibiotics.

EPIDEMIOLOGY:

Staphylococcus aureus. *Staphylococcus aureus,* which is second only to coagulase-negative staphylococci as a cause of episodes of nosocomial bacteremia, is equal to *Pseudomonas aeruginosa* as the most common cause of nosocomial pneumonia and is responsible for most nosocomial wound infections. *Staphylococcus aureus* colonizes skin and mucous membranes of 30% to 50% of healthy adults and children. The anterior nares, axilla, and perineum are the more dominant sites of colonization. The anterior nares are colonized most densely, and colonization may persist for years in 10% to 20% of affected persons. From 25% to 50% of nasal carriers also carry the organism on their hands and skin. Rates of carriage of more than 50% occur in children with desquamating skin disorders or burns and in persons with frequent needle use (eg, diabetes mellitus, hemodialysis, recreational drug use, allergy shots).

Transmission of* S aureus *in Hospitals. *Staphylococcus aureus* is transmitted most commonly by direct contact. Health care personnel also may be colonized with *S aureus* in the nares and on the skin and can serve as an important reservoir for transmission of *S aureus* to patients. Health care personnel also may acquire transient hand colonization while caring for one patient and then transmit the organism to another patient. Infants colonized shortly after birth can serve as a reservoir for transmission to other infants. The role of clothing, gowns, and environmental surfaces in the transmission of *S aureus* is unclear. Airborne transmission by droplets may occur when patients have draining wounds, burns, or areas of dermatitis that are colonized or infected. Changing dressings or linens may cause these organisms to become airborne. Patients with tracheostomies also may produce droplet nuclei that may remain suspended in the air for prolonged periods. Environmental dissemination of *S aureus* from persons, including infants, with nasal carriage is increased markedly during viral upper respiratory tract infections. Additional risk factors for nosocomial acquisition of *S aureus* include location on a high-risk ward, such as a newborn nursery, intensive care or burn unit, surgical procedures, prolonged hospitalization, and the presence of indwelling vascular catheters or prosthetic devices. Previous antibiotic therapy increases the risk of acquiring an antibiotic-resistant strain.

Staphylococcus aureus *Colonization and Disease.* Nasal and skin carriage are the primary reservoirs for *S aureus.* Patients who carry *S aureus* in the nose preoperatively are more likely to develop surgical site infections than patients who are not carriers. Heavy cutaneous colonization of the insertion site is the single most important predictor of catheter-related infections for short-term percutaneously inserted catheters. For patients with *S aureus* skin colonization who receive hemodialysis, the incidence of vascular-access bacteremia is 6-fold higher than for patients without skin colonization. After head trauma, nasal carriers of *S aureus* are more likely to develop a *S aureus* pneumonia than are noncolonized patients.

***Methicillin-resistant* S aureus.** Methicillin-resistant *S aureus* (MRSA) accounts for one quarter of nosocomial *S aureus* infections. Strains of MRSA are resistant to all ß-lactam and cephalosporin antibiotics, as well as to many antibiotics of other classes. Methicillin-susceptible *S aureus* (MSSA) strains are heterogeneous for methicillin resistance (see Diagnostic Tests, p 518). When ß-lactamase–resistant antibiotics are used to treat MSSA infections, the MSSA organisms are killed; the MRSA organisms are selected and allowed to grow. Risk factors for nasal carriage of MRSA include recent hospitalization, recent (within the previous 60 days) antibiotic use, prolonged hospital stay, frequent contact with a health care environment, presence of an intravascular catheter or tracheostomy, increased number of surgical procedures, and hospitalization before the onset of infection. After discharge from a hospital, a patient known to have been colonized with MRSA should be assumed to have continued MRSA colonization when rehospitalized. Nasal carriage can be prolonged for years.

Epidemic Strains of MRSA. Most nosocomial MRSA infections result from the patient's own organism or from endemic strains transmitted to the patient by the hands of health care personnel. On occasion, an epidemic strain of MRSA will be introduced into a hospital environment where it spreads rapidly despite measures that contain the spread of other strains. This spread seems to be the result of a unique virulence factor. It is important to identify these epidemic MRSA strains using pulsed-field gel electrophoresis (PFGE) because containment of epidemic MRSA strains requires strict adherence to and enhancement of infection control policies.

Overall, MRSA and methicillin-resistant coagulase-negative staphylococci are responsible for the majority of nosocomial infections. These strains are particularly difficult to treat because they usually are multidrug-resistant and predictably susceptible only to vancomycin.

Community-acquired MRSA. Strains of MRSA increasingly are responsible for infections in healthy children and adults from the community who have no risk factors for MRSA (ie, no contact with hospitals, previously hospitalized patients or health care personnel). The antibiotic susceptibility patterns of these strains in children may be unique because they are resistant to methicillin but usually are not multidrug-resistant. Recent isolation of "community" strains of MRSA from persons without risk factors from several countries, cities, and child care centers suggests that MRSA strains are moving from the hospital setting to the community, as happened with penicillin-resistant *S aureus*.

***Vancomycin-intermediate* S aureus.** Strains of MRSA with intermediate susceptibility to vancomycin (minimum inhibitory concentration [MIC], >4 µg/mL and ≤16 µg/mL) were isolated from 4 adults in the United States from 1996 to 1999. All had received multiple courses of vancomycin for MRSA infections. Strains of MRSA can be heterogeneous for vancomycin resistance (see Diagnostic Tests, p 518), and extensive vancomycin use allows the vancomycin-intermediate *S aureus* strains to grow. Rapid and aggressive attention should be focused on containing a vancomycin-intermediate *S aureus* strain to prevent potential rapid spread. Recently recommended measures from the Centers for Disease Control and Prevention (CDC) have included more rapid diagnostic tests to determine susceptibility, restricted vancomycin use, and strict infection control measures for the infected patient and the institution. Communicability persists for as long as lesions or the carrier state are present.

Coagulase-negative Staphylococci. Coagulase-negative staphylococci are common inhabitants of the skin and mucous membranes. Virtually all infants are colonized at multiple sites by 2 to 4 days of age. Different species colonize specific areas of the body. *Staphylococcus epidermidis* is the most frequent skin colonizer, while *S haemolyticus* is found on areas of skin with numerous apocrine glands, and

S capitis is found on the scalp. The frequency of nosocomial coagulase-negative staphylococcal infections has increased steadily during the past 2 decades. Infants and children in intensive care units, including high-risk nurseries, have the highest incidence of bloodstream infections. Coagulase-negative staphylococci colonizing the skin may be introduced at the time of medical device placement or through mucous membrane or skin breaks. Less often, the hands of health care personnel, colonized with environmental coagulase-negative staphylococci, may transmit the organism. The roles of the environment, fomites, and airborne modes of coagulase-negative staphylococcal transmission are not known.

Methicillin-resistant Coagulase-negative Staphylococci. Methicillin-resistant coagulase-negative staphylococci now account for the majority of nosocomial coagulase-negative staphylococcal infections. Most methicillin-susceptible strains have heterogeneous resistance to methicillin (see Diagnostic Tests, below) because there are subpopulations with varying resistance to methicillin. Treatment of an infection with methicillin or other semisynthetic penicillins or cephalosporins allows methicillin-resistant populations to become the predominant isolate. Methicillin-resistant strains are resistant to all ß-lactam drugs, including the cephalosporins, and usually several other drug classes. Once these strains become endemic to a hospital, eradication is difficult even when strict infection control techniques are followed.

Vancomycin-intermediate Coagulase-negative Staphylococci. Methicillin-resistant coagulase-negative staphylococci also are heterogeneous for vancomycin resistance. Use of vancomycin to treat methicillin-resistant coagulase-negative staphylococcal infections selects for the emergence of strains with intermediate susceptibility to vancomycin. Although uncommon, infections caused by these strains have been described and may become more frequent. To prevent or delay development of resistance, the CDC has published recommendations for the prudent use of vancomycin (see Judicious Use of Antimicrobial Agents, p 647).

For the toxin-mediated scalded skin syndrome, the **incubation period** is usually 1 to 10 days. For other staphylococcal infections, the incubation period is extremely variable. A long delay can occur between acquisition of the organism and the onset of disease.

DIAGNOSTIC TESTS: Gram-stained smears of material from lesions can provide presumptive evidence of infection. Isolation of organisms from culture of an otherwise sterile body fluid is definitive. *Staphylococcus aureus* is not a contaminant when isolated from a blood culture. Isolation of coagulase-negative staphylococci from a blood culture frequently is dismissed as "a contaminant." In a neonate, immunocompromised person, or a patient with a prosthetic implant, repeated isolation of the same phenotypic strain of coagulase-negative staphylococci from blood cultures facilitates interpretation. For catheter-related bacteremia, quantitative cultures from the catheter will have 5 to 10 times more organisms than cultures from a peripheral vessel. Criteria that may be used to distinguish whether coagulase-negative staphylococci is a contaminant or a pathogen include the following: (1) growth generally within 24 hours, (2) multiple positive blood cultures, (3) symptoms of infection in the patient, (4) an intravascular catheter that has been in place for 3 days or more, and (5) multidrug resistance of the coagulase-negative staphylococcal strain.

Quantitative antimicrobial susceptibility testing should be performed for all staphylococci, including coagulase-negative staphylococci, isolated from normally sterile sites. Some community-acquired *S aureus* strains will be methicillin-resistant, and some hospital-acquired *S aureus* and most hospital-acquired coagulase-negative staphylococci will be methicillin- and multidrug resistant. Detection of vancomycin-intermediate *S aureus* is critical (see Table 3.51, p 520).

Staphylococci have several mechanisms mediating resistance to the ß-lactam antibiotics. ß-Lactamase production breaks down the nonsemisynthetic penicillins. Resistance to the ß-lactamase–resistant semisynthetic penicillins is mediated by a novel cell wall penicillin-binding protein called PBP2a. PBP2a has a decreased affinity for ß-lactam antibiotics and cephalosporins. PBP2a is coded for by the gene *mecA.* Clinical isolates of coagulase-negative staphylococci and of *S aureus* carrying the *mecA* gene vary widely in their resistance to methicillin based on the number of organisms of different susceptibilities and on the culture conditions (methicillin MICs of ≤4 µg/mL to ≥1000 µg/mL). This phenomenon is known as **heterogeneous resistance.** Coagulase-negative staphylococci and *S aureus* strains with heterogeneous resistance may have MICs to methicillin or vancomycin indicating susceptibility after 24 hours of incubation. However, if these strains are incubated overnight on plates of increasing concentrations of methicillin or vancomycin, a small fraction of the total population will be able to grow at much higher antibiotic concentrations. If these highly resistant subclones are recultured, they may maintain this high level of resistance, suggesting a mutant strain. However, in some cases, the highly resistant subclone will revert to methicillin or vancomycin susceptibility when replated, even though it was grown from a single colony. There is no satisfactory model that can explain the mechanism governing heterogeneous resistance. Strains of coagulase-negative staphylococci and *S aureus* with heterogeneous resistance are stable in the absence of antibiotic selective pressure. These strains may constitute 10% to 15% of any coagulase-negative staphylococci or *S aureus* collection of isolates.

The MIC breakpoints for coagulase-negative staphylococci are based on the presence of the *mecA* gene and, therefore, the potential for the organism to develop methicillin resistance. The coagulase-negative staphylococcal MICs no longer represent an interpretation of MIC breakpoints as determined by growth in medium.

The mechanism for vancomycin-intermediate resistance of *S aureus* and coagulase-negative staphylococci is unknown. Vancomycin-intermediate *S aureus* and vancomycin-intermediate coagulase-negative staphylococcal strains have thickened cell walls as shown by electron microscopy. Vancomycin resistance may be related to an increased ability of these organisms to bind vancomycin at sites other than those to which they normally bind.

Staphylococcus aureus and coagulase-negative staphylococcal strain typing has become a useful adjunct for determining whether several isolates from one patient or from different patients are the same or different. Typing will allow accurate identification of the source, extent, and mechanism of transmission of an outbreak. Antimicrobial susceptibility testing is the most readily available method for typing using a phenotypic characteristic. Multilocus enzyme electrophoresis is another phenotypic tool for use in typing. Typing by genotype has proven to be highly discriminatory and highly effective for identifying epidemiologically related isolates.

Table 3.51. Recommendations for Detecting and Preventing the Spread of *Staphylococcus aureus* With Reduced Susceptibility to Vancomycin*

Strategies for selection of strains for additional testing:

- Select isolates with vancomycin MICs of ≥4 µg/mL. This is based on the apparent heterogeneity of strains because organisms with MICs of ≥4 µg/mL have subpopulations with higher MICs. Clinical treatment failures have occurred with vancomycin in infections with these isolates.
- Select isolates with vancomycin MICs of ≥8 µg/mL (based on National Committee for Clinical Laboratory Standards [NCCLS] breakpoints[†]).
- Select all methicillin-resistant *S aureus* (MRSA). All identified isolates of *S aureus* with reduced susceptibility to vancomycin have been MRSA.
- Select all *S aureus* isolates. Because little is known about the extent of this resistance, any *S aureus* potentially could have reduced susceptibility to vancomycin.

Testing and confirmation:

- Primary testing of *S aureus* against vancomycin requires 24 hours of incubation time.
- Disk diffusion is not an acceptable method for vancomycin susceptibility testing of *S aureus.* None of the known strains of *S aureus* with reduced susceptibility to vancomycin have been detected by this method.
- An MIC susceptibility testing method should be used to confirm vancomycin test results.

Infection control: To minimize spread and prevent development of an endemic strain

- Isolate patient in a private room and begin one-on-one care by specified personnel using contact transmission precautions and including masks.
- Initiate epidemiologic and laboratory investigations with assistance of state health departments and CDC.
- Educate health care personnel about epidemiologic implications and necessary infection control procedures.
- Monitor and strictly enforce compliance with contact precautions and other measures.
- Perform baseline cultures of hands and nares of:
  - those with recent direct patient contact
  - the patient's health care providers
  - the patient's roommates
- Assess efficacy of precautions by monitoring personnel for acquisition of staphylococci with reduced susceptibility to vancomycin.
- Consult with state health department and CDC before discharging and/or transferring the patient, *and* notify receiving institution or unit of presence of *S aureus* with reduced susceptibility to vancomycin and of appropriate precautions.

* Centers for Disease Control and Prevention. Laboratory capacity to detect antimicrobial resistance, 1998. *MMWR Morb Mortal Wkly Rep.* 2000;48:1167–1171. MIC indicates minimum inhibitory concentration; CDC, Centers for Disease Control and Prevention.

† NCCLS MIC breakpoints for vancomycin are as follows: susceptible, ≤4 µg/mL; intermediate, 8–16 µg/mL; and resistant, ≥32 µg/mL.

TREATMENT: Serious staphylococcal infections require intravenous therapy with a penicillinase-resistant penicillin, such as nafcillin or oxacillin, because most *S aureus* strains in the community or in hospitals produce penicillinase and are resistant to penicillin and ampicillin (see Table 3.52, p 521). First- or second-generation cephalosporins (eg, cephalothin or cefuroxime) and clindamycin also

Table 3.52. **Antibiotic Choices for Bacteremia and Other Serious Staphylococcal Infections***

Susceptibility	Antibiotic	Comments
I. Methicillin-susceptible *Staphylococcus aureus* and penicillin-resistant *S aureus*		
Drugs of choice:	• Nafcillin or oxacillin	...
Alternatives:	• Cefazolin	...
	• Vancomycin	...
	• Ampicillin + sulbactam	...
	• Amoxicillin + clavulanate	...
	• Clindamycin	...
	• Imipenem	...
	• Meropenem	...
II. Methicillin-resistant (MRSA) *S aureus*[†]		
Drugs of choice:	• Vancomycin ± gentamicin ± rifampin	...
Alternatives: Susceptibility testing should be done before alternative drugs used	• TMP-SMX	...
	• Minocycline	Not recommended for pregnant women or children younger than 8 years of age
	• Fluoroquinolones	Not recommended for persons younger than 18 years of age
	• Clindamycin	...
	• Quinupristin-dalfopristin	...
		...
III. Vancomycin-intermediate *S aureus* (MIC >4 µg/mL and ≤16 µg/mL)		
Drug of choice:	• Unknown	...
Alternatives:	• Vancomycin + ß-lactam	...
	• Vancomycin + gentamicin	...

Table 3.52. **Antibiotic Choices for Bacteremia and Other Serious Staphylococcal Infections,* continued**

Susceptibility	Antibiotic	Comments
III. Vancomycin-intermediate *S aureus*, continued		
Alternatives, continued:	• Vancomycin + rifampin	…
	• Linezolid	…
	• Rifampin + TMP-SMX	• Investigational oxazolidinone
	• Investigational oxazolidinone	…
IV. Initial empiric therapy to be used only until susceptibility pattern is available (organism of unknown susceptibility)		
Drugs of choice:	• Nafcillin or oxacillin + vancomycin + gentamicin	• For life-threatening infections (ie, septicemia, endocarditis, pneumonia, meningitis); some experts would not add nafcillin or oxacillin
	• Nafcillin or oxacillin	• For non–life-threatening infection, without signs of sepsis (eg, osteomyelitis, pyarthrosis, skin infection, cellulitis)
		• Community-acquired infection in children when rate of MRSA in community is low
	• Nafcillin or oxacillin + clindamycin	• Community-acquired infections in communities with increased rate of MRSA colonization and infections
	• Vancomycin + nafcillin	• Hospital-acquired infections, not life-threatening
	• Vancomycin + quinupristin-dalfopristin	• For life-threatening infection in patient who has received several recent courses of vancomycin

* CSF indicates cerebrospinal fluid; and TMP-SMX, trimethoprim-sulfamethoxazole. PBP2a is a cell wall penicillin-binding protein.

† Many strains that are resistant to penicillinase-resistant penicillins (eg, nafcillin) are also resistant to cephalosporins, imipenem, and meropenem.

are effective. The expanded-spectrum cephalosporins usually are not as active in vitro against *S aureus* or coagulase-negative staphylococci, and some may be ineffective in infections. Patients who are allergic to penicillin can be treated with a cephalosporin (if the patient is not also allergic to cephalosporins), clindamycin, or vancomycin. For staphylococcal strains resistant to the penicillinase-resistant penicillins (ie, MRSA), intravenous vancomycin is indicated. A penicillinase-resistant penicillin (a parenteral formulation of nafcillin or oxacillin) should be used for susceptible strains rather than vancomycin to minimize the emergence of vancomycin-resistant strains. Vancomycin-intermediate *S aureus* and vancomycin-intermediate coagulase-negative staphylococcal strains rarely have been isolated. Potential therapeutic options for these organisms based on in vitro studies are outlined in Table 3.52 (p 521).

Duration of therapy for serious invasive infections depends on the site of infection and usually is 3 weeks or more. After the initial parenteral therapy and clinical response of the patient, completion of the recommended antimicrobial course with an oral drug can be considered if appropriate compliance can be assured. In addition, monitoring therapeutic blood concentrations of the antimicrobial agent should be considered. For endocarditis, parenteral therapy should be maintained. Drainage of abscesses is desirable and usually required.

Skin and soft tissue infections, such as impetigo or cellulitis due to *S aureus,* usually can be treated with oral penicillinase-resistant ß-lactam drugs, such as cloxacillin, dicloxacillin, or a first- or second-generation cephalosporin. For localized superficial skin lesions, topical antibacterial therapy with mupirocin or bacitracin and local hygiene may be sufficient.

The duration of therapy for central venous line infections is controversial and depends on consideration of a number of factors, including the organism (*S aureus* vs coagulase-negative staphylococci), the type and location of the catheter, the site of infection (exit site vs tunnel vs bacteremia), the feasibility of using an alternative vessel at a later date, and the presence or absence of a catheter-related thrombosis. Infections are more difficult to treat when associated with a thrombosed vessel or an intra-atrial thrombus. If a catheter can be removed and bacteremia resolves promptly, a 3- to 5-day course of therapy seems appropriate. A longer course of 2 to 3 weeks is suggested when the organism is *S aureus.* If the patient needs a new catheter, it is optimal to wait several days before insertion. If a tunneled catheter is needed for ongoing care, in situ treatment of the infection can be attempted. If the patient responds to antibiotics with resolution of the bacteremia, the antibiotics can be continued for 7 to 10 days parenterally. If the blood cultures remain positive for staphylococci for more than 3 to 5 days, the catheter should be removed and the patient evaluated for metastatic foci of infection. If the patient develops hypotension at any time during therapy for a catheter-related infection, the catheter should be removed immediately. Vegetation or a thrombus in the heart or great vessels always should be considered when an intravascular catheter becomes infected. Transesophageal echocardiography is the most sensitive technique for identifying vegetation.

ISOLATION OF THE HOSPITALIZED PATIENT: For patients with exposed lesions, eg, draining wounds, scalded skin syndrome, burns, bullous impetigo, and abscesses caused by MSSA, standard and contact transmission precautions should be implemented for the duration of illness. For MSSA pneumonia, droplet transmission precautions are recommended for the first 24 hours of antimicrobial therapy. Droplet transmission precautions should be maintained throughout the illness for MSSA and MRSA tracheitis with a tracheostomy tube in place.

Patients infected or colonized with MRSA should be managed with contact transmission precautions for multidrug-resistant organisms for the duration of illness, because MRSA carriage can persist for weeks to months. To reduce transmission of vancomycin-intermediate *S aureus,* the CDC has issued specific infection recommendations that should be followed (see Table 3.51, p 520). For methicillin-resistant coagulase-negative staphylococci, standard precautions should be used. For vancomycin-intermediate coagulase-negative staphylococci, contact transmission precautions for multidrug-resistant organisms should be used.

Control Measures:

Coagulase-negative Staphylococci. Prevention and control of coagulase-negative staphylococcal infections have focused on prevention of intraoperative contamination by skin flora and the sterile insertion of intravascular and intraperitoneal catheters and other prosthetic devices. Prophylactic administration of antibiotics intraoperatively lowers the incidence of infection after cardiac surgery and the implantation of synthetic vascular grafts and prosthetic devices. There is no consensus about the role of intraoperative antibiotics at the time of cerebrospinal fluid shunt placement.

Staphylococcus aureus. Measures to prevent and control *S aureus* infections can be considered separately for the individual patient and for the institution.

Individual Patient.

Community-acquired *S aureus* infections in immunocompetent hosts cannot be prevented because the organism is ubiquitous and there is no vaccine. Frequent hand washing, treatment, and maintaining cleanliness of skin abrasions may prevent hematogenous spread. For patients with disorders of neutrophil function or with chronic skin conditions, who are predisposed to *S aureus* infections, a variety of techniques have been used to prevent infection. These may include scrupulous attention to skin hygiene and to the types of clothing and bed linen used to minimize sweating. Eradication of nasal carriage, if present, early use of antibiotics, and, in some cases, the prolonged use of trimethoprim-sulfamethoxazole also may be helpful.

Nosocomial *S aureus* infections may be prevented or controlled for the individual patient by general measures, intraoperative antibiotic prophylaxis, and eradication of nasal carriage.

General Measures. The published recommendations of the CDC Hospital Infection Control Practices Advisory Committee (HICPAC) for prevention of all nosocomial pneumonia should be effective for reducing the incidence of *S aureus* pneumonia. Careful preparation of the skin before surgery and before placement of intravascular catheters will decrease the incidence of *S aureus* wound and catheter infections. Meticulous surgical technique with minimal trauma to tissues, maintenance of good oxygenation, and minimal hematoma and dead space formation will minimize infection of the wound. Good hand washing, including before and after use of gloves, by health care personnel and strict adherence to contact transmission precautions are of paramount importance.

Intraoperative Antibiotic Prophylaxis. Bacteria are inoculated into wounds between the start and closure of the surgical incision. Antimicrobial agents can be given to achieve and maintain high concentrations of antibiotics in the blood and tissues during this critical period. This pharmacologic defense can kill some inoculated bacteria directly and facilitate neutrophil killing of bacteria. The efficacy of antibiotic prophylaxis for clean surgery is established. The antibiotics are started immediately before or at the start of the operation, and high levels are maintained throughout the procedure. A total duration of therapy of less than 24 hours is recommended. Staphylococci are the most important pathogens for several surgical procedures; thus, prophylaxis is recommended for most cardiac, general thoracic, vascular, orthopedic, and neurosurgical procedures. Cefazolin has become the most popular drug. For situations in which vancomycin is appropriate for use in prophylaxis, see Principles of Judicious Use of Vancomycin, p 649.

Eradication of Nasal Carriage. Detection and eradication of nasal carriage using mupirocin twice a day for 1 to 5 days has been shown to reduce the incidence of *S aureus* infections after cardiothoracic, general, and neurosurgical procedures in adults. The use of intermittent or continuous intranasal mupirocin for eradication of nasal carriage also has been shown to reduce the incidence of invasive *S aureus* infections in adult patients undergoing long-term hemodialysis or ambulatory peritoneal dialysis. Eradication of nasal carriage of *S aureus* may be difficult.

Institutions.

Measures to control the spread of *S aureus* within hospitals or hospital units involves use and careful monitoring of HICPAC guidelines published in 1996.* Strategies for controlling nosocomial transmission of MRSA vary widely among hospitals, and the guidelines recommend that hospitals individualize their recommendations. When a patient or health care worker is found to be a chronic carrier of *S aureus,* including MRSA, topical mupirocin therapy may effectively eradicate carriage. Although an increasing number of MRSA strains are resistant in vitro to mupirocin, concentrations used topically (2% or 20 000 µg/mL) are high enough to be effective even for these strains. Reduction of overuse of antimicrobial agents will reduce the emergence of vancomycin-intermediate *S aureus.* Restriction and cycling of antibiotics should be considered. Recommendations for containment of the recently identified strains of vancomycin-intermediate *S aureus* have been published by the CDC (Table 3.51, p 520).† Ongoing review and restriction of vancomycin use is critical to attempt to control the emergence of vancomycin-intermediate *S aureus* (see Judicious Use of Antimicrobial Agents, p 647). To date, catheters impregnated with various antibacterial agents to prevent nosocomial infections have not been used extensively in children.

Newborn Nurseries. Outbreaks of *S aureus* infections in newborn nurseries require unique measures for control. Application of triple dye, iodophor ointment,

---

* The Hospital Infection Control Practices Advisory Committee. Guideline for isolation precautions in hospitals [published correction appears in *Infect Control Hosp Epidemiol.* 1996;17:214]. *Infect Control Hosp Epidemiol.* 1996;17:53–80

† Centers for Disease Control and Prevention. Interim guidelines for the prevention and control of staphylococcal infection associated with reduced susceptibility to vancomycin. *MMWR Morb Mortal Wkly Rep.* 1997;46:626–628, 635

or hexachlorophene powder to the umbilical stump has been used to delay or prevent colonization. For full-term infants only, 3% hexachlorophene can be used for bathing followed by thorough rinsing. Other measures recommended during outbreaks include cohorting of infants and staff, alleviating overcrowding and understaffing, and an emphasis on hand washing. Soaps containing antimicrobial agents are preferred during an outbreak. Culturing the umbilicus and nares of infants and nares and skin lesions of personnel for *S aureus* can help establish the extent of the outbreak. Pulsed-field gel electrophoresis should be used to determine strain identity. Epidemiologically implicated personnel may be treated for nasal carriage with mupirocin.

Group A Streptococcal Infections

Clinical Manifestations: The most common clinical illness produced by group A streptococcal (GAS) infection is acute pharyngitis or tonsillitis. In some patients, who usually are untreated, purulent complications, including otitis media, sinusitis, peritonsillar and retropharyngeal abscesses, and suppurative cervical adenitis develop. The significance of streptococcal upper respiratory tract disease relates particularly to its acute morbidity and nonsuppurative sequelae, ie, acute rheumatic fever and acute glomerulonephritis. Scarlet fever occurs most commonly in association with pharyngitis and, rarely, with pyoderma or an infected surgical or traumatic wound. Scarlet fever has a characteristic confluent erythematous sandpaper-like rash, which is caused by one or more of the several erythrogenic exotoxins produced by GAS strains. Severe scarlet fever with systemic toxic effects occurs rarely. Other than the occurrence of rash, the epidemiologic features, symptoms, sequelae, and treatment of scarlet fever are the same as those of streptococcal pharyngitis.

Toddlers (1 to 3 years of age) with GAS respiratory tract infection may present with moderate fever and serous rhinitis and may have a protracted illness with fever, irritability, and anorexia (streptococcal fever). The classic clinical presentation of streptococcal upper respiratory tract infection as acute pharyngitis is uncommon in children younger than 3 years of age. Rheumatic fever also is uncommon at this age.

The second most common site of GAS infection is the skin. Streptococcal skin infections (ie, pyoderma or impetigo) can result in acute glomerulonephritis, which occasionally occurs in epidemics, but acute rheumatic fever is not a sequela of streptococcal skin infection.

Other GAS infections include erysipelas, perianal cellulitis, vaginitis, bacteremia, pneumonia, endocarditis, pericarditis, septic arthritis, cellulitis, necrotizing fasciitis, osteomyelitis, myositis, puerperal sepsis, surgical wound infection, and neonatal omphalitis. Necrotizing fasciitis and other invasive GAS infections in children often occur as complications of varicella. Bacteremic GAS infections can be severe, with or without an identified focus of local infection, and can be associated with streptococcal toxic shock syndrome. The portal of entry of invasive infections often is the skin or soft tissue and may follow minor or unrecognized trauma.

The toxic shock syndrome caused by GAS infection is reviewed in the chapter Toxic Shock Syndrome (p 576).

ETIOLOGY: More than 100 distinct M-protein types of group A ß-hemolytic streptococci *(Streptococcus pyogenes)* have been identified. Epidemiologic studies suggest an association between certain serotypes (eg, types 1, 3, 5, 6, 18, 19, and 24) and rheumatic fever, but a specific rheumatogenic factor has not been identified. Several serotypes (eg, types 49, 55, 57, and 59) are associated with pyoderma and acute glomerulonephritis. Pharyngitis-associated nephritis often is associated with other serotypes (eg, types 1, 6, and 12). Groups C and G streptococci have been associated with pharyngitis and, occasionally, acute nephritis but do not cause rheumatic fever.

EPIDEMIOLOGY: Pharyngitis usually results from contact with a person who has streptococcal pharyngitis. Fomites and household pets, such as dogs, are not vectors of GAS infection. Transmission of GAS infection, including school outbreaks of pharyngitis, almost always follows contact with respiratory tract secretions. Pharyngitis and impetigo (and their nonsuppurative complications) may be associated with crowding, which often is present in socioeconomically disadvantaged populations. The close contact that occurs in schools, child care, and military installations facilitates transmission. Foodborne outbreaks have occurred and are a consequence of human contamination of food in conjunction with improper preparation or refrigeration procedures.

Streptococcal pharyngitis occurs at all ages, but it is most common among school-age children. Group A streptococcal pharyngitis and pyoderma are less common in adults than in children except during epidemics.

Geographically, streptococcal pharyngitis and pyoderma are ubiquitous. Pyoderma is more common in tropical climates and in warm seasons, presumably in part because of antecedent insect bites and other minor skin trauma. Streptococcal pharyngitis occurs more frequently in the late autumn, winter, and spring in temperate climates, presumably because of the close person-to-person contact that occurs in schools. Communicability of patients with streptococcal pharyngitis is highest during the acute infection and, in untreated persons, gradually diminishes during a period of weeks. Patients are no longer contagious within 24 hours of the initiation of appropriate antimicrobial therapy.

Throat culture surveys of asymptomatic children during school outbreaks of pharyngitis have yielded GAS prevalence rates as high as 15% to 50%. These include children with asymptomatic infections and pharyngeal carriers with no subsequent immune response to GAS cellular or extracellular antigens. Carriage of GAS may persist for many months, but the risk of transmission to others is not appreciable, perhaps because of diminished numbers of organisms in the pharynx or the disappearance of bacteria from nasal secretions.

The incidence of acute rheumatic fever in the United States has decreased sharply over several decades, but outbreaks of rheumatic fever in the 1990s in school-age children in various geographic areas demonstrated that acute rheumatic fever remains a risk. Although the reason(s) for these local outbreaks is not clear, their occurrence reemphasizes the importance of diagnosing GAS pharyngitis and of compliance with the recommended duration of antimicrobial therapy.

In streptococcal impetigo, the organism usually is acquired from a person with impetigo, possibly by direct physical contact. Colonization of healthy skin by GAS usually precedes development of skin infection. Impetiginous lesions occur at the site of open lesions (eg, insect bites, traumatic wounds, or burns) since GAS organisms do not penetrate intact skin. After development of impetiginous lesions, the upper respiratory tract often becomes colonized. Infections of surgical wounds and postpartum (puerperal) sepsis usually result from contact transmission via hand carriage. At times, anal or vaginal carriers and persons with pyoderma or local suppurative infections can transmit GAS to surgical and obstetrical patients resulting in nosocomial outbreaks. Infections in neonates can result from intrapartum or contact transmission; in the latter situation, infection often begins with omphalitis.

In recent years, the incidence of severe invasive GAS infections, including bacteremia, streptococcal toxic shock syndrome, and necrotizing fasciitis, has increased. The incidence seems to be highest in the very young and in older persons. Varicella is the most commonly identified risk factor in children. Other risk factors include intravenous drug use, human immunodeficiency virus infection, diabetes mellitus, and chronic cardiac or pulmonary disease. Results from studies of the possible association between the use of nonsteroidal anti-inflammatory drugs and invasive GAS infections in children with varicella are conflicting. Additional studies are needed to establish whether there is a causal relationship. The portal of entry is unknown in almost 50% of invasive GAS infections; in most cases, it is believed to be skin or mucous membrane. Such infections rarely follow GAS pharyngitis.

The **incubation period** for streptococcal pharyngitis is 2 to 5 days. For impetigo, a 7- to 10-day period between the acquisition of GAS on healthy skin and development of lesions has been demonstrated.

DIAGNOSTIC TESTS: Laboratory confirmation of GAS is recommended for children with pharyngitis because reliable clinical differentiation of viral and GAS pharyngitis is not possible. A specimen should be obtained by vigorous swabbing of the tonsils and posterior pharynx. Culture on sheep blood agar can confirm GAS infection, and latex agglutination, fluorescent antibody, coagglutination, and precipitation techniques performed on colonies growing on the agar plate can differentiate group A from other ß-hemolytic streptococci. Appropriate use of bacitracin-susceptibility disks (containing 0.04 units) allows presumptive identification of GAS but is a less accurate method of diagnosis. False-negative cultures occur in fewer than 10% of symptomatic patients when a throat swab specimen is obtained properly and cultured. Recovery of GAS from the pharynx does not distinguish patients with bona fide streptococcal infection (defined by a serologic antibody response) from streptococcal carriers who have an intercurrent pharyngitis caused by a different organism (eg, a virus). The number of colonies of GAS on the agar culture plate does not accurately differentiate bona fide infection from carriage. Cultures that are negative for GAS after 24 hours should be incubated for a second day to optimize recovery of GAS.

Several rapid diagnostic tests for GAS pharyngitis are available. Most are based on nitrous acid extraction of group A carbohydrate antigen from organisms obtained by throat swab. Although the methods for these tests vary, their sensitivities and specificities, in general, are similar when carefully performed, including rigorous attention to technique and use of controls. The specificities of these tests generally are very high, but the reported sensitivities vary considerably. As with throat cultures, the accuracy of these tests is highly dependent on the quality of the throat swab specimen, which must contain pharyngeal and/or tonsillar secretions, and on the experience of the person performing the test. Therefore, when a patient suspected on clinical grounds of having GAS pharyngitis has a negative rapid streptococcal test, a throat culture should be obtained to ensure that the patient does not have GAS infection. Because of the very high specificity of these rapid tests, a positive test result does not require throat culture confirmation. Rapid diagnostic tests using new techniques, such as optical immunoassay and chemiluminescent DNA probes, have been developed. Published data suggest that these tests may be as sensitive as standard throat cultures on sheep blood agar and more sensitive than other rapid tests for GAS. Some experts believe that the optical immunoassay test is sufficiently sensitive to be used without throat culture backup. Physicians who use this test without culture backup may wish to compare their results with those of culture to validate adequate sensitivity in their practice.

Indications for GAS Testing. Factors to be considered in the decision to obtain a throat swab for testing in children with pharyngitis are the patient's age, clinical signs and symptoms, the season, and the family and community epidemiology, including contact with a case of GAS infection, presence in the family of a person with acute rheumatic fever, or history thereof, or with poststreptococcal glomerulonephritis. Group A streptococcal infection is less common in children younger than 3 years of age, but outbreaks of streptococcal pharyngitis rarely have been reported in young children in child care settings. The risk of acute rheumatic fever is so remote in developed countries in such young children that diagnostic studies for streptococcal pharyngitis are not recommended routinely for children younger than 3 years of age. Children with manifestations highly suggestive of viral infection, such as coryza, conjunctivitis, hoarseness, cough, anterior stomatitis, discrete ulcerative lesions, or diarrhea, are unlikely to have GAS as the cause of their pharyngitis and should not be swabbed for GAS. Children with acute onset of sore throat, fever, headache, pain on swallowing, abdominal pain, nausea, vomiting, and enlarged tender anterior cervical lymph nodes are much more likely to have GAS as the cause of their pharyngitis and should be tested.

Indications for testing contacts for GAS vary according to circumstances. Testing asymptomatic household contacts for GAS usually is not recommended except during outbreaks or when contacts are at increased risk for developing sequelae of GAS infection. Siblings and all other household contacts of a child who has acute rheumatic fever or poststreptococcal glomerulonephritis should have their throats swabbed and, if test results are positive, should be treated regardless of whether they are currently or were recently symptomatic. Household contacts of an index case with streptococcal pharyngitis who have recent or current symptoms suggestive of streptococcal infection also should be tested. Pyoderma lesions should be cultured in families with one or more cases of acute nephritis or streptococcal toxic shock syndrome so that antibiotic therapy can be administered to eradicate GAS.

Posttreatment throat swab cultures are indicated only for patients at particularly high risk for rheumatic fever or who are still or again symptomatic. Repeated courses of antimicrobial therapy are not indicated for asymptomatic patients who remain GAS positive after appropriate antibiotic therapy; the exceptions are persons who have had, or whose family members have had, rheumatic fever or rheumatic heart disease or in other unique epidemiologic circumstances, such as outbreaks of rheumatic fever or acute poststreptococcal glomerulonephritis.

Patients in whom repeated episodes of pharyngitis occur at short intervals with GAS documented by culture or antigen detection test present a special problem. Often these persons are long-term GAS carriers who are experiencing frequent viral illnesses. In assessing such patients, inadequate compliance with oral treatment also should be considered. Although rare, in some areas, erythromycin resistance may occur, resulting in treatment failures. Such strains also are resistant to other macrolides, such as clarithromycin and azithromycin. Testing asymptomatic household members usually is not helpful. However, if multiple household members have symptomatic pharyngitis or other GAS infection, such as pyoderma, simultaneous cultures of all household members and treatment of all persons with positive cultures may be of value.

In schools, child care centers, or other environments in which large numbers of persons are in close contact, the prevalence of GAS pharyngeal carriage in healthy children can be as high as 15% in the absence of an outbreak of streptococcal disease. Therefore, classroom or more widespread culture surveys are not indicated routinely and should be considered only if multiple cases of rheumatic fever, glomerulonephritis, or severe invasive GAS disease have occurred.

Cultures of impetiginous lesions are not indicated routinely since they often yield both streptococci and staphylococci, and determination of the primary pathogen may not be possible.

In suspected invasive GAS infections, cultures of blood and focal sites of possible infection are indicated. In necrotizing fasciitis, magnetic resonance imaging can be helpful for confirming the anatomic diagnosis.

TREATMENT:

Pharyngitis.

- Penicillin V is the drug of choice for treatment of GAS pharyngitis, except in penicillin-allergic persons. A clinical isolate of group A streptococci resistant to penicillin has never been documented. Ampicillin or amoxicillin often is used in place of penicillin V, but these drugs have no microbiologic advantage over penicillin. However, preliminary data suggest that orally administered amoxicillin given as a single dose for 10 days is as effective as orally administered penicillin V given 3 times per day for 10 days. Penicillin therapy prevents acute rheumatic fever even when therapy is started as long as 9 days after the onset of the acute illness, shortens the clinical course, reduces the risk of transmission, and decreases the risk of suppurative sequelae. For patients examined early in their illness, a brief delay for processing of the throat culture before therapy is started does not increase the risk of rheumatic fever. For all patients with acute rheumatic fever, a complete course of penicillin or other appropriate antibiotic for GAS pharyngitis should be given to eradicate GAS from the throat, even though the organism may not be recovered in the initial throat culture.

  The dose of orally administered penicillin V is 400 000 U (250 mg), 2 to 3 times per day for 10 days for children and 500 mg 2 to 3 times per day for adolescents and adults. To prevent acute rheumatic fever, oral treatment with penicillin should be given for the full 10 days, regardless of the promptness of clinical recovery. Although different preparations of oral penicillin vary in absorption, their clinical efficacy is similar. Treatment failures may occur more frequently with oral penicillin than with intramuscularly administered benzathine penicillin G as a result of inadequate compliance with oral therapy.

- Intramuscular benzathine penicillin G (BPG) is appropriate therapy. It ensures adequate blood concentrations and avoids the problem of compliance, but administration is painful. For children who weigh less than 60 lb (27 kg), BPG is given in a single dose of 600 000 U; for larger children and adults, the dose is 1.2 million U. Discomfort is less if the preparation of benzathine penicillin G is brought to room temperature before intramuscular injection. Mixtures containing shorter acting penicillins (eg, procaine penicillin) in addition to BPG have not been demonstrated to be more effective than BPG alone but are less painful when administered. Although supporting data are limited, the combination of 900 000 U of BPG and 300 000 U of procaine penicillin G is satisfactory therapy for most children; however, the efficacy of this combination for heavier patients, such as adolescents and adults, has not been demonstrated.
- Orally administered erythromycin is indicated for patients allergic to penicillin. Treatment should be given for 10 days. Erythromycin estolate (20 to 40 mg/kg per day in 2 to 4 divided doses) or erythromycin ethyl succinate (40 mg/kg per day in 2 to 4 divided doses) is effective for treating streptococcal pharyngitis; the maximal dose is 1 g/d. Other macrolides, such as clarithromycin for 10 days or azithromycin for 5 days (a regimen approved by the US Food and Drug Administration) are also effective. Although GAS strains resistant to erythromycin and other macrolides have been prevalent in some areas of the world (eg, Japan and Finland) and have resulted in treatment failures, they remain uncommon in most areas of the United States.
- A 10-day course of a narrow-spectrum (first-generation), oral cephalosporin is an acceptable alternative, particularly for persons allergic to penicillin. However, as many as 15% of penicillin-allergic persons also are allergic to cephalosporins. Patients with immediate, anaphylactic-type hypersensitivity to penicillin should not be treated with a cephalosporin. A number of reports have suggested that a 5-day course of certain oral cephalosporins is similar to a 10-day course of oral penicillin in eradicating GAS from the upper respiratory tract. However, additional studies are warranted to expand and confirm these observations before these regimens can be recommended. The additional cost of cephalosporins and their wider range of antibacterial activity compared with penicillin preclude recommending them for routine use in persons with GAS pharyngitis who are not allergic to penicillin.
- Tetracyclines and sulfonamides should **not** be used for treating GAS pharyngitis. Many strains are resistant to tetracycline, and sulfonamides do not eradicate GAS, even though they are effective for continuous prophylaxis for recurrent rheumatic fever (see Secondary Prophylaxis for Rheumatic Fever, p 534).

Children who have a recurrence of GAS pharyngitis shortly after completing a 10-day course of a recommended oral antimicrobial agent can be retreated with that antimicrobial agent; given an alternative oral drug; or given an intramuscular dose of benzathine penicillin G, especially if inadequate compliance with oral therapy is likely. Alternative drugs include a cephalosporin, amoxicillin-clavulanate, clindamycin, erythromycin, or other macrolide. Expert opinions differ about the most appropriate therapy in this circumstance.

Management of a patient who has repeated and frequent episodes of acute pharyngitis associated with a positive laboratory test for GAS is problematic. To determine whether the patient is a long-term streptococcal pharyngeal carrier who is experiencing repeated episodes of intercurrent viral pharyngitis (which is the situation in the majority of cases), the following should be determined: (1) whether the clinical findings are more suggestive of a GAS or a viral cause, (2) whether epidemiologic factors in the community are more suggestive of a GAS or a viral cause, (3) the nature of the clinical response to the antimicrobial therapy (in bona fide GAS pharyngitis, this usually is rapid), (4) whether laboratory tests are positive for GAS between episodes of acute pharyngitis, and (5) whether a serologic response to GAS extracellular antigens (eg, antistreptolysin O) has occurred. Serotyping of GAS isolates generally is available only in research laboratories, but if performed, repeated isolation of the same serotype suggests carriage, while isolation of differing serotypes indicates repeated infections.

Pharyngeal Carriers. Antimicrobial therapy is not indicated for most GAS pharyngeal carriers. Exceptions, ie, specific situations in which eradication of carriage may be indicated, include the following: (1) during an outbreak of acute rheumatic fever or poststreptococcal glomerulonephritis, (2) during an outbreak of GAS pharyngitis in a closed or semiclosed community, (3) when a family history of rheumatic fever exists, (4) when multiple episodes of documented symptomatic GAS pharyngitis continue to occur within a family during a period of many weeks despite appropriate therapy, (5) when a family has excessive anxiety about GAS infections, (6) when tonsillectomy is considered only because of chronic GAS carriage, and (7) when a case of GAS toxic shock syndrome or necrotizing fasciitis has occurred in a household contact.

Streptococcal carriage can be difficult to eradicate with conventional antibiotic therapy. A number of antimicrobial agents, including clindamycin, amoxicillin-clavulanate, and a combination of rifampin and either penicillin V or benzathine penicillin G, have been demonstrated to be more effective than penicillin in eliminating chronic streptococcal carriage. Of these drugs, oral clindamycin given as 20 mg/kg per day in 3 doses (maximum, 1.8 g/d) for 10 days has been reported to be the most effective. Documented eradication of the carrier state is helpful in the evaluation of subsequent episodes of acute pharyngitis; however, long-term carriage may recur after reacquisition of GAS.

Streptococcal Impetigo.

- Local antibacterial preparations, such as bacitracin or mupirocin ointment, may be useful for limiting person-to-person spread of GAS impetigo and for eradicating localized disease. With multiple lesions or with impetigo in multiple family members, child care groups, or athletic teams, impetigo should be treated with antibiotic regimens administered systemically. Because episodes of what seems to be GAS impetigo frequently are caused by *Staphylococcus aureus,* children with impetigo usually should be treated with an antibiotic active against both GAS and *S aureus.*

Other Infections.

- High-dose parenteral antimicrobial therapy is required for severe infections, such as endocarditis, pneumonia, septicemia, meningitis, arthritis, osteomyelitis, necrotizing fasciitis, and streptococcal toxic shock syndrome. Treatment often is prolonged (2 to 6 weeks).
- For treatment of patients with severe invasive GAS infection, including toxic shock syndrome, see the chapter Toxic Shock Syndrome (p 576).

Prevention of Sequelae. Acute rheumatic fever and acute glomerulonephritis are serious nonsuppurative sequelae of GAS infections. During epidemics of GAS infections on military bases in the 1950s, rheumatic fever developed in 3% of untreated patients with acute streptococcal pharyngitis. The current attack rate after endemic infections is not known, but it is believed to be substantially lower. The risk of rheumatic fever virtually can be eliminated by adequate treatment of the antecedent GAS infection; however, rare cases of rheumatic fever have occurred even after apparently appropriate therapy. The effectiveness of antimicrobial therapy for preventing acute poststreptococcal glomerulonephritis after pyoderma has not been established. Suppurative sequelae, such as peritonsillar abscesses and cervical adenitis, usually are prevented by therapy of the primary infection.

ISOLATION OF THE HOSPITALIZED PATIENT: In addition to standard precautions, droplet precautions are recommended for children with pharyngitis or pneumonia until 24 hours after initiation of appropriate therapy. For burns with secondary GAS infection and extensive or draining cutaneous infections that cannot be covered or contained adequately by dressings, contact precautions should be used for at least 24 hours after the start of appropriate therapy.

CONTROL MEASURES: The most important means of controlling GAS disease and its sequelae is prompt identification and treatment of infections.

School and Child Care. Children with streptococcal pharyngitis or skin infections should not return to school or child care until at least 24 hours after beginning appropriate antimicrobial therapy. Close contact with other children during this time should be avoided, if possible.

Care of Exposed Persons. Persons who are contacts of documented cases of streptococcal infection and who have recent or current clinical evidence of a GAS infection should undergo appropriate laboratory tests and should be treated if test results are positive. Rates of GAS acquisition are higher among sibling contacts than among parent contacts in nonepidemic settings; rates as high as 50% for sibling contacts and 20% for parent contacts have been reported during epidemics. More than half of the contacts who acquire the organism will become ill. Asymptomatic acquisition of GAS may pose some risk of nonsuppurative complications; studies indicate that as many as one third of patients with rheumatic fever had no history of recent streptococcal infection, and another third had minor respiratory tract symptoms that were not brought to medical attention. However, laboratory evaluation of asymptomatic household contacts usually is not indicated except during outbreaks or when the contacts are at increased risk for developing sequelae of infection (see Indications for GAS Testing, p 529). Short courses (<10 days) of antibiotics for contacts are inappropriate. In rare circumstances, such as a large family with documented, repeated, intrafamily transmission resulting in frequent episodes of GAS pharyngitis during a prolonged period, physicians may elect to treat all family members. Laboratory tests should be obtained in these unusual circumstances to identify the persons harboring GAS.

Some experts recommend oral penicillin prophylaxis during the period of the year of greatest risk for children with repeated episodes of GAS pharyngitis. However, this approach should be limited because of concerns about selecting resistant organisms (not GAS).

Limited data suggest that household contacts of patients with severe invasive GAS disease, including streptococcal toxic shock syndrome, may be at increased risk for development of severe invasive GAS disease compared with the general population. The data currently available about the risk of secondary invasive GAS infections are limited, and the effectiveness of chemoprophylaxis is uncertain. Therefore, no recommendations for the routine use of chemoprophylaxis can be made. Physicians contemplating chemoprophylaxis for household contacts should consider factors including the severity of disease in the index case, the extent of contact with the index case, underlying conditions in contacts that may increase the risk of disease or mortality (eg, advanced age, immunosuppression, diabetes mellitus, varicella infection), and the costs and potential adverse effects of chemoprophylaxis. Because of the rarity of subsequent cases and the low risk of invasive GAS infections in children in general, chemoprophylaxis is not recommended in schools or child care facilities.

Secondary Prophylaxis for Rheumatic Fever. Patients who have a well-documented history of acute rheumatic fever (including cases manifested solely by Sydenham chorea) and patients who have documented evidence of rheumatic heart disease should be given continuous antibiotic prophylaxis to prevent recurrent attacks (secondary prophylaxis), because asymptomatic and symptomatic GAS infections can result in a rheumatic recurrence. Continuous prophylaxis should be initiated as soon as the diagnosis of acute rheumatic fever or rheumatic heart disease is made.

Duration. Secondary prophylaxis should be long-term, perhaps for life, for patients with rheumatic heart disease (even after prosthetic valve replacement because these patients remain at risk for recurrence of rheumatic fever). The risk of recurrence declines as the interval from the most recent episode lengthens, and patients without rheumatic heart disease are at a lower risk of recurrence than are patients with cardiac involvement. These considerations influence the duration of secondary prophylaxis in adults but should not alter the practice of secondary prophylaxis for children and adolescents. Secondary prophylaxis for all patients who have had rheumatic fever should be continued for at least 5 years or until the person is 21 years of age, whichever is longer (see Table 3.53, p 535). Prophylaxis also should be continued if the risk of contact with persons with GAS infection is high, such as for parents with school-age children and teachers.

Table 3.53. Duration of Prophylaxis for Persons Who Have Had Rheumatic Fever: Recommendations of the American Heart Association*

Category	Duration
Rheumatic fever without carditis	5 y or until age 21 y, whichever is longer
Rheumatic fever with carditis but without residual heart disease (no valvular disease†)	10 y or well into adulthood, whichever is longer
Rheumatic fever with carditis and residual heart disease (persistent valvular disease†)	At least 10 y since last episode and at least until age 40 y; sometimes lifelong prophylaxis

* Modified from Dajani A, Taubert K, Ferrieri P, Peter G, Shulman S. Treatment of acute streptococcal pharyngitis and prevention of rheumatic fever: a statement for health professionals: Committee on Rheumatic Fever, Endocarditis, and Kawasaki Disease of the Council on Cardiovascular Disease in the Young, The American Heart Association. *Pediatrics.* 1995;96:758–764

† Clinical or echocardiographic evidence.

When streptococcal infections occur in family members of patients with rheumatic fever, infected persons should be treated promptly with an appropriate antibiotic (see Indications for GAS Testing, p 529, and Treatment, p 530).

The drug regimens in Table 3.54 (p 536) are effective for secondary prophylaxis. The intramuscular regimen has been shown to be the most reliable because the success of oral prophylaxis depends primarily on patient compliance; however, inconvenience and the pain of injection may cause some patients to discontinue intramuscular prophylaxis. In some countries and in situations in which the risk of GAS infection is particularly high, benzathine penicillin G is given every 3 weeks because of greater effectiveness. In the United States, administration every 4 weeks seems adequate in most circumstances. Oral sulfadiazine is as effective as oral penicillin for secondary prophylaxis but may not be readily available in the United States. By extrapolating from data demonstrating effectiveness of sulfadiazine, sulfisoxazole has been deemed an appropriate alternative.

Allergic reactions to oral penicillin are similar to those with intramuscular penicillin, but they usually are less severe and occur less frequently. These reactions also occur less often in children than in adults. Anaphylaxis is rare in patients receiving oral penicillin. Severe allergic reactions in patients receiving continuous benzathine penicillin G prophylaxis also are rare. The rare reports of anaphylaxis and death generally have involved patients older than 12 years of age with severe rheumatic heart disease. Most of these severe reactions seem to represent vasovagal responses rather than anaphylaxis. Reactions include a serum sickness–like reaction characterized by fever and joint pains, which can be mistaken for recurrence of acute rheumatic fever.

Reactions to continuous sulfadiazine or sulfisoxazole prophylaxis are infrequent and usually minor; evaluation of blood cell counts may be advisable after 2 weeks of prophylaxis, since leukopenia has been reported. Prophylaxis with a sulfonamide during late pregnancy is contraindicated because of interference with fetal bilirubin metabolism. Febrile mucocutaneous syndromes (erythema multiforme, Stevens-Johnson syndrome, or toxic epidermal necrolysis) have been associated with penicillin and with sulfonamides. When an adverse event occurs with any of these therapeutic

Table 3.54. **Chemoprophylaxis for Recurrences of Rheumatic Fever***

Drug	Dose	Route
Benzathine penicillin G	1 200 000 U every 4 wk†	Intramuscular
OR		
Penicillin V	250 mg twice a day	Oral
OR		
Sulfadiazine or sulfisoxazole	0.5 g once a day for patients ≤27 kg (60 lb) 1.0 g once a day for patients >27 kg (60 lb)	Oral
For persons allergic to penicillin and sulfonamide drugs		
Erythromycin	250 mg twice a day	Oral

* Modified from Dajani A, Taubert K, Ferrieri P, Peter G, Shulman S. Treatment of acute streptococcal pharyngitis and prevention of rheumatic fever: a statement for health professionals: Committee on Rheumatic Fever, Endocarditis, and Kawasaki Disease of the Council on Cardiovascular Disease in the Young, The American Heart Association. *Pediatrics.* 1995;96:758–764

† In high-risk situations, administration every 3 weeks is recommended.

regimens, the drug should be stopped immediately and an alternative drug selected. For the rare patient allergic to both penicillins and sulfonamides, erythromycin is recommended. Newer macrolides, such as azithromycin or clarithromycin, also should be acceptable; they have less gastrointestinal intolerance but increased costs.

Poststreptococcal Reactive Arthritis. After an episode of acute GAS pharyngitis, reactive arthritis may develop in the absence of sufficient clinical manifestations and laboratory findings to fulfill the Jones criteria for the diagnosis of acute rheumatic fever. This syndrome has been termed poststreptococcal reactive arthritis (PSRA). The precise relationship of PSRA to acute rheumatic fever is unclear. In contrast with the arthritis of acute rheumatic fever, the arthritis of PSRA does not respond dramatically to nonsteroidal anti-inflammatory agents. Because some patients with PSRA apparently may have silent or delayed-onset carditis, patients should be observed carefully for several months for the subsequent development of carditis. Some experts recommend prophylaxis for these patients for several months to a year if carditis does not develop; if carditis occurs, the patient should be considered to have had rheumatic fever, and prophylaxis should be continued (see Secondary Prophylaxis for Rheumatic Fever, p 534).

Infective Endocarditis Prophylaxis. Patients with rheumatic valvular heart disease also require additional short-term antibiotic prophylaxis at the time of certain procedures (including dental and surgical procedures) to prevent the possible development of infective endocarditis (see Prevention of Bacterial Endocarditis, p 735). Patients who have had rheumatic fever without evidence of valvular heart disease do not need prophylaxis for prevention of endocarditis. Penicillin, ampicillin, and amoxicillin should not be used for endocarditis prophylaxis for patients who are receiving oral penicillin for secondary rheumatic fever prophylaxis because of relative penicillin and aminopenicillin resistance among viridans streptococci in the oral cavity in such patients. Clindamycin, azithromycin, and clarithromycin are the alternative antibiotics recommended for such patients.

Group B Streptococcal Infections

CLINICAL MANIFESTATIONS: Group B streptococci (GBS) are a major cause of perinatal bacterial infections, including bacteremia, endometritis, amnionitis, and urinary tract infections in parturient women and systemic and focal infections in infants from birth until 3 or more months of age. Invasive disease in young infants is categorized into 2 entities based on time of onset after birth. Early-onset disease usually occurs within the first 24 hours of life (range, 0 to 6 days) and is characterized by respiratory distress, apnea, shock, pneumonia, and, less often, meningitis (5%–10% of cases). Late-onset disease, which typically occurs at 3 to 4 weeks of age (range, 7 days to 3 months), frequently is manifested as occult bacteremia or meningitis; other focal infections, such as osteomyelitis, septic arthritis, and cellulitis, also can occur. Group B streptococci also cause chorioamnionitis and postpartum endometritis and systemic infections in nonpregnant adults, particularly adults with diabetes mellitus, chronic liver or renal disease, malignant neoplasm, or other immunocompromising conditions.

ETIOLOGY: Group B streptococci *(Streptococcus agalactiae)* are divided into the following serotypes based on capsular polysaccharides: Ia, Ib, II, and III through VIII. All serotypes may cause infections in newborn infants and in adults, but serotypes Ia, II, III, and V account for approximately 90% of cases in the United States. Serotype III is the predominant cause of early-onset meningitis and all late-onset infections in newborns.

EPIDEMIOLOGY: Group B streptococci are common inhabitants of the gastrointestinal and the genitourinary tracts. Less commonly, they colonize the pharynx. The colonization rate in pregnant women and newborn infants ranges from 5% to 35%. Colonization during pregnancy usually is constant but can be intermittent. Before recommendations for prevention of early-onset GBS disease by maternal intrapartum antibiotic prophylaxis (see Control Measures, p 539), the incidence was 1 to 4 cases per 1000 live births. Now the incidence varies considerably among hospitals. Without maternal prophylaxis, early-onset disease accounts for approximately 75% of infant cases and occurs in approximately 1 infant per 100 to 200 colonized women. Case fatality ratios range from 5% to 8% but are higher in preterm neonates. Transmission from mother to infant occurs shortly before or during delivery. After delivery, person-to-person transmission can occur. Although uncommon, GBS can be acquired in the nursery from colonized infants or hospital personnel (probably via hand contamination) or in the community. The risk of early-onset disease is increased in preterm infants born at less than 37 weeks of gestation, in infants born after the amniotic membranes have been ruptured 18 hours or more, and in infants born of women with high genital GBS inoculum, intrapartum fever, chorioamnionitis, or GBS bacteriuria. A low or an absent concentration of serotype-specific serum antibody also is a predisposing factor. Other risk factors are maternal age younger than 20 years and African American ethnicity. The period of communicability is unknown but may extend throughout the duration of colonization or of disease. Infants can remain colonized for several months after birth and after treatment for symptomatic infection. Recurrent GBS disease affects an estimated 1% of appropriately treated infants.

The **incubation period** of early-onset disease is less than 6 days. In late-onset disease, the incubation period from GBS acquisition to disease is unknown. Onset usually occurs from 7 days to 3 months of age, but up to 10% of pediatric cases occur beyond early infancy.

DIAGNOSTIC TESTS: Gram-positive cocci in fluids that ordinarily are sterile (such as cerebrospinal, pleural, or joint fluid) provide presumptive evidence of infection. Cultures of blood or body fluids are necessary to establish the diagnosis. Serotype identification is available in reference laboratories. Rapid tests that identify group B streptococcal antigen in body fluids other than cerebrospinal fluid (CSF) are not recommended.

TREATMENT:

- Ampicillin plus an aminoglycoside is the initial treatment of choice for a newborn infant with presumptive, invasive infection with GBS.
- Penicillin G alone can be given when GBS has been identified as the cause of the infection and when clinical and microbiologic responses have been documented. Some experts advise determination of the susceptibility of the organism to penicillin, especially for CSF isolates.
- For infants with meningitis due to GBS, the recommended dosage of penicillin G for infants 7 days of age or younger is 250 000 to 450 000 U/kg per day intravenously in 3 divided doses; for infants older than 7 days of age, 450 000 U/kg per day intravenously in 4 divided doses is recommended. For ampicillin, the recommended dosage for infants with meningitis age 7 days of age or younger is 200 to 300 mg/kg per day intravenously in 3 divided doses; for infants older than 7 days of age, 300 mg/kg per day in 4 to 6 divided doses is recommended.
- For meningitis, some experts believe that a second lumbar puncture approximately 24 to 48 hours after initiation of therapy assists in management and prognosis. Additional lumbar punctures and other studies often are indicated if response to therapy is in doubt. Consultation with a specialist in pediatric infectious diseases may be useful.
- For infants with bacteremia without a defined focus, treatment should be continued for 10 days. For infants with uncomplicated meningitis, 14 days of treatment usually is satisfactory, but longer periods of treatment may be necessary for infants with prolonged or complicated courses. Osteomyelitis or ventriculitis requires treatment for 4 weeks. Treatment duration in all cases should be guided by the patient's clinical and bacteriologic responses.
- Because of the reported risk of coinfection, the twin, triplets, or any multiples of an index case with early- or late-onset disease should be observed carefully and evaluated and treated empirically for suspected systemic infection if any manifestations of illness occur.

ISOLATION OF THE HOSPITALIZED PATIENT: Standard precautions are recommended except during a nursery outbreak of disease due to GBS (see Control Measures, p 539).

CONTROL MEASURES:

Chemoprophylaxis. Recommendations for prevention of early-onset neonatal GBS infection are as follows:

- Obstetric care practitioners should adopt a strategy for prevention of early-onset GBS disease. Patients should be informed about the available strategies for prevention of GBS. Individual patient requests about GBS cultures should be honored.
- Regardless of the prevention strategy used, women should be managed as follows:
  - Women found to have symptomatic or asymptomatic GBS bacteriuria during pregnancy should be treated at diagnosis. Because such women usually have heavy GBS colonization, they also should receive intrapartum chemoprophylaxis.
  - Intrapartum chemoprophylaxis should be administered to women who previously have given birth to an infant with disease due to GBS; prenatal culture screening is unnecessary.
- Until further data become available to define the most effective prevention strategy, either of the following strategies is appropriate:
  1. *Screening-based Strategy Using Cultures*
     - All pregnant women at 35 to 37 weeks of gestation should be screened for vaginal and rectal GBS colonization. All women identified as GBS carriers by culture should be offered intrapartum chemoprophylaxis even if a risk factor is not present.
     - If the results of GBS cultures are not known at the onset of labor or rupture of membranes, intrapartum antimicrobial prophylaxis should be administered if one of the following is present: gestation of less than 37 weeks, rupture of membranes for 18 hours or longer, or a temperature of 38.0°C (100.4°F) or greater.
     - Culture techniques that maximize the likelihood of GBS recovery should be used. The optimal method for GBS screening is collection of 1 swab or 2 separate swabs of the distal vagina and anorectum followed by inoculation into selective broth medium, overnight incubation, and subculture onto solid blood agar medium.
     - Oral antimicrobial agents should *not* be used to treat women who are found to have GBS colonization during prenatal screening. Such treatment is ineffective for eliminating carriage or preventing neonatal disease.

  These recommendations are summarized in Figure 3.1, p 540.

  2. *Risk Factor–based Strategy*
     - A prevention strategy based on the presence of intrapartum risk factors without culture screening (eg, gestation of less than 37 weeks, duration of membrane rupture 18 hours or more, or temperature of 38°C [100°F] or greater) is an acceptable alternative to the culture-based strategy.

  These recommendations are summarized in Figure 3.2, p 541.
- For intrapartum chemoprophylaxis, intravenous penicillin G (5 million U initially and 2.5 million U every 4 hours) is the drug of choice. Intravenous

Figure 3.1. **Prevention strategy for early-onset group B streptococcal (GBS) disease using prenatal culture screening at 35 to 37 weeks of gestation. Plus sign indicates positive culture results; minus sign, negative culture results.**

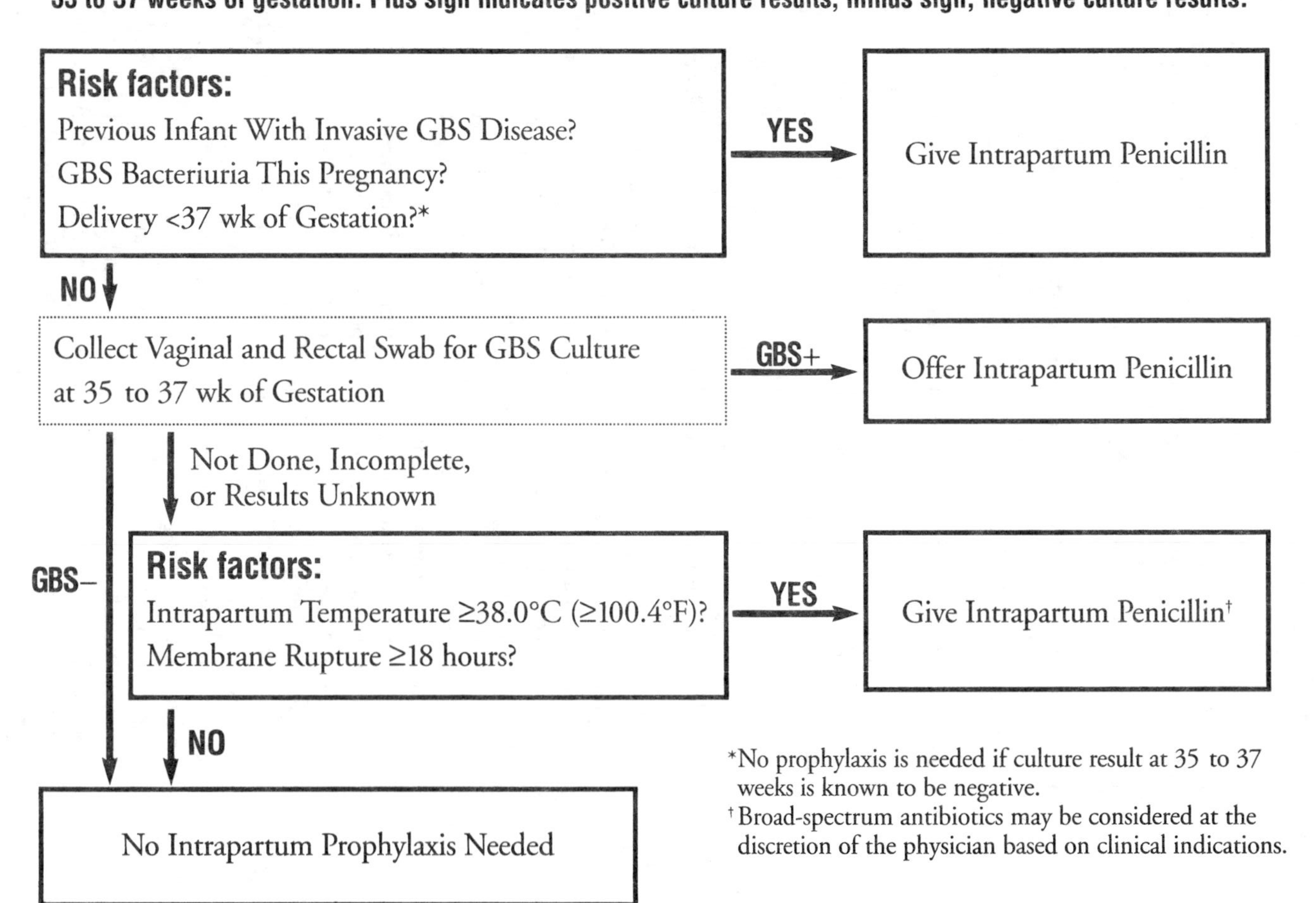

Risk factors:
Previous Infant With Invasive GBS Disease?
GBS Bacteriuria This Pregnancy?
Delivery <37 wk of Gestation?*
YES
Give Intrapartum Penicillin
NO
Collect Vaginal and Rectal Swab for GBS Culture at 35 to 37 wk of Gestation
GBS+
Offer Intrapartum Penicillin
Not Done, Incomplete, or Results Unknown
GBS–
Risk factors:
Intrapartum Temperature ≥38.0°C (≥100.4°F)?
Membrane Rupture ≥18 hours?
YES
Give Intrapartum Penicillin†
NO
No Intrapartum Prophylaxis Needed

*No prophylaxis is needed if culture result at 35 to 37 weeks is known to be negative.

†Broad-spectrum antibiotics may be considered at the discretion of the physician based on clinical indications.

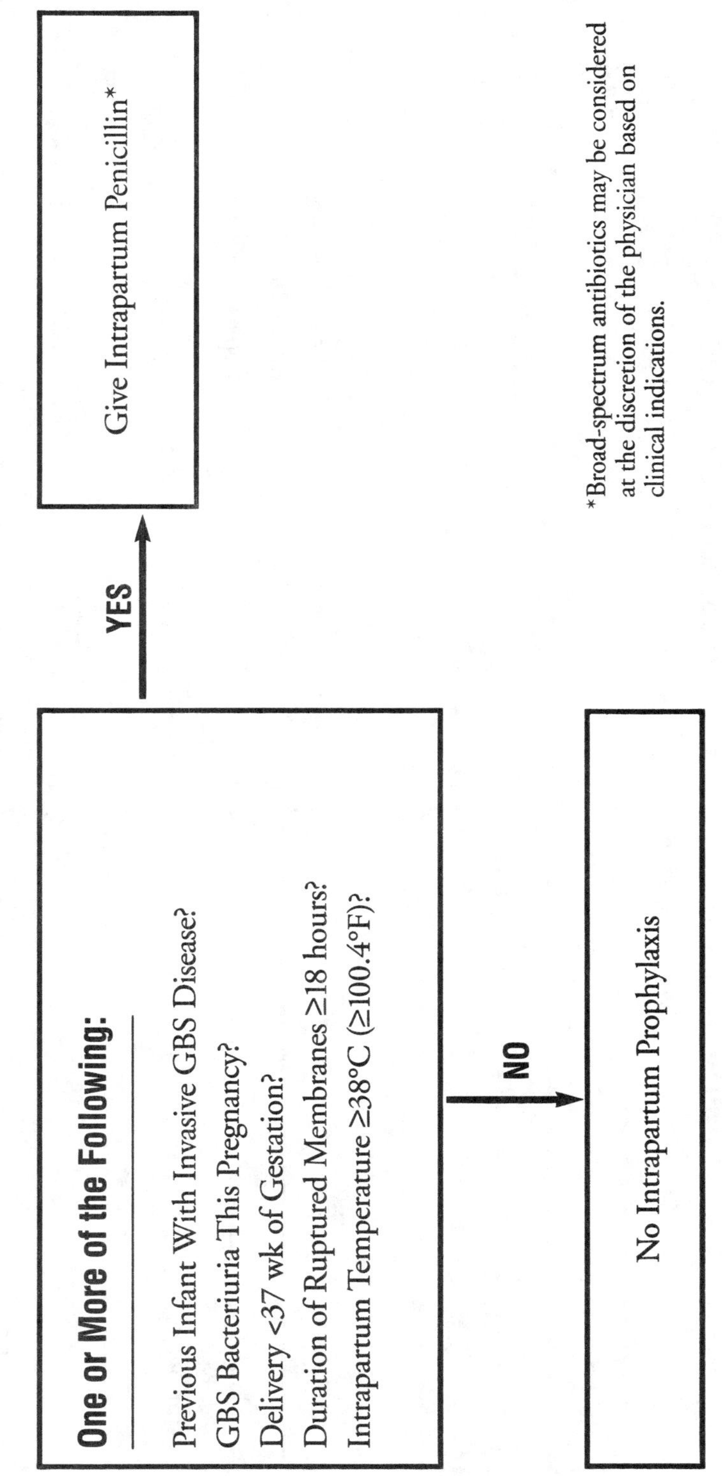
One or More of the Following:
Previous Infant With Invasive GBS Disease?
GBS Bacteriuria This Pregnancy?
Delivery <37 wk of Gestation?
Duration of Ruptured Membranes ≥18 hours?
Intrapartum Temperature ≥38°C (≥100.4°F)?
YES
Give Intrapartum Penicillin*
NO
No Intrapartum Prophylaxis
*Broad-spectrum antibiotics may be considered at the discretion of the physician based on clinical indications.

Figure 3.2. **Prevention strategy for early-onset group B streptococcal (GBS) disease using risk factors without prenatal culture screening.**

Fig 3.3. **Empiric management of a neonate born to a mother who received intrapartum antimicrobial prophylaxis (IAP) for prevention of early-onset group B streptococcal (GBS) disease.**

This algorithm is a suggested but is not an exclusive approach to management.

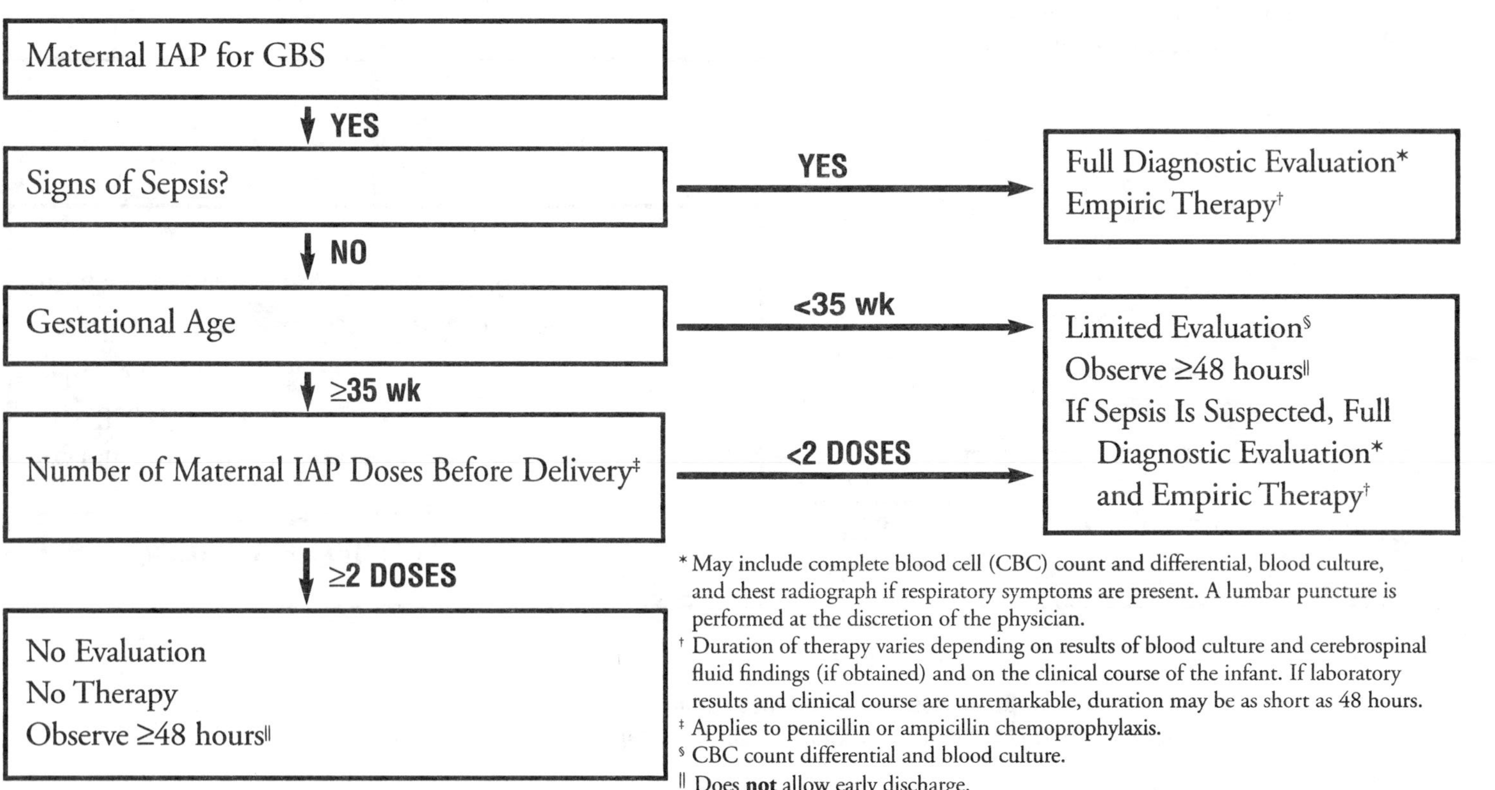

* May include complete blood cell (CBC) count and differential, blood culture, and chest radiograph if respiratory symptoms are present. A lumbar puncture is performed at the discretion of the physician.

† Duration of therapy varies depending on results of blood culture and cerebrospinal fluid findings (if obtained) and on the clinical course of the infant. If laboratory results and clinical course are unremarkable, duration may be as short as 48 hours.

‡ Applies to penicillin or ampicillin chemoprophylaxis.

§ CBC count differential and blood culture.

|| Does **not** allow early discharge.

ampicillin (2 g initially followed by 1 g every 4 hours until delivery) is an acceptable alternative, but penicillin G is preferred because it has a narrow spectrum and it is theoretically less likely to select for antibiotic-resistant organisms. Intravenous clindamycin, erythromycin, or a first-generation cephalosporin may be used for women allergic to penicillin. The number of doses of antibiotics received and the duration of intrapartum chemoprophylaxis are considered important factors in the prevention of early-onset infection. Controlled clinical trials have not been performed, but it seems that prophylaxis administered 4 or more hours before delivery (2 or more doses of penicillin or ampicillin) is more effective than prophylaxis administered for a shorter interval.

- Routine use of prophylactic antimicrobial agents for infants born to mothers who have received adequate intrapartum chemoprophylaxis is not recommended. However, therapeutic use of these agents is appropriate for infants with clinically suspected systemic infection. The duration of therapy in symptomatic infants varies depending on the results of laboratory evaluation and clinical course. If the laboratory evaluation and clinical course are inconsistent with a diagnosis of invasive infection, the duration of empiric therapy should be as short as 48 hours.
- Guidelines about management of asymptomatic infants born to women given intrapartum chemoprophylaxis are empiric. The following suggested approach is not an exclusive course of management. Other treatment modalities that consider individual circumstances and individual physician or institutional preferences may be appropriate.
  - For asymptomatic infants whose mothers have received intrapartum prophylaxis and for infants with gestations less than 35 weeks, a limited diagnostic evaluation (eg, complete blood cell count [and differential] and blood culture) should be performed, and the infants should be observed without antimicrobial therapy in the hospital for at least 48 hours. If, during observation, signs of systemic infection develop, a complete diagnostic evaluation should be performed, and antimicrobial therapy should be initiated.
  - In asymptomatic infants with a gestational age of 35 weeks or longer, the number of doses of intravenous intrapartum prophylaxis before delivery determines subsequent management. If 2 or more doses of maternal antibiotic were given before delivery, no laboratory evaluation or antimicrobial therapy is recommended. These infants should be observed in the hospital for at least 48 hours (ie, does not allow for early discharge). If only 1 dose of maternal prophylaxis was given before delivery, infants should undergo a limited evaluation and at least 48 hours of observation before hospital discharge.

These recommendations are summarized in Figure 3.3.

Studies designed to evaluate and compare these and other strategies are needed urgently to assess outcomes, including the incidence of neonatal disease due to GBS, occurrence of adverse reactions to antimicrobial prophylaxis, and the emergence of perinatal infections due to penicillin-resistant organisms. Characterization of prevention failures also is important.

Neonatal Infection Control. Routine cultures of infants to determine colonization with GBS are not recommended. Epidemiologic evaluation of late-onset cases in a special care nursery may be required to exclude a nosocomial source.

Nursery Outbreak. Placing ill and colonized infants in cohorts and the use of contact isolation during an outbreak are recommended. Other methods of control (eg, treatment of asymptomatic carriers with penicillin) are impractical or ineffective. Routine hand washing by personnel caring for infants colonized or infected with GBS is the best way to prevent spread to other infants.

Non–Group A or B Streptococcal and Enterococcal Infections

CLINICAL MANIFESTATIONS: Streptococci of groups other than A or B may be associated with invasive disease in newborn infants, older children, and adults. Urinary tract infection, endocarditis, upper and lower respiratory tract infections, and meningitis are the principal clinical syndromes.

ETIOLOGY: Streptococci of groups C and G and *Enterococcus* species are common pathogens. The two most common enterococcal species are *Enterococcus faecalis* and *Enterococcus faecium*. Streptococci belonging to groups D, F, H, and K also can be pathogens. Nongroupable streptococci, such as viridans and anaerobic streptococci (peptostreptococci), also can cause infections.

EPIDEMIOLOGY: The common habitats in humans of these streptococcal groups are skin (C, F, and G), oropharynx (C, F, G, H, and K), gastrointestinal tract (D, F, and G and *Enterococcus* species), and vagina (C, D, F, and G and *Enterococcus* species). The normal habitats of different species of viridans streptococci include the oropharynx, dental surfaces, skin, and genitourinary tract. Intrapartum transmission probably is responsible for most cases of early-onset neonatal infection. Environmental contamination or transmission via the hands of health care personnel can lead to colonization of patients.

The **incubation period** and the period of communicability are unknown.

DIAGNOSTIC TESTS: Microscopic examination of fluids that ordinarily are sterile can yield presumptive evidence of infections by gram-positive cocci. The diagnosis is established by culture and serogrouping of the isolate, using group-specific antisera. Identification of the species of enterococci may be useful to predict antimicrobial susceptibility. In addition, in some circumstances, biochemical testing may be necessary to accurately identify the organism. Antibiotic susceptibility testing of enterococci from sterile sites is important to determine ampicillin and vancomycin susceptibility, as well as gentamicin susceptibility for synergy. Some automated methods may not detect vancomycin resistance.

TREATMENT: Enterococci and occasional streptococcal strains are less susceptible to penicillin than are most streptococcal isolates. Enterococci are not susceptible to cephalosporins, and strains resistant to ampicillin and vancomycin have been identified. In invasive enterococcal infections, including endocarditis and meningitis, ampicillin or vancomycin in combination with an aminoglycoside (usually gentamicin), for possible synergy and for bactericidal activity, should be administered until in vitro susceptibility is known and appropriate combination therapy can be selected. The combination quinupristin/dalfopristin (Synercid) has been approved for adults for treatment of infections due to vancomycin-resistant *E faecium*. This compound is not effective against *E faecalis*. Combination therapy with ampicillin and gentamicin may be required for optimum treatment of severe infections due to groups C, F, and G. In other infections, penicillin G or ampicillin alone is sufficient.

Endocarditis. Guidelines for antimicrobial therapy in adults have been formulated by the American Heart Association and should be consulted for regimens that may be appropriate for children and adolescents.*

ISOLATION OF THE HOSPITALIZED PATIENT: Standard precautions are recommended. The exception is for patients with vancomycin-resistant enterococcal infection or colonization, for whom standard and contact precautions are indicated until the patient is no longer receiving antibiotics and culture results from multiple body sites (including stool or rectal swab, perineal area, axilla or umbilicus, wound, and indwelling urinary catheter or colostomy, sites if present) are negative on at least 3 separate occasions (more than 1 week apart).

CONTROL MEASURES: Patients with valvular or congenital heart disease should receive antimicrobial prophylaxis to prevent streptococcal and enterococcal endocarditis at the time of dental and selected other surgical procedures (see Prevention of Bacterial Endocarditis, p 735). Vancomycin use and use of broad-spectrum antibiotics are risk factors for colonization and infection with vancomycin-resistant enterococci. Hospitals should develop institution-specific guidelines for the proper use of vancomycin.†

Strongyloidiasis

(Strongyloides stercoralis)

CLINICAL MANIFESTATIONS: Eosinophilia can be the only manifestation of infection. Hence, strongyloidiasis warrants consideration whenever eosinophilia (>500/µL), without an obvious clinical correlation, occurs in a patient who has resided in an endemic area. Infective larvae first entering the body can produce transient pruritic papules at the site of penetration of the skin, usually on the feet. Larval migration through the lungs can cause pneumonitis with a cough productive of blood-streaked sputum. The intestinal phase of infection can be accompanied by vague abdominal pain, distention, vomiting, and diarrhea that consists of mucoid

* Wilson WR, Karchmer AW, Dajani AS, et al. Antibiotic treatment of adults with infective endocarditis due to streptococci, enterococci, staphylococci, and HACEK microorganisms. *JAMA.* 1995;274: 1706–1713

† Centers for Disease Control and Prevention: Recommendations for preventing the spread of vancomycin resistance: recommendations of the Hospital Infection Control Practices Advisory Committee (HICPAC). *MMWR Morb Mortal Wkly Rep.* 1995;44(RR-12):1–13

voluminous stools. Malabsorption has been reported. Larval migration from defecated stool can result in pruritic skin lesions in the perianal area, buttocks, and upper thighs. The lesions may present as migrating, pruritic, serpiginous, erythematous tracks called *cutaneous larva currens.* In immunocompromised patients, particularly those receiving corticosteroids, those who are malnourished, and those who are alcoholic, complications include disseminated strongyloidiasis (caused by hyperinfection), diffuse pulmonary infiltrates, and septicemia from gram-negative bacilli.

ETIOLOGY: *Strongyloides stercoralis* is a nematode (roundworm).

EPIDEMIOLOGY: Strongyloidiasis is endemic in the tropics and subtropics, including the southern and southwestern United States, wherever suitable moist soil and improper disposal of human waste coexist. Humans are the principal hosts. Dogs, cats, and other animals also can be reservoirs. Transmission involves penetration of the skin by infective larvae, either from contact with infected soil or autoinfection. Infections rarely can be acquired from intimate skin contact or from inadvertent coprophagy, such as from ingestion of contaminated food scavenged from garbage. Because some larvae mature into the infective forms in the colon, autoinfection can occur. Asymptomatic infection, especially in healthy hosts, is common. In immunocompromised patients, autoinfection is more frequent, resulting in disseminated strongyloidiasis wherein organs and tissues are hyperinfected with larvae, and the number of adult worms in the small intestine is high. In addition, because these larvae penetrate the wall of the colon, bacteremia and meningitis caused by enteric flora can occur. Immunosuppression induced by treatment with corticosteroids is the most common factor predisposing to hyperinfection. The period of communicability lasts as long as the patient is infected, which can be several decades.

The **incubation period** in humans is unknown.

DIAGNOSTIC TESTS: Stool examination may disclose the characteristic larvae, but several fresh stool specimens may need to be examined before a positive one is found. Stool concentration procedures may be required. Examination of duodenal contents obtained by a commercially available string test (Entero-test*) or a direct aspirate may demonstrate larvae. Serodiagnosis can be helpful but is available only in a few reference laboratories, and false-negative results occur. The enzyme immunoassay test for antibodies is positive in approximately 85% of infected people; however, cross-reaction with the antigens of filarial worms also occurs and limits the specificity of serodiagnosis. Eosinophilia (>500/µL) is common. In disseminated strongyloidiasis, larvae can be found in the sputum.

TREATMENT: Treatment with ivermectin, thiabendazole, or albendazole is curative in most patients, but none of these drugs are recommended for use during pregnancy. Side effects of nausea, vomiting, and malaise are common. If treatment is required for heavy infection in pregnancy, ivermectin or albendazole would be the drug of choice. Treatment may need to be repeated or prolonged in the hyperinfection syndrome or in immunocompromised patients. Relapses occur and should be treated.

---

* HDC Corporation, San Jose, Calif.

ISOLATION OF THE HOSPITALIZED PATIENT: Standard precautions are recommended.

CONTROL MEASURES: Sanitary disposal measures for human waste should be followed. Education about the risk of infection through bare skin is important.

For a patient who has an immunologic defect or who requires immunosuppressive therapy and is from an endemic region, examination of stool and, possibly, duodenal fluid and respiratory tract secretions for *S stercoralis* should be considered before immunosuppressive therapy is started. Serologic tests seem to be the most sensitive for diagnosis, but they do not distinguish between past and current infection, and results from a reference laboratory may not be available immediately. If a patient's status requires the initiation of immunosuppressive therapy before the results of diagnostic tests can be obtained, the risks of empiric antiparasitic therapy for strongyloidiasis must be weighed against the risks of a disseminated infection.

Syphilis

CLINICAL MANIFESTATIONS:

Congenital Syphilis. Infection can result in stillbirth, hydrops fetalis, or prematurity; at birth, infants may or may not have signs of disease or they may present up to 2 years of age with hepatosplenomegaly, snuffles, lymphadenopathy, mucocutaneous lesions, osteochondritis and pseudoparalysis, edema, rash, hemolytic anemia, and thrombocytopenia. Some infected infants who are asymptomatic, if untreated or inadequately treated, may develop these signs within the first weeks of life. Untreated infants, regardless of whether they have early manifestations, may develop late manifestations, which usually appear after 2 years of age and involve the central nervous system (CNS), bones and joints, teeth, eyes, and skin. Some consequences of intrauterine infection may not become apparent until many years after birth, such as interstitial keratitis (5 to 20 years), eighth cranial nerve deafness (10 to 40 years), anterior bowing of the shins, frontal bossing, mulberry molars, Hutchinson teeth, saddle nose, rhagades, and Clutton joints.

Acquired Syphilis. Infection can be divided into 3 stages. The primary stage appears as one or more painless indurated ulcers (chancre) of the skin and mucous membranes at the site of inoculation, most commonly on the genitalia. The secondary stage, beginning 1 to 2 months later, is characterized by a polymorphic rash that most frequently is maculopapular and generalized and classically includes the palms and soles. In moist areas around the vulva or anus, hypertrophic papular lesions (condyloma latum) can occur. Generalized lymphadenopathy, fever, malaise, splenomegaly, sore throat, headache, and arthralgia can be present. A variable latent period follows but sometimes is interrupted during the first few years by recurrences of symptoms of secondary syphilis. Latent syphilis is defined as the periods after infection when patients are seroreactive but demonstrate no other evidence of disease. Latent syphilis acquired within the preceding year is referred to as *early latent syphilis;* all other cases of latent syphilis are *late latent syphilis* or *syphilis of unknown* *duration.* The tertiary stage refers to gumma and cardiovascular syphilis but not to neurosyphilis. The tertiary stage can be marked by aortitis or gummatous changes of the skin, bone, or viscera, occurring from years to decades after the primary infection. Neurosyphilis occurs when there is evidence of CNS infection with *Treponema pallidum.* The various manifestations of neurosyphilis can occur in any stage, especially in persons infected with the human immunodeficiency virus (HIV).

ETIOLOGY: *Treponema pallidum* is a thin motile spirochete that is extremely fragile, surviving only briefly outside the host. The organism has not been cultivated successfully on artificial media.

EPIDEMIOLOGY: Syphilis, which is rare in much of the industrialized world, persists in the United States and in developing countries. The incidence of acquired and congenital syphilis increased dramatically in the United States during the late 1980s and early 1990s but subsequently declined in all areas, but the rates remain disproportionately high in large urban areas and the rural South of the United States. In adults, syphilis is more likely among persons with HIV infection in whom the risk of neurologic complications may be increased.

Congenital syphilis is contracted from an infected mother via transplacental transmission of *T pallidum* at any time during pregnancy or at birth. Among women with untreated early syphilis, 40% of pregnancies result in spontaneous abortion, stillbirth, or perinatal death. Infection can be transmitted to the fetus at any stage of disease; the rate of transmission is 60% to 100% during the secondary stage and slowly decreases with time. The moist secretions of congenital syphilis are highly infectious. Organisms rarely are found in lesions more than 24 hours after treatment has begun.

Acquired syphilis is contracted almost always through direct sexual contact with ulcerative lesions of the skin or mucous membranes of infected persons. Sexual abuse must be suspected in any young child with acquired syphilis. Open moist lesions of the primary or secondary stages are highly infectious. Relapses with infectious mucocutaneous lesions of secondary syphilis can occur up to 4 years later.

The **incubation period** for acquired primary syphilis typically is 3 weeks but ranges from 10 to 90 days after exposure.

DIAGNOSTIC TESTS: Definitive diagnosis is achieved by identifying spirochetes by microscopic darkfield examination or direct fluorescent antibody tests of lesion exudate or tissue, such as placenta or umbilical cord. Specimens should be scraped from moist mucocutaneous lesions or aspirated from a regional lymph node. Since false-negative microscopic results are common, serologic testing, follow-up, and, often, repeated testing are necessary. Specimens from mouth lesions require direct fluorescent antibody (DFA-TP) techniques to distinguish *T pallidum* from nonpathogenic treponemes. Polymerase chain reaction tests and immunoglobulin (Ig) M immunoblotting have been developed but are not yet available commercially.

Presumptive diagnosis is possible using 2 types of serologic tests: (1) nontreponemal tests and (2) treponemal tests. The use of only 1 type of test is insufficient for diagnosis because of false-positive nontreponemal test results that occur in various medical conditions and false-positive treponemal test results that occur in other spirochetal diseases.

The standard nontreponemal tests for syphilis include the VDRL slide test, the rapid plasma reagin (RPR), and the automated reagin test (ART). These tests measure antibody directed against lipoidal antigen from *T pallidum,* antibody interaction with host tissues, or both. These tests are inexpensive, rapidly performed, and provide quantitative results, which are helpful indicators of disease activity and useful to monitor the response to treatment. Nontreponemal test results may be falsely negative, ie, nonreactive, in early primary syphilis, latent acquired syphilis of long duration, and late congenital syphilis. Occasionally, a nontreponemal test performed on serum samples containing high concentrations of antibody against *T pallidum* will be weakly reactive or falsely negative, a reaction termed the *prozone* phenomenon. This reaction usually can be detected by experienced laboratory technicians, and diluting the serum will result in a positive test result. When these tests are used to monitor treatment response, the same type of test (eg, VDRL, RPR, or ART) must be used throughout the follow-up period, preferably by the same laboratory so that results can be compared appropriately.

A reactive nontreponemal test from a patient with typical lesions indicates the need for treatment. However, any reactive nontreponemal test must be confirmed by one of the specific treponemal tests to exclude a false-positive test result, which can be caused by certain viral infections (eg, infectious mononucleosis, hepatitis, varicella, and measles), lymphoma, tuberculosis, malaria, endocarditis, connective tissue disease, pregnancy, abuse of injection drugs, or laboratory or technical error, or by Wharton jelly contamination when cord blood specimens are used. Treatment should not be delayed pending the treponemal test results in symptomatic patients or patients at high risk of infection. A sustained 4-fold decrease in titer of the nontreponemal test result after treatment demonstrates adequate therapy; a 4-fold titer increase after treatment suggests reinfection or relapse. The quantitative nontreponemal test result usually becomes nonreactive after successful therapy within 1 year in low titer (≤1:8) early (primary or secondary) syphilis and within 2 years in high titer early and congenital syphilis but may remain positive despite treatment in latent or tertiary syphilis (the "serofast" state).

Treponemal tests currently in use are the fluorescent treponemal antibody absorption (FTA-ABS) test and the microhemagglutination test for *T pallidum* (MHA-TP). Positive FTA-ABS and MHA-TP test results usually remain reactive for life, even after successful therapy. Treponemal test antibody titers correlate poorly with disease activity and should not be used to assess treatment response.

Treponemal tests also are not 100% specific for syphilis; positive reactions variably occur in patients with other spirochetal diseases, such as yaws, pinta, leptospirosis, rat-bite fever, relapsing fever, and Lyme disease. Nontreponemal tests can be used to differentiate Lyme disease from syphilis because the VDRL uniformly is nonreactive in Lyme disease.

Usually a serum nontreponemal test is obtained initially, and, if it is reactive, a treponemal test is performed. The probability of syphilis is high in a sexually active person whose serum is reactive on both nontreponemal and treponemal tests. Differentiating syphilis treated in the past from reinfection often is difficult unless the nontreponemal titer is known to be rising.

In summary, the nontreponemal antibody tests (VDRL, RPR, and ART) are useful for screening; the treponemal tests (FTA-ABS and MHA-TP) are used to establish a presumptive diagnosis. Quantitative nontreponemal antibody tests are used to assess the adequacy of therapy and to detect reinfection and relapse.

Cerebrospinal Fluid Tests. For evaluation of possible neurosyphilis, the VDRL test should be performed on cerebrospinal fluid (CSF). In addition to CSF VDRL testing, evaluation of CSF protein and cell count is used to assess the likelihood of CNS involvement. Some experts also use the FTA-ABS, believing it to be more sensitive although less specific than CSF VDRL testing for neurosyphilis. Fewer data exist for the MHA-TP on CSF, and none for the RPR; these tests should not be used for CSF evaluation. VDRL test results should be interpreted cautiously because a negative CSF VDRL test result does not exclude a diagnosis of neurosyphilis.

Testing During Pregnancy. All women should be screened serologically for syphilis early in pregnancy with a nontreponemal test (eg, VDRL or RPR) and preferably again at delivery. In areas of high prevalence and in patients considered at high risk for syphilis, a nontreponemal serum test at the beginning of the third trimester (28 weeks) also is indicated. For women treated during pregnancy, follow-up serologic testing is necessary to assess the efficacy of therapy. Low-titer nontreponemal antibody test results that are false-positive occasionally occur in pregnancy. The nontreponemal antibody test result should be confirmed as false-positive with a treponemal antibody test (eg, FTA-ABS). When a pregnant woman has a reactive nontreponemal test result and a persistently negative treponemal test result, a false-positive test is confirmed.

Evaluation of Newborn Infants for Congenital Infection. No newborn infant should be discharged from the hospital without determination of the mother's serologic status for syphilis. Testing of cord blood or an infant serum sample is inadequate for screening because these test results can be nonreactive when the mother is positive. All infants born to seropositive mothers require a careful examination and a quantitative nontreponemal syphilis test. The test performed on the infant should be the same as that performed on the mother to enable comparison of titer results.

An infant should be evaluated further for congenital syphilis if the infant is born to a mother with positive nontreponemal test results confirmed by a positive treponemal test result and if the mother has one or more of the following conditions:

- Syphilis untreated or inadequately treated or treatment not documented (see Treatment, p 552)
- Syphilis during pregnancy treated with a nonpenicillin regimen, such as erythromycin
- Syphilis during pregnancy treated with an appropriate penicillin regimen, but the expected decrease in nontreponemal antibody titer after therapy did not occur (ie, a 4-fold decrease after treatment of early (primary, secondary, or early latent syphilis), or high-titer syphilis (see p 554)
- Syphilis treated less than 1 month before delivery (since treatment failures occur, and the efficacy of treatment cannot be assumed)
- Syphilis treated before pregnancy, but with insufficient serologic follow-up to assess the response to treatment and current infection status
- Infants also need evaluation if the maternal titer has increased 4-fold or the infant titer is 4-fold greater than the mother's titer or if the infant is symptomatic

Evaluation for syphilis in an infant should include the following:

- Physical examination
- Quantitative nontreponemal and a treponemal serologic test for syphilis on the infant's serum sample (not on cord blood because false-positive and false-negative results can occur)
- If available, determination of antitreponemal IgM antibody by a testing method recognized by the Centers for Disease Control and Prevention as a standard or provisional method
- Cerebrospinal fluid VDRL, analysis for cells, and protein concentration
- Long-bone radiographs (unless the diagnosis has been otherwise established)
- Complete blood cell count and platelet count
- Other clinically indicated tests (eg, chest radiograph and liver function tests)

Pathologic examination of the placenta or umbilical cord using specific fluorescent antitreponemal antibody staining, if available, also is recommended.

A guide for interpretation of the results of nontreponemal and treponemal serologic tests is given in Table 3.55, p 552. Note that an infected infant's test may be reactive or nonreactive, depending on the timing of maternal and fetal infection, thus the emphasis on screening maternal blood. Conversely, transplacental transmission of nontreponemal and treponemal antibodies to the fetus can occur in a mother who has been treated appropriately for syphilis during pregnancy, resulting in positive test results in the uninfected newborn infant. The neonate's nontreponemal test titer in these circumstances usually reverts to negative in 4 to 6 months, whereas a positive FTA-ABS or MHA-TP test result from passively acquired antibody may not become negative for 1 year or longer.

In an infant with clinical or tissue findings suggestive of congenital syphilis, a positive nontreponemal test result on serum strongly supports the diagnosis regardless of the therapy the mother received during the pregnancy.

CSF Testing. Cerebrospinal fluid should be examined in all infants who are evaluated for congenital syphilis if the infant has any of the following: (1) abnormal physical examination findings consistent with congenital syphilis; (2) a serum quantitative nontreponemal titer that is 4-fold greater than the mother's; or (3) a positive darkfield or fluorescent antibody test result on body fluid(s) (see Evaluation of Newborn Infants for Congenital Infection, p 550). Cerebrospinal fluid also should be examined in all patients with suspected neurosyphilis or with acquired untreated syphilis of more than 1 year's duration. Abnormalities in CSF in patients with neurosyphilis include increased protein concentration and leukocyte cell count and a reactive VDRL. Some experts also use the FTA-ABS, believing it to be more sensitive but less specific than CSF VDRL testing for neurosyphilis. Because of the wide range of normal values for CSF cell counts and protein concentrations in the newborn infant, interpretation often is difficult. Normal values differ by gestational age and are higher in preterm infants. White blood cell counts as high as 25/µL and a protein level of 150 mg/dL might occur among normal neonates; some experts, however, recommend that lower values, ie, a white blood cell count of 5/µL and a protein concentration of 40 mg/dL be considered the upper limits of normal. A negative CSF VDRL test result or a negative CSF FTA-ABS test result does not

Table 3.55. **Guide for Interpretation of the Syphilis Serology of Mothers and Their Infants***

Nontreponemal Test (eg, VDRL, RPR, ART)		Treponemal Test (eg, MHA-TP, FTA-ABS)		
Mother	Infant	Mother	Infant	Interpretation†
−	−	−	−	No syphilis or incubating syphilis in the mother and infant or prozone phenomenon
+	+	−	−	No syphilis in mother (false-positive nontreponemal test with passive transfer to infant)
+	+ or −	+	+	Maternal syphilis with possible infant infection; or mother treated for syphilis during pregnancy; or mother with latent syphilis and possible infection of infant‡
+	+	+	+	Recent or previous syphilis in the mother; possible infection in infant
−	−	+	+	Mother successfully treated for syphilis before or early in pregnancy; or mother with Lyme disease, yaws, or pinta (ie, false-positive serology)

* RPR indicates rapid plasma reagin; ART, automated reagin test; MHA-TP, microhemagglutination test for *Treponema pallidum;* FTA-ABS, fluorescent treponemal antibody absorption; plus sign, reactive; and minus sign, nonreactive.

† Table presents a guide and not the definitive interpretation of serologic tests for syphilis in mothers and their newborn infants. Maternal history is the most important aspect for interpretation of test results. Factors that should be considered include the timing of maternal infection, the nature and timing of maternal treatment, quantitative maternal and infant titers, and serial determination of nontreponemal test titers in both mother and infant.

‡ Mothers with latent syphilis may have nonreactive nontreponemal tests.

exclude congenital neurosyphilis. If CSF test results cannot exclude infection in an infant evaluated for congenital syphilis, the infant should be treated. Other causes of elevated values also should be considered when an infant is being evaluated for congenital syphilis. In patients beyond the neonatal period, normal CSF findings differentiate latent syphilis from asymptomatic neurosyphilis in persons with acquired untreated syphilis of more than 1 year's duration.

Treatment: Parenteral penicillin G remains the preferred drug for treatment of syphilis at any stage. Recommendations for penicillin G and duration of therapy vary, depending on the stage of the disease and clinical manifestations. Parenteral penicillin G is the only documented effective therapy for patients who have neurosyphilis, congenital syphilis, or syphilis during pregnancy, and is strongly recommended for HIV-infected patients. Such patients should always be treated with penicillin, after desensitization for penicillin allergy if necessary, or should be managed in consultation with a specialist. If penicillin G cannot be obtained, alternate treatment recommendations can be found at: www.cdc.gov/nchstp/dstd/penicillinG.htm/.

Penicillin Allergy. Skin testing for penicillin hypersensitivity with the major and minor determinants can reliably identify persons at high risk for reacting to penicillin; currently, only the major determinant (penicilloyl-polylysine) and penicillin G are available commercially. Testing with the major determinant of penicillin G is estimated to miss 3% to 6% of penicillin-allergic patients who are at risk for serious or fatal reactions. Thus, a cautious approach to penicillin therapy is advised when the patient cannot be tested with all of the penicillin skin test reagents. An oral or intravenous desensitization protocol for patients with a positive skin test is available and should be done in a hospital setting.* Oral desensitization is regarded as safer and easier to perform. Desensitization usually can be completed in approximately 4 hours, after which the first dose of penicillin can be given.

Congenital Syphilis: Newborn Infants (see also Table 3.56, p 555). Infants should be treated for congenital syphilis if they have proven or probable disease, as is demonstrated by the following: (1) they have physical, laboratory, or radiographic evidence of active disease; (2) the placenta or umbilical cord is positive for treponemes using DFA-TP staining or darkfield test; (3) their CSF VDRL test result is reactive or the CSF cell count and/or protein concentration is abnormal (or uninterpretable due to blood contamination); or (4) their serum quantitative nontreponemal titer is at least 4 times higher than the mother's titer. Note, if the mother's titer is 4 times higher than that of the infant, congenital syphilis can still be present. When an infant warrants evaluation for congenital syphilis (see Evaluation of Newborn Infants for Congenital Infection, p 550), the infant should be treated if test results cannot exclude infection, if the infant cannot be evaluated fully, or if adequate follow-up cannot be assured.

In infants with proven or probable disease, aqueous crystalline penicillin G is preferred. The dosage should be based on chronologic, not gestational, age (Table 3.56, p 555). Alternatively, some experts recommend procaine penicillin G for treatment of congenital syphilis; however, adequate CSF concentrations may not always be achieved by this regimen. If more than 1 day of therapy is missed, the entire course should be restarted. Data supporting the use of ampicillin for the treatment of congenital syphilis are not available.

Infants born to mothers with syphilis who have received no treatment require evaluation and treatment. The infant may be asymptomatic and test results may be inconclusive, and yet the infant may have early syphilis; thus, treatment is required.

Asymptomatic infants are at minimal risk for syphilis if they are born to mothers who received appropriate penicillin treatment for syphilis more than 4 weeks before delivery and, in early or high-titer syphilis, responded with a documented 4-fold or greater decrease in their VDRL, RPR, or ART titer; or, in latent low-titer syphilis, the titers remained stable and low. Although a full workup may be unnecessary, these infants should be examined carefully, preferably monthly, until their nontreponemal

* Centers for Disease Control and Prevention. 1998 guidelines for treatment of sexually transmitted diseases. *MMWR Morb Mortal Wkly Rep.* 1998;47(RR-1):1–111

serologic test results are negative. If this is not possible, many experts would treat such infants with a single injection of benzathine penicillin.

Infants whose mothers received inadequate treatment for syphilis require special consideration. Maternal treatment for syphilis is deemed inadequate for this purpose in the following circumstances: (1) the mother's penicillin dose is unknown, undocumented, or inadequate; (2) the mother received erythromycin or any other nonpenicillin regimen during pregnancy for syphilis; (3) treatment was given within 30 days of the infant's birth; or (4) the mother's response to treatment of early or high-titer syphilis has not been established by demonstrating a 4-fold decrease in titer by nontreponemal serologic testing for syphilis.

Asymptomatic infants born to mothers whose treatment for syphilis may have been inadequate, as defined by one or more of these criteria, should be fully evaluated, including CSF examination (see Evaluation of Newborn Infants for Congenital Infection, p 550). Some experts would treat all such infants with aqueous crystalline penicillin G (or aqueous procaine penicillin G) for 10 days since physical examination and laboratory test results cannot reliably exclude the diagnosis in all cases. However, if the infant's physical examination, CSF findings, radiographs of long bones, and complete blood cell count with platelet count are normal, some experts would treat infants in the specific circumstances given in Table 3.56 (p 555) only with a single dose of 50 000 U/kg of benzathine penicillin G intramuscularly. In the case in which maternal response to treatment has not been demonstrated (eg, nontreponemal antibody titer has not decreased 4-fold) but the mother received an appropriate regimen of penicillin therapy more than 1 month before delivery, the infant's evaluation is normal, and both clinical and serologic follow-up can be ensured, some experts would give a single dose of benzathine penicillin G and continue to observe the infant.

Congenital Syphilis: Older Infants and Children. Since establishing the diagnosis of neurosyphilis is difficult, infants older than 4 weeks of age who possibly have congenital syphilis or who have neurologic involvement should be treated with aqueous crystalline penicillin, 200 000 to 300 000 U/kg per day intravenously (administered every 6 hours) for 10 days. This regimen also should be used to treat children older than 1 year of age who have late and previously untreated congenital syphilis. Some experts also suggest giving such patients benzathine penicillin G, 50 000 U/kg intramuscularly in 3 weekly doses following the 10-day course of intravenous aqueous penicillin. If the patient has minimal clinical manifestations of disease, the CSF examination is normal, and the CSF VDRL test result is negative, some experts would treat with 3 weekly doses of benzathine penicillin G, 50 000 U/kg intramuscularly.

Syphilis in Pregnancy. Regardless of the stage of pregnancy, patients should be treated with penicillin according to the dosage schedules appropriate for the stage of syphilis as recommended for nonpregnant patients. For women with early acquired syphilis, some experts recommend 2 doses of benzathine penicillin (2.4 million U intramuscularly) given 1 week apart, rather than 1 dose. For penicillin-allergic patients, no proven alternative therapy has been established. A pregnant woman with a history of penicillin allergy should be treated with penicillin after desensitization. In some patients, skin testing may be helpful. Desensitization should be performed

Table 3.56. **Recommended Treatment of Neonates (≤4 Weeks of Age) With Proven or Possible Congenital Syphilis**

Clinical Status	Antimicrobial Therapy*
Proven or highly probable disease†	Aqueous crystalline penicillin G 100 000–150 000 U/kg per day, administered as 50 000 U/kg per dose IV every 12 h during the first 7 d of life, and every 8 h thereafter for a total of 10 d **OR** Procaine penicillin G 50 000 U/kg per dose IM a day in a single dose for 10 d
Asymptomatic; normal CSF examination results, CBC, platelet count, and radiographic examination; and follow-up is certain with the following maternal treatment history:	
None or inadequate penicillin treatment,‡ undocumented, failed, or reinfected	Aqueous crystalline penicillin G, IV, for 10 to 14 d† **OR** Clinical, serologic follow-up, and benzathine penicillin G, 50 000 U/kg IM in a single dose
Adequate therapy but given less than 1 mo before delivery, mother's response to treatment is not demonstrated by a 4-fold decrease in titer of a nontreponemal serologic test, or erythromycin therapy	Clinical, serologic follow-up, and benzathine penicillin G, 50 000 U/kg IM in a single dose§

* See text for details. IV indicates intravenously; IM, intramuscularly; CSF, cerebrospinal fluid; and CBC, complete blood cell count.

† If more than 1 day of therapy is missed, the entire course should be restarted.

‡ See text for definition (includes those in whom sequential serologic tests on the mother do not demonstrate a 4-fold or greater decrease in a nontreponemal antibody titer). If any part of the infant's evaluation is abnormal or not done or if the CSF is uninterpretable, the 10-day course of penicillin is required.

§ Some experts recommend aqueous crystalline penicillin G as for proven or highly probable disease.

in consultation with a specialist and only in facilities where emergency assistance is available (see Penicillin Allergy, p 553).

Erythromycin or any other nonpenicillin treatment of syphilis during pregnancy cannot be considered reliable to cure infection in the fetus. Tetracycline is not recommended for pregnant women because of potential adverse effects on the fetus.

Early Acquired Syphilis (Primary, Secondary, Early Latent Syphilis). A single dose of benzathine penicillin G intramuscularly is the preferred treatment for children and adults (Table 3.57, p 556). All children should have a CSF examination before treatment to exclude a diagnosis of neurosyphilis. Evaluation of CSF in adolescents and adults is necessary only if clinical signs or symptoms of neurologic or

Table 3.57. **Recommended Therapy for Syphilis***

	Children	Adults
Primary, secondary, and early latent syphilis†	Benzathine penicillin G 50 000 U/kg IM, up to the adult dose of 2.4 million U in a single dose	Benzathine penicillin G 2.4 million U IM in a single dose **OR** *If allergic to penicillin and not pregnant,* Doxycycline 100 mg orally twice a day for 14 d **OR** Tetracycline 500 mg orally 4 times a day for 14 d
Late latent syphilis or latent syphilis of unknown duration	Benzathine penicillin G 50 000 U/kg IM, up to the adult dose of 2.4 million U, administered as 3 doses at 1-wk intervals (total 150 000 U/kg up to the adult dose of 7.2 million U)	Benzathine penicillin G 7.2 million U total, administered as 3 doses of 2.4 million U IM each at 1-wk intervals **OR** *If allergic to penicillin and not pregnant,* Doxycycline 100 mg orally twice a day for 4 wk **OR** Tetracycline 500 mg orally 4 times a day for 4 wk
Tertiary	...	Benzathine penicillin G 7.2 million U total, administered as 3 doses of 2.4 million U IM at 1-wk intervals
Neurosyphilis‡	Aqueous crystalline penicillin G 200 000 to 300 000 U/kg per day given every 4 to 6 h for 10 to 14 d in doses not to exceed the adult dose	Aqueous crystalline penicillin G 18-24 million U a day, administered as 3-4 million U IV every 4 h for 10-14 d **OR** Procaine penicillin 2.4 million U IM daily **PLUS** probenecid 500 mg orally 4 times a day, both for 10-14 d

* IM indicates intramuscularly; IV, intravenously.

† Early latent syphilis is defined as being acquired within the preceding year.

‡ Patients allergic to penicillin should be desensitized.

ophthalmic involvement are present. Neurosyphilis should be considered in the differential diagnosis of neurologic disease in HIV-infected persons.

For nonpregnant patients allergic to penicillin, doxycycline or tetracycline should be given for 14 days. The clinical experience with doxycycline is less, but patient adherence to a regimen requiring twice-a-day doses is likely to be better. Tetracycline or doxycycline should not be given to children younger than 8 years of age unless the benefits of therapy are greater than the risks of dental staining (see Antimicrobial Agents and Related Therapy, p 646). Drugs other than penicillin and tetracycline do not have proven efficacy in the treatment of syphilis. Single-dose therapy with ceftriaxone is not effective. For nonpregnant, penicillin-allergic patients, if follow-up can be ensured, erythromycin (500 mg orally 4 times a day) for 14 days, or ceftriaxone regimens of 8 to 10 days, in consultation with an expert, can be given. When follow-up cannot be ensured, especially for children younger than 8 years of age, consideration must be given to hospitalization and desensitization followed by administration of penicillin G (see Penicillin Allergy, p 553).

Syphilis of More Than 1 Year's Duration (Except Neurosyphilis). Benzathine penicillin G should be given intramuscularly, weekly for 3 successive weeks (Table 3.57, p 556). In patients who are allergic to penicillin, doxycycline or tetracycline for 4 weeks should be given only if a CSF examination has excluded neurosyphilis. Tetracycline or doxycycline should not be given to children younger than 8 years of age unless the benefits of therapy are greater than the risks of dental staining (see Antimicrobial Agents and Related Therapy, p 646). Testing of CSF VDRL, protein concentration, and cell count is mandatory for persons with suspected or symptomatic neurosyphilis, persons who have concurrent HIV infection, persons who have failed treatment, and persons receiving antimicrobial agents other than penicillin.

Neurosyphilis. The recommended regimen for adults is aqueous crystalline penicillin G, intravenously for 10 to 14 days (Table 3.57, p 556). If compliance with therapy can be assured, patients may be treated with an alternative regimen of procaine penicillin plus probenecid, both for 10 to 14 days. Some experts recommend following this regimen with a single dose of benzathine penicillin G, 2.4 million U intramuscularly. For children, aqueous crystalline penicillin G for 10 to 14 days, in doses not to exceed the adult dose, is recommended, possibly followed by a single dose of benzathine penicillin, 50 000 U/kg per dose (not to exceed 2.4 million U) in 3 weekly doses.

If the patient has a history of allergy to penicillin, consideration should be given to desensitization, and the patient should be managed in consultation with a specialist (see Penicillin Allergy, p 553).

Other Considerations.

- Mothers of infants with congenital syphilis should be tested for other sexually transmitted diseases (STDs) including gonorrhea, *Chlamydia trachomatis,* HIV, and hepatitis B virus infection. Because of lifestyle, the mother also may be at risk for hepatitis C virus infection.
- All recent sexual contacts of persons with acquired syphilis should be evaluated for other STDs, as well as for syphilis (see Control Measures, p 559).

- All patients with syphilis should be tested for other STDs, including HIV. Patients who have primary syphilis should be retested for HIV after 3 months if the first HIV test result was negative.
- For HIV-infected patients with syphilis, careful follow-up is essential. Patients infected with HIV who have early syphilis may be at increased risk for neurologic complications and higher rates of treatment failure with the currently recommended regimens. Nevertheless, such risk, although not precisely defined, is probably small. No therapy, however, has been demonstrated to be more effective for preventing development of neurosyphilis than that recommended for patients without HIV infection.

Follow-up and Retreatment.

Congenital Syphilis. Treated infants should have careful follow-up evaluations at 1, 2, 3, 6, and 12 months of age. Serologic nontreponemal tests should be performed 3, 6, and 12 months after conclusion of treatment or until results become nonreactive. Nontreponemal antibody titers should decline by 3 months of age and should be nonreactive by 6 months of age if the infant were adequately treated or not infected and the initially positive serologic test result reflected transplacentally acquired maternal antibody. Patients with increasing titers or with persistent stable titers, including those with low titers at 6 to 12 months of age should be evaluated and considered for retreatment.

Treated infants with congenital neurosyphilis and initially positive CSF VDRL test results or abnormal or uninterpretable CSF cell counts and/or protein concentrations should undergo repeated clinical evaluation and CSF examination at 6-month intervals until their CSF examination is normal. A reactive CSF VDRL test result at the 6-month interval is an indication for retreatment. If cell counts are still abnormal at 2 years or are not decreasing at each examination, retreatment is indicated.

Early Acquired Syphilis. Treated pregnant women with syphilis should have quantitative nontreponemal serologic tests performed monthly for the remainder of their pregnancy. Other patients with early acquired syphilis should return for repeated quantitative nontreponemal tests at 3, 6, and 12 months after the conclusion of treatment. Patients with syphilis for more than 1 year should also undergo serologic testing 24 months after treatment. Careful follow-up serologic testing is particularly important for patients treated with antimicrobial agents other than penicillin.

Retreatment. In the following circumstances, retreatment is indicated.

- The clinical signs or symptoms of syphilis persist or recur.
- A 4-fold increase in the titer of a nontreponemal test occurs.
- An initially high-titer nontreponemal test fails to decrease 4-fold within 6 months.
- In a pregnant woman with high-titer (>1:8) syphilis, the nontreponemal test titer fails to decrease 4-fold within a 3- to 6-month period.
- In a pregnant woman with low-titer primary or secondary syphilis, the nontreponemal test titer fails to decrease 4-fold by delivery.

Retreated patients should be treated with the schedules recommended for patients with syphilis for more than 1 year. In general, only 1 retreatment course is indicated. The possibility of reinfection or concurrent HIV infection always should be considered when retreating patients with early syphilis.

The CSF should be examined before retreatment unless evidence indicates that the patient has been reinfected and again requires treatment for early syphilis. Patients with neurosyphilis must have periodic serologic testing, clinical evaluation at 6-month intervals, and repeated CSF examinations for at least 3 years or until CSF examination is normal.

Isolation of the Hospitalized Patient: Standard precautions are recommended for all patients, including infants with suspected or proven congenital syphilis. However, in addition, for infants with suspected or proven congenital syphilis, parents, visitors, hospital personnel, and medical staff should use gloves when handling the infant until therapy has been administered for at least 24 hours. Because moist open lesions and possibly blood are contagious in all patients with syphilis, these precautions also are required for patients with primary and secondary syphilis with skin and mucous membrane lesions.

Control Measures:

- All women should be screened for syphilis early in pregnancy and preferably at delivery. Women at high risk for syphilis also should be screened at 28 weeks (see p 550).
- Education about STDs, treatment of sexual contacts, reporting of each case to local public health authorities for contact investigation and appropriate follow-up, and serologic screening of high-risk populations are indicated.
- All recent sexual contacts of a person with acquired syphilis should be identified, examined, serologically tested, and treated appropriately. Sexual contacts within the last 3 months who are seronegative are at high risk for early syphilis and should be treated for early acquired syphilis. Every effort, including physical examination and serologic testing, should be made to establish a diagnosis in these patients.
- All persons, including hospital personnel, who have had close unprotected contact with a patient with early congenital syphilis before identification of the disease or during the first 24 hours of therapy should be examined clinically for the presence of lesions 2 to 3 weeks after contact. Serologic testing should be performed and repeated 3 months after contact or sooner if symptoms occur. If the degree of exposure is considered significant, immediate treatment should be considered.

Tapeworm Diseases

(Taeniasis and Cysticercosis)

CLINICAL MANIFESTATIONS:

Taeniasis. Mild gastrointestinal tract symptoms, such as nausea, diarrhea, and pain, can occur. Tapeworm segments can be seen migrating from the anus or feces.

Cysticercosis. Manifestations depend on the location and numbers of pork tapeworm cysts and the host response. Cysts may be found anywhere in the body. The most common and serious manifestations usually are caused by those in the central nervous system. Cysts of *Taenia solium* in the brain (neurocysticercosis) can cause seizures, behavioral disturbances, obstructive hydrocephalus, and other neurologic signs and symptoms. Neurocysticercosis can be a leading cause of epilepsy, depending on epidemiologic circumstances. The host reaction to degenerating cysts can produce signs and symptoms of meningitis. Cysts in the spinal column can cause gait disturbance, pain, or transverse myelitis. Subcutaneous cysts produce palpable nodules, and ocular involvement can cause visual impairment.

ETIOLOGY: Taeniasis is caused by intestinal infection by the adult tapeworm, *Taenia saginata* (beef tapeworm) or *T solium* (pork tapeworm). Usually only 1 adult worm is present in the intestine. Human cysticercosis is caused only by the larvae of *T solium (Cysticercus cellulosae).*

EPIDEMIOLOGY: These tapeworm diseases have worldwide distribution, and prevalence rates are high in areas with poor sanitation and human fecal contamination in areas where cattle graze or swine are fed. Most cases of *T solium* infection in the United States are imported from Mexico, Central and South America, Africa, Asia, Spain, and Portugal. High rates of *T saginata* infection also occur in Mexico, Argentina, Africa (especially Ethiopia), and central Europe. Taeniasis is acquired by eating undercooked beef *(T saginata)* or pork *(T solium)* that contains encysted larvae. Infection often is asymptomatic.

Cysticercosis is transmitted by fecal-oral contact by ingesting eggs of the pork tapeworm, *T solium,* either by heteroinfection from a contact harboring the adult tapeworm or by autoinfection. The eggs are found in human feces only, since humans are the only definitive host. The eggs liberate oncospheres in the intestine that migrate to tissues throughout the body, including the central nervous system where cysts form. Although most cases of cysticercosis in the United States have been imported from Mexico and Central and South America, cysticercosis in the United States can be acquired from index cases who recently immigrated from an endemic area and still have *T solium* intestinal stage infection.

The **incubation period** for taeniasis, the time from ingestion of the larvae until segments are passed in the feces, is 2 to 3 months. For cysticercosis, it is months to years.

DIAGNOSIS: Diagnosis of taeniasis (adult tapeworm infection) is based on demonstration of the proglottids or ova in feces or the perianal region. Species identification of the parasite is based on the different structures of the terminal gravid segments. Diagnosis of neurocysticercosis is based primarily on computed tomography (CT) or magnetic resonance imaging (MRI). Enhanced CT may be helpful for identifying spinal and intraventricular lesions. The enzyme immunotransfer blot assay to detect serum and cerebrospinal fluid (CSF) antibody to *T solium* is the antibody test of choice and is available through the Centers for Disease Control and Prevention. The test is more sensitive with serum samples than with CSF specimens. The serum antibody assay results often are negative in children with solitary parenchymal lesions but usually are positive in patients with multiple inflamed lesions.

TREATMENT:

Taeniasis. Praziquantel is highly effective for eradicating infection with the adult tapeworm.

Cysticercosis. Neurocysticercosis treatment should be individualized based on whether cysts are nonviable or active, which usually can be assessed by neuroimaging studies (MRI or CT), and where they are located. For patients with only nonviable cysts (eg, only calcifications on CT scan), management should be symptomatic and include anticonvulsants for patients with seizures and shunting for patients with hydrocephalus. There is no consensus on the role of antiparasitic drugs for patients with parenchymal cysts and inflammation (seen as ring enhancement on neuro-imaging). Two antiparasitic drugs are available, albendazole (15 mg/kg per day with a maximum of 800 mg given for 8 or more days) and praziquantel (50–100 mg/kg per day for 15 or more days). Although both drugs are taeniacidal and hasten radio-logic resolution of cysts, symptoms seem to result from the host inflammatory response and may be exacerbated by treatment. In some clinical trials, patients treated with albendazole had better radiologic and clinical responses than those treated with low doses of praziquantel. However, neither drug has been proven better than placebo in controlled trials. Some clinicians strongly favor the use of antiparasitic drugs in all cases. Coadministration of corticosteroids for the first 2 to 3 days of therapy is common to decrease adverse effects. Other clinicians note excel-lent clinical responses in patients with parenchymal disease treated symptomatically. Corticosteroids are indicated for all patients with multiple cysts and associated cere-bral edema ("cysticercal encephalitis"). Antiparasitic therapy should be deferred until cerebral edema is controlled.

Seizures may recur for months and will require anticonvulsant medication until patients demonstrate neuroradiologic evidence of resolution and they have been seizure free for 1 to 2 years. Calcification of cysts may require the indefinite use of anticonvulsants. Intraventricular cysts and hydrocephalus usually require surgical therapy and often placement of intraventricular shunts. Adjunctive chemotherapy with antiparasitic agents and corticosteroids can reduce the rate of subsequent shunt failure. Ocular cysticercosis also is treated by surgical excision of the cysts, but not usually with antihelmintic drugs, which could exacerbate ocular inflammation.

ISOLATION OF THE HOSPITALIZED PATIENT: Standard precautions are recommended.

CONTROL MEASURES: Eating raw or undercooked beef or pork should be avoided. Persons known to harbor the adult tapeworm of *T solium* should be treated immediately and use careful hand washing and care in the disposal of fecal material.

Stool examination of food handlers who recently have emigrated from endemic countries for detection of eggs and proglottids is advisable. Persons traveling to developing countries with high endemic rates of cysticercosis should avoid eating uncooked vegetables and fruits that cannot be peeled.

Other Tapeworm Infections
(Including Hydatid Disease)

Ingestion of certain cestode (tapeworm) eggs or accidental contact with certain larval forms can lead to tissue infection. Most infections are asymptomatic, but nausea, abdominal pain, and diarrhea have been observed in persons who are heavily infested.

Hymenolepis nana. This tapeworm, also called dwarf tapeworm because it is the smallest of the adult tapeworms, has its entire cycle within humans. Therefore, person-to-person transmission is possible. More problematic is autoinfection, which tends to perpetuate the infection in the host because the eggs can hatch within the intestine and reinitiate the cycle, leading to development of new worms and a large worm burden. This cycle makes eradicating the infection with praziquantel difficult. For that reason, higher-than-usual doses are required. If infection persists after treatment, retreatment with praziquantel is indicated.

Dipylidium caninum. This tapeworm is the most common and widespread adult tapeworm of dogs and cats. *Dipylidium caninum* infects children when they inadvertently swallow a dog or cat flea, which serves as the intermediate host. Diagnosis is made by finding the characteristic eggs or tapeworm segments in stool. Therapy with praziquantel or niclosamide is effective.

Diphyllobothrium latum *(and related species).* This tapeworm, also called fish tapeworm, has fish as one of its intermediate hosts. Consumption of infected, raw, freshwater fish (including salmon) leads to the infection. Three to 5 weeks are needed for the adult tapeworm to mature and begin to lay eggs. The worm sometimes causes mechanical obstruction of the bowel, diarrhea, abdominal pain, or megaloblastic anemia secondary to vitamin B_{12} deficiency. The diagnosis is made by recognition of the characteristic eggs or proglottids passed in stool. Therapy with praziquantel is effective. Hydroxocobalamin injections and folic acid supplements may be required.

Echinococcus granulosus *and* Echinococcus multilocularis. The larval forms of these tapeworms are the causes of hydatid disease. The distribution of *E granulosus* is related to sheep or cattle herding. Countries with the highest prevalence include Argentina, China, Greece, Italy, Lebanon, Romania, South Africa, Spain, Syria, Turkey, and the countries in the former Soviet Union. In the United States, small endemic foci exist in Arizona, California, New Mexico, and Utah, and a strain adapted to wolves, moose, and caribou occurs in Alaska and Canada. Dogs, coyotes, wolves, dingoes, and jackals can become infected by swallowing protoscolices of the parasite within hydatid cysts in the organs of sheep or other intermediate hosts. Dogs pass embryonated eggs in their stools, and sheep become infected by swallowing the eggs. If humans swallow *Echinococcus* eggs, they can become inadvertent intermediate hosts, and cysts can develop in various organs, such as the liver, lungs, kidney, and spleen. These cysts grow slowly (1 cm in diameter per year) and eventually can contain several liters of fluid. If a cyst ruptures, anaphylaxis and multiple secondary cysts from seeding of protoscolices can result. Clinical diagnosis frequently is difficult. A history of contact with dogs in an endemic area is helpful. Space-occupying lesions can be demonstrated by radiographs, ultrasonography, or computed tomography of various organs. Serologic tests, available at the Centers for Disease Control and Prevention, are helpful, but false-negative results can occur. Surgical treatment is indicated for some patients and requires meticulous care to prevent spillage of cyst contents. Injection of scolecidal solutions into the cyst before attempted removal can minimize the risk of dissemination if spillage occurs. Treatment with albendazole for several months is of benefit in many cases.

Echinococcus multilocularis, a species for which the life cycle involves foxes and rodents, causes the alveolar form of hydatid disease, which is characterized by invasive growth of the larvae in the liver with occasional metastatic spread. The alveolar form of hydatid disease is limited to the northern hemisphere and usually is diagnosed in persons 50 years of age or older. The preferred treatment is surgical extirpation of the entire larval mass. In nonresectable cases, continuous treatment with mebendazole or albendazole has been associated with clinical improvement.

ISOLATION OF THE HOSPITALIZED PATIENT: Standard precautions are recommended.

CONTROL MEASURES:

Preventive measures for *H nana* include educating the public about personal hygiene and sanitary disposal of feces.

Infection with *D caninum* is prevented by keeping dogs and cats free of fleas and worms.

Thorough cooking of freshwater fish (56°C [133°F] for 5 minutes) or freezing for 24 hours at −18°C (0°F) or irradiation ensures protection from *D latum.*

Control measures for prevention of *E granulosus* and *E multilocularis* include educating the public about good hand washing and about avoiding exposure to dog feces. Prevention and control of the infection in dogs decreases the risk.

Tetanus

(Lockjaw)

CLINICAL MANIFESTATIONS: Generalized tetanus (lockjaw) is a neurologic disease manifested by trismus and severe muscular spasms. Tetanus is caused by the neurotoxin produced by the anaerobic bacterium, *Clostridium tetani,* in a contaminated wound. Onset is gradual, occurring over 1 to 7 days, and progresses to severe generalized muscle spasms, which frequently are aggravated by any external stimulus. Severe spasms persist for 1 week or more and subside in a period of weeks in those who recover. Neonatal tetanus, a common cause of neonatal mortality in developing countries but rare in the United States, arises from contamination of the umbilical stump.

Localized tetanus is manifested by local muscle spasms in areas contiguous to a wound. Cephalic tetanus is a dysfunction of the cranial nerves associated with infected wounds on the head and neck. Both conditions may precede generalized tetanus.

ETIOLOGY: *Clostridium tetani,* the tetanus bacillus, is a spore-forming, anaerobic, gram-positive bacillus. The vegetative form produces a potent plasmid-encoded exotoxin (tetanospasmin), which binds to gangliosides at the myoneural junction of skeletal muscle and on neuronal membranes in the spinal cord, blocking inhibitory pulses to motor neurons. The action of tetanus toxin on the brain and sympathetic nervous system is less well documented. *Clostridium tetani* is a wound contaminant; it causes neither tissue destruction nor an inflammatory response.

EPIDEMIOLOGY: Tetanus occurs worldwide and is more frequent in warmer climates and warmer months, in part because of the frequency of contaminated wounds. In the United States, fewer than 60 cases have been reported annually for the past 5 years. The organism, a normal inhabitant of soil and of animal and human intestines, is ubiquitous in the environment, especially where contamination by excreta is frequent. Wounds, recognized or unrecognized, are the sites at which the organism multiplies and elaborates toxin. Contaminated wounds, those with devitalized tissue and deep-puncture trauma, are at greatest risk. Neonatal tetanus is common in many developing countries where women are not immunized appropriately against tetanus and nonsterile umbilical cord–care practices are followed. Widespread active immunization against tetanus has modified the epidemiology of the disease in the United States. Tetanus is not transmissible from person to person.

The **incubation period** ranges from 2 days to months, with most cases occurring within 14 days. In neonates, the incubation period is usually 5 to 14 days. Shorter incubation periods have been associated with more heavily contaminated wounds, more severe disease, and a worse prognosis.

DIAGNOSTIC TESTS: The offending wound should be cultured. However, confirmation of the causative organism is made infrequently by culture. The diagnosis is made clinically by excluding other possibilities, such as hypocalcemic tetany, phenothiazine reaction, strychnine poisoning, and hysteria.

TREATMENT:

- Tetanus Immune Globulin (human) (TIG) is recommended for treatment. A single total dose of 3000 to 6000 U is recommended for children and adults. The optimum therapeutic dose, has not yet been established, and doses as small as 500 U have been effective in treatment of infants with tetanus neonatorum. Available preparations must be given intramuscularly. Some authorities recommend infiltration of part of the dose locally around the wound, although the efficacy of this approach has not been proven. Results of studies on the benefit from intrathecal TIG are conflicting. The TIG formulation in use in the United States is not licensed or appropriate for intrathecal or intravenous use.
- In countries where TIG is not available, equine tetanus antitoxin may be available. This product is no longer available in the United States. Tetanus

antitoxin is administered as a single dose of 50 000 to 100 000 U after appropriate testing for sensitivity and desensitization if necessary (see Sensitivity Tests for Reactions to Animal Sera, p 48, and Desensitization to Animal Sera, p 49). Part of this dose (20 000 U) should be given intravenously. Doses as small as 10 000 U may be as effective as larger doses.

- Immune Globulin Intravenous contains antibodies to tetanus and can be considered for treatment if TIG is not available. Approval by the US Food and Drug Administration has not been given for this use, and the dosage has not been determined.
- All wounds should be properly cleaned and débrided, especially if extensive necrosis is present. In neonatal tetanus, wide excision of the umbilical stump is not indicated.
- Supportive care and pharmacotherapy to control tetanic spasms are of major importance.
- Oral (or intravenous) metronidazole (30 mg/kg per day, given at 6-hour intervals) is effective in reducing the number of vegetative forms of *C tetani* and is the antibiotic of choice. Parenteral penicillin G (100 000 U/kg per day, given at 4- to 6-hour intervals) is an alternative treatment. Therapy for 10 to 14 days is recommended.

ISOLATION OF THE HOSPITALIZED PATIENT: Standard precautions are recommended.

CONTROL MEASURES:

Care of Exposed Persons (see Table 3.58, p 566). Fewer than 1% of the recently reported cases of tetanus in the United States have occurred in persons with adequate, up-to-date immunization. After primary immunization with tetanus toxoid, antitoxin persists at protective levels in most persons for at least 10 years and for a longer time after a booster immunization.

- The use of tetanus toxoid and TIG or antitoxin in the management of wounds depends on the nature of the wound and the history of immunization with tetanus toxoid as described in Table 3.58.
- While any open wound is a potential source of tetanus, wounds contaminated with dirt, feces, soil, or saliva are at increased risk. Wounds containing devitalized tissue, including necrotic or gangrenous wounds, frostbite, crush and avulsion injuries, and burns, are particularly prone to contamination with *C tetani.*
- If tetanus immunization is incomplete at the time of wound treatment, a dose of vaccine should be given, and the immunization series should be completed according to the primary immunization schedule. Tetanus Immune Globulin should be administered for tetanus-prone wounds in patients infected with the human immunodeficiency virus, regardless of the history of tetanus immunizations.
- In usual practice, when tetanus toxoid is required for wound prophylaxis in a child 7 years of age or older, the use of adult-type diphtheria and tetanus toxoids (dT) instead of tetanus toxoid alone is advisable so that diphtheria immunity also is maintained. When a booster injection is indicated for wound

Table 3.58. **Guide to Tetanus Prophylaxis in Routine Wound Management**

History of Absorbed Tetanus Toxoid (Doses)	Clean, Minor Wounds dT[†]	TIG[‡]	All Other Wounds* dT[†]	TIG[‡]
Unknown or <3	Yes	No	Yes	Yes
≥3[§]	No[‖]	No	No[¶]	No

* Such as, but not limited to, wounds contaminated with dirt, feces, soil, and saliva; puncture wounds; avulsions; and wounds resulting from missiles, crushing, burns, and frostbite.

† For children younger than 7 years of age, diphtheria and tetanus toxoids and acellular pertussis vaccine (DTaP) is recommended; if pertussis vaccine is contraindicated, DT is given. For persons 7 years of age or older, dT is recommended. dT indicates adult-type diphtheria and tetanus toxoids; TIG, tetanus immune globulin (human).

‡ Equine tetanus antitoxin should be used when TIG is not available.

§ If only 3 doses of fluid toxoid have been received, a fourth dose of toxoid, preferably an adsorbed toxoid, should be given. Although licensed, fluid tetanus toxoid is rarely used.

‖ Yes, if more than 10 years since last dose.

¶ Yes, if more than 5 years since last dose. More frequent boosters are not needed and can accentuate adverse effects.

prophylaxis in a child younger than 7 years of age, diphtheria and tetanus toxoids and acellular pertussis vaccine (DTaP) should be used unless pertussis vaccine is contraindicated (see Pertussis, p 435), in which case immunization with diphtheria and tetanus toxoids (DT) is recommended.

- When TIG is required for wound prophylaxis, it is given intramuscularly in a dose of 250 U. Equine tetanus antitoxin is recommended if TIG is unavailable; the dose is 3000 to 5000 U intramuscularly, after appropriate testing of the patient for sensitivity (see Sensitivity Tests for Reactions to Animal Sera, p 48). If tetanus toxoid and TIG or equine tetanus antitoxin are given concurrently, separate syringes and sites should be used. Administration of TIG or equine tetanus antitoxin does not preclude initiation of active immunization with tetanus toxoid. Efforts should be made to initiate immunization and arrange for its completion.
- Regardless of immunization status, dirty wounds should be properly cleaned and débrided if dirt or necrotic tissue is present. Wounds should receive prompt surgical treatment to remove all devitalized tissue and foreign material as an essential part of tetanus prophylaxis. It is not necessary or appropriate to extensively débride puncture wounds.

Immunization. Active immunization with tetanus toxoid is indicated for all persons. For all indications, tetanus immunization is administered with diphtheria toxoid–containing vaccines. Vaccine is given intramuscularly and may be given concurrently with other vaccines (see Simultaneous Administration of Multiple Vaccines, p 26). *Haemophilus influenzae* type b conjugate vaccines containing tetanus toxoid (PRP-T) are not substitutes for tetanus toxoid immunization. Recommendations for use of tetanus and diphtheria toxoid–containing vaccines are summarized in Fig 1.1 (p 22) and Table 1.5 (p 24) are as follows:

- Immunization for children from 2 months of age to the seventh birthday (see Fig 1.1 and Table 1.5, p 22 and p 24) should consist of 5 doses of tetanus and diphtheria toxoid–containing vaccine. The initial 3 doses are given as

DTaP administered at 2-month intervals beginning at approximately 2 months of age. A fourth dose is recommended 6 to 12 months after the third dose, usually at 15 to 18 months of age (see Pertussis, p 435). An additional dose of DTaP is necessary before school entry (kindergarten or elementary school) at 4 to 6 years of age, unless the fourth dose was given after the fourth birthday. DTaP can be given concurrently with other vaccines (see Simultaneous Administration of Multiple Vaccines, p 26).

Immunization against tetanus and diphtheria for children younger than 7 years of age in whom pertussis immunization is contraindicated (see Pertussis, p 435) should be accomplished with DT instead of DTaP, as follows:

- For children younger than 1 year of age, 3 doses of DT are given at 2-month intervals; a fourth dose should be given 6 to 12 months after the third dose, and the fifth dose should be given before school entry at 4 to 6 years of age.
- For children 1 through 6 years of age who have not received prior doses of DT, DTaP, or diphtheria and tetanus toxoids and pertussis vaccine (DTP), 2 doses of DT approximately 2 months apart should be given, followed by a third dose 6 to 12 months later to complete the initial series. DT can be given concurrently with other vaccines. An additional dose is necessary before school entry at 4 to 6 years of age, unless the preceding dose was given after the fourth birthday.
- For children 1 through 6 years of age who have received 1 or 2 doses of DTaP, DTP, or DT during the first year of life and for whom further pertussis immunization is contraindicated, additional doses of DT should be given until a total of 5 doses of diphtheria and tetanus toxoids are received by the time of school entry. The fourth dose is administered 6 to 12 months after the third dose. The preschool (fifth) dose is omitted if the fourth dose was given after the fourth birthday.
- For children who have received fewer than the recommended number of doses of pertussis vaccine but who have received the recommended number of DT doses for their age (ie, those in whom immunization was started with DT and who were then given DTaP [or DTP]), dose(s) of DTaP should be given to complete the recommended pertussis immunization schedule (see Pertussis, p 435). However the total number of doses of diphtheria and tetanus toxoids (as DT, DTaP, or DTP) should not exceed 6 before the fourth birthday.

Other recommendations for tetanus and diphtheria immunization, including those for older children, are as follows:

- For children after their seventh birthday (see Table 1.5, p 24), tetanus immunization should consist of dT, ie, adult-type diphtheria and tetanus toxoids. The dT preparation contains not more than 2 Lf (flocculation units) of diphtheria toxoid per dose, compared with 6.7 to 25.0 Lf per dose in the DTaP and DT preparations for use in infants and younger children. Because of the lower dose of diphtheria toxoid, the dT vaccine is less likely than DTaP or DT to produce reactions in older children and adults. Two doses are given 1 to 2 months apart; a third dose should be given 6 to 12 months after the second.
- After the initial immunization series is completed at 4 to 6 years of age, a booster dose of diphtheria and tetanus toxoids (given as dT) is recommended at 11 to 12 years of age and should be given no later than by 16 years of age

and every 10 years thereafter. This 10-year period is determined from the time that the last dose was administered, irrespective of whether it was given earlier in routine childhood immunization or as part of wound management. Since the immunity conferred by absorbed preparations of tetanus toxoid has proved to be of long duration, routine boosters more frequently than every 10 years are not indicated and may be associated with an increased incidence and severity of reactions.

- If more than 5 years have elapsed since the last dose, a booster of dT should be considered for persons who are going on wilderness expeditions where tetanus boosters may not be readily available.
- Prevention of neonatal tetanus can be accomplished by prenatal immunization of the previously unimmunized mother. Pregnant women who have not completed their primary series should do so before delivery if time permits. If there is insufficient time, 2 doses of dT should be administered at least 4 weeks apart, and the second dose should be given at least 2 weeks before delivery. Immunization with tetanus toxoid or dT is not contraindicated during pregnancy.
- Active immunization against tetanus should always be undertaken during convalescence from tetanus because this exotoxin-mediated disease usually does not confer immunity.

Adverse Events, Precautions, and Contraindications. Severe anaphylactic reactions, Guillain-Barré syndrome (GBS), and brachial neuritis attributable to tetanus toxoid have been reported but are rare. No increased risk of GBS has been observed with use of DTaP vaccine in children, and, therefore, no special precautions are recommended when immunizing children with a history of GBS.

An immediate anaphylactic reaction to tetanus and diphtheria toxoid–containing vaccine (ie, DTaP, DT, or dT) is a contraindication to further doses unless the patient can be desensitized to these toxoids (see Pertussis, p 435). Because of uncertainty about which vaccine component (ie, diphtheria, tetanus, or pertussis) might be responsible and the importance of tetanus immunization, persons who experience anaphylactic reactions may be referred to an allergist for evaluation and possible desensitization.

Other Control Measures. Sterilization of hospital supplies will prevent the infrequent instances of tetanus that may occur in a hospital from contaminated sutures, instruments, or plaster casts.

For prevention of neonatal tetanus, preventive measures (in addition to maternal immunization) include community immunization programs for adolescent girls and women of childbearing age and appropriate training of midwives in recommendations for immunization and sterile technique.

Tinea Capitis
(Ringworm of the Scalp)

CLINICAL MANIFESTATIONS: Fungal infection of the scalp may present with one of the following distinct clinical syndromes:

- Patchy areas of dandruff-like scaling, with subtle or extensive hair loss, which easily is confused with dandruff, seborrheic dermatitis, or atopic dermatitis
- Discrete areas of hair loss studded by the stubs of broken hairs, which is referred to as *black-dot ringworm*
- Numerous discrete pustules or excoriations with little hair loss or scaling
- Kerion, a boggy inflammatory mass surrounded by follicular pustules, is a hypersensitivity reaction to the fungal infection. Kerion may be accompanied by fever and local lymphadenopathy and frequently is misdiagnosed as impetigo, cellulitis, or an abscess of the scalp.

A pruritic, fine, papulovesicular eruption (dermatophytid or id reaction) involving the trunk, hands, or face, caused by a hypersensitivity response to the infecting fungus, may accompany the scalp lesions.

Tinea capitis may be confused with many other diseases, including seborrheic dermatitis, atopic dermatitis, psoriasis, alopecia areata, trichotillomania, folliculitis, impetigo, and lupus erythematosus.

ETIOLOGY: *Trichophyton tonsurans* is the cause of tinea capitis in more than 90% of cases in North and Central America. *Microsporum canis, Microsporum audouinii,* and *Trichophyton mentagrophytes* are less common. The causative agents may vary in different geographic areas.

EPIDEMIOLOGY: Infection of the scalp with *T tonsurans* is the result of person-to-person transmission. This organism remains viable on combs, hairbrushes, couches, and sheets for long periods. Occasionally, *T tonsurans* is cultured from the scalps of asymptomatic children and is cultured readily from asymptomatic family members of infected persons. Persons who harbor the organism are thought to have a significant role as reservoirs for infection and reinfection within families, schools, and communities. Tinea capitis due to *T tonsurans* occurs most commonly in children between the ages of 3 and 9 years and seems to be more common in African American children.

Microsporum canis infection results from transmission from animals to humans. Infection frequently is the result of contact with household pets.

The **incubation period** is unknown.

DIAGNOSTIC TESTS: Hairs may be obtained by gentle scraping of a moistened area of the scalp with a curved scalpel, toothbrush, or cotton-tip applicator for potassium hydroxide wet mount examination and for culture. In black-dot ringworm, broken hairs should be obtained for diagnosis. In cases of *T tonsurans* infection, microscopic examination of a potassium hydroxide wet mount preparation will disclose numerous arthroconidia within the hair shaft. In *Microsporum* infection, spores surround the hair shaft. Use of dermatophyte test medium also is a reliable, simple, and inexpensive method of diagnosing tinea capitis. Skin scrapings, brushings, or hairs from lesions are inoculated directly onto the culture medium and incubated at room temperature. After 1 to 2 weeks, a phenol red indicator in the agar will turn from yellow to red in the area surrounding a dermatophyte colony. When necessary, the diagnosis also may be confirmed by culture on Sabouraud dextrose agar.

Wood's light examination of the hair of patients with *Microsporum* infection results in brilliant green fluorescence. However, because *T tonsurans* does not fluoresce under Wood's light, this diagnostic test is not helpful for most patients with tinea capitis.

TREATMENT: Topical antifungal medications are not effective for the treatment of tinea capitis. Tinea capitis requires systemic antifungal therapy. Microsize griseofulvin is given orally, 15 to 20 mg/kg per day (maximum 1 g) once daily. The dose of ultramicrosize griseofulvin is 5 to 10 mg/kg per day (maximum 750 mg) once daily. Optimally, griseofulvin is given after a meal containing fat (eg, peanut butter or ice cream). Treatment for 4 to 6 weeks usually is required and should be continued 2 weeks beyond clinical resolution. Some children may require higher doses of microsize griseofulvin (20 to 25 mg/kg per day) or the ultramicrosize drug formulation to achieve clinical cure. Treatment with oral itraconazole, oral terbinafine, or oral fluconazole also is effective for tinea capitis, but these products have not been approved by the US Food and Drug Administration for this indication. Selenium sulfide shampoo, either 1% or 2.5%, used twice a week, decreases fungal shedding and may help curb the spread of infection.

Kerion is treated with griseofulvin. Corticosteroid therapy consisting of prednisone or prednisolone given orally in dosages of 1.5 to 2 mg/kg per day may be used in addition. Treatment with corticosteroids should be continued for approximately 2 weeks, with tapering doses toward the end of therapy. Antibiotics and surgery are not indicated.

ISOLATION OF THE HOSPITALIZED PATIENT: Standard precautions are recommended.

CONTROL MEASURES: Early treatment of infected persons is indicated, as is examination of siblings and other household contacts for evidence of tinea capitis. Ribbons, combs, and hairbrushes should not be shared by family members.

Children receiving treatment for tinea capitis may attend school. Hair cuts, shaving of the head, or wearing a cap during treatment are unnecessary.

Tinea Corporis

(Ringworm of the Body)

CLINICAL MANIFESTATIONS: Superficial tinea infections of the nonhairy (glabrous) skin may involve the face, trunk, or limbs but not the scalp, beard, groin, hands, or feet. The lesion generally is circular (hence, the term "ringworm"), slightly erythematous, and well demarcated with a scaly, vesicular, or pustular border. Pruritus is common. Lesions often are mistaken for atopic dermatitis, seborrheic dermatitis, or contact dermatitis. A frequent source of confusion in diagnosis is an alteration in the appearance of lesions resulting from application of a topical corticosteroid preparation. This atypical presentation has been termed "tinea incognita." In patients with diminished T-lymphocyte function (eg, human immunodeficiency virus infection), the rash may appear as grouped papules or pustules unaccompanied by scaling or erythema.

A pruritic, fine, papulovesicular eruption (dermatophytid or id reaction) involving the trunk, hands, or face, caused by a hypersensitivity response to the infecting fungus, may accompany the rash.

ETIOLOGY: The prime causes of the disease are fungi of the genus *Trichophyton,* especially *Trichophyton rubrum, Trichophyton mentagrophytes,* and *Trichophyton tonsurans;* the genus *Microsporum,* especially *Microsporum canis;* and *Epidermophyton floccosum.*

EPIDEMIOLOGY: The fungi occur worldwide and are transmissible by direct contact with infected humans, animals, or fomites. Fungi in the lesions are communicable.

The **incubation period** is unknown.

DIAGNOSIS: The fungi responsible for tinea corporis can be detected by microscopic examination of a potassium hydroxide wet mount of skin scrapings. Use of dermatophyte test medium also is a reliable, simple, and inexpensive method of diagnosis. Skin scrapings from lesions are inoculated directly onto the culture medium and incubated at room temperature. After 1 to 2 weeks, a phenol red indicator in the agar will turn from yellow to red in the area surrounding a dermatophyte colony. When necessary, the diagnosis also can be confirmed by culture on Sabouraud dextrose agar.

TREATMENT: Topical application of miconazole, clotrimazole, terbinafine, tolnaftate, naftifine, or ciclopirox preparation twice a day, or of econazole, ketoconazole, oxiconazole, butenafine, or sulconazole preparation once a day, is recommended (see Topical Drugs for Superficial Fungal Infections, p 673). Although clinical resolution may be evident within 2 weeks of therapy, a minimum duration of 4 weeks generally is indicated. Topical preparations of antifungal medication mixed with high-potency corticosteroids should not be used because corticosteroids can cause striae and atrophy of the skin.

If the lesions are extensive or unresponsive to topical therapy, griseofulvin is administered orally for 4 weeks (see Tinea Capitis, p 569). Oral itraconazole, oral fluconazole, and oral terbinafine are effective alternative therapies for tinea corporis, but these products are not approved by the US Food and Drug Administration for this indication.

ISOLATION OF THE HOSPITALIZED PATIENT: Standard precautions are recommended.

CONTROL MEASURES: Direct contact with known or suspected sources of infection should be avoided. Periodic inspections of contacts for early lesions and prompt therapy are recommended.

Tinea Cruris

(Jock Itch)

CLINICAL MANIFESTATIONS: Tinea cruris is a common superficial fungal disorder of the groin and upper thighs. The eruption is sharply marginated and usually is bilaterally symmetric. Involved skin is erythematous and scaly and varies from red to brown; occasionally, the eruption is accompanied by central clearing and a vesiculopapular border. In chronic infections, the margin may be subtle, and lichenification may be present. Tinea cruris skin lesions may be extremely pruritic. These lesions should be differentiated from intertrigo, seborrheic dermatitis, psoriasis, primary irritant dermatitis, allergic contact dermatitis (generally caused by the therapeutic agents applied to the area), or erythrasma, which is a superficial bacterial infection of the skin caused by *Corynebacterium minutissimum.*

ETIOLOGY: The fungi *Epidermophyton floccosum, Trichophyton rubrum,* and *Trichophyton mentagrophytes* are the most common causes.

EPIDEMIOLOGY: Tinea cruris occurs predominantly in adolescent and adult males. Moisture, close-fitting garments, friction, and obesity are predisposing factors. Direct or indirect person-to-person transmission may occur. This infection commonly occurs in association with tinea pedis.

The **incubation period** is unknown.

DIAGNOSTIC TESTS: The fungi responsible for tinea cruris may be detected by microscopic examination of a potassium hydroxide wet mount of scales. Use of dermatophyte test medium also is a reliable, simple, and inexpensive method of diagnosing tinea cruris. Skin scrapings from lesions are inoculated directly onto the culture medium and incubated at room temperature. After 1 to 2 weeks, a phenol red indicator in the agar will turn from yellow to red in the area surrounding a dermatophyte colony. When necessary, the diagnosis also can be confirmed by culture on Sabouraud dextrose agar. A characteristic coral-red fluorescence under Wood's light can identify the presence of erythrasma and, thus, exclude tinea cruris.

TREATMENT: Topical application for 4 to 6 weeks of clotrimazole, haloprogin, miconazole, terbinafine, tolnaftate, or ciclopirox preparation gently rubbed into the affected areas and surrounding skin twice daily, or topical econazole, ketoconazole, naftifine, oxiconazole, butenafine, or sulconazole preparation once daily is effective (see Topical Drugs for Superficial Fungal Infections, p 673). Tinea pedis, if present, should be treated concurrently (see Tinea Pedis, p 573).

Topical preparations of antifungal medication mixed with high-potency corticosteroids should not be used because the corticosteroids can cause striae and atrophy of the skin. Loose-fitting, washed, cotton underclothes to reduce chafing, as well as the use of a bland absorbent powder can be helpful adjuvants to therapy. Griseofulvin orally for 2 to 6 weeks may be effective in unresponsive cases (see Tinea Capitis, p 569). Oral itraconazole and oral terbinafine are effective alternative therapies, but these products are not approved by the US Food and Drug Administration for treatment of tinea cruris, and they usually are unnecessary.

Isolation of the Hospitalized Patient: Standard precautions are recommended.

Control Measures: Infections should be treated promptly. Potentially involved areas should be kept dry, and loose undergarments should be recommended. Patients should be advised to dry the groin area before drying their feet to avoid inoculating dermatophytes of tinea pedis into the groin area.

Tinea Pedis

(Athlete's Foot, Ringworm of the Feet)

Clinical Manifestations: Tinea pedis is manifest by fine vesiculopustular or scaly lesions that frequently are pruritic. The lesions can involve all areas of the foot, but usually they are patchy in distribution, with a predisposition to fissures and scaling between the toes, particularly in the third and fourth interdigital spaces. Toenails may be infected and can be dystrophic (tinea unguium). Tinea pedis must be differentiated from dyshidrotic eczema, atopic dermatitis, contact dermatitis, juvenile plantar dermatosis, and erythrasma (a superficial bacterial infection caused by *Corynebacterium minutissimum*). Tinea pedis commonly occurs in association with tinea cruris.

Tinea pedis and many other fungal infections can be accompanied by a hypersensitivity reaction to the fungi (the dermatophytid or id reaction), with resulting vesicular eruptions on the palms and the sides of the fingers, and, occasionally, by an erythematous vesicular eruption on the extremities and trunk.

Etiology: The fungi *Trichophyton rubrum, Trichophyton mentagrophytes,* and *Epidermophyton floccosum* are the most common causes.

Epidemiology: Tinea pedis is a common infection worldwide in adolescents and adults but is relatively uncommon in young children. The fungi are acquired by contact with skin scales containing fungi or with fungi in damp areas, such as swimming pools, locker rooms, and shower rooms. Tinea pedis in a family member tends to spread throughout the household. It is communicable for as long as the infection is present. The rapid growth of fingernails and toenails makes fungal infection of the nail plate uncommon in children.

The **incubation period** is unknown.

Diagnosis: Tinea pedis usually is diagnosed by clinical manifestations and may be confirmed by microscopic examination of a potassium hydroxide wet mount of the cutaneous scrapings. Use of dermatophyte test medium is a reliable, simple, and inexpensive method of diagnosis in complicated or unresponsive cases. Skin scrapings or nail clippings are inoculated directly onto the culture medium and incubated at room temperature. After 1 to 2 weeks, a phenol red indicator in the agar will turn from yellow to red in the area surrounding a dermatophyte colony. When necessary, the diagnosis also can be confirmed by culture on Sabouraud dextrose agar. Infection of the nail can be verified by fungal culture of desquamated subungual material.

TREATMENT: Topical application of miconazole, haloprogin, clotrimazole, ciclopirox, terbinafine, butenafine, or tolnaftate preparation twice a day, or of econazole, ketoconazole, naftifine, oxiconazole, or sulconazole preparation once a day for 2 to 3 weeks, can be used for active infections (see Topical Drugs for Superficial Fungal Infections, p 673). Acute vesicular lesions may be treated with intermittent use of open wet compresses (eg, with Burrow solution, 1:80). Tinea cruris, if present, should be treated concurrently (see Tinea Cruris, p 572).

Griseofulvin administered orally for 6 to 8 weeks may be necessary for treatment of severe, chronic, or recalcitrant tinea pedis. Oral itraconazole and oral terbinafine also are effective alternative therapies for tinea pedis unresponsive to topical therapy, but these products have not been approved by the US Food and Drug Administration for this indication. Id reactions (eg, hypersensitivity response) are treated by wet compresses, topical corticosteroids, occasionally systemic corticosteroids, and eradication of the primary source of infection.

Recurrence is prevented by proper foot hygiene, which includes keeping the feet dry and cool, gentle cleaning, drying between the toes, the use of absorbent antifungal foot powder, frequent airing of affected areas, and avoidance of occlusive footwear and nylon socks or other fabrics that interfere with dissipation of moisture.

In the past, most nail infections, particularly toenail infections, have been highly resistant to oral griseofulvin therapy. Studies in adult patients have demonstrated a high cure rate after therapy with oral itraconazole or oral terbinafine. Further studies on the safety and efficacy of these drugs in children are necessary before either drug can be recommended. Recurrences are common. Removal of the nail plate followed by use of oral therapy during the period of regrowth can help to effect a cure in resistant cases.

ISOLATION OF THE HOSPITALIZED PATIENT: Standard precautions are recommended.

CONTROL MEASURES: Treatment of patients with active infections should reduce transmission. Public areas conducive to transmission (eg, swimming pools) should not be used by those with active infection. Chemical foot baths are of no value and can facilitate spread of infection. Because recurrence after treatment is common, proper foot hygiene is important (as described in Treatment). Patients should be advised to dry the groin area before drying their feet to avoid inoculating tinea pedis dermatophytes into the groin area.

Tinea Versicolor

(Pityriasis Versicolor)

CLINICAL MANIFESTATIONS: Tinea (pityriasis) versicolor is a common superficial yeast infection of the skin characterized by multiple, scaling, oval, and patchy macular lesions, usually distributed over the upper portions of the trunk, proximal areas of the arms, and neck. Facial involvement is particularly common in children. The lesions may be hypopigmented or hyperpigmented (fawn colored or brown) and may be somewhat lighter than the surrounding skin. The lesions fail to tan during the summer and during the winter are relatively darker, hence the term *versicolor*. Common conditions confused with this disorder include pityriasis alba, postinflammatory hypopigmentation, vitiligo, melasma, seborrheic dermatitis, pityriasis rosea, and secondary syphilis.

ETIOLOGY: *Malassezia furfur* is the cause. This dimorphic lipid-dependent yeast exists on healthy skin in the yeast phase and causes clinical lesions only when substantial growth of hyphae occurs. Moist heat and lipid-containing sebaceous secretions encourage rapid overgrowth.

EPIDEMIOLOGY: Tinea versicolor occurs worldwide but is more common in tropical areas. Although primarily a disorder of adolescents and young adults 15 to 30 years of age, tinea versicolor also may occur in prepubertal children and infants. The yeast is transmitted by personal contact during periods of scaling.

The **incubation period** is unknown.

DIAGNOSIS: The clinical appearance usually is diagnostic. Involved areas are yellow fluorescent under Wood's light. Scale scrapings examined microscopically in a potassium hydroxide wet mount preparation or stained with methylene blue or May-Grünwald-Giemsa stain disclose the pathognomonic clusters of yeast cells and hyphae ("spaghetti and meatball" appearance). Growth of this yeast on culture requires a source of long-chain fatty acids, which may be accomplished by overlaying Sabouraud dextrose agar medium with sterile olive oil.

TREATMENT: Topical treatment with selenium sulfide as 2.5% lotion or 1% shampoo is the treatment of choice. These preparations are applied in a thin layer covering the body surface from the face to the knees daily for 30 minutes for a week, followed by monthly applications for 3 months (to help prevent recurrences). Other topical preparations with therapeutic efficacy include sodium hyposulfite or thiosulfate in 15% to 25% concentrations (eg, Tinver lotion) applied twice a day for 2 to 4 weeks. Small focal infections may be treated with topical antifungal agents, such as clotrimazole, econazole, haloprogin, ketoconazole, miconazole, or naftifine (see Topical Drugs for Superficial Fungal Infections, p 672).

Oral antifungal therapy has the advantages over topical therapy of ease of administration and shorter duration of treatment, but it is more expensive and associated with a greater risk of adverse reactions. A single dose of ketoconazole (400 mg orally) or fluconazole (400 mg orally) or a 5-day course of itraconazole (200 mg orally once a day) has been effective in adults. Some experts recommend that children receive 3 days of ketoconazole therapy rather than the single dose given adults. For pediatric dosage recommendations for ketoconazole, fluconazole, and itraconazole, see Recommended Doses of Parenteral and Oral Antifungal Drugs, p 670. These drugs have not been tested extensively in children for this disorder and are not yet approved by the US Food and Drug Administration for this indication. Exercise to increase sweating and skin concentrations of medication may enhance the effectiveness of systemic therapy. Patients should be warned that repigmentation may not occur for several months after successful treatment.

ISOLATION OF THE HOSPITALIZED PATIENT: Standard precautions are recommended.

CONTROL MEASURES: Infected persons should be treated.

Toxic Shock Syndrome

CLINICAL MANIFESTATIONS: Toxic shock syndrome (TSS) may be caused by *Staphylococcus aureus* or *Streptococcus pyogenes* (group A streptococci). Both organisms cause an acute illness characterized by fever, rapid-onset hypotension, rapidly accelerated renal failure, and multisystem organ involvement (see Tables 3.59, p 577, and 3.60, p 578). Profuse watery diarrhea, vomiting, generalized erythroderma, conjunctival infection, and severe myalgias frequently are present with *S aureus*–mediated TSS but are less common with *S pyogenes*–mediated TSS. Evidence of local soft tissue infection (eg, cellulitis, abscess, myositis, or necrotizing fasciitis) associated with severe increasing pain is common with *S pyogenes*–mediated TSS, but not with *S aureus*–mediated TSS. The presence of a foreign body at the site of infection is common with *S aureus*–mediated TSS, but not with *S pyogenes*–mediated TSS. Both forms of TSS may occur without a readily identifiable focus of infection. Both forms of TSS also may be associated with more invasive infections, such as pneumonia, osteomyelitis, bacteremia, pyarthrosis, or endocarditis. Patients with *S aureus*–mediated TSS, especially menses associated, are at risk for a recurrent episode of TSS. Recurrent episodes have not been reported for *S pyogenes*–mediated TSS. Toxic shock syndrome can be confused with meningococcemia, Rocky Mountain spotted fever, septic shock, Kawasaki disease, ehrlichiosis, scarlet fever, measles, systemic lupus erythematosus, and other febrile mucocutaneous diseases.

ETIOLOGY: *Staphylococcus aureus*–mediated TSS usually is caused by strains producing toxic-shock syndrome toxin-1 (TSST-1). Most of these strains also produce at least one of the staphylococcal enterotoxins. Some TSST-1 negative strains of *S aureus* have been implicated in nonmenstrual cases of TSS. Most cases of *S pyogenes*–mediated TSS are caused by strains producing at least 1 of 5 protein superantigenic exotoxins: streptococcal pyrogenic exotoxins A, B, or C; mitogenic factor; or streptococcal superantigen.

EPIDEMIOLOGY:

Staphylococcus aureus*–Mediated TSS.* This syndrome was first recognized in 1978. A marked increase in the number of cases in 1979 and 1980 resulted in the finding that greater than 90% of cases were associated with tampon use in menstruating women, with a particular predilection for adolescents and young women with no circulating antibody to TSST-1. Changes in tampon composition and a decrease in absorbency during the past 2 decades have resulted in a significant decrease in the proportion of cases associated with menstruation. In 1996, menstrual cases accounted for fewer than 50% of reported cases. Risk factors for nonmenstrual TSS are outlined in Table 3.61, p 579.

Table 3.59. Staphylococcal Toxic Shock Syndrome: Clinical Case Definition*

- Fever: temperature ≥38.9°C (102.0°F)
- Rash: diffuse macular erythroderma
- Desquamation: 1–2 wk after onset, particularly palms and soles
- Hypotension: systolic blood pressure ≤90 mm Hg for adults; lower than fifth percentile by age for children younger than 16 years of age; orthostatic drop in diastolic blood pressure of ≥15 mm Hg from lying to sitting; orthostatic syncope or orthostatic dizziness
- Multisystem involvement: 3 or more of the following:
  - Gastrointestinal: vomiting or diarrhea at onset of illness
  - Muscular: severe myalgia or creatinine phosphokinase level greater than twice the upper limit of normal
  - Mucous membrane: vaginal, oropharyngeal, or conjunctival hyperemia
  - Renal: serum urea nitrogen or serum creatinine level greater than twice the upper limit of normal or urinary sediment with ≥5 white blood cells per high-power field in the absence of a urinary tract infection
  - Hepatic: total bilirubin, aspartate aminotransferase, or alanine aminotransferase level greater than twice the upper limit of normal
  - Hematologic: platelet count, $<100 \times 10^9$/L ($<100 \times 10^3/\mu L$)
  - Central nervous system: disorientation or alterations in consciousness without focal neurologic signs when fever and hypotension are absent
- Negative results on the following tests, if obtained:
  - Blood, throat, or cerebrospinal fluid cultures; blood culture may be positive for *Staphylococcus aureus*
  - Serologic tests for Rocky Mountain spotted fever, leptospirosis, or measles

Case Classification

Probable:	a case with 5 of the 6 aforementioned clinical findings
Confirmed:	a case with all 6 of the clinical findings, including desquamation. If the patient dies before desquamation could have occurred, the other 5 criteria constitute a definitive case.

* Adapted from Wharton M, Chorba TL, Vogt RL, Morse DL, Buehler JW. Case definitions for public health surveillance. *MMWR Morb Mortal Wkly Rep.* 1990;39(RR-13):1–43

In adults, TSST-1–producing strains of *S aureus* may be part of the normal flora of the anterior nares and the vagina. Colonization is believed to produce antibody formation and immunity, and more than 90% of adults have antibodies to TSST-1. Persons in whom *S aureus*–mediated TSS with TSST-1 producing strains develops usually do not have antibodies to TSST-1. Person-to-person transmission of TSS is rare. Nosocomial cases are uncommon and most often have followed surgical procedures. In postoperative cases, the organism almost certainly originates from the patient's own flora. The **incubation period** for postoperative TSS can be as short as 12 hours. Menses-related cases generally develop on the third or fourth day of menses. The mortality rate is less than 5% overall and is highest in men and women older than 45 years of age.

Table 3.60. Streptococcal Toxic Shock Syndrome: Clinical Case Definition*

I. Isolation of group A ß-hemolytic streptococci
   A. From a normally sterile site (eg, blood, cerebrospinal fluid, peritoneal fluid, tissue biopsy specimen)
   B. From a nonsterile site (eg, throat, sputum, vagina)

II. Clinical signs of severity
   A. Hypotension: systolic blood pressure ≤90 mm Hg in adults or lower than the fifth percentile for age in children

   AND

   B. Two or more of the following signs:
   - Renal impairment: creatinine level, ≥177 µmol/L (≥2 mg/dL) for adults or two times or more the upper limit of normal for age
   - Coagulopathy: platelet count, ≤100 × 10^9/L (≤100 × 10^3/µL) or disseminated intravascular coagulation
   - Hepatic involvement: alanine aminotransferase, aspartate aminotransferase, or total bilirubin levels two times or more the upper limit of normal for age
   - Adult respiratory distress syndrome
   - A generalized erythematous macular rash that may desquamate
   - Soft tissue necrosis, including necrotizing fasciitis or myositis, or gangrene

* An illness fulfilling criteria IA and II A and II B can be defined as a *definite* case. An illness fulfilling criteria IB and IIA and IIB can be defined as a *probable* case if no other cause for the illness is identified. Adapted from The Working Group on Severe Streptococcal infections. Defining the group A streptococcal toxic shock syndrome: rationale and consensus definition. *JAMA*. 1993;269:390–391

Streptococcus pyogenes*–Mediated TSS.* The incidence of *S pyogenes*–mediated TSS seems to be highest among young children, particularly those with varicella, and the elderly. Of all cases of severe invasive streptococcal infections in children, fewer than 10% are associated with TSS, compared with almost one third of such infections in persons older than 75 years of age. Other persons at increased risk include those with diabetes mellitus, chronic cardiac or pulmonary disease, human immunodeficiency virus infection, and intravenous drug and alcohol use. The risk of severe invasive infection in contacts has been estimated to be 200 times greater than for the general population, but is still rare. Most contacts will have asymptomatic colonization.

Mortality rates are higher for adults than for children and depend on whether the *S pyogenes*–mediated TSS is associated only with bacteremia or with a specific organ infection (eg, necrotizing fasciitis, myositis, or pneumonia).

The **incubation period** is not defined clearly and may depend on the route of inoculation. The incubation period has been as short as 14 hours in cases associated with the accidental subcutaneous inoculation of infected blood, such as during childbirth or following penetrating trauma.

DIAGNOSTIC TESTS:

Staphylococcus aureus*–Mediated TSS.* Diagnosis of *S aureus*–mediated TSS remains a clinical diagnosis. Blood cultures are positive for *S aureus* in fewer than 5% of

Table 3.61. **Risk Factors for Nonmenstrual Staphylococcal Toxic Shock Syndrome**

I. Colonization with or introduction of toxin-producing *Staphylococcus aureus*

II. Absence of protective antitoxin antibody

III. Infected site

- Primary *S aureus* infection

Carbuncle	Endocarditis	Peritonitis	Pyomyositis
Cellulitis	Folliculitis	Peritonsillar abscess	Sinusitis
Dental abscess	Mastitis	Pneumonia	Tracheitis
Empyema	Osteomyelitis	Pyarthrosis	

- Postoperative wound infection

Abdominal	Ear, nose, and throat	Cesarean section	Neurosurgical
Breast	Genitourinary	Dermatologic	Orthopedic

- Skin or mucous membrane disruption

Burns (eg, chemical, scald)	Viral infection
Dermatitis	Influenza
Postpartum (vaginal delivery)	Pharyngitis
Superficial or penetrating trauma (eg, insect bite, needle stick)	Varicella

- Surgical or nonsurgical foreign body placement

Augmentation mammoplasty	Sponge (contraceptive)
Catheters	Surgical prostheses, stents, packing material, or sutures
Diaphragm	Tampons

- No obvious focus of infection (vaginal or pharyngeal colonization)

patients with *S aureus*–mediated TSS. Cultures usually are positive from the site of infection and should be obtained as soon as the site is identified. Once *S aureus* is isolated in the laboratory, it is important to obtain antimicrobial susceptibilities because methicillin-resistant *S aureus* strains have caused TSS, although rarely. Because 33% of isolates of *S aureus* from nonmenstrual cases do not produce TSST-1, and TSST-1 producing organisms can be present as part of the normal flora of the anterior nares and vagina, production of TSST-1 by an isolate of *S aureus* is not helpful diagnostically.

Streptococcus pyogenes*–Mediated TSS.* Blood cultures are positive for *S pyogenes* in more than 50% of patients with *S pyogenes*–mediated TSS. Cultures from the site of infection usually are positive and may remain positive for several days after appropriate antibiotics have been initiated. *Streptococcus pyogenes* is uniformly susceptible to ß-lactam antibiotics. Antimicrobial susceptibilities should be determined for the non–ß-lactam antibiotics, clindamycin and erythromycin, to which *S pyogenes* may be resistant. A significant increase in antibody titers to antistreptolysin O, antideoxyribonuclease B, or other streptococcal extracellular product 4 to 6 weeks after infection may help confirm the diagnosis if culture results were negative.

Table 3.62. **Management of Staphylococcal or Streptococcal Toxic Shock Syndrome *Without* Necrotizing Fasciitis**

- Fluid management to maintain adequate venous return and cardiac filling pressures to prevent end-organ damage
- Anticipatory management of multisystem organ failure
- Parenteral antimicrobial therapy at maximal doses for age
  - Kill organism with bactericidal cell wall inhibitor (eg, ß-lactamase–resistant antistaphylococcal antimicrobials)
  - Stop enzyme, toxin, or cytokine production with protein synthesis inhibitor (eg, clindamycin)
- Immune Globulin Intravenous may be considered for infection refractory to several hours of aggressive therapy, presence of an undrainable focus, or persistent oliguria with pulmonary edema

For both forms of TSS, laboratory studies may reflect multisystem organ involvement and disseminated intravascular coagulation.

TREATMENT: As outlined in Tables 3.62 (above) and 3.63 (p 581), most aspects of management are the same for TSS caused by *S aureus* and *S pyogenes.* The first priority always is rapid and aggressive fluid replacement, as well as management of respiratory or cardiac failure or arrhythmias if present. Because it may be impossible to distinguish the two forms of TSS, initial empiric antimicrobial therapy should include a ß-lactamase–resistant antistaphylococcal antibiotic and a protein synthesis–inhibiting antibiotic, such as clindamycin. Both should be given parenterally at maximal doses for age. In mice, clindamycin is more effective than penicillin for treating well-established *S pyogenes* infections because of 3 properties of clindamycin: (1) unlike the ß-lactam antibiotics, the antimicrobial activity of clindamycin is not affected by inoculum size, (2) it has a long postantibiotic effect, and (3) it acts on bacteria by inhibiting protein synthesis. This inhibition of protein synthesis results in suppression of synthesis of the *S pyogenes* antiphagocytic M protein and the bacterial toxins. Erythromycin also inhibits protein synthesis, but was not as effective as clindamycin in the animal model. Clindamycin should not be used alone as initial empiric therapy, because in the United States, 1% to 2% of *S pyogenes* strains are resistant to clindamycin. Methicillin-resistant *S aureus* has caused fewer than 1% of cases of TSS. Thus, vancomycin should not be used routinely as initial empiric therapy.

Once the organism has been identified, antibiotic therapy can be changed to penicillin and clindamycin for *S pyogenes*–mediated TSS. For *S aureus*–mediated TSS, the most appropriate parenteral ß-lactam antibiotic based on susceptibility testing should be given with clindamycin.

For *S aureus*–mediated TSS, antimicrobial therapy should be continued for a minimum of 10 to 14 days to eradicate the organism, thus preventing recurrent disease. The antimicrobial may be changed to high-dose oral therapy once the patient's condition is stable hemodynamically and clearly improved, and the patient is receiv-

Table 3.63. Management of Streptococcal Toxic Shock Syndrome *With* Necrotizing Fasciitis

- Principles outlined in Table 3.62 (p 580)
- Immediate evaluation by surgery
  - Exploration or incisional biopsy for diagnosis and culture
  - Immediate resection of all necrotic tissue
- Repeated resection of tissue may be needed if infection persists or progresses

ing oral alimentation. The total duration of therapy should be based on the usual duration established for the underlying focus, such as osteomyelitis or pneumonia.

For *S pyogenes*–mediated TSS, intravenous therapy should be continued until the patient is afebrile, is in hemodynamically stable condition, and negative blood cultures have been documented. The total duration of therapy should be based on the duration established for infection of the underlying focus.

Aggressive drainage and irrigation of accessible sites of infection should be performed as soon as possible. Concerted efforts should be made to identify a foreign body at the site of infection, and all foreign bodies, including those recently inserted during surgery, should be removed if possible. If necrotizing fasciitis is suspected, immediate surgical exploration or biopsy is crucial to identify a deep soft tissue infection that should be débrided immediately.

The use of Immune Globulin Intravenous (IGIV) may be considered in the treatment of either form of TSS. The mechanism of action of IGIV is unclear but may be related to neutralization of circulating bacterial toxins. For *S pyogenes*–mediated TSS, in vitro data, case reports, and a comparative observational study from Canada support a potential role for IGIV, but further studies are needed. A potential role also is supported by the high rate of positive blood culture results and the high mortality rate. For *S aureus*–mediated TSS, IGIV may be considered for patients who remain unresponsive to all other therapeutic measures and for patients with infection in an area that cannot be drained. Various regimens of IGIV, including 150 to 400 mg/kg per day for 5 days and a single dose of 1 to 2 g/kg, have been used, but at this time, the optimal regimen is not known. As the clearance of IGIV may be as short as 4 to 6 days in these patients, more than 1 dose may be needed.

ISOLATION OF THE HOSPITALIZED PATIENT: Standard precautions, as well as droplet and contact transmission precautions. are recommended for all patients with TSS due to *S pyogenes.* Because person-to-person transmission of *S aureus*–mediated TSS is uncommon, only standard precautions may be needed.

CONTROL MEASURES: The control measures for *S pyogenes*–mediated TSS are the same as those for other forms of severe, invasive, group A streptococcal infections (see p 533).

For *S aureus*–mediated TSS, the control measures are the same as those for other forms of severe staphylococcal diseases (see p 524).

Toxocariasis

(Visceral Larva Migrans, Ocular Larva Migrans)

CLINICAL MANIFESTATIONS: The severity of the symptoms depends on the number of larvae ingested and the degree of allergic response. Most persons who are lightly infected are asymptomatic. Visceral larva migrans (VLM) typically occurs in children 1 to 4 years of age with a history of pica, but VLM can occur in older children. Characteristic manifestations include fever, leukocytosis, persistent eosinophilia, hypergammaglobulinemia, and hepatomegaly. Other manifestations include malaise, anemia, cough, and, in rare instances, pneumonia, myocarditis, and encephalitis. When ocular invasion (endophthalmitis or retinal granulomas) occurs, other evidence of infection usually is lacking, suggesting that the visceral and ocular manifestations are distinct syndromes. Atypical forms of presentation include hemorrhagic rash and seizures.

ETIOLOGY: Toxocariasis is caused by *Toxocara* species, which are common roundworms of dogs and cats (especially puppies or kittens), specifically *Toxocara canis* and *Toxocara cati* in the United States; most cases are caused by *T canis.* Other nematodes of animals also can cause this syndrome, although rarely.

EPIDEMIOLOGY: Humans are infected by ingestion of soil containing infective eggs of the parasite. A history of pica, particularly eating soil, is common. Direct contact with dogs is of secondary importance because eggs are not infective immediately when shed in the feces. Most reported cases involve children. Toxocariasis is endemic to Puerto Rico and the contiguous United States. Eggs may be found wherever dogs and cats defecate.

The **incubation period** is unknown.

DIAGNOSTIC TESTS: Hypereosinophilia and hypergammaglobulinemia associated with elevated titers of isohemagglutinin to the A and B blood group antigens are presumptive evidence of infection. Microscopic identification of the larvae in a liver biopsy specimen is diagnostic, but this finding is infrequent. A liver biopsy negative for larvae therefore does not exclude the diagnosis. An enzyme immunoassay for *Toxocara* antibodies in serum, available at the Centers for Disease Control and Prevention and some private laboratories, can provide presumptive evidence of toxocariasis. This assay is specific and sensitive for the diagnosis of VLM but is less sensitive for the diagnosis of ocular larva migrans.

TREATMENT: Mebendazole and albendazoleare the recommended drugs for treatment of toxocariasis. Albendazole has been approved by the US Food and Drug Administration, but not for this indication. In severe cases with myocarditis or involvement of the central nervous system, corticosteroid therapy is indicated. Correcting the underlying causes of pica helps prevent reinfection.

Treatment of ocular larva migrans may not be effective. Inflammation may be reduced by injection of corticosteroids, and secondary damage may be aided by surgery.

ISOLATION OF THE HOSPITALIZED PATIENT: Standard precautions are recommended.

CONTROL MEASURES: Proper disposal of cat and dog feces is essential. Treatment of puppies and kittens with anthelmintics at 2, 4, 6, and 8 weeks of age prevents excretion of eggs by worms acquired transplacentally or through mother's milk. Covering sandboxes when not in use is helpful. No specific management of exposed persons is recommended.

Toxoplasma gondii Infections

(Toxoplasmosis)

CLINICAL MANIFESTATIONS: Infants with congenital infection are asymptomatic at birth in 70% to 90% of cases, although visual impairment, learning disabilities, or mental retardation will become apparent in a large percentage of children several months to years later. Signs of congenital toxoplasmosis present at birth can include a maculopapular rash, generalized lymphadenopathy, hepatomegaly, splenomegaly, jaundice, and thrombocytopenia. As a consequence of intrauterine meningoencephalitis, cerebrospinal fluid (CSF) abnormalities, hydrocephalus, microcephaly, chorioretinitis, and seizures can develop. Some of the severely affected die in utero or within a few days of birth. Cerebral calcifications may be demonstrated by radiography, ultrasonography, or computed tomography of the head.

Toxoplasma gondii infection acquired after birth usually is asymptomatic. When symptoms develop, they are nonspecific and include malaise, fever, sore throat, and myalgia. Lymphadenopathy, frequently cervical, is the most common sign. Occasionally, patients may present with a mononucleosis-like illness associated with a macular rash and hepatosplenomegaly. The clinical course usually is benign and self-limited. Myocarditis, pericarditis, and pneumonitis are rare complications.

Isolated ocular toxoplasmosis most often occurs as a result of congenital infection and less frequently can result from acquired infection. Acute ocular involvement presents as new onset of blurred vision with characteristic retinal infiltrates. Ocular disease can become reactivated years after the initial infection in healthy and in immunocompromised persons.

In chronically infected immunodeficient patients, such as those with human immunodeficiency virus (HIV) infection, reactivated infection can result in encephalitis, pneumonitis, or, less commonly, systemic toxoplasmosis. Although rare, infants who are born to HIV-infected mothers or mothers immunocompromised for other reasons and who have chronic infection with *T gondii* may acquire congenital toxoplasmosis as a result of reactivated maternal parasitemia.

ETIOLOGY: *Toxoplasma gondii,* a protozoan parasite, is the only known species of *Toxoplasma* that is pathogenic for humans.

EPIDEMIOLOGY: *Toxoplasma gondii* is worldwide in distribution and infects most species of warm-blooded animals. Members of the cat family are the definitive hosts. Cats generally acquire the infection by feeding on infected animals, such as mice or uncooked household meats. The parasite replicates sexually in the feline small intestine. Cats may begin to excrete oocysts in their stools 3 to 30 days after primary infection and may shed oocysts for 7 to 14 days. After excretion, oocysts require a maturation phase (sporulation) of 24 to 48 hours in temperate climates before they are infective by the oral route. Intermediate hosts (including sheep, pigs, and cattle) can have tissue cysts in the brain, myocardium, skeletal muscle, and other organs. These cysts remain viable for the lifetime of the host. Humans become infected primarily either by consumption of poorly cooked meat that contains cysts or by accidental ingestion of sporulated oocysts from soil or in contaminated food. A large outbreak epidemiologically linked to contamination of a municipal water supply also has been reported. Transmission of *T gondii* has been documented to result from blood or blood product transfusion and organ (eg, heart) or bone marrow transplantation from a seropositive donor with latent infection. Congenital transmission in the overwhelming majority of cases occurs as a result of primary maternal infection during gestation. The frequency of congenital toxoplasmosis in the United States has been estimated to be 1 in 1000 to 1 in 10 000 live births. Rarely, infection has occurred as a result of a laboratory accident.

The **incubation period** of acquired infection, based on a well-studied outbreak, is estimated to be approximately 7 days, with a range of 4 to 21 days.

DIAGNOSTIC TESTS: Serologic tests are the primary means of diagnosis, but results must be interpreted carefully. Immunoglobulin (Ig) G–specific antibodies (eg, measured by indirect immunofluorescence or enzyme immunoassay) achieve a peak concentration 1 to 2 months after infection and remain positive indefinitely. For patients with seroconversion or a 4-fold rise in IgG antibody titer, specific IgM antibody determinations should be performed by a reference laboratory to confirm acute infection. The presence of *T gondii*–specific IgM antibodies may indicate acute or recent infection. Enzyme immunoassay tests are the more sensitive assays for IgM, while indirect fluorescent antibody tests are the least sensitive to detect IgM. IgM-specific antibodies can be detected 2 weeks after infection, achieve peak concentrations in 1 month, decline thereafter, and usually become undetectable within 6 to 9 months but uncommonly persist for as long as 2 years, hindering the differentiation of acute vs remote infection. Tests to detect IgA and IgE antibodies, which decline to undetectable concentrations sooner than do IgM antibodies, are useful for the diagnosis of congenital infections and infections in other patients for whom more precise information about the duration of infection is needed, such as pregnant women. *Toxoplasma gondii*–specific IgA and IgE antibody tests are available commercially but are not used frequently in routine laboratories.

Special Situations.

Prenatal. A definitive diagnosis of congenital toxoplasmosis can be made prenatally by detecting the parasite in fetal blood or amniotic fluid or documenting the presence of *T gondii* IgM or IgA antibodies in fetal blood. The parasite rarely can be isolated by mouse inoculation. Detection of *T gondii* DNA in amniotic fluid by polymerase chain reaction (PCR) in a reference laboratory has been shown to be a safe and accurate method of diagnosis. Serial fetal ultrasonographic examinations should be performed in cases of suspected congenital infection to detect any increase in size of the lateral ventricles of the central nervous system or other signs of fetal infection.

Postnatal. Infants who are born to women who have evidence of primary *T gondii* infection during gestation or women who are infected with HIV *and* have serologic evidence of past infection with *T gondii* should be assessed for congenital toxoplasmosis.

If the diagnosis for an infant is unclear at the time of delivery, workup of the infant should include ophthalmologic, auditory, and neurologic examinations, lumbar puncture, and computed tomography of the head. An attempt should be made to isolate *T gondii* from the placenta, umbilical cord, or infant blood by mouse inoculation. Alternatively, the peripheral blood white blood cells, CSF, and amniotic fluid should be assayed for *T gondii* by PCR in a reference laboratory.

The serologic diagnosis of congenital infection is based on a positive IgM or IgA assay within the first 6 months of life or persistently positive IgG titers beyond the first 12 months of life. The sensitivity of *T gondii*–specific IgM by the double-sandwich enzyme immunoassay or an immunosorbent assay is 75% to 80%. The indirect florescent assay for IgM should not be relied on to diagnose congenital infection. In an uninfected infant, a continuous decline in IgG titer without IgM or IgA will occur. Transplacentally transmitted IgG antibody usually will become undetectable by 6 to 12 months of age.

HIV Infection. Patients with HIV infection who are infected latently with *T gondii* have variable titers of IgG antibody to *T gondii* but rarely have IgM antibody. While seroconversion and 4-fold rises in IgG antibody titers may occur, the ability to diagnose active disease in patients with acquired immunodeficiency syndrome commonly is impaired by immunosuppression. In HIV-infected patients who are seropositive for *T gondii* IgG, a presumptive diagnosis of *T gondii* encephalitis is based on the presence of the characteristic clinical and radiographic findings. If the infection does not respond to an empiric trial of anti–*T gondii* therapy, demonstration of *T gondii* organisms, antigen, or DNA in biopsied tissue, blood, or cerebrospinal fluid may be necessary to confirm the diagnosis.

Infants born to women who are infected simultaneously with HIV and *T gondii* should be evaluated for congenital toxoplasmosis because of an increased likelihood of reactivation in this setting.

Diagnosis of ocular toxoplasmosis is based on observation of characteristic retinal lesions in conjunction with serum *T gondii*–specific IgG or IgM antibodies.

TREATMENT: Most cases of acquired infection do not require specific antimicrobial therapy. When indicated (eg, chorioretinitis or significant organ damage), the combination of pyrimethamine and sulfadiazine,* which is synergistic against *T gondii,* is the most widely accepted regimen for children and adults with acute symptomatic disease (see Drugs for Parasitic Infections, p 693). Alternatively, pyrimethamine can be used in combination with clindamycin if the patient does not tolerate sulfadiazine. The use of corticosteroids for the management of ocular complications and central nervous system disease is controversial.

Patients infected with HIV who have had toxoplasmic encephalitis should receive lifelong suppressive therapy. Regimens for primary treatment also are effective for suppressive therapy.

---

* Available from Eon Labs, Laurelton, NY (800-526-0225).

For HIV-infected adults, primary chemoprophylaxis with trimethoprim-sulfamethoxazole against toxoplasmosis has been recommended for persons who are *T gondii*–seropositive and have CD4+ T-lymphocyte counts less than 100 × 10^6/L (<100/µL) by the US Public Health Services and Infectious Diseases Society of America Prevention of Opportunistic Infections Working Group.* Current data are insufficient for formulation of specific guidelines for children; in some circumstances, chemoprophylaxis should be considered and is recommended by some experts.

For symptomatic and asymptomatic congenital infection, pyrimethamine combined with sulfadiazine (supplemented with folinic acid) also is recommended as the initial therapy. Duration of therapy is prolonged and often is 1 year. However, the optimal dosage and duration are not established definitively and should be determined in consultation with appropriate specialists.

Treatment of primary *T gondii* infection in pregnant women, including those with HIV infection, is recommended. Appropriate specialists should be consulted for management. Spiramycin treatment of primary infection during gestation is used in an attempt to reduce transmission of *T gondii* from the mother to the fetus. Maternal therapy will not prevent sequelae in the fetus once congenital toxoplasmosis has occurred. Spiramycin is available only as an investigational drug in the United States. It may be obtained from the manufacturer with authorization from the US Food and Drug Administration.† If fetal infection is confirmed after 17 weeks of gestation or if the mother acquires infection during the third trimester, consideration should be given to starting therapy with pyrimethamine and sulfadiazine.

ISOLATION OF THE HOSPITALIZED PATIENT: Standard precautions are recommended.

CONTROL MEASURES: Pregnant women whose serostatus for *T gondii* is negative or unknown should avoid activities that potentially expose them to cat feces (such as changing litter boxes, gardening, and landscaping), or they should wear gloves and wash their hands after changing the litter box if such activities are unavoidable. Daily changing of cat litter will reduce the chance of infection because oocysts are not infective during the first 1 to 2 days after passage. Domestic cats can be protected from infection by feeding commercially prepared cat food and preventing them from eating undercooked kitchen scraps and hunting wild rodents.

Oral ingestion of *T gondii* oocysts can be avoided by the following measures: (1) cooking meat, particularly pork, lamb, and venison to 65.5°C (150°F) (no longer pink) before consumption (smoked meat and meat cured in brine are considered safe); (2) washing fruits and vegetables; (3) washing hands and cleaning kitchen surfaces after handling fruits, vegetables, and raw meat; (4) washing hands after gardening or other contact with soil; and (5) preventing contamination of food. All HIV-infected persons and pregnant women should be counseled about the various sources of toxoplasmic infection.

---

* Centers for Disease Control and Prevention. 1999 US Public Health Service–Infectious Diseases Society of America guidelines for the prevention of opportunistic infections in persons infected with human immunodeficiency virus. *MMWR Morb Mortal Wkly Rep.* 1999;48(RR-10):1–59, 61–66

† Division of Special Pathogen and Immunologic Drug Products: telephone, 301-827-2127; fax, 301-927-2475.

Trichinosis

(Trichinella spiralis)

CLINICAL MANIFESTATIONS: The clinical spectrum of infection ranges from inapparent infection to fulminating, fatal illness, but most infections are inapparent. The severity of the disease is proportional to the infective dose. During the first week after ingesting infected meat, a person may experience abdominal discomfort, nausea, vomiting, and/or diarrhea. Two to 8 weeks later, as larvae migrate into tissues, fever, myalgia, periorbital edema, urticarial rash, and conjunctival and subungual hemorrhages may develop. Larvae may remain viable in tissues for years; calcification of larvae in skeletal muscle usually occurs within 6 to 24 months and may be detected on radiographs. In severe infections, myocardial failure, neurologic involvement, and pneumonitis can follow in 1 or 2 months.

ETIOLOGY: Infection is caused by nematodes of *Trichinella*. Five species capable of infecting only warm-blooded animals have been identified. *Trichinella spiralis* is the most common cause of human infection.

EPIDEMIOLOGY: The infection is enzootic worldwide in many carnivores, especially scavengers. Infection occurs as a result of ingestion of raw or insufficiently cooked meat containing encysted larvae of *T spiralis*. Adult worms live in the mucosa of the small intestine. The usual source of human infections is pork, but horse meat and wild carnivorous game, such as bear, seal, and walrus meat in North America, can be sources. Feeding pigs uncooked garbage perpetuates the cycle of infection. In the United States, the incidence of infection in humans has declined considerably, but infection occurs sporadically, often within a family or among friends who have prepared uncooked sausage from fresh pork. The disease is not transmitted from person to person.

The **incubation period** is usually 1 to 2 weeks.

DIAGNOSTIC TESTS: Eosinophilia approaching 70%, in conjunction with compatible symptoms and dietary history, suggests the diagnosis. Encapsulated larvae in a skeletal muscle biopsy specimen (particularly deltoid and gastrocnemius) can be visualized microscopically, beginning 2 weeks after infection. Fresh tissue, compressed between 2 microscope slides, should be examined. Digestion of muscle tissue in artificial gastric juice followed by examination of the sediment for larvae is more sensitive. Identification of larvae in suspect meat can be the most rapid source of diagnostic information. Serologic tests are available through state laboratories and at the Centers for Disease Control and Prevention. Serum antibody titers rarely become positive before the third week of illness. Testing paired acute and convalescent serum samples usually is diagnostic.

TREATMENT: Albendazole and mebendazole have comparable efficacy for treatment of trichinosis. Coadministration of corticosteroids with mebendazole or albendazole is often recommended. Corticosteroids alleviate symptoms of the inflammatory reaction and can be lifesaving when the central nervous system or heart is involved.

ISOLATION OF THE HOSPITALIZED PATIENT: Standard precautions are recommended.

CONTROL MEASURES: Transmission to pigs can be reduced by not feeding pigs garbage and by active rat control. People should be educated about the necessity of cooking pork thoroughly (until the meat is no longer pink). Freezing pork at −23°C (−10°F) for 10 days kills larvae. However, *Trichinella* organisms in Arctic wild animals can survive this procedure. Persons known to recently have ingested contaminated meat should be treated with mebendazole (or thiabendazole).

Trichomonas vaginalis Infections

(Trichomoniasis)

CLINICAL MANIFESTATIONS: Infection with *Trichomonas vaginalis* frequently is asymptomatic. The usual clinical picture in symptomatic postmenarcheal female patients consists of a frothy vaginal discharge and mild vulvovaginal itching. Dysuria and, rarely, lower abdominal pain can occur. The vaginal discharge usually is pale yellow to gray-green and has a musty odor. Symptoms frequently are more severe just before or after menstruation. The vaginal mucosa often is deeply erythematous, and the cervix is friable and diffusely inflamed, sometimes covered with numerous petechiae ("strawberry cervix"). Urethritis and, more rarely epididymitis, or prostatitis can develop in infected males, but the majority are asymptomatic. Reinfection is common.

ETIOLOGY: *Trichomonas vaginalis* is a flagellated protozoan, slightly larger than a granulocyte.

EPIDEMIOLOGY: *Trichomonas vaginalis* infection primarily is transmitted sexually and frequently coexists with other such infections, particularly gonococcal infections. The presence of *T vaginalis* in a prepubertal child should raise suspicion of sexual abuse. *Trichomonas vaginalis* acquired during birth by newborn infants can cause a vaginal discharge during the first weeks of life.

The **incubation period** averages 1 week but may vary from 4 to 28 days.

DIAGNOSTIC TESTS: Diagnosis usually is established by examination of a wet-mount preparation of the vaginal discharge. Lashing of the flagella and jerky motility of the organism are distinctive. Positive preparations, found more frequently in women who have symptoms, are related directly to the number of organisms but are identified in only 40% to 80% of cases. Culture of the organism and antibody tests using an enzyme immunoassay and immunofluorescence techniques for demonstration of the organism are more sensitive than wet-mount preparations but generally are not required for diagnosis. Culture for *T vaginalis* is positive in more than 95% of cases. Polymerase chain reaction test for *T vaginalis* is sensitive and specific but is available only as a research diagnostic test.

TREATMENT: Metronidazole is the treatment of choice, resulting in cure rates of approximately 95%. For prepubertal girls, 15 mg/kg per day in 3 divided doses (maximum daily dose, 2 g for 7 days), 500 mg twice a day for 7 days, or 40 mg/kg (maximum, 2 g) in a single dose is recommended. In adolescents and adults, treatment is a single dose of 2 g. The sexual partner should be treated concurrently, even if asymptomatic. Patients should abstain from alcohol for 48 hours because of the disulfiram-like effects of the drug. During pregnancy, patients can be treated with a 2-g single dose of metronidazole.

Patients whose infections do not respond to treatment should be retreated with metronidazole (1 g in 2 divided doses for adolescents and adults) for 7 days. Repeated failure to respond should be treated with metronidazole, 2 g, once a day for 3 to 5 days. *Trichomonas* strains with reduced susceptibility to metronidazole have been reported. In the event of treatment failure to therapies recommended, consultation with an expert is advised.

Persons infected with *T vaginalis* should be evaluated for the presence of other sexually transmitted diseases, including syphilis, *Neisseria gonorrhoeae, Chlamydia trachomatis,* hepatitis B virus, and human immunodeficiency virus infection.

ISOLATION OF THE HOSPITALIZED PATIENT: Standard precautions are recommended.

CONTROL MEASURES: Measures to prevent sexually transmitted diseases, particularly the consistent use of condoms, are indicated.

Trichuriasis

(Whipworm Infection)

CLINICAL MANIFESTATIONS: Abdominal pain, tenesmus, and bloody diarrhea with mucus can occur. Children with heavy infections can develop a *Trichuris trichiura* dysentery syndrome or chronic *T trichiura* colitis. *Trichuris trichiura* colitis can mimic other forms of inflammatory bowel disease and lead to physical growth retardation. Chronic infection associated with heavy infection also can be associated with rectal prolapse.

ETIOLOGY: *Trichuris trichiura,* the whipworm, is the causative agent. Adult worms are 30- to 50-mm long with a large thread-like anterior end that is embedded in the mucosa of the large intestine.

EPIDEMIOLOGY: The parasite has a worldwide distribution but is more common in the tropics and in areas of poor sanitation. In some areas of Asia, the prevalence is 50%. In the United States, trichuriasis generally has been limited to rural areas of the southeast and to migrants from tropical areas. Infections usually are asymptomatic. Eggs require a minimum of 10 days of incubation in the soil before they are infectious. The disease is not communicable from person to person.

The **incubation period** is unknown. However, the time required for mature worms to begin laying eggs that are passed in feces is about 90 days after ingestion of the eggs.

DIAGNOSTIC TESTS: Eggs may be found on direct examination of the stool or by using concentration techniques.

TREATMENT: Mebendazole for 3 days usually is effective in eradicating most of the worms. Albendazole also is effective.

ISOLATION OF THE HOSPITALIZED PATIENT: Standard precautions are recommended.

CONTROL MEASURES: Proper disposal of fecal material is indicated.

African Trypanosomiasis

(African Sleeping Sickness)

CLINICAL MANIFESTATIONS: The rapidity and severity of clinical manifestations vary with the infecting species. With *Trypanosoma brucei gambiense* (West African) infection, a cutaneous nodule or chancre may appear at the site of parasite inoculation within a few days of a bite by an infected tsetse fly. Systemic illness is chronic, occurring months to years later, and is characterized by intermittent fever, posterior cervical lymphadenopathy (Winterbottom sign), and multiple nonspecific complaints, including malaise, weight loss, arthralgia, rash, pruritus, and edema. If the central nervous system (CNS) is involved, chronic meningoencephalitis with behavioral changes, cachexia, headache, hallucinations, delusions, and somnolence can occur. In contrast, *Trypanosoma brucei rhodesiense* (East African) infection is acute; generalized illness develops days to weeks after parasite inoculation with acute manifestations, including high fever, cutaneous chancre, myocarditis, hepatitis, anemia, thrombocytopenia, and laboratory evidence of disseminated intravascular coagulation. Clinical meningoencephalitis can develop as early as 3 weeks after onset of the untreated systemic illness. *Trypanosoma brucei rhodesiense* infection has a high fatality rate; without treatment, infected patients usually die within days to months after clinical onset of disease.

ETIOLOGY: The West African (Gambian) form of sleeping sickness is caused by *T brucei gambiense,* whereas the East African (Rhodesian) form is caused by *T brucei rhodesiense.* Both are extracellular protozoan hemoflagellates that live in the blood and tissue of the human host.

EPIDEMIOLOGY: Approximately 20 000 human cases occur annually worldwide, although only 1 or 2 cases, acquired in Africa, are reported every year in the United States. Transmission is confined to an area in Africa between the latitudes of 15° north and 20° south, corresponding precisely with the distribution of the tsetse fly vector (*Glossina* species). In East Africa, wild animals, such as antelope, bushbuck, and hartebeest, constitute the major reservoir of *T brucei rhodesiense.* Domestic pigs and dogs have been found as incidental reservoirs. Humans are the only important reservoir of *T brucei gambiense* in West and Central Africa.

The **incubation period** for *T brucei rhodesiense* infection is 3 to 21 days, usually 5 to 14 days; for *T brucei gambiense* infection, the incubation period is usually longer and variable, ranging from several months to years.

DIAGNOSTIC TESTS: Diagnosis is made by identification of trypomastigotes in blood, cerebrospinal fluid (CSF), or fluid aspirated from a chancre or lymph node or by inoculation of susceptible laboratory animals (mice) with heparinized blood. Examination of the CSF is critical to management and should be performed using the double-centrifugation technique. Concentration and Giemsa staining of the buffy coat layer of peripheral blood also can be helpful. *Trypanosoma brucei gambiense* is more likely to be found in lymph node aspirates. Although an increased concentration of immunoglobulin M in serum or CSF is considered characteristic of African trypanosomiasis, polyclonal hyperglobulinemia is common.

TREATMENT: When no evidence of CNS involvement is present (including absence of trypanosomes and CSF pleocytosis), the drug of choice for the acute hemolymphatic stage of infection due to either subspecies of *T brucei* is pentamidine. For treatment of hemolymphatic and CNS disease, see Drugs for Parasitic Infections, p 693. Because of the risk of relapse, patients should undergo repeated CSF examinations for 2 years when CNS involvement has occurred.

ISOLATION OF THE HOSPITALIZED PATIENT: Standard precautions are recommended.

CONTROL MEASURES: Travelers to endemic areas should avoid known foci of sleeping sickness and tsetse fly infestation and minimize fly bites by the use of protective clothing, bed netting, and insect repellents. Infected patients should not breastfeed or donate blood.

American Trypanosomiasis

(Chagas Disease)

CLINICAL MANIFESTATIONS: Patients can present with acute or chronic disease. The early phase of this disease frequently is asymptomatic. However, children are more likely to exhibit symptoms than adults. In some patients, a red nodule known as a *chagoma* develops at the site of the original inoculation, usually on the face or arms. The surrounding skin becomes indurated and, later, hypopigmented. Unilateral firm edema of the eyelids, known as Romaña sign, is the earliest indication of the infection but is not always present. The edematous skin is violaceous and associated with conjunctivitis and enlargement of the ipsilateral preauricular lymph node. A few days after the appearance of Romaña sign, fever, generalized lymphadenopathy, and malaise can develop. Acute myocarditis, hepatosplenomegaly, edema, and meningoencephalitis can follow. Serious sequelae, consisting of cardiomyopathy and heart failure (the major cause of death), megaesophagus, and/or megacolon, can develop many years after the initial manifestations in the chronic phase of disease. Congenital disease is characterized by low birth weight, hepatomegaly, and meningoencephalitis, with seizures and tremors.

ETIOLOGY: *Trypanosoma cruzi,* a protozoan hemoflagellate, is the cause.

EPIDEMIOLOGY: Parasites are transmitted through feces of the insects of the triatomine family, usually of an infected reduviid (cone-nose or kissing) bug. These insects defecate during or after taking blood. The bitten person is inoculated by inadvertently rubbing the insect feces containing the parasite into the site of the bite or mucous membranes of the eye or the mouth. The parasite also can be transmitted congenitally, during organ transplantation, and through blood transfusion. Accidental laboratory infections can result from handling blood from infected persons or laboratory animals or consumption of the vector or the vector's excreta. The disease is limited to the Western hemisphere, predominantly Mexico and Central and South America. Although some small mammals in the southern and southwestern United States harbor *T cruzi,* vector-borne transmission to humans is rare in the United States. Several transfusion-associated cases have been documented in the United States. Infection is common in immigrants from Central and South America. The disease is a leading cause of death in South America, where between 7 and 15 million people are infected.

The **incubation period** for the acute phase of disease is 1 to 2 weeks or longer. The chronic manifestations do not appear for years to decades.

DIAGNOSTIC TESTS: During the acute disease, the parasite is demonstrable in blood, either by Giemsa staining or by direct wet-mount preparation. In chronic infections, which are characterized by low-level parasitemia, recovery of the parasite by culture on special media or identification by xenodiagnosis should be undertaken. Serologic tests include indirect hemagglutination, indirect immunofluorescence, and enzyme immunoassay.

TREATMENT: The acute phase of Chagas disease is treated with nifurtimox or benznidazole. The effectiveness of these therapies during the latent and chronic phases of disease is being evaluated.

ISOLATION OF THE HOSPITALIZED PATIENT: Standard precautions should be followed.

CONTROL MEASURES: Travelers to endemic areas should avoid contact with reduviid insects by avoiding habitation in buildings that do not have control measures for these insects, particularly buildings constructed of mud, palm thatch, or adobe brick, and especially those with cracks in the walls or roof. The use of bed netting also may be beneficial, especially for travelers to highly endemic areas who plan to camp or sleep outdoors. Blood and serologic examinations should be performed on members of households with an infected patient if they have had exposure to the vector similar to that of the patient. Serologic testing before and after travel should be considered for travelers visiting highly endemic areas with poor control measures where contact with vectors may be unavoidable.

Education about the mode of spread and the methods of prevention is warranted in endemic areas. Homes should be examined for the presence of the vectors, and, if found, thorough disinfection is indicated. Vector control is recommended through the use of effective control of the rodent population on which the vectors feed, use of insecticides, elimination of habitats of the vectors, and using screens on windows and doors to exclude the insect vectors.

Blood donors in endemic areas should be screened by serologic tests (see Blood Safety, p 88). Infected patients should not donate blood. Blood recipients can be protected in endemic areas by treatment of the donated blood with gentian violet at a dilution of 1:4000.

Tuberculosis

CLINICAL MANIFESTATIONS: Most tuberculosis infections in children and adolescents usually are asymptomatic when the tuberculin skin test (TST) result is positive. The primary complex of infection usually is not evident on chest radiograph, and primary infection in most immunocompetent children does not progress rapidly to disease. Early clinical manifestations occurring 1 to 6 months after initial infection can include fever, weight loss, cough, night sweats, and chills. Pulmonary radiographic findings include lymphadenopathy of the hilar, mediastinal, cervical, or other nodes; involvement of a segment or lobe, occasionally with atelectasis or infiltrate; pleural effusion; cavitary lesions; and miliary disease. Meningitis also can occur. Extrapulmonary manifestations that can occur 12 months or more after the initial infection include disease of the middle ear and mastoid, bones, joints, and skin. Tuberculosis of a kidney and reactivation or adult-type pulmonary tuberculosis are rare in young children but can occur in adolescents. Manifestations in patients with drug-resistant tuberculosis are indistinguishable from the manifestations in patients with drug-susceptible disease.

ETIOLOGY: The agent is *Mycobacterium tuberculosis,* an acid-fast bacillus. Pulmonary or abdominal disease caused by *Mycobacterium bovis,* the cause of bovine tuberculosis, occurs occasionally in the United States, while *Mycobacterium africanum* is rare.

DEFINITIONS:

- **Positive TST.** A positive TST (see Table 3.64, p 594) indicates likely infection with *M tuberculosis.* Tuberculin reactivity appears 2 to 12 weeks after initial infection; the median interval is 3 to 4 weeks (see Tuberculin Testing, p 596).
- **Exposed person** refers to a patient who has had recent contact with a person with suspected or confirmed, contagious, pulmonary tuberculosis and who has a negative TST result, normal physical examination findings, and chest radiographic findings that are negative. Some exposed persons have infection (and subsequently develop a positive TST result) and some do not; the two groups at this stage cannot be distinguished.
- **Latent tuberculosis infection (LTBI)** is defined as an infection in a person who has a positive TST, no physical findings of disease, and a chest radiograph

Table 3.64. Definitions of Positive Tuberculin Skin Test (TST) Results in Infants, Children, and Adolescents*

TSTs should be read at 48 to 72 hours after placement

Induration ≥5 mm

Children in close contact with known or suspected contagious cases of tuberculosis disease:

- Households with active or previously active cases if treatment cannot be verified as adequate before exposure, treatment was initiated after the child's contact, or reactivation of latent tuberculosis infection is suspected

Children suspected to have tuberculosis disease:

- Chest radiograph consistent with active or previously active tuberculosis
- Clinical evidence of tuberculosis disease†

Children receiving immunosuppressive therapy‡ or with immunosuppressive conditions, including HIV infection

Induration ≥10 mm

Children at increased risk of disseminated disease:

- Young age: younger than 4 years of age
- Other medical conditions, including Hodgkin disease, lymphoma, diabetes mellitus, chronic renal failure, or malnutrition (see Table 3.65, p 597)

Children with increased exposure to tuberculosis disease:

- Born or whose parents were born in high-prevalence regions of the world
- Frequently exposed to adults who are HIV-infected, homeless, users of illicit drugs, residents of nursing homes, incarcerated or institutionalized persons, and migrant farm workers
- Travel and exposure to high-prevalence regions of the world

Induration ≥15 mm

Children 4 years of age or older without any risk factors

* These definitions apply regardless of previous bacille Calmette-Guérin (BCG) immunization (see also Interpretation of TST Results in Prior Recipients of BCG, p 598); erythema at TST site does not indicate a positive test. HIV indicates human immunodeficiency virus.

† Evidence by physical examination or laboratory assessment that would include tuberculosis in the working differential diagnosis (eg, meningitis).

‡ Including immunosuppressive doses of corticosteroids (see Corticosteroids, p 607).

that is either normal or reveals only granulomas or calcification in the lung, regional lymph nodes, or both.

- **Tuberculosis disease** is defined as disease in a person with infection in whom symptoms, signs, and/or radiographic manifestations caused by *M tuberculosis* are apparent; disease may be pulmonary, extrapulmonary, or both.
- **Directly observed therapy (DOT)** is defined as treatment provided directly to the patient by a health care worker or trained third party (not a relative or friend) to document that the patient takes each dose of medication.

EPIDEMIOLOGY: Case rates of tuberculosis disease for all ages are highest in urban, low-income areas and in nonwhite racial and ethnic groups, among whom more than two thirds of reported cases in the United States now occur. Some rural areas also have high rates. In recent years, foreign-born children have accounted for almost one quarter of newly diagnosed pediatric cases. Specific groups with the highest rates of LTBI and disease include first-generation immigrants from high-risk countries (eg, Asia, Africa, and Latin America), the homeless, and residents of correctional facilities.

Infants and postpubertal adolescents are at increased risk of progression of infection to tuberculosis disease. Other predictive factors for development of disease include recent TST conversion; immunodeficiency, including human immunodeficiency virus (HIV) infection; immunodeficiency due to immunosuppressive drugs, such as prolonged or high-dose corticosteroid therapy or chemotherapy; intravenous drug use; and certain diseases or medical conditions, including Hodgkin disease, lymphoma, diabetes mellitus, chronic renal failure, and malnutrition.

A diagnosis of tuberculosis infection or disease in a child is a sentinel event representing recent transmission of *M tuberculosis* in the community. Transmission of *M tuberculosis* usually is airborne, with inhalation of droplet nuclei produced by an adult or adolescent with contagious, cavitary, pulmonary tuberculosis. The duration of contagiousness of an adult receiving effective treatment depends on drug susceptibilities of the organism, the number of organisms in sputum, and frequency of cough. Although contagiousness usually lasts only a few weeks after initiation of effective drug therapy, it may last longer, especially when the adult patient does not adhere to medical therapy or is infected with a resistant strain. If the sputum is negative for organisms on 3 smears and if coughing has ceased, the person is considered noncontagious. Children younger than 12 years of age with primary pulmonary tuberculosis usually are not contagious because their pulmonary lesions are small, cough is minimal or nonexistent, and there is little or no expulsion of bacilli.

The **incubation period** from infection to development of a positive TST result is 2 to 12 weeks. The risk of developing tuberculosis disease is highest during the 6 months after infection and remains high for 2 years; however, many years may elapse between LTBI and disease.

DIAGNOSTIC TESTS: Isolation of *M tuberculosis* by culture from gastric aspirates, sputum, pleural fluid, cerebrospinal fluid (CSF), urine, other body fluids, or a biopsy specimen establishes the diagnosis. The best specimen for the diagnosis of pulmonary tuberculosis in any young child or in any older child or adolescent in whom the cough is nonproductive or absent is an early morning gastric aspirate. Gastric aspirate specimens should be obtained with a nasogastric tube upon awakening the child and before ambulation or feeding. Three aspirates should be submitted. Regardless of the results of the smears for acid-fast bacilli (AFB), each specimen should be cultured.

Because *M tuberculosis* is slow growing, detection of this organism may take as long as 10 weeks using solid media and 2 to 6 weeks by the radiometric method. Even with optimal culture techniques, organisms are isolated from fewer than 50% of children and 75% of infants with pulmonary tuberculosis. Identification of isolates by culture can be more rapid if a DNA probe is used. Attempts should be made to demonstrate AFB in sputum, body fluids, or both by the Ziehl-Neelsen method or by auramine-rhodamine staining and with fluorescence microscopy. Fluorescent methods are superior and, if available, preferred. Histologic examination for and demonstration of AFB in biopsy specimens from lymph node, pleura, liver, bone marrow, or other tissues can be valuable for diagnosis, but *M tuberculosis* cannot be reliably distinguished from other mycobacteria in stained specimens.

Nucleic acid amplification tests, including polymerase chain reaction, for rapid diagnosis are of limited availability, expensive, and approved only for smear-positive respiratory tract specimens. Restriction fragment length polymorphism analysis for epidemiologic investigation is available in research and reference laboratories. Both tests should be ordered in consultation with a specialist in tuberculosis.

Identification of a source case should be actively pursued to support the presumptive diagnosis, define drug susceptibility if *M tuberculosis* is isolated from this source case, clarify resistance patterns that will affect the choice of drugs for the contact, and identify all persons with LTBI or disease. These activities should be coordinated with the local health department.

Culture material should be obtained from children with evidence of tuberculosis disease, especially when (1) an isolate from a source case is not available; (2) the child is immunocompromised, including children with HIV infection; or (3) the child has extrapulmonary disease.

Tuberculin Testing.* The TST is the only practical tool for diagnosing tuberculosis infection in asymptomatic persons. The Mantoux test containing 5 tuberculin units (TU) of purified protein derivative (PPD), administered intradermally, is the recommended TST. Other strengths of Mantoux skin tests (1 or 250 TU) should not be used. Multiple puncture tests are not recommended because they lack adequate sensitivity and specificity.

The American Academy of Pediatrics recommends a TST for children who are at increased risk of acquiring tuberculosis infection and disease (see Tuberculin Skin Test [TST] Recommendations for Infants, Children, and Adolescents, Table 3.65, p 597). Routine TST administration, including school-based programs that include populations at low risk, that has either a low yield of positive results or a large number of false-positive results represents an inefficient use of health care resources. Children without risk factors, including children who are younger than 1 year of age, do not need routine TSTs.

A TST can be administered during the same visit that immunizations are given, including live-virus vaccines. Previous immunization with bacille Calmette-Guérin (BCG) is not a contraindication to TST skin testing.

Administration of TSTs and interpretation of results should be performed by experienced health care professionals who have been trained in the proper methods because administration and interpretation by unskilled persons are unreliable. The TST is administered by injecting 0.1 mL of 5 TU of PPD intradermally (Mantoux method) into the volar aspect of the forearm using a 27-gauge needle and a tuberculin syringe. When a physician is unavailable to interpret the TST, it can be interpreted by specifically trained staff of an after-hours clinic or local public health clinic, school-based nurses, home health care staff, or emergency department personnel. The primary care physician should be notified of the result promptly.

---

* For further information see American Academy of Pediatrics Committee on Infectious Diseases. Screening for tuberculosis in infants and children. *Pediatrics.* 1994;93:131–134; and American Academy of Pediatrics Committee on Infectious Diseases. Update on tuberculosis skin testing of children. *Pediatrics.* 1996;97:282–284

Table 3.65. **Tuberculin Skin Test (TST) Recommendations for Infants, Children, and Adolescents***

Children for whom immediate TST is indicated:

- Contacts of persons with confirmed or suspected infectious tuberculosis (contact investigation); this includes children identified as contacts of family members or associates in jail or prison during the last 5 years
- Children with radiographic or clinical findings suggesting tuberculosis disease
- Children immigrating from endemic countries (eg, Asia, Middle East, Africa, Latin America)
- Children with travel histories to endemic countries and/or significant contact with indigenous persons from such countries

Children who should have annual TST[†]:

- Children infected with HIV or living in household with HIV-infected persons.
- Incarcerated adolescents

Children who should be tested every 2–3 years[†]:

- Children exposed to the following persons: HIV-infected, homeless, residents of nursing homes, institutionalized adolescents or adults, users of illicit drugs, incarcerated adolescents or adults, and migrant farm workers; foster children with exposure to adults in the preceding high-risk groups are included

Children who should be considered for TST at 4–6 and 11–16 years of age:

- Children whose parents immigrated (with unknown TST status) from regions of the world with high prevalence of tuberculosis; continued potential exposure by travel to the endemic areas and/or household contact with persons from the endemic areas (with unknown TST status) should be an indication for a repeated TST
- Children without specific risk factors who reside in high-prevalence areas; in general, a high-risk neighborhood or community does not mean an entire city is at high risk; rates in any area of the city may vary by neighborhood or even from block to block; physicians should be aware of these patterns when determining the likelihood of exposure; public health officials or local tuberculosis experts should help physicians identify areas with appreciable tuberculosis rates

Children at increased risk for progression of infection to disease: Those with other medical conditions, including diabetes mellitus, chronic renal failure, malnutrition, and congenital or acquired immunodeficiencies deserve special consideration. Without recent exposure, these persons are not at increased risk of acquiring tuberculosis infection. Underlying immune deficiencies associated with these conditions theoretically would enhance the possibility for progression to severe disease. Initial histories of potential exposure to tuberculosis should be included for all of these patients. If these histories or local epidemiologic factors suggest a possibility of exposure, immediate and periodic TST should be considered. An initial TST should be performed before initiation of immunosuppressive therapy for any child with an underlying condition that necessitates immunosuppressive therapy.

* Bacille Calmette-Guérin immunization is not a contraindication to TST. HIV indicates human immunodeficiency virus.

† Initial TST is at the time of diagnosis or circumstance, beginning at 3 months of age.

The recommended time for assessing the TST result (ie, measurement of the size of induration by the ballpoint pen technique) is 48 to 72 hours after administration. The diameter of induration in millimeters is measured transversely to the long axis of the forearm. Positive test results, as defined in Table 3.64 (p 594), can persist for up to 1 week.

A negative TST result never excludes tuberculosis infection or disease. Approximately 10% of immunocompetent children with culture-documented disease do not react initially to a TST. Host-related factors, such as young age, poor nutrition, immunosuppression, other viral infections (especially measles, varicella, and influenza), and severe disseminated tuberculosis can decrease TST reactivity. Many children and adults coinfected with HIV and *M tuberculosis* often are anergic and do not react to TST. Control skin tests to assess cutaneous anergy are no longer recommended.

Interpretation of TST Results (see Table 3.64, p 594). The classification of TST results is based on epidemiologic and clinical factors. The appropriate cutoff size for induration in millimeters for a positive result varies with the person tested and the associated epidemiologic factors. In areas of the United States where nontuberculous mycobacteria are common, only 5% of children in the general population who have a 5- to 9-mm area of induration from TST are infected with *M tuberculosis.* However, a child with the same reaction who has had contact with an adult with contagious tuberculosis has an almost 50% chance of having tuberculosis infection.

Current guidelines from the Centers for Disease Control and Prevention (CDC), American Thoracic Society, and the American Academy of Pediatrics accept 15 mm or greater of induration as a positive TST result for any person. Interpretation of 5 mm or more or 10 mm or more induration from a TST is summarized in Table 3.64 (p 594). The physician is aided by knowledge of the tuberculosis case rates and characteristics of tuberculosis within the community, information that should be available from the local health department.

Interpretation of TST Results in Prior Recipients of BCG Vaccine. Generally, interpretation of TST results in BCG recipients is the same as for those who have not received BCG. After BCG immunization, distinguishing between a positive TST result caused by *M tuberculosis* infection and that caused by BCG can be difficult. Reactivity of the TST after receipt of BCG may not occur in some persons. The size of the TST reaction (ie, induration) after receipt of BCG depends on many factors, including age at BCG immunization, quality and strain of BCG used, number of doses of BCG received, nutritional and immunologic status of the vaccine recipient, and frequency of TST administration. A BCG immunization given a few months or more after birth induces a larger reaction than when given immediately after birth.

Infection with *M tuberculosis* should be strongly suspected in any symptomatic person with a positive TST result, regardless of history of BCG immunization. When evaluating an asymptomatic child who has a positive TST result but who possibly received BCG, verification of prior BCG immunization by written documentation or identification of the typical BCG immunization scar should be undertaken. While a positive TST result can never be proven to be due to BCG, certain factors, such as documented receipt of multiple BCG immunizations (as evidenced by multiple BCG scars), decrease the likelihood that the positive TST result is due to tuberculosis infection. Factors that increase the probability that a positive TST result is due to infection with *M tuberculosis* include known contact with a person with contagious tuberculosis, a family history of tuberculosis, immigration from a country with a high prevalence of tuberculosis, and a long interval since the last BCG immunization.

Radiographic evaluation of all children with a positive TST reaction is recommended, regardless of the child's BCG immunization status. In most situations, an asymptomatic BCG-immunized child with a positive TST result will have a normal chest radiograph. In such children, LTBI should be assumed, and antituberculosis therapy should be initiated to prevent progression to *M tuberculosis* disease. In selected instances, such as a child recently immunized with BCG, documented multiple BCG immunizations, and/or immigration from a country with a low prevalence of tuberculosis, treatment may not be indicated. In such cases, follow-up should include education and awareness of the signs and symptoms of tuberculosis disease.

Recommendations for TST Administration. The most reliable strategies for preventing tuberculosis infection and disease in children are based on aggressive, expedient contact investigations rather than routine TST screening of large populations. Household investigation is indicated whenever a TST result of a parent or child converts from negative to positive (indicating recent infection). Specific recommendations for TST use are found in Table 3.65 (p 597). All children need routine health care evaluations that include an assessment of their risk of exposure to tuberculosis. Only children deemed to have increased risk of contact with persons with contagious tuberculosis or those with suspected tuberculosis disease should be considered for a TST.

HIV Testing. Persons with tuberculosis disease should be tested for HIV infection, including counseling before and after testing.

TREATMENT (SEE TABLE 3.66, P 600):

Specific Drugs. Antituberculosis drugs kill *M tuberculosis* or inhibit its multiplication, thereby arresting progression of tuberculosis and preventing most complications of early primary disease. Chemotherapy does not cause rapid disappearance of already caseous or granulomatous lesions (eg, mediastinal lymphadenitis with endobronchial breakthrough). Dosage recommendations and possible adverse reactions of major antituberculosis drugs are summarized in Tables 3.67 and 3.68, p 600 and p 602).

Isoniazid is bactericidal, rapidly absorbed, and well tolerated and penetrates well into body fluids, including CSF. Isoniazid is metabolized in the liver and excreted primarily through the kidneys. Hepatotoxic effects are rare in children. In children and adolescents given recommended doses, peripheral neuritis or seizures caused by inhibition of pyridoxine metabolism are rare, and most do not need pyridoxine supplements. Pyridoxine is recommended for children and adolescents on meat- and milk-deficient diets, those with nutritional deficiencies including all symptomatic HIV-infected children, breastfeeding infants and their mothers, and pregnant adolescents and women. For infants and young children, isoniazid tablets can be pulverized because the liquid preparation is difficult to administer because of its taste.

Rifampin is a bactericidal agent that is absorbed rapidly and penetrates well into body fluids, including CSF. It is metabolized by the liver and can alter the

Table 3.66. **Recommended Treatment Regimens for Drug-Susceptible Tuberculosis in Infants, Children, and Adolescents***

Infection or Disease Category	Regimen	Remarks
Latent tuberculosis infection (positive TST, no disease):		
• Isoniazid-susceptible	9 mo of isoniazid once a day	If daily therapy is not possible, therapy twice a week DOT may be used for 9 mo; HIV-infected children should be treated for 9–12 mo.
• Isoniazid-resistant	6 mo of rifampin once a day	
• Isoniazid-rifampin-resistant†	Consult a tuberculosis specialist	
Pulmonary	**6-mo regimens**	
	2 mo of isoniazid, rifampin, and pyrazinamide once a day, followed by 4 mo of isoniazid and rifampin daily	If possible drug resistance is a concern (see text), another drug (ethambutol or streptomycin) is added to the initial 3-drug therapy until drug susceptibilities are determined.
	OR	
	2 mo of isoniazid, rifampin, and pyrazinamide daily, followed by 4 mo of isoniazid and rifampin twice a week	Drugs can be given 2 or 3 times per wk under DOT in the initial phase if nonadherence is likely.
	9-mo regimens	
	9-mo alternative regimens (for hilar adenopathy only):	Regimens consisting of 6 mo of isoniazid and rifampin once a day, and 1 mo of isoniazid and rifampin once a day, followed by 5 mo of isoniazid and rifampin DOT twice a week have been successful in areas where drug resistance is rare.
	9 mo of isoniazid and rifampin once a day	
	OR	
	1 mo of isoniazid and rifampin once a day, followed by 8 mo of isoniazid and rifampin twice a week	

Table 3.66. **Recommended Treatment Regimens for Drug-Susceptible Tuberculosis in Infants, Children, and Adolescents,* continued**

Infection or Disease Category	Regimen	Remarks
Extrapulmonary: meningitis, disseminated (miliary), bone or joint disease	2 mo of isoniazid, rifampin, pyrazinamide, and streptomycin once a day, followed by 7–10 mo of isoniazid and rifampin once a day (9–12 mo total)	Streptomycin is given with initial therapy until drug susceptibility is known.
	OR	
	2 mo of isoniazid, rifampin, pyrazinamide, and streptomycin once a day, followed by 7–10 mo of isoniazid and rifampin twice a week (9–12 mo total)	For patients who may have acquired tuberculosis in geographic areas where resistance to streptomycin is common, capreomycin (15–30 mg/kg per day) or kanamycin (15–30 mg/kg per day) may be used instead of streptomycin.
Other (eg, cervical lymphadenopathy)	Same as for pulmonary disease	See **Pulmonary**

* TST indicates tuberculin skin test; DOT, directly observed therapy.

† Duration of therapy is longer for human immunodeficiency virus (HIV)-infected persons, and additional drugs may be indicated (see Tuberculosis Disease and HIV Infection, p 607).

Table 3.67. **Commonly Used Drugs for the Treatment of Tuberculosis in Infants, Children, and Adolescents**

Drugs	Dosage Forms	Daily Dosage, mg/kg per Day	Twice a Week Dosage, mg/kg per Dose	Maximum Dose	Adverse Reactions
Ethambutol	Tablets 100 mg 400 mg	15–25	50	2.5 g	Optic neuritis (usually reversible), decreased red-green color discrimination, gastrointestinal tract disturbances, hypersensitivity
Isoniazid*	Scored tablets 100 mg 300 mg Syrup 10 mg/mL	10–15†	20–30	Daily, 300 mg Twice a week, 900 mg	Mild hepatic enzyme elevation, hepatitis,† peripheral neuritis, hypersensitivity
Pyrazinamide*	Scored tablets 500 mg	20–40	50	2 g	Hepatotoxic effects, hyperuricemia
Rifampin*	Capsules 150 mg 300 mg Syrup formulated in syrup from capsules	10–20	10–20	600 mg	Orange discoloration of secretions or urine, staining of contact lenses, vomiting, hepatitis, influenza-like reaction, thrombocytopenia; oral contraceptives may be ineffective
Streptomycin (intramuscular administration)	Vials 1 g 4 g	20–40	20–40	1 g	Auditory and vestibular toxic effects, nephrotoxic effects, rash

* Rifamate is a capsule containing 150 mg of isoniazid and 300 mg of rifampin. Two capsules provide the usual adult (>50 kg body weight) daily doses of each drug. Rifater is a capsule containing 50 mg of isoniazid, 120 mg of rifampin, and 300 mg of pyrazinamide.

† When isoniazid in a dosage exceeding 10 mg/kg per day is used in combination with rifampin, the incidence of hepatotoxic effects may be increased.

Table 3.68. Less Commonly Used Drugs for Treatment of Drug-Resistant Tuberculosis in Infants, Children, and Adolescents*

Drugs	Dosage Forms	Daily Dosage, mg/kg per Day	Maximum Dose	Adverse Reactions
Capreomycin	Vials, 1 g	15–30 (intramuscular administration)	1 g	Ototoxic and nephrotoxic effects
Ciprofloxacin†	Tablets 250 mg 500 mg 750 mg	Adults 500–1500 mg total per day (twice a day)	1.5 g	Theoretical effect on growing cartilage, gastrointestinal tract disturbances, rash, headache
Cycloserine	Capsules, 250 mg	10–20	1 g	Psychosis, personality changes, seizures, rash
Ethionamide	Tablets, 250 mg	15–20 given in 2 or 3 divided doses	1 g	Gastrointestinal tract disturbances, hepatotoxic effects, hypersensitivity reactions
Kanamycin	Vials 75 mg/2 mL 500 mg/2 mL 1 g/3 mL	15–30 (intramuscular administration)	1 g	Auditory and vestibular toxic effects, nephrotoxic effects
Ofloxacin†	Tablets 200 mg 300 mg 400 mg	Adults 400–800 mg total per day (twice a day)	0.8 g	Theoretical effect on growing cartilage, gastrointestinal tract disturbances, rash, headache
Levofloxacin†	Tablets 250 mg 500 mg Vials 25 mg/mL	Adults 500–1000 mg (once daily)	1 g	Theoretical effect on growing cartilage, gastrointestinal tract disturbances, rash, headache
Para-amino salicylic acid (PAS)	Tablets, 500 mg	200–300 (3 or 4 times a day)	10 g	Gastrointestinal tract disturbances, hypersensitivity, hepatotoxic effects

* These drugs should be used in consultation with a specialist in tuberculosis.

† Fluoroquinolones currently are not approved for use in persons younger than 18 years of age; their use in younger patients necessitates assessment of the potential risks and benefits (see Antimicrobial Agents and Related Therapy, p 645).

pharmacokinetics and serum concentrations of many other drugs. Hepatotoxic effects occur rarely. Rifampin is excreted in bile and urine and can cause orange urine, sweat, and tears and discoloration of soft contact lenses and can make oral contraceptives ineffective. Blood dyscrasia accompanied by influenza-like symptoms can occur if doses are taken sporadically or at intervals of 1 week or more. For infants and young children, the contents of the capsules can be suspended in wild cherry–flavored syrup or sprinkled on applesauce. *Mycobacterium tuberculosis* that is resistant to rifampin is uncommon in most areas of the United States.

Pyrazinamide is bactericidal, attains therapeutic CSF concentrations, is detectable in macrophages, is administered orally, and is metabolized by the liver. In doses of 30 mg/kg per day or less, pyrazinamide seldom has hepatotoxic effects and is well tolerated by children. Some adolescents and many adults develop arthralgia because of inhibition of uric acid excretion.

Streptomycin is a bactericidal drug that is administered by the intramuscular route and excreted by the kidneys. Therapeutic CSF concentrations are achieved only in patients with meningitis. Streptomycin usually is prescribed only for 4 to 8 weeks and for no longer than 12 weeks because the incidence of vestibular and cochlear damage correlates with total dose. If streptomycin is not available, kanamycin, capreomycin, or amikacin are alternatives. Resistance to streptomycin is common, particularly among *M tuberculosis* isolates from developing areas of the world, such as Southeast Asia.

Ethambutol is well absorbed after oral administration, diffuses well into tissues including CSF, and is excreted in urine. At 15 mg/kg per day, ethambutol is bacteriostatic only, and its primary therapeutic role is to prevent emergence of drug-resistant organisms. A dose of 25 mg/kg per day is necessary for bactericidal activity. Since ethambutol may cause reversible optic neuritis, recipients should be monitored monthly for visual acuity, visual fields, and red-green color discrimination. Because cooperation is essential for performance of these tests, use of ethambutol in young children whose visual acuity cannot be monitored requires careful consideration of risks and benefits.

The less commonly used antituberculosis drugs, their doses, and adverse effects are listed in Table 3.68 (p 603). These drugs have limited usefulness because of minimal effectiveness and toxic properties and should be used only in consultation with a specialist. Ethionamide is an orally administered antituberculosis drug that is well tolerated by children, achieves therapeutic CSF concentrations, and may be useful for treatment of persons with drug-resistant tuberculosis. Fluoroquinolones (ofloxacin, levofloxacin, and ciprofloxacin) have antituberculosis activity and can be used in special circumstances. Since these drugs are approved by the US Food and Drug Administration for use only in persons 18 years of age and older, their use in younger patients necessitates careful assessment of the potential risks and benefits (see Antimicrobial Agents and Related Therapy, p 645). In cases of multiple drug-resistant tuberculosis, these drugs should be considered for therapy.

Therapy for LTBI. Isoniazid given to adults who have LTBI (ie, no clinical or radiographic manifestations) provides substantial protection (54% to 88% protection) against development of tuberculosis disease for at least 20 years. Among children, efficacy approaches 100% with appropriate adherence to therapy. All infants, children, and adolescents who have a positive TST result but no evidence of tuberculosis disease and who have never received antituberculosis therapy should receive isoniazid alone unless resistance to isoniazid is suspected or a specific contraindication exists. Isoniazid in this circumstance is therapeutic and prevents development of disease. A chest radiograph should be obtained at the time therapy is initiated; if radiographic findings are normal, the child remains asymptomatic, and treatment is completed, the radiograph need not be repeated.

Contacts. Isoniazid therapy often is indicated for recent contacts of persons with contagious tuberculosis when clinical disease has been excluded, even if the TST result is negative, especially for infants and young children and those who are HIV-infected (see Therapy for Contacts, p 611).

Duration of Therapy for LTBI. The optimal duration for therapy remains unknown. In early studies, children received isoniazid for 1 year with efficacy that approached 100%. Data for adults indicate that a 6-month regimen resulted in a 65% reduction in disease compared with a 75% reduction with a 12-month regimen. The CDC recommends a 2-month daily regimen of rifampin and pyrazinamide in adults as an alternative to isoniazid for 9 months; this alternative regimen is not recommended for children.

For most infants and children, the recommended duration of isoniazid therapy is 9 months. Potential exceptions are patients with HIV infection or other immunocompromising conditions for whom some experts recommend a minimum of 12 months of therapy. Isoniazid is given daily, 10 mg/kg (maximum, 300 mg), in a single dose. When adherence with daily therapy cannot be assured, twice-a-week DOT with isoniazid can be considered, preferably after completion of 1 month of daily therapy. Each dose of isoniazid in the twice-a-week DOT regimen is 20 to 30 mg/kg, not to exceed a daily maximum of 900 mg.

Therapy for Contacts of Patients With Isoniazid-Resistant *M tuberculosis*. Possible isoniazid resistance always should be considered, particularly in children who are members of a population in which the prevalence of drug-resistant tuberculosis is high (eg, persons born in countries with a high prevalence, defined as >4% isoniazid resistance, or who have other risk factors listed in Table 3.69, see p 606). Rifampin in addition to isoniazid should be given to these patients. If the source case is found to have isoniazid-resistant organisms, isoniazid should be discontinued and rifampin given for a total course of at least 6 months. Optimal therapy for children with tuberculosis infection caused by organisms with resistance to isoniazid and rifampin is unknown. In these circumstances, multidrug regimens have been used. Drugs to consider include pyrazinamide, a fluoroquinolone, and/or ethambutol, depending on susceptibility of the isolate. Consultation with a tuberculosis specialist is indicated.

Treatment of Tuberculosis Disease. The goal of treatment is to achieve sterilization of the tuberculous lesion in the shortest possible time. Achievement of this goal reduces treatment cost and minimizes the possibility of development of resistant organisms. The major problem limiting successful treatment is poor adherence to prescribed treatment regimens. The use of DOT decreases relapse rates, treatment failures, and drug resistance rates, and, therefore, **DOT is recommended for treatment of people with tuberculosis in the United States.**

The encouraging results of 6- and 9-month treatment regimens for infants, children, and adolescents with pulmonary and extrapulmonary tuberculosis have led to

Table 3.69. **Persons at Increased Risk for Drug-Resistant Tuberculosis Infection or Disease**

- Persons with a history of treatment for active tuberculosis (or whose source case for the contact received such treatment)
- Contacts of a patient with drug-resistant contagious tuberculosis disease
- Foreign-born persons
- Residents of areas where the prevalence of drug-resistant *Mycobacterium tuberculosis* is documented to be high (defined by most experts as isoniazid resistance rates ≥4%)
- Persons whose source case has positive smears for acid-fast bacilli or cultures after 2 months of appropriate antituberculosis therapy

use of these shorter regimens. Shorter treatment regimens also can be used for adolescents with adult-type disease, especially those with radiographic evidence of reactivation disease.

A 6-month regimen consisting of isoniazid, rifampin, and pyrazinamide for the first 2 months and isoniazid and rifampin for the remaining 4 months is recommended for treatment of drug-susceptible *M tuberculosis* disease, including pulmonary, pulmonary with hilar adenopathy, and hilar adenopathy disease in infants, children, and adolescents. For children with hilar adenopathy in whom drug resistance is not a consideration, a 6-month regimen of only isoniazid and rifampin is adequate.

When drug resistance is suspected (see Table 3.69, above), initial therapy should include a fourth drug, either ethambutol or streptomycin, until drug susceptibility results are available. If an isolate from the pediatric case under treatment is not available, drug susceptibilities can be determined by the susceptibility pattern of isolates from the adult source case. If this information is not available, local endemic rates of single and multiple drug resistance can be helpful. Data may not be available for foreign-born children or in circumstances of foreign travel. **If this information is not available, a 4-drug initial regimen is recommended.**

In the 6-month regimen with triple-drug therapy, isoniazid, rifampin, and pyrazinamide are given once a day for the first 2 weeks to 2 months. After this initial period, a DOT regimen of isoniazid and rifampin given twice a week is acceptable (see Table 3.66, p 601, for doses). Several alternative regimens with differing durations of daily therapy and total therapy have been used successfully in adults and children. These alternative regimens should be prescribed and managed with a specialist in tuberculosis.

Therapy for Drug-Resistant Tuberculosis Disease. In North America, the incidence of drug resistance in previously untreated patients has increased in recent years, and, in certain areas, the incidence of resistance to isoniazid can be as high as 10% to 20%. Drug resistance is most common in the following: (1) foreign-born persons from areas such as Asia, Africa, and Latin America; (2) New York City and several other cities where hospital- and community-based outbreaks of drug-resistant tuberculosis have been documented; (3) the homeless; (4) persons previously treated for tuberculosis; and (5) contacts, especially children, with tuberculosis whose source case is a person from one of these groups (see also Table 3.69, p 606). If a child is at risk for or has isoniazid-resistant tuberculosis disease, at least 2 drugs to which the isolate is susceptible should be given. For cases of drug-resistant tuberculosis, an initial treatment regimen should include 4 antituberculosis drugs. Treatment should include at least 2 bactericidal drugs, such as isoniazid and rifampin, pyrazinamide, and either streptomycin or another aminoglycoside (also bactericidal) or high-dose ethambutol (25 mg/kg per day). In cases of tuberculosis with isoniazid- or rifampin-resistant strains, 6-month drug regimens are not recommended. Twice-a-week regimens also are not recommended for drug-resistant disease; 12 to 18 months of therapy usually are necessary to effect a cure. To cure children with drug-resistant tuberculosis and prevent emergence of further resistance, DOT is critical.

Extrapulmonary Tuberculosis. In general, extrapulmonary tuberculosis, including cervical lymphadenopathy, can be treated with the same regimens as pulmonary tuberculosis. Exceptions are bone and joint disease, miliary disease, and meningitis, for which current data in children are too limited to support a 6-month course of therapy. For these severe forms of drug-susceptible extrapulmonary tuberculosis, daily treatment with isoniazid, rifampin, pyrazinamide, and, usually, streptomycin for the first 1 or 2 months, followed by isoniazid and rifampin once a day or twice a week by DOT is recommended for a total of 9 to 12 months. Some experts would treat all extrapulmonary tuberculosis for no more than 9 months. For life-threatening tuberculosis, 4 drugs are given initially because of the possibility of drug resistance and the severe consequences of treatment failure (see Therapy for Drug-Resistant Tuberculosis Disease, p 606).

Pyrazinamide is useful for disseminated and meningeal tuberculosis because it achieves better CSF concentrations than streptomycin or ethambutol. In cases of severe tuberculosis with vomiting or obtundation, isoniazid or rifampin can be given parenterally. The dose is the same as that recommended for oral therapy.

Corticosteroids. Adjuvant treatment with corticosteroids for children with tuberculosis is controversial. Corticosteroids are indicated for children with tuberculous meningitis. Dexamethasone has lowered mortality and long-term neurologic impairment. Corticosteroids also may be considered for children with pleural and pericardial effusions (to hasten reabsorption of fluid), severe miliary disease (to mitigate alveolocapillary block), and endobronchial disease (to relieve obstruction and atelectasis). Corticosteroids should be given only when accompanied by appropriate antituberculosis therapy. Most experts consider 1 to 2 mg/kg per day of prednisone or its equivalent for 6 to 8 weeks to be appropriate.

Tuberculosis Disease and HIV Infection. Adults and children with HIV infection have an increased incidence of tuberculosis disease. Hence, testing for HIV is indicated for all persons with tuberculosis disease. The clinical manifestations and radiographic appearance of tuberculosis in children with HIV infection tend to be similar to those in immunocompetent children, but manifestations in these children can be unusual and can include extrapulmonary involvement of multiple organs. In HIV-infected patients, a TST result of 5-mm induration or more is considered positive (see Table 3.64, p 594); however, a negative TST result due to HIV-related immunosuppression also can occur. Specimens for culture should be obtained from all HIV-infected children with suspected tuberculosis.

Most HIV-infected adults with drug-susceptible tuberculosis respond well to antituberculosis drugs when appropriate therapy is given early. However, optimal therapy for tuberculosis in children with HIV infection has not been established. Therapy always should include at least 3 drugs initially and be continued for at least 9 months. Isoniazid, rifampin, and pyrazinamide with or without ethambutol or streptomycin should be given for at least the first 2 months. A fourth drug is indicated for disseminated disease and whenever drug-resistant disease is suspected. Consultation with a specialist who has experience in managing HIV-infected patients with tuberculosis is advised.

Evaluation and Monitoring of Therapy in Children and Adolescents. Careful monthly monitoring of the clinical and bacteriological responses to therapy is important. With DOT, clinical evaluation is an integral component of each visit for drug administration. For patients with pulmonary tuberculosis, chest radiographs should be obtained 2 to 3 months into therapy to help evaluate response. Even with successful 6-month regimens, however, hilar adenopathy may require as long as 2 to 3 years for radiographic resolution, and a normal radiograph is not a necessary criterion to discontinue therapy. Follow-up chest radiographs beyond the termination of successful therapy usually are not necessary unless clinical deterioration occurs.

If therapy has been interrupted, the date for completion should be extended. Although guidelines cannot be provided for every situation, factors to consider when establishing the date for completion include the following: (1) length of interruption of therapy; (2) time during therapy (early or late) when interruption occurred; and (3) patient's clinical, radiographic, and bacteriologic status before, during, and after interruption of therapy. Consultation with a specialist is advised.

Untoward effects of isoniazid therapy in otherwise healthy infants, children, and adolescents, including severe hepatitis, are rare. Routine determination of serum aminotransferase concentrations is not recommended. However, for children with severe tuberculosis, especially meningitis or disseminated disease, aminotransferase concentrations should be monitored approximately monthly during the first several months of treatment. Other indications for testing include the following: (1) concurrent or recent liver disease; (2) high daily dose of isoniazid (more than 10 mg/kg per day) in combination with rifampin, pyrazinamide, or both; (3) pregnancy or first 6 weeks postpartum; (4) clinical evidence of hepatotoxic effects; (5) hepatobiliary tract disease from other causes; or (6) concurrent use of other hepatotoxic drugs (especially anticonvulsants). In most other circumstances, monthly clinical evaluations for 3 months, followed by evaluation every 1 to 3 months to observe for signs or symptoms of hepatitis and other adverse effects of drug therapy without routine monitoring of aminotransferase levels, is an appropriate schedule for follow-up. In all cases, regular physician-patient contact to assess drug adherence, efficacy, and toxic effects is an important aspect of management.

Immunizations. Patients who are receiving treatment for tuberculosis can be given measles and other live-virus vaccines unless they are receiving high-dose corticosteroids, are severely ill, or have other specific vaccine contraindications to immunization.

Tuberculosis During Pregnancy and Breastfeeding. Tuberculosis during pregnancy should be managed on a case-by-case basis because of the complexity of management decisions. During pregnancy, if tuberculosis disease is diagnosed, a regimen of isoniazid, rifampin, and ethambutol is recommended. Pyrazinamide frequently is used in a 3- or 4-drug regimen, but safety in pregnancy has not been established. At least 6 months of therapy is indicated for drug-susceptible disease. Prompt initiation of therapy is mandatory to protect mother and fetus.

Asymptomatic pregnant women with a positive TST result, a normal chest radiograph, and recent contact with an infectious person should receive isoniazid therapy. The recommended duration of therapy is 9 months. Therapy in these circumstances should begin after the first trimester. Although no harmful effects of isoniazid to the fetus have been observed, some experts delay therapy until after delivery in the absence of HIV infection, immunosuppression, recent tuberculosis infection, or other illness, such as diabetes mellitus. Pyridoxine is indicated for all pregnant women receiving isoniazid.

Isoniazid, ethambutol, and rifampin seem to be relatively safe for the fetus. The benefit of ethambutol and rifampin for therapy of tuberculosis disease in the mother outweighs the risk to the infant. Because streptomycin can cause ototoxic effects in the fetus, it should not be used unless administration is essential to treat the maternal disease.

Women who are receiving isoniazid and are breastfeeding should receive pyridoxine. While isoniazid is secreted in human milk, no adverse effects of isoniazid on nursing infants have been demonstrated (see Human Milk, p 98).

Congenital Tuberculosis. Women who have only pulmonary tuberculosis are not likely to infect the fetus but may infect their infant after delivery. Congenital tuberculosis is rare, but in utero infections can occur after maternal *M tuberculosis* bacillemia.

If a newborn is suspected of having congenital tuberculosis, a TST, chest radiograph, lumbar puncture, and appropriate cultures should be performed promptly. The TST result usually is negative in newborn infants with congenital or perinatally acquired infection. Hence, regardless of the TST results, treatment of the infant should be initiated promptly with isoniazid, rifampin, pyrazinamide, and streptomycin or kanamycin. The placenta should be examined histologically and cultured for *M tuberculosis.* The mother should be evaluated for the presence of pulmonary or extrapulmonary, including uterine, tuberculosis. If the maternal physical examination or chest radiograph support the diagnosis of tuberculosis disease, the newborn infant should be treated with regimens recommended for tuberculous meningitis, excluding corticosteroids. If meningitis is confirmed, corticosteroids should be given (see Corticosteroids, p 607). Drug susceptibilities of the organism recovered from the mother, infant, or both should be determined.

Management of the Newborn Infant Whose Mother (or Other Household Contact) Has LTBI or Disease. Management of the newborn infant is based on categorization of the maternal (or household contact) infection. While protection of the infant from infection is of paramount importance, separation of the infant from the mother (or household contact) should be avoided when possible. Differing circumstances and resulting recommendations are as follows:

- ***Mother (or household contact) has a normal chest radiograph.*** If the mother (or household contact) is asymptomatic, no separation is required. The mother usually is a candidate for treatment of LTBI. The newborn infant needs no special evaluation or therapy. Because the positive TST result could be a marker of an unrecognized case of contagious tuberculosis within the household, other household members should have a TST and further evaluation.

- ***Mother (or household contact) has an abnormal chest radiograph.*** If the radiograph is abnormal, the mother (or household contact) and infant should be separated until the mother (or household contact) has been evaluated and, if tuberculosis disease is found, until the mother or contact is receiving appropriate antituberculosis therapy. Other household members should have a TST and further evaluation.
- ***Mother (or household contact) has an abnormal chest radiograph but no evidence of tuberculosis disease.*** If the chest radiograph of the mother (or household contact) is abnormal, but the history, physical examination, sputum smear, and radiograph indicate no evidence of tuberculosis disease, the infant can be assumed to be at low risk for *M tuberculosis* infection and need not be separated from the mother. The mother and her infant should receive follow-up care. Other household members should have a TST and further evaluation.
- ***Mother (or household contact) has clinical or radiographic evidence of possibly contagious tuberculosis.*** The case in the mother (or household contact) should be reported immediately to the local health department so that health department investigation of all household members can be performed within several days. All contacts should have a TST, chest radiograph, and physical examination. The infant should be evaluated for congenital tuberculosis (see Congenital Tuberculosis, p 609) and tested for HIV infection. If the infant is receiving isoniazid, separation is not necessary. Other household members should have a TST and further evaluation.

If congenital tuberculosis is excluded, isoniazid is given until the infant is 3 or 4 months of age, at which time the TST should be repeated. If the TST result is positive, the infant should be reassessed for tuberculosis disease. If disease is not present, isoniazid should be continued for at least 9 months. If the PPD is negative and the mother and other household contacts with tuberculosis have good adherence and response to treatment and are no longer contagious, isoniazid may be discontinued. The infant should be evaluated at monthly intervals during treatment.

If the mother (or household contact) has disease due to multiple drug-resistant *M tuberculosis* or has poor adherence to treatment and DOT is not possible, the infant should be separated from the ill mother or household member and BCG immunization should be considered for the infant. Since the response to BCG in infants may be delayed and inadequate for prevention of tuberculosis, DOT for the mother or household contact and infant is preferred.

ISOLATION OF THE HOSPITALIZED PATIENT: Most children with tuberculosis are not contagious and require only standard precautions. Precautions for tuberculosis (TB) or AFB precautions are indicated until effective therapy has been initiated, sputum smears demonstrate a diminishing number of organisms, and cough is abating, for children with the following: (1) cavitary pulmonary tuberculosis, (2) positive sputum AFB smears, (3) laryngeal involvement, or (4) extensive pulmonary infection. Children with no cough and negative sputum AFB smears can be hospitalized on an open ward. Infection control measures for hospital personnel in contagious cases should include the use of personally "fitted" and "sealed" particulate respirators for all patient contacts (see Infection Control for Hospitalized Children, p 127).

The major concern in infection control relates to adult household members and contacts who may be the source case. Appropriate evaluation with a TST and chest radiograph is warranted. Household members should be managed with TB or AFB precautions when visiting until they are demonstrated not to have contagious tuberculosis. Nonadherent household contacts should be excluded from hospital visitation until evaluation is complete and tuberculosis is excluded or treatment has rendered source cases noncontagious.

Control Measures:

The control of tuberculosis in the United States necessitates access to health care, obtaining a thorough history of exposure(s) to persons with contagious tuberculosis, timely and effective contact investigations, proper interpretation of a TST result, and appropriate antituberculosis therapy, including DOT. Variations in the epidemiology of tuberculosis in different locations reinforce the importance of communication with local public health officials, regional experts on tuberculosis, or both.

Management of Contacts, Including Epidemiologic Investigation. Children with a positive TST result or tuberculosis disease should be the starting point for epidemiologic investigation, which is best accomplished by assistance from the local health department. Close contacts of a TST-positive child should have a TST, and persons with a positive TST result or symptoms consistent with tuberculosis disease should be investigated further. Since children with primary tuberculosis usually are not contagious, their contacts are not likely to be infected unless they also have been in contact with the same adult source case. After the presumptive adult source of the child's tuberculosis is identified, other contacts of that adult should be evaluated, including a TST, and chest radiograph for those with a positive TST result to identify persons who need antituberculosis therapy.

Therapy for Contacts. Persons exposed within the previous 3 months to a potentially contagious case of tuberculosis, especially contacts with impaired immunity (eg, HIV-infected) and all household contacts younger than 4 years of age who are exposed to any adult with tuberculosis disease, should have a TST and a chest radiograph and be given isoniazid therapy, even if the TST result is negative, once clinical disease is excluded (see Therapy for LTBI, p 604). Other candidates for therapy if the TST result is negative include recent contacts and household contacts of any age, especially if they are from a population with a high prevalence of tuberculosis. Infected persons can have a negative TST result because cellular reactivity has not yet developed or because of cutaneous anergy. Persons with a negative TST result should be retested 12 weeks after the last contact. If the TST is still negative, isoniazid can be discontinued. If the TST result becomes positive, isoniazid is continued for a total of 9 months.

Child Care and Schools. Children with tuberculosis infection or disease can attend school or child care if they are receiving therapy (see Children in Out-of-Home Child Care, p 105). They can return to regular activities as soon as effective therapy has been instituted, adherence to therapy has been documented, and clinical symptoms have disappeared.

BCG Vaccine. The BCG vaccine is a live vaccine prepared from attenuated strains of *M bovis*. Use of BCG is recommended by the Expanded Programme on Immunization of the World Health Organization (WHO) for administration at birth (see Table 1.3, p 7), and currently is used in more than 100 countries. Use of BCG is primarily in young infants, in an attempt to prevent disseminated and other life-threatening manifestations of *M tuberculosis* disease. However, BCG does not prevent infection with *M tuberculosis.* The various BCG vaccines used throughout the world differ because of genetic changes in the bacterial strains that have occurred over many years. Efficacy of different BCG vaccines seems to be highly variable.

Two meta-analyses of published clinical trials and case-control studies concerning the efficacy of BCG vaccines concluded that BCG has relatively high protective efficacy (approximately 80%) against meningeal and miliary tuberculosis in children. The protective efficacy against pulmonary tuberculosis, however, differed significantly among the studies, precluding a specific conclusion. Protection afforded by BCG in one meta-analysis was estimated to be 50%. As of December 1999, BCG vaccines manufactured by Organon Teknika Corporation, Durham, NC, and Connaught Laboratories, Willowdale, Ontario, are licensed in the United States. Comparative evaluations of these and other BCG vaccines have not been performed.

Indications. In the United States, administration of BCG should be considered only in limited and select circumstances, such as unavoidable risk of exposure to *M tuberculosis* and failure or infeasibility of other methods of control of tuberculosis. Recommendations for use of BCG for control of tuberculosis among children and health care workers have been published by the Advisory Committee on Immunization Practices (ACIP) and the Advisory Council for the Elimination of Tuberculosis of the CDC.* For infants and children, BCG immunization should be considered only for persons with a negative TST result who are not infected with HIV in the following circumstances:

- The child is exposed continually to a person or persons with contagious pulmonary tuberculosis resistant to isoniazid and rifampin and the child cannot be removed from this exposure.
- The child is exposed continually to a person or persons with untreated or ineffectively treated contagious pulmonary tuberculosis and the child cannot be removed from such exposure or given antituberculosis therapy.

Vaccination with BCG also should be considered for health care workers in certain high-risk settings (see ACIP recommendation*).

Careful assessment of the potential risks and benefits of BCG vaccine and consultation with personnel in local area control programs for tuberculosis is strongly recommended before use of BCG.

When BCG vaccine is given, care should be taken to observe precautions and directions for administration in the product label. Healthy infants from birth to 2 months of age may be given BCG without TST testing; thereafter, BCG is given only to children with a negative TST result.

Adverse Reactions. Uncommonly (1% to 2% of vaccinations), BCG can result in local adverse reactions, such as subcutaneous abscess and lymphadenopathy, which generally are not serious. One rare complication, osteitis affecting the epiphysis of long bones, may occur as long as several years after BCG immunization.

---

* Centers for Disease Control and Prevention. The role of BCG vaccine in the prevention and control of tuberculosis in the United States: a joint statement by the Advisory Committee for the Elimination of Tuberculosis and the Advisory Committee on Immunization Practices. *MMWR Morb Mortal Wkly Rep.* 1996;45(RR-4):1–18

Disseminated fatal disease occurs rarely (approximately 2 in 1 million persons), primarily in persons with severely impaired immune systems. Antituberculosis therapy, except for pyrazinamide, is recommended to treat osteitis and disseminated disease caused by BCG. Some experts also recommend treatment of chronic suppurative lymphadenitis caused by BCG. Persons with complications caused by BCG should be referred, if possible, to a tuberculosis expert for management.

Contraindications. Persons with burns, skin infections, and primary or secondary immunodeficiencies, including HIV infection, should not receive BCG. However, in populations of the world in which the risk of tuberculosis is high, the WHO recommends BCG immunization for asymptomatic HIV-infected children. Use of BCG also is contraindicated for persons receiving immunosuppressive medications, including high-dose corticosteroids (see Corticosteroids, p 607). Although no untoward effects of BCG on the fetus have been observed, immunization during pregnancy is not recommended.

Reporting of Cases. Reporting of suspected and confirmed cases of tuberculosis is mandated by law in all states. **A diagnosis of tuberculosis infection or disease in a child is a sentinel event representing recent transmission of *M tuberculosis* in the community.** Physicians should assist in the search for a source case and others infected by the source case. Usually adults or adolescents, such as members of the household (including relatives, baby-sitters, boarders, domestic workers, and frequent visitors) or other adults with whom the child has frequent contact, are source cases.

Diseases Caused By Nontuberculous Mycobacteria

(Atypical Mycobacteria, Mycobacteria Other Than *Mycobacterium tuberculosis*)

CLINICAL MANIFESTATIONS: Several syndromes are caused by nontuberculous mycobacteria (NTM). In children, the most common of these syndromes is cervical lymphadenitis. Less common infections are cutaneous infection, osteomyelitis, otitis media, and pulmonary disease. Disseminated infections almost always are associated with immunodeficiency characterized by impaired cell-mediated immunity, such as congenital immune defects or human immunodeficiency virus (HIV) infection. Manifestations of disseminated NTM infections depend on the species and route of infection and include fever, night sweats, weight loss, abdominal pain, fatigue, diarrhea, and anemia.

ETIOLOGY: Of the many species of NTM that have been identified, only a small number account for most human infections. The species most frequently encountered in children are *Mycobacterium avium* complex (MAC) (including *Mycobacterium avium* and *Mycobacterium intracellulare*), *Mycobacterium scrofulaceum, Mycobacterium fortuitum, Mycobacterium kansasii,* and *Mycobacterium marinum* (see Table 3.70, p 614). Infection in patients with HIV usually is caused by MAC. *Mycobacterium fortuitum, Mycobacterium chelonae,* and *Mycobacterium abscessus* frequently are referred to as "rapidly growing" mycobacteria because they grow sufficiently in the laboratory to be identified within 3 to 7 days, whereas other NTM and *Mycobacterium tuberculosis* often require weeks to grow in the laboratory.

Table 3.70. Diseases Caused by Nontuberculous Mycobacterial Species*

Clinical Disease	Common Species	Less Common Species
Cutaneous infection	*Mycobacterium chelonae, Mycobacterium fortuitum, Mycobacterium abscessus, Mycobacterium marinum*	*Mycobacterium ulcerans,*† *Mycobacterium haemophilum*
Lymphadenitis	MAC, *Mycobacterium scrofulaceum*	*M kansasii, M fortuitum, Mycobacterium malmoense*†
Otologic infection	*M abscessus*	*M fortuitum*
Pulmonary infection	MAC, *Mycobacterium kansasii*	*Mycobacterium xenopi, M abscessus, M malmoense,*† *Mycobacterium szulgai, M fortuitum, Mycobacterium simiae*
Catheter-associated infection	*M chelonae, M fortuitum*	*M abscessus*
Skeletal infection	*M kansasii,* MAC	*M fortuitum, M chelonae, M marinum, M abscessus*
Disseminated	MAC	*M kansasii, Mycobacterium genavense*

* MAC indicates *Mycobacterium avium* complex.

† Found primarily outside of the United States.

Rapidly growing mycobacteria occasionally have been implicated in wound, soft tissue, bone, pulmonary, and middle-ear infections. Other mycobacterial species, which usually are not pathogenic, have caused infections in immunocompromised hosts or have been associated with the presence of a foreign body.

EPIDEMIOLOGY: Because infections caused by NTM are not reportable, fewer systematically collected data about their incidence and distribution are available than for infections caused by *M tuberculosis.* In the past, as the incidence of tuberculosis decreased, the relative proportion of mycobacterial infections caused by NTM increased. Since the epidemic of HIV infection, however, tuberculosis and MAC infections have increased in incidence.

Many NTM species are ubiquitous and are found in soil, food, water, and animals. Although many persons are exposed to NTM, only a few of these exposures result in chronic infection or disease. *Mycobacterium avium* complex in the respiratory or gastrointestinal tract is common in persons with HIV infection. Nontuberculous mycobacteria, usually MAC, also can be recovered from 10% to 20% of adolescents and young adults with cystic fibrosis. The usual portals of entry for NTM infection are believed to be abrasions in the skin (eg, for the cutaneous lesions caused by *M marinum*), the oropharyngeal mucosa (the presumed portal for cervical lymphadenitis), the gastrointestinal or respiratory tract for MAC, and the respiratory tract (including tympanostomy tubes) for otitis media and rare cases of mediastinal adenitis and of endobronchial disease. Most infections remain localized at the portal of entry or in regional lymph nodes. Severe pulmonary disease and dissemination to distal sites primarily occur in immunocompromised hosts, especially in persons with acquired immunodeficiency syndrome (AIDS). No definitive evidence for person-to-person transmission of NTM exists; however, clustering of patients with the same *M avium* strain has been reported and may represent a common environmental exposure or person-to-person spread. Cases of otitis media caused by *M abscessus* have been associated with use of contaminated equipment and water. A waterborne route of transmission has been suspected for MAC infection in immunodeficient hosts.

The **incubation period** is unknown.

DIAGNOSTIC TESTS: Definitive diagnosis of disease caused by NTM requires isolation of the organism. However, because these organisms commonly are found in the environment, contamination of cultures or transient colonization can occur. Therefore, caution must be exercised in the interpretation of cultures obtained from sites that are not sterile, such as gastric washings, a draining sinus tract, a single sputum specimen, or a urine specimen. Caution in ascribing illness to NTM also is warranted if the species cultured usually is nonpathogenic (eg, *Mycobacterium gordonae*) and if only a few colonies are recovered from a single specimen. Repeated isolation of numerous colonies of a single species is more likely to indicate disease than culture contamination or transient colonization. Recovery of NTM from sites that usually are sterile, such as cerebrospinal fluid, pleural fluid, bone marrow, blood, lymph node aspirates, middle ear or mastoid aspirates, or surgically excised tissue, is the most reliable diagnostic test. With the radiometric broth or lysis-centrifugation techniques, blood cultures are highly sensitive in recovery of MAC and other blood-borne NTM species. Disseminated MAC disease should prompt a search for underlying immunosuppression, usually HIV infection.

Patients with NTM infection can have false-positive PPD skin test results, since this preparation, derived from *M tuberculosis,* shares a number of antigens with NTM species. These false-positive PPD reactions usually measure less than 10 mm of induration and occur in otherwise healthy children who have no history of exposure to *M tuberculosis* but have been sensitized by exposure to NTM in the environment.

TREATMENT: Many NTM are relatively resistant in vitro to antituberculosis drugs. In vitro resistance, however, does not necessarily correlate with clinical response. Only limited controlled therapeutic trials have been performed in patients with NTM infections. The approach to therapy should be dictated by the following: (1) the species causing the infection, (2) the results of drug-susceptibility testing, (3) the site(s) of infection, (4) the patient's underlying disease (if any), and (5) the need to treat a patient presumptively for tuberculosis while awaiting culture reports that subsequently reveal NTM.

For the common problem of NTM lymphadenitis in otherwise healthy children, especially when the disease is caused by *M scrofulaceum* or MAC, complete surgical excision almost always is effective treatment. Antituberculosis chemotherapy usually offers little benefit, but specific therapy may be beneficial for some children, especially when surgical excision is incomplete (see Table 3.71, p 616).

Isolates of rapid-growing mycobacteria (*M fortuitum, M abscessus,* and *M chelonae*) should be tested in vitro against antituberculosis agents, as well as against other drugs (such as amikacin, imipenem, cefoxitin, ciprofloxacin, clarithromycin, and doxycycline) to which they frequently are susceptible and that have been used with

Table 3.71. Treatment of Nontuberculous Mycobacteria Infections in Children*

Organism	Disease	Treatment
Mycobacterium avium complex (MAC)	Lymphadenitis	Complete excision; if excision incomplete or disease recurs, clarithromycin
	Pulmonary infection	Clarithromycin or azithromycin plus another drug† (pulmonary resection in some patients)
	Disseminated	See text
Mycobacterium fortuitum complex	Lymphadenitis	Complete excision (see MAC)
	Cutaneous infection	Excision of tissue; initial therapy is amikacin plus cefoxitin IV followed by erythromycin, clarithromycin, doxycycline, or ciprofloxacin orally
	Catheter infection	Catheter removal and amikacin plus cefoxitin IV; clarithromycin, doxycycline, or ciprofloxacin orally
Mycobacterium kansasii	Lymphadenitis	Complete excision
	Pulmonary infection	Isoniazid plus rifampin with or without ethambutol
	Osteomyelitis	Surgical débridement and prolonged antimicrobial therapy
Mycobacterium marinum	Cutaneous infection	None, if minor; rifampin, trimethoprim-sulfamethoxazole, clarithromycin, or doxycycline for moderate disease; extensive lesions may require surgical débridement

* IV indicates intravenously.

† Agents to be considered are ethambutol, rifabutin, ciprofloxacin, rifampin, or amikacin.

some success. Clarithromycin plus at least one other agent seems to be the treatment of choice for cutaneous (disseminated) infections due to *M chelonae.* Details about choice of drugs, dosages, and duration should be reviewed with a consultant experienced in the management of these infections.

In patients with AIDS and in other immunocompromised persons with disseminated MAC infection, multidrug therapy is indicated. Single-dose therapy results in frequent development of antimicrobial resistance. Clinical isolates of MAC usually are resistant to many of the approved antituberculosis drugs, including isoniazid, but often are susceptible in vitro to clarithromycin, azithromycin, ethambutol, rifabutin, rifampin, clofazimine, amikacin, and fluoroquinolones. The optimal regimen has yet to be determined. Treatment of disseminated MAC infection should be done in consultation with an expert. In addition, the following treatment guidelines should be considered:

- Unless there is clinical or laboratory evidence of macrolide resistance, treatment regimens should contain clarithromycin or azithromycin with at least one other drug (ie, ethambutol or rifabutin).
- Many clinicians have added one or more of the following as a third or fourth agent: rifampin, ciprofloxacin, or, in some situations, amikacin.

- Patients receiving protease inhibitor antiretroviral therapy generally should not be treated with rifabutin. However, if coadministration of rifabutin and a protease inhibitor is necessary, indinavir and nelfinavir are the preferred protease inhibitors, and the dose of rifabutin should be decreased by 50%.
- Clofazimine is ineffective for the treatment of MAC disease and should not be used.
- Patients with HIV infection who are treated for disseminated MAC disease should continue to receive full therapeutic doses of antimycobacterial agents for life.
- Patients receiving therapy should be monitored. Considerations are as follows:
  - Clinical manifestations of disseminated MAC infection, such as fever, weight loss, and night sweats, should be monitored several times during the initial weeks of therapy. Microbiologic response, as assessed by blood culture every 4 weeks during initial therapy, also can be helpful for interpreting the efficacy of a therapeutic regimen.
  - Most patients who ultimately respond show substantial clinical improvement in the first 4 to 6 weeks of therapy. Elimination of the organisms from blood cultures may take somewhat longer, often requiring 4 to 12 weeks.
  - Patients receiving clarithromycin plus rifabutin or high-dose rifabutin (with another drug) should be observed for the rifabutin-related development of uveitis, polyarthralgias, and pseudojaundice.

Chemoprophylaxis. According to the 1999 guidelines of the US Public Health Service/Infectious Diseases Society of America Prevention of Opportunistic Infections Working Group, to prevent the first MAC episode, prophylaxis with azithromycin or clarithromycin should be considered for HIV-infected adults and adolescents with CD4+ T-lymphocyte counts of less than 50 cells × 10^6/L (50 cells/µL).* Rifabutin is an alternative prophylactic agent but should not be used until active tuberculosis has been excluded to avoid the development of rifampin-resistant tuberculosis. Also, disseminated MAC disease should be excluded by a negative blood culture result before prophylaxis is initiated.

Prophylaxis for prevention of a first MAC infection should be offered to HIV-infected children younger than 13 years with the following CD4+ T-lymphocyte counts: children 6 years of age or older, less than 50 cells × 10^6/L (<50/µL); children 2 to 6 years of age, less than 75 cells × 10^6/L (<75/µL); children 1 to 2 years of age, less than 500 cells × 10^6/L (<500/µL); and children younger than 12 months of age, less than 750 cells × 10^6/L (<750/µL).

Oral suspensions of clarithromycin and azithromycin are available commercially in the United States. No pediatric formulation of rifabutin is available, but a dosage of 5 mg/kg per day seems appropriate. Rifabutin should be used only for children older than 6 years of age.

ISOLATION OF THE HOSPITALIZED PATIENT: Standard precautions are recommended.

* Centers for Disease Control and Prevention. 1999 USPHS/IDSA guidelines for the prevention of opportunistic infections in persons infected with human immunodeficiency virus. *MMWR Morb Mortal Wkly Rep.* 1999;48(RR-10):1–59, 61–66

Control Measures: The only control measures are chemoprophylaxis for certain patients with HIV infection (see Treatment, p 617) and use of sterile equipment for middle-ear instrumentation, including otoscopic equipment for prevention of *M abscessus* otitis media. Since MAC organisms are common in environmental sources, such as food and water, current information does not support specific recommendations about avoidance of exposure for HIV-infected persons.

Tularemia

Clinical Manifestations: Most patients with tularemia experience an abrupt onset of fever, chills, myalgia, and headache. Illness usually conforms to one of the several tularemic syndromes. Most common is the ulceroglandular syndrome, which is characterized by the following: (1) a primary, painful, maculopapular lesion at the portal of bacterial entry, with subsequent ulceration and slow healing; and (2) painful, acutely inflamed, regional lymph nodes, which may drain spontaneously. Less common disease syndromes are the following: (1) glandular (regional lymphadenopathy with no ulcer), (2) oculoglandular (severe conjunctivitis and preauricular lymphadenopathy), (3) oropharyngeal (severe exudative stomatitis, pharyngitis, or tonsillitis and cervical lymphadenopathy), (4) typhoidal (high fever, hepatomegaly, and splenomegaly), (5) intestinal (intestinal pain, vomiting, and diarrhea), and (6) pneumonic (primary pleuropulmonary disease).

Etiology: *Francisella tularensis,* the causative agent of tularemia, is a gram-negative pleomorphic coccobacillus.

Epidemiology: Sources of the organism include approximately 100 species of wild mammals (eg, rabbits, hares, muskrats, and voles); at least 9 species of domestic animals (eg, sheep, cattle, and cats); blood-sucking arthropods that bite these animals (eg, ticks, deerflies, and mosquitoes); and water and soil contaminated by infected animals. In the United States, rabbits and ticks are major sources of human infection. Infected animals and arthropods, especially ticks, are infective for prolonged periods; frozen killed rabbits can remain infective for more than 3 years. Persons at risk are those with occupational or recreational exposure to infected animals or their habitat, such as rabbit hunters and trappers, persons exposed to certain ticks or biting insects, and laboratory technicians working with *F tularensis,* which is a highly infectious agent in a laboratory setting. In the United States, ticks are the most important arthropod vectors. Infection also may be acquired by direct contact with infected animals, ingestion of contaminated water or inadequately cooked meat, or inhalation of contaminated particles. Person-to-person transmission has not been documented. Organisms may be present in blood during the first 2 weeks of disease and in cutaneous lesions for as long as 1 month if untreated.

The **incubation period** usually is 3 to 5 days with a range of 1 to 21 days.

DIAGNOSTIC TESTS: Diagnosis is established most frequently by serologic testing. A 4-fold or greater change in *F tularensis* agglutinin titer frequently is evident after the second week of illness and is considered diagnostic. A single convalescent titer of 1:160 or greater is consistent with recent or past infection. Slide agglutination tests are less reliable than plate or tube agglutination tests; nonspecific cross-agglutination with *Brucella, Proteus,* and heterophil antibodies can cause false-positive antibody titers to *F tularensis.* The indirect fluorescent antibody test of ulcer exudate or aspirate material can be useful as a rapid and specific screening test. Polymerase chain reaction–based assays have been developed for detection of *F tularensis* DNA in clinical materials, but this assay is not available in most clinical laboratories. Isolation of the organism from blood, skin, ulcers, lymph node drainage, gastric washings, or respiratory tract secretions is best made by inoculation of cysteine-enriched media or laboratory mice, but work with cultures should be attempted only by personnel who have been immunized against *F tularensis.* Supplemented chocolate agar or modified charcoal-yeast agar (used for culture of *Legionella* organisms) can support growth of *F tularensis.* Laboratory personnel always should be informed that *F tularensis* is suspected because of the potential hazard to laboratory personnel and the need to use special media.

TREATMENT: Streptomycin has been the recommended drug of choice for treatment of tularemia; however, gentamicin is a highly effective alternative. Duration of therapy usually is 6 to 10 days; the longer course is given for more severe illness.

Alternative drugs include a tetracycline, which should not be given to children younger than 8 years of age unless the benefits of therapy are greater than the risks (see Antimicrobial Agents and Related Therapy, p 646), and chloramphenicol. Clinical relapses are frequent in patients treated with either of these drugs. Ciprofloxacin (which ordinarily should not be given to patients younger than 18 years of age) has been reported to be effective in a limited number of patients.

ISOLATION OF THE HOSPITALIZED PATIENT: Standard precautions are recommended for cutaneous and pulmonary infection.

CONTROL MEASURES:

- Persons should protect against arthropod bites by wearing protective clothing, by frequent inspection for and removal of ticks from the skin and scalp, and by using insect repellents (see Prevention of Tick-Borne Infections, p 159).
- Children should be instructed not to handle sick or dead animals.
- Rubber gloves should be worn by hunters, trappers, and food preparers when handling the carcasses of wild rabbits and other potentially infected animals.
- Game meats should be cooked thoroughly.
- Face masks and rubber gloves should be worn by those working with cultures or infective material in the laboratory, and the work should be performed in a biologic safety cabinet.
- Standard precautions should be used for handling clinical materials.

- A live-attenuated vaccine is recommended for laboratory technicians who work with the organism. It is available from the US Army Medical Research and Material Command.*

Endemic Typhus

(Flea-borne Typhus or Murine Typhus)

CLINICAL MANIFESTATIONS: Flea-borne typhus resembles epidemic (louse-borne) typhus but usually is milder, may have a less abrupt onset, and has less severe systemic symptoms. In young children, the disease is mild. Fever can be accompanied by persistent headache and myalgias. The rash typically is macular or maculopapular, appears on days 4 to 7 of illness, lasts 4 to 8 days, and tends to remain discrete, with sparse lesions and no hemorrhage. The illness seldom lasts longer than 2 weeks; visceral involvement usually does not occur. The disease rarely is fatal.

ETIOLOGY: Flea-borne typhus is caused by *Rickettsia typhi* (formerly *Rickettsia mooseri*) and *Rickettsia felis*.

EPIDEMIOLOGY: Rats, in which infection is inapparent, are the natural hosts. Opossums and domestic cats and dogs also can be infected and serve as a reservoir. The vector for transmission among rats and to humans is the rat flea (usually *Xenopsylla cheopis*). Infected flea feces are rubbed into broken skin or mucous membranes or inhaled as an aerosol. The disease is worldwide in distribution, affects all races, tends to occur more commonly in adults and in males, and is most common during April to October. The disease is rare in the United States; most cases occur in focal areas in southern California, the southeastern Gulf Coast and southern border states, and Hawaii. Exposure to rats and their fleas is the major risk factor, although a history of such exposure frequently is absent in infected patients. In some localized regions, the classic rat-flea-rat cycle has been replaced by a peridomestic cycle involving cats, dogs, opossums, and their fleas.

The **incubation period** is 6 to 14 days.

DIAGNOSTIC TESTS: Indirect fluorescent antibody assay, enzyme immunoassay (EIA), latex agglutination, or complement fixation antibody concentrations peak at a similar or slightly later time. A 4-fold titer change between acute and convalescent serum specimens is diagnostic but also can occur in patients with epidemic (louse-borne) typhus. An EIA specific for immunoglobulin M antibody may aid in confirmation of clinical diagnoses. Serologic differentiation between these diseases by antibody absorption is possible but is not available routinely. Isolation of the organism in culture is possible but is not attempted routinely because it is hazardous and requires specialized facilities.

* Attn: SGRD-UMB, Fort Detrich, Frederick, MD 21702-5009 (www.usamriid.army.mil/html).

TREATMENT: A single dose of doxycycline is the treatment of choice. Although repeated doses of doxycycline generally are not recommended for children younger than 8 years of age, the risk of dental staining from a single dose of doxycycline is minimal (see Antimicrobial Agents and Related Therapy, p 646). Other tetracyclines, chloramphenicol, and a fluoroquinolone, which is not approved for persons younger than 18 years of age, also are effective drugs.

ISOLATION OF THE HOSPITALIZED PATIENT: Standard precautions are recommended.

CONTROL MEASURES: Rat fleas should be controlled by appropriate insecticides, preferably before the use of rodenticides, because the flea will seek alternative hosts when rats are not available. Rat populations should be controlled by appropriate means. A vaccine no longer is available in the United States. No treatment is recommended for exposed persons. The disease should be reported to personnel in local or state public health departments.

Epidemic Typhus

(Louse-borne Typhus)

CLINICAL MANIFESTATIONS: In epidemic louse-borne typhus, the onset of high fever, chills, and myalgias, accompanied by severe headache and malaise, usually is abrupt. Influenza-like illness frequently is suspected. The rash appears 4 to 7 days later, beginning on the trunk and spreading to the limbs. A concentrated eruption is present in the axillae. The rash is maculopapular, becomes petechial or hemorrhagic, then develops into brownish pigmented areas. The face, palms, and soles usually are not affected. Changes in mental status are common, and delirium or coma often occurs. Myocardial and renal failure occur when the disease is severe. Illness varies from moderately severe to fatal. When untreated, the illness typically lasts 2 weeks and ends by lysis of fever and subsidence of symptoms in persons who recover. In untreated cases, mortality is uncommon in children but increases with advancing age. Brill-Zinsser disease is a relapse of epidemic louse-borne typhus that occurs years after the initial episode. Factors that reactivate the rickettsiae are unknown. The recrudescent illness is similar to the primary infection but generally is milder and of shorter duration.

ETIOLOGY: *Rickettsia prowazekii* is the cause.

EPIDEMIOLOGY: Humans are the major source of the organism, which is transmitted from person to person by the body louse, *Pediculus humanus* subsp *corporis*. Infected louse feces are rubbed into broken skin or mucous membranes or inhaled as an aerosol. All ages and races and both sexes are affected. Poverty, crowding, poor sanitary conditions, lack of bathing, and poor personal hygiene contribute to the spread of lice, and, hence, the disease. Currently, cases of typhus rarely are reported but have occurred throughout the world, including Asia, Africa, some parts of

Europe, and Central and South America. Typhus is common during the winter when conditions favor person-to-person transmission of the vector, the body louse. Rickettsiae are present in the blood and tissues of patients during the early febrile phase but are not found in secretions. Direct person-to-person spread of the disease does not occur in the absence of the vector. Cases in humans have been associated with contact with infected flying squirrels in the United States, their nests, or their ectoparasites. Flying squirrel–related disease is a milder illness than epidemic louse-borne typhus.

The **incubation period** is 1 to 2 weeks.

DIAGNOSTIC TESTS: *Rickettsia prowazekii* can be isolated from blood by inoculation into guinea pigs and mice or the yolk sac of embryonated hens' eggs, but isolation is dangerous and is attempted rarely. Definitive diagnosis requires visualization of rickettsiae in tissues, isolation of the organism, detecting rickettsiae by polymerase chain reaction, or testing of serum specimens obtained during the acute and convalescent phases of disease. Serum specimens can be tested for specific antibodies to typhus rickettsiae by any of several methods. The indirect fluorescent antibody test is preferred, but an enzyme immunoassay, microagglutination, and latex agglutination also are available. A 4-fold change in antibody titer between serum specimens obtained during the acute and convalescent phases of disease is diagnostic of endemic flea-borne or epidemic louse-borne typhus. An antibody absorption test often can differentiate the 2 diseases but is not available routinely. An immunohistochemical assay for *R prowazekii* in formalin-fixed tissue specimens is available at the Centers for Disease Control and Prevention.

TREATMENT: Tetracyclines given intravenously or orally, chloramphenicol given intravenously, or a fluoroquinolone is the treatment of choice for epidemic louse-borne typhus. Therapy is given until the patient is afebrile for at least 72 hours; the usual duration of therapy is 7 to 10 days. Tetracycline antibiotics generally are not recommended for children younger than 8 years of age, but the risk of dental staining with a single course is minimal (see Antimicrobial Agents and Related Therapy, p 646). Fluoroquinolones are not recommended for persons younger than 18 years of age. Cream and gel pediculicides containing pyrethrins (0.16% to 0.33%), piperonyl butoxide (2% to 4%), crotamiton (10%), or lindane (1%) can be used for delousing.

ISOLATION OF THE HOSPITALIZED PATIENT: Standard precautions are recommended.

CONTROL MEASURES: Thorough delousing in epidemic situations, particularly among exposed contacts of cases, is recommended. Several applications may be needed because the lice eggs are resistant to most insecticides. Washing clothes in hot water kills lice and eggs. During epidemics, insecticides dusted onto clothes of louse-infested populations are effective in louse control efforts. In some circumstances, preventing flying squirrels from living in human dwellings by sealing their access ports is recommended. A vaccine no longer is available in the United States. Cases should be reported to the regional public health department.

Ureaplasma urealyticum Infections

CLINICAL MANIFESTATIONS: The most common syndrome associated with *Ureaplasma urealyticum* infection is nongonococcal urethritis (NGU). While NGU most frequently is caused by *Chlamydia trachomatis, U urealyticum* seems to be responsible for a significant proportion of the remainder of cases (20% to 30%). Without treatment, the disease usually resolves within 1 to 6 months, although asymptomatic infection may persist thereafter. In women, salpingitis, endometritis, and chorioamnionitis can occur. Prostatitis and epididymitis have been associated with *U urealyticum* infection in men.

Ureaplasma urealyticum has been isolated from the lower respiratory tract and lung biopsy specimens of preterm infants and may contribute to pneumonia and chronic lung disease of prematurity. Although the organism also has been recovered from respiratory tract secretions of infants 3 months of age or younger with pneumonia, its role in the development of lower respiratory tract disease in otherwise healthy young infants is controversial. *Ureaplasma urealyticum* has been isolated from cerebrospinal fluid of newborns with meningitis, hydrocephalus, and intraventricular hemorrhage. The contribution of *U urealyticum* to the outcome of these newborn infants is unclear given the confounding effects of prematurity and intraventricular hemorrhage.

Isolated cases of *U urealyticum* arthritis, osteomyelitis, pericarditis, and progressive sinopulmonary disease in immunocompromised patients have been reported.

ETIOLOGY: The genera *Ureaplasma* and *Mycoplasma* form the family Mycoplasmataceae. The genus *Ureaplasma* contains a single species, *U urealyticum,* which includes at least 16 serotypes.

EPIDEMIOLOGY: The principal reservoir of human *U urealyticum* is the genital tract of sexually active adults. Colonization occurs in approximately half of sexually active women; the incidence in sexually active men is lower. Colonization is uncommon in prepubertal children and in adolescents who are not active sexually. Transmission during delivery is likely from an asymptomatic colonized mother to her newborn. *Ureaplasma urealyticum* may colonize the throat, eyes, umbilicus, and perineum of newborn infants and may persist for several months after birth.

Since *U urealyticum* frequently is isolated from the lower female genital tract and neonatal respiratory tract in the absence of disease, a positive culture does not establish its causative role in an acute infection.

The **incubation period** for NGU after sexual transmission is 10 to 20 days.

DIAGNOSTIC TESTS: If a specimen for culture is obtained, specific *Ureaplasma* transport media with refrigeration at 4°C (39°F) is necessary. The use of cotton swabs should be avoided. A rapid, sensitive, polymerase chain reaction test for detection of *U urealyticum* has been developed but is not available routinely. The *U urealyticum* organism can be cultured in urea-containing broth in 1 to 2 days. Serologic testing for *U urealyticum* antibodies is of limited value and should not be used for routine diagnosis.

TREATMENT: A positive culture does not indicate need for therapy if the patient is asymptomatic. For symptomatic older children, adolescents, and adults, doxycycline (100 mg orally twice a day for 7 days) is the drug of choice. Recurrences are common. Erythromycin is the preferred antimicrobial agent for children younger than 8 years of age and for men with urethritis caused by tetracycline-resistant strains. Studies in adult men with NGU indicate that single-dose azithromycin (1 g orally in a single dose) also is effective. Antibiotic efficacy studies have been performed only in adult patients with NGU. Definitive evidence of efficacy of antimicrobial agents in the treatment of pulmonary or central nervous system (CNS) infections in infants and children is lacking. If therapy for CNS infection is considered for infants, antimicrobial agents with better CNS penetration than oral erythromycin should be considered, such as treatment with intravenous erythromycin, doxycycline, or chloramphenicol. An association between orally administered erythromycin and infantile hypertrophic pyloric stenosis has been reported in infants younger than 6 weeks of age (see Chlamydial Infections, p 205).

ISOLATION OF THE HOSPITALIZED PATIENT: Standard precautions are recommended.

CONTROL MEASURES: Partners of infected sexually active persons should be notified so they can be offered treatment.

Varicella-Zoster Infections

CLINICAL MANIFESTATIONS: Primary infection results in chickenpox, manifested by a generalized, pruritic, vesicular rash typically consisting of 250 to 500 lesions and mild fever and systemic symptoms. Complications include bacterial superinfection of skin lesions, thrombocytopenia, arthritis, hepatitis, cerebellar ataxia, encephalitis, meningitis, or glomerulonephritis. Invasive group A streptococcal disease has been reported increasingly as a complication. The disease can be more severe in adolescents and adults. Reye syndrome can follow some cases of chickenpox, although the incidence of Reye syndrome has declined dramatically with the decline in use of aspirin during varicella or influenza-like illness. In immunocompromised children, progressive severe varicella characterized by continuing eruption of lesions and a high fever into the second week of the illness, as well as encephalitis, hepatitis, or pneumonia, can develop. Hemorrhagic varicella is more common among immunocompromised patients. Pneumonia is relatively less common among immunocompetent children but is the most common complication in adults. In children with human immunodeficiency virus (HIV) infection, chronic or recurrent varicella (disseminated herpes zoster) can develop with new lesions appearing for months. Varicella is one of the most important risk factors for severe invasive group A streptococcal disease. Severe and even fatal varicella has been reported in otherwise healthy children receiving intermittent courses of corticosteroids for treatment of asthma and other illnesses. The risk is especially dangerous when corticosteroids are given during the incubation period for chickenpox.

The virus establishes latency in the dorsal root ganglia during primary infection. Reactivation results in herpes zoster ("shingles"). Grouped vesicular lesions appear in the distribution of 1 to 3 sensory dermatomes, sometimes accompanied by pain localized to the area. *Postherpetic neuralgia* is defined as pain that persists beyond 1 month. Systemic symptoms are few. Zoster occasionally can become disseminated in immunocompromised patients, with lesions appearing outside the primary dermatomes and with visceral complications.

Fetal infection after maternal varicella during the first or early second trimester of pregnancy occasionally results in varicella embryopathy, which is characterized by limb atrophy and scarring of the skin of the extremity (the congenital varicella syndrome). Central nervous system and eye manifestations also can occur. Children exposed to varicella-zoster virus in utero during the second 20 weeks of pregnancy can develop inapparent varicella and subsequent zoster early in life without having had extrauterine varicella. Varicella infection can be fatal for an infant if the mother develops varicella from 5 days before to 2 days after delivery. When varicella develops in a mother more than 5 days before delivery and gestational age is 28 weeks or more, the severity of disease in the newborn is modified by transplacental transfer of varicella-zoster virus (VZV)-specific maternal immunoglobulin (Ig) G antibody.

ETIOLOGY: Varicella-zoster virus is a member of the herpesvirus family.

EPIDEMIOLOGY: Humans are the only source of infection for this highly contagious virus. Humans are infected when the virus comes in contact with the mucosa of the upper respiratory tract or the conjunctiva. Person-to-person transmission occurs primarily by direct contact with patients with varicella or zoster and occasionally occurs by airborne spread from respiratory tract secretions and, rarely, from zoster lesions. In utero infection also can occur as a result of transplacental passage of virus during maternal varicella infection and, occasionally, with zoster. Varicella-zoster virus infection in a household member usually results in infection of almost all susceptible persons in that household. Children who acquire their infection at home (secondary family cases) may have more severe disease than that in the index case. Nosocomial transmission is well documented in pediatric units, but transmission is rare in newborn nurseries.

In temperate climates, varicella is a childhood disease that is most common during the late winter and early spring. In tropical climates, the epidemiology of varicella seems to differ; seasonality is described less clearly, and a higher proportion of adults are susceptible to varicella compared with adults in temperate climates. Most cases of varicella in the United States occur in children younger than 10 years of age. Immunity generally is lifelong. Cellular immunity is more important than humoral immunity, both for limiting the extent of primary infection with VZV and for preventing reactivation of virus with herpes zoster. Symptomatic reinfection is thought to be uncommon in immunocompetent persons, although asymptomatic reinfection occurs. Asymptomatic primary infection is unusual, but since some cases are mild, they may not be recognized.

Immunocompromised persons with primary (varicella) or recurrent (zoster) infection are at increased risk of severe disease. Disseminated chickenpox and zoster are more likely to develop in children with congenital T-cell defects or acquired immunodeficiency syndrome than in children with B-cell abnormalities. Other groups of pediatric patients who may experience more severe or complicated disease include infants, adolescents, patients with chronic cutaneous or pulmonary disorders, and patients receiving systemic corticosteroids or long-term salicylate therapy. The attack rate for congenital varicella syndrome in infants born to mothers with varicella between 0 and 12 weeks of gestation is 0.4% and is 2% when infection occurs between 13 and 20 weeks of gestation. In 1 study, zoster during infancy or early childhood occurred in 0.8% of infants with intrauterine exposure to VZV between 13 and 24 weeks of gestation and in 1.7% of infants with exposure between 25 and 36 weeks of gestation.

Patients are most contagious for 1 to 2 days before and shortly after the onset of the rash. Contagiousness, however, can persist until crusting of lesions. In immunocompromised patients with progressive varicella, contagiousness probably lasts throughout the period of eruption of new lesions.

The **incubation period** usually is 14 to 16 days, occasionally as early as 10 or as late as 21 days after contact. It may be prolonged for as long as 28 days by use of Varicella-Zoster Immune Globulin (VZIG) and shortened in immunocompromised patients. Varicella can develop between 1 and 16 days of life in infants born to mothers with active varicella; the usual interval from onset of rash in a mother to onset in her neonate is 9 to 15 days.

DIAGNOSTIC TESTS: Diagnostic tests for VZV are summarized in Table 3.72, p 627. Varicella virus can be isolated from scrapings of vesicle base during the first 3 to 4 days of the eruption but rarely from other sites, including respiratory tract secretions. A significant increase in serum varicella IgG antibody by any standard serologic assay can retrospectively confirm a diagnosis. These antibody tests are reliable for determining immune status in healthy hosts after natural infection but are not necessarily reliable in immunocompromised persons (see Care of Exposed Persons, p 629). Many commercially available tests are not sufficiently sensitive to demonstrate a vaccine-induced antibody response.

TREATMENT: Varicella and zoster may be treated with intravenous or oral acyclovir, valacyclovir, famciclovir, and foscarnet. The decision to use therapy and the duration and route of therapy should be determined by specific host factors, extent of infection, and initial response to therapy. Antiviral drugs have a limited window of opportunity to affect outcome of varicella-zoster infection. In immunocompetent hosts, most virus replication has stopped by 72 hours after onset of rash; the duration is extended in immunocompromised hosts. Oral acyclovir is not recommended for routine use in otherwise healthy children with varicella. Administration within 24 hours of the onset of rash results in only a modest decrease in symptoms. Oral acyclovir should be considered for otherwise healthy persons at increased risk of moderate to severe varicella, such as persons older than 12 years of age, persons with chronic cutaneous or pulmonary disorders, persons receiving long-term salicylate therapy, and persons receiving short, intermittent, or aerosolized courses of corticosteroids. For recommendations on dosage and duration of therapy, see Antiviral Drugs for Non-HIV Infections (p 675). Some experts also recommend the use of oral acyclovir for secondary household cases in which the disease usually is more severe.

Table 3.72. **Diagnostic Tests for Varicella-Zoster Virus (VZV) Infection***

	Specimen	Advantages and Disadvantages
Tissue cultures	Vesicle base	• Distinguish VZV from HSV • Cost, limited availability
DFA	Vesicle scraping	• Distinguish VZV from HSV • More rapid and sensitive than culture
Tzanck smear	Vesicle scraping	• See multinucleated giant cells with inclusion • Not specific for VZV • Less sensitive and accurate than DFA
EIA	Acute and convalescent serum samples for IgG	• Requires special equipment • May not be sensitive enough to identify vaccine-induced immunity
LA	Acute and convalescent serum samples for IgG	• Rapid (15 min), special equipment not needed • More sensitive than EIA
IFA	Acute and convalescent serum samples for IgG	• Requires special equipment • Good sensitivity, specificity
FAMA	Acute and convalescent serum samples for IgG	• Very sensitive and specific but not widely available
CF	Acute and convalescent serum samples for IgG	• Poor sensitivity
PCR	Body fluid or tissue	• Can distinguish wild type strains from vaccine virus • Very sensitive

* HSV indicates herpes simplex virus; DFA, direct fluorescent antigen; EIA, enzyme immunoassay; IgG, immunoglobulin G; LA, latex agglutination; IFA, indirect fluorescent antibody; FAMA, fluorescent antibody to membrane assay; CF, complement fixation; and PCR, polymerase chain reaction

Oral acyclovir is not recommended routinely for the pregnant adolescent or adult with uncomplicated varicella, since the risks and benefits to the fetus and mother are unknown. Some experts, however, recommend oral acyclovir for pregnant women with varicella, especially during the second and third trimesters. Intravenous acyclovir is recommended for the pregnant patient with serious complications of varicella.*

Intravenous therapy is recommended for immunocompromised patients. Therapy initiated early in the course of the illness, especially within 24 hours of rash onset (<48–72 hours) maximizes efficacy. Oral acyclovir usually should not be used to treat immunocompromised children with varicella because of poor oral

* Burroughs Welcome Company, in conjunction with the Centers for Disease Control and Prevention, maintains an Acyclovir in Pregnancy Registry to monitor fetal-maternal outcomes of pregnant women given systemic acyclovir. Physicians are encouraged to register pregnant women treated with acyclovir by calling 800-722-9292, extension 39437.

bioavailability. However, some experts have used oral high-dose acyclovir in highly selected immunocompromised patients perceived to be at lower risk of developing severe varicella, such as HIV-infected patients with relatively normal concentrations of CD4+ T-lymphocytes and children with leukemia in whom careful follow-up is assured. Although VZIG given shortly after exposure can prevent or modify the course of disease, it is not effective once disease is established (see Care of Exposed Persons, p 629).

Famciclovir and valacyclovir have been licensed for treatment of zoster in adults. Famciclovir is converted to penciclovir, which has an extended half-life in infected cells. Valacyclovir is converted to acyclovir and produces 4-fold greater serum levels than acyclovir. No pediatric formulation is available, and insufficient data exist on the use or dose of these drugs in children to recommend them for therapy in children. Infections caused by acyclovir-resistant VZV strains should be treated with parenteral foscarnet therapy.

Children with varicella should not receive salicylates because administration of salicylates to such children increases the risk of subsequent Reye syndrome. Acetaminophen may be used for control of fever. Recent studies indicate that some nonsteroidal anti-inflammatory agents may increase the risk for more severe varicella in healthy children. Until further studies clarify this situation, it would be reasonable to use acetaminophen for control of fever.

ISOLATION OF THE HOSPITALIZED PATIENT: In addition to standard precautions, airborne and contact precautions are recommended for patients with varicella for a minimum of 5 days after the onset of the rash and as long as the rash remains vesicular, which in immunocompromised patients can be a week or longer. For exposed susceptible patients, airborne and contact precautions from 8 until 21 days after onset of the rash in the index patient also are indicated; these precautions should be maintained until 28 days after exposure for those who received VZIG.

Airborne and contact precautions are recommended for neonates born to mothers with varicella and, if still hospitalized, continued until 21 days of age, or 28 days of age if they received VZIG. Infants with varicella embryopathy do not require isolation.

Immunocompromised patients who have zoster (localized or disseminated) and immunocompetent patients with disseminated zoster require airborne and contact precautions for the duration of illness. For immunocompetent patients with localized zoster, contact precautions are indicated until all lesions are crusted.

CONTROL MEASURES:

Child Care and School. Children with uncomplicated chickenpox who have been excluded from school or child care may return when the rash has crusted, which may be several days in mild cases and several weeks in severe cases or in immunocompromised children. In mild cases with only a few lesions and rapid resolution, children may return sooner if all lesions are crusted. Immunocompromised and other children with a prolonged course should be excluded for the duration of the vesicular eruption.

Exclusion of children with zoster whose lesions cannot be covered is based on similar criteria. Those who are excluded may return after the lesions have crusted. Lesions that are covered seem to pose little risk to susceptible persons. Older children and staff members with zoster should be instructed to wash their hands if they touch potentially infectious lesions.

Care of Exposed Persons:

Potential interventions for susceptible persons exposed to a person with varicella include VZIG (1 dose up to 4 days after exposure) or varicella vaccine (1 dose up to 72 hours after exposure).

Hospital Exposure. If an inadvertent exposure in the hospital by an infected patient, health care professional, or visitor occurs, the following control measures are recommended:

- Personnel and patients who have been exposed (see Table 3.73, p 630) and are susceptible to varicella should be identified.
- Varicella-Zoster Immune Globulin should be administered to appropriate candidates (see Table 3.74, p 631).
- All exposed susceptible patients should be discharged as soon as possible.
- All exposed susceptible patients who cannot be discharged should be placed in strict isolation from day 8 to day 21 after exposure to the index patient. For those who have received VZIG, strict isolation should be continued until day 28.
- All susceptible exposed staff should be furloughed or excused from patient contact from day 8 to day 21 after exposure to an infectious patient. The interval is until day 28 for those who have received VZIG (see Active Immunization, p 632).
- For the management of immunized personnel, serologic testing for immunity is not considered necessary because 99% of adults are seropositive after the second vaccine dose. However, since seroconversion does not always result in complete protection against disease, testing vaccine recipients for seropositivity immediately after exposure and retesting 5 to 6 days later for an anamnestic response is a potentially effective strategy for identifying those who remain at risk for varicella. For more information, see the recommendations of the Advisory Committee on Immunization Practices (ACIP) of the Centers for Disease Control and Prevention (CDC).*
- Varicella immunization is recommended for susceptible staff if varicella does not develop from the exposure.

Postexposure Immunization. The American Academy of Pediatrics recommends administration of varicella vaccine to susceptible children within 72 hours and possibly up to 120 hours after varicella exposure to prevent or significantly modify disease. If exposure to varicella does not cause infection, postexposure immunization with varicella should result in protection against subsequent exposure. Physicians should advise parents and their children in these circumstances that the vaccine may not protect against disease and that some children may have been exposed at the same time as the index case. The vaccine will not protect in the latter instance, and moderate or severe varicella may develop in some children within a few days after

* Centers for Disease Control and Prevention. Prevention of varicella: recommendations of the Advisory Committee on Immunization Practices (ACIP). *MMWR Morb Mortal Wkly Rep*. 1996;45(RR-11):1–36

Table 3.73. **Types of Exposure to Varicella or Zoster for Which VZIG Is Indicated for Susceptible Persons***

- Household: Residing in the same household
- Playmate: Face-to-face† indoor play
- Hospital:
  - Varicella: In same 2- to 4-bed room or adjacent beds in a large ward, face-to-face† contact with an infectious staff member or patient, or visit by a person deemed contagious
  - Zoster: Intimate contact (eg, touching or hugging) with a person deemed contagious.
- Newborn infant: Onset of varicella in the mother 5 d or less before delivery or within 48 h after delivery; VZIG is not indicated if the mother has zoster

* Patients should meet criteria of both significant exposure and candidacy for receiving Varicella-Zoster Immune Globulin (VZIG), as given in Table 3.74, (p 631). Varicella-Zoster Immune Globulin should be administered as soon as possible, and no later than 96 hours after exposure.

† Experts differ in the duration of face-to-face contact that warrants administration of VZIG. However, the contact should be nontransient. Some experts suggest a contact of 5 or more minutes as constituting significant exposure for this purpose; others define close contact as more than 1 hour.

immunization in such situations. There is no evidence that administration of varicella vaccine during the presymptomatic or prodromal stage of illness increases the risk for vaccine-associated adverse events or more severe natural disease.

Chemoprophylaxis. Oral acyclovir is not recommended.

Passive Immunoprophylaxis. Susceptible persons at high risk for developing severe varicella should be given VZIG within 96 hours; for maximum effectiveness, it should be given as soon as possible after exposure. VZIG can be obtained by contacting the local American Red Cross Blood Services or FFF Enterprises (41093 County Center, Temecula, CA 92591; telephone, 1-800-843-7477). The Red Cross has contracted with FFF Enterprises to handle distribution.

The decision to administer VZIG depends on 3 factors: (1) the likelihood that complications of varicella will develop if the person is infected; (2) the probability that a given exposure to varicella or zoster will result in infection; and (3) the likelihood that the exposed person is susceptible to varicella.

Household exposure to varicella poses an almost certain risk of infection; exposure to an immunocompetent contact with varicella whose rash has been present for more than 5 days is low risk. Persons with a history of varicella usually are considered immune. However, persons without such a history also may be immune. In deciding whether an adolescent or young adult with no history of varicella infection is likely to be immune, careful questioning about the following can be helpful: (1) history of varicella in other siblings (particularly younger siblings), (2) whether the patient attended an urban school, (3) previous exposure to persons with chickenpox or zoster, and (4) childhood in temperate climates and other clues, such as clinical description of disease.

In immunocompetent persons, serologic testing to determine immune status is reliable, but in immunocompromised patients, the use of serologic tests to determine immune status may not be reliable. A carefully obtained history of varicella

Table 3.74. **Candidates for VZIG, Provided Significant Exposure Has Occurred***

- Immunocompromised children[†] without history of chickenpox[‡]
- Susceptible pregnant women
- Newborn infant whose mother had onset of chickenpox within 5 d before delivery or within 48 h after delivery
- Hospitalized premature infant (≥28 wk of gestation) whose mother lacks a reliable history of chickenpox or serologic evidence of protection against varicella
- Hospitalized premature infants (<28 wk of gestation or ≤1000 g), regardless of maternal history of varicella or varicella-zoster virus serostatus

* VZIG indicates Varicella-Zoster Immune Globulin. See text and Table 3.73 (p 630) for additional discussion.

† Including those who are infected with the human immunodeficiency virus.

‡ Immunocompromised adolescents and adults known to be susceptible also should receive VZIG.

should be the primary consideration in the determination of immunity in immunocompromised patients. Administration of VZIG to exposed immunocompromised children with no history of varicella, regardless of serologic results, usually is advised. Some experts, however, do not recommend administration of VZIG when the child is seropositive if determined by a sensitive assay (eg, latex agglutination [LA] or enzyme immunoassay [EIA]) and has not received a blood product that could have provided the passive antibody.

Patients receiving monthly high-dose Immune Globulin Intravenous (IGIV) (400 mg/kg) are likely to be protected and probably do not require VZIG if the last dose of IGIV was given 3 weeks or less before exposure.

Administration and Dose. Varicella-Zoster Immune Globulin is given by intramuscular (IM) injection. VZIG contains between 10% and 18% globulin; VZIG does not contain thimerosal. One vial (approximate volume, 1.25 mL) containing 125 U is given for each 10 kg of body weight and is the minimal dose. The suggested maximal dose of VZIG is 625 U (ie, 5 vials).

Local discomfort after IM injection, the most frequent adverse effect, is common and can be lessened if the VZIG is at room temperature when administered. Use of VZIG for patients with a bleeding diathesis should be avoided, as with other IM injections, if possible. Immune Globulin Intravenous would be an acceptable alternative in this situation. VZIG never should be given intravenously.

Indications for VZIG. Tables 3.73 (p 630) and 3.74 (above) indicate susceptible persons who should receive VZIG, including immunocompromised persons, susceptible pregnant women, and certain newborn infants.

For healthy, full-term infants exposed postnatally to varicella, including infants whose mother's rash developed more than 48 hours after delivery, VZIG is not indicated. Some experts advise use of VZIG for any exposed susceptible newborn who has severe skin disease.

- ***Healthy adults.*** Varicella-Zoster Immune Globulin can be given to healthy susceptible adults after exposure to varicella, but VZIG is not recommended routinely. A 7-day course of acyclovir may be given to susceptible adults beginning 7 to 9 days after varicella exposure if vaccine is contraindicated or to persons with late presentations. For adults with no history of chickenpox or with an uncertain history, most have a high probability of immunity.

- ***Subsequent exposures and follow-up of VZIG recipients.*** Since administration of VZIG can cause varicella infection to be asymptomatic, testing of recipients 2 months or later after administration of VZIG to ascertain their immune status may be helpful in the event of subsequent exposure of a recipient in whom varicella did not develop. Some experts, however, would advise VZIG administration regardless of serologic results because of the unreliability of serologic testing in immunocompromised persons and the uncertainty about whether asymptomatic infection after VZIG administration confers lasting protection.

The duration for which VZIG recipients are protected against varicella is unknown. If a second exposure occurs more than 3 weeks after administration of VZIG in a recipient in whom varicella did not develop, another dose of VZIG should be given.

*Active Immunization.**

Vaccine. Varicella vaccine is a live-attenuated preparation of the serially propagated and attenuated wild Oka strain. The product contains trace amounts of neomycin and gelatin. The vaccine was licensed in March 1995 by the US Food and Drug Administration for use in healthy persons 12 months of age or older who have not had varicella.

Dose and Administration. The recommended dose of the vaccine is 0.5 mL, which provides at least 1350 plaque-forming units of VZV. Subcutaneous administration is recommended, although IM administration has been demonstrated to result in similar rates of seroconversion.

Immunogenicity. More than 95% of immunized healthy children between 12 months and 12 years of age develop humoral and cell-mediated immune response to VZV after a single dose of varicella vaccine. In persons 13 years of age and older, seroconversion rates are 78% to 82% after 1 dose and 99% after 2 doses.

Effectiveness. The currently licensed product is 85% to 90% effective for the prevention of varicella in children during outbreaks and 100% effective for prevention of moderate or severe disease. Each year after varicella immunization, a mild varicella-like syndrome develops in 1% to 4% of immunized children. Neither the rate nor the severity of varicella increases with time after immunization. Varicella in vaccine recipients has been milder than that occurring in unimmunized children, with a median of 15 to 32 vesicles, lower rate of fever (10% with temperature ≥39°C [≥102°F]), and rapid recovery. At times, the disease is so mild that it is not easily recognizable as varicella because the skin lesions may resemble insect bites. In contrast, the median number of lesions in unimmunized children with varicella is more than 250. Nevertheless, vaccine recipients with mild disease potentially may be infectious to susceptible persons.

Duration of Immunity. Although there has been concern about waning immunity, follow-up evaluations of children immunized during prelicensure clinical trials

---

* American Academy of Pediatrics Committee on Infectious Diseases. Recommendations for the use of live attenuated varicella vaccine. *Pediatrics.* 1995;95:791–796 and American Academy of Pediatrics Committee on Infectious Diseases. Varicella vaccine update. *Pediatrics.* 2000,105:136–141

in the United States reveal protection for at least 11 years, and studies in Japan indicate protection for at least 20 years. However, these studies were during a period when a substantial amount of wild-type VZV was present in the community, with many opportunities for boosting of immunity by subclinical infection in immunized persons. Experience with other live virus vaccines (eg, measles, rubella) suggests that immunity remains high throughout life; the primary reason for second doses of measles vaccine is to induce protection in children without an adequate response to the first dose, not because of waning immunity. Follow-up studies of clinical trials in children are being performed to determine the need, if any, for additional doses of varicella vaccine.

Simultaneous Administration With Other Vaccines. Varicella vaccine may be given simultaneously with measles-mumps-rubella (MMR) vaccine, but separate syringes and injection sites must be used. If not given simultaneously, the interval between administration of varicella vaccine and MMR should be at least 4 weeks. Although further immunogenicity studies are needed on the use of varicella vaccine administered simultaneously with DTaP (diphtheria and tetanus toxoids and acellular pertussis), poliovirus, hepatitis B, or *Haemophilus influenzae* type b vaccine, no reason exists to suspect that varicella vaccine will affect the immune response to these other vaccines. When necessary, varicella vaccine may be given simultaneously or at any interval after or before these vaccines.

Adverse Events. Varicella vaccine is safe; reactions generally are mild and occur with an overall frequency of approximately 5% to 35%. Approximately 20% of immunized persons will experience minor injection site reactions (eg, pain, redness, swelling). In approximately 3% to 5% of immunized children, a localized rash develops, and in an additional 3% to 5%, a generalized varicella-like rash develops. These rashes typically consist of 2 to 5 lesions and may be maculopapular rather than vesicular; lesions usually appear 5 to 26 days after immunization. However, most varicelliform rashes that occur within the first 2 weeks after varicella immunization are due to wild-type VZV. Although a temperature higher than 39°C (102°F) has been observed from 1 to 42 days after immunization in 15% of healthy immunized children, fever also occurs in a similar percentage of children receiving placebo and is not considered to be a significant adverse event of immunization. A temperature higher than 38°C (100°F) has been reported in 10% of adolescents and adults who are immunized with the vaccine. Serious adverse events, such as encephalitis, ataxia, erythema multiforme, Stevens-Johnson syndrome, pneumonia, thrombocytopenia, seizures, neuropathy, and death, have been reported rarely in temporal association with varicella vaccine. In very rare instances, a causal relationship between the varicella vaccine and some of these serious adverse events has been established. In some cases, wild-type VZV or another causal agent has been identified. In the vast majority of cases, data are insufficient to determine a causal association.

Herpes Zoster After Immunization. The varicella vaccine virus has caused herpes zoster in immunocompetent and immunocompromised persons within 25 to 722 days after immunization. Data from postlicensure surveillance indicate that the age-specific risk of herpes zoster seems to be lower among immunocompetent children immunized with varicella vaccine than among children who have had natural infection. A population-based study indicated that the incidence of herpes zoster after natural varicella infection among immunocompetent children younger than

20 years of age was 68 per 100 000 person years, while the reported rate of herpes zoster after varicella immunization among immunocompetent persons was approximately 2.6 per 100 000 vaccine doses distributed (CDC, unpublished data). However, these rates should be compared cautiously because the former rates are based on populations monitored actively for longer periods than the passive surveillance after immunization. Wild-type VZV also has been identified in persons with herpes zoster after immunization, indicating that herpes zoster in immunized persons also may result from antecedent natural varicella infection.

Transmission of Vaccine-Associated Virus. Experience since 1995 with more than 14 million doses of varicella vaccine distributed in the United States indicates that vaccine-associated virus transmission to contacts is extremely rare (only 3 well-documented cases) and occurs only if the immunized person develops a rash (Merck and Company, Inc, unpublished data).

The role of VZIG or acyclovir as prophylaxis for high-risk persons exposed to immunized persons with lesions will be difficult to evaluate given the rarity of transmission. If contact inadvertently occurs, the routine use of VZIG is not recommended because transmission is rare and disease, if it were to develop, would be expected to be mild. However, some experts believe that immunocompromised persons in whom skin lesions develop, possibly related to vaccine virus, should receive acyclovir treatment.

Storage. The lyophilized vaccine should be stored in a frost-free freezer at an average temperature of –15°C (+5°F) or colder. Vaccine may be stored at refrigerator temperature of 2°C to 8°C (36°F–46°F) for up to 72 continuous hours before administration. The diluent used for reconstitution should be stored separately in a refrigerator or at room temperature. Once the vaccine has been reconstituted, it should be injected as soon as possible and discarded if not used within 30 minutes. For further information, see the package insert.

Recommendations for Immunization. Universal immunization of infants and immunization of susceptible older children and adolescents without a contraindication is recommended based on the frequency of serious complications and deaths after infection with wild varicella, the excessive cost to the family and society incurred by varicella infection, and the efficacy and safety of the live-attenuated varicella vaccine. Susceptibility is defined by lack of proof of varicella immunization, lack of a reliable history of varicella, or absence of serologic evidence of varicella. Age-specific recommendations are as follows:

- **Age 12 months to the 13th birthday:**

  Age 12 to 18 months. One dose of varicella vaccine is recommended for universal immunization for all immunocompetent children who lack a reliable history or serologic evidence of varicella.

  Age 19 months to the 13th birthday. Immunization of susceptible children is recommended, and immunization may be given any time during childhood but before the 13th birthday because of the potential increased severity of natural varicella after this age.
- **Healthy adolescents and young adults.** Healthy adolescents past their 13th birthday who are susceptible should be immunized against varicella by administration of 2 doses of vaccine 4 to 8 weeks apart. Longer intervals

between doses do not necessitate a third dose but may leave the person unprotected during the intervening months.

- **Adults.** Recommendations for the use of varicella vaccine in adults have been issued by the ACIP of the CDC.* Varicella immunization of susceptible adults is encouraged. Priority, according to the ACIP, should be given to immunization of persons in the following high-risk groups:
  - Persons who live or work in environments where transmission of VZV is likely (eg, teachers of young children, child care employees, and residents and staff members in institutional settings)
  - Persons who live and work in environments where transmission can occur (eg, college students, inmates and staff members of correctional institutions, and military personnel)
  - Nonpregnant women of childbearing age
  - Adolescents and adults living in households with children
  - International travelers

Serologic Testing Before and After Immunization

An adult, adolescent, or child with a reliable history of varicella can be assumed to be immune, and immunization is unnecessary. Because approximately 70% to 90% of persons 18 years of age or older without a reliable history of varicella also will be immune, it may be cost-effective to perform serologic tests on persons 13 years of age or older and immunize those who are seronegative. If serologic testing is performed, a tracking system for seronegative persons should be developed to assure that susceptible persons are immunized. However, serologic testing is not required because varicella vaccine is well tolerated by persons immune from earlier disease. In some situations, universal immunization may be easier to implement than serologic testing and tracking. Most children younger than 3 years of age without a reliable history of varicella should be considered susceptible and immunized without serologic testing. However, data from some populations indicate that a large proportion of 9- to 12-year old children with an uncertain history of varicella will be immune and that serologic testing before deciding about immunization may be cost-effective. Seroconversion rates after 1 dose of varicella vaccine in children younger than 13 years of age and after 2 doses in adolescents and adults are so high that serologic testing after immunization is unnecessary.

Whole-cell EIA is the most commonly used commercially available serologic test for VZV. The sensitivity of this test is sufficient to determine immunity after natural varicella, but it may not be sensitive enough to determine vaccine-induced immunity. Tests such as the fluorescent antibody to membrane antigen (FAMA) and LA tests are more sensitive, but the FAMA assay is not commercially available, and the LA assay is not convenient for mass testing.

Booster Immunization. Reimmunization is not recommended currently, but the need for reimmunization will be reassessed with time.

---

* Centers for Disease Control and Prevention. Prevention of varicella: recommendations of the Advisory Committee on Immunization Practices (ACIP). *MMWR Morb Mortal Wkly Rep.* 1996;45(RR-11): 1–36

Contraindications and Precautions.

Intercurrent Illness. As with other vaccines, varicella vaccine should not be administered to persons who have moderate or severe illnesses, with or without fever (see Vaccine Safety and Contraindications, p 30).

Immunocompromised Patients.

General recommendations. Varicella vaccine should not be administered routinely to children who have T-lymphocyte immunodeficiency, including persons with leukemia, lymphoma, other malignant neoplasms affecting the bone marrow or lymphatic systems, and congenital T-cell abnormalities (see Immunocompromised Children, p 56). Exceptions include children with acute lymphocytic leukemia (ALL) to whom vaccine may be given in study conditions (see Acute lymphocytic leukemia) and certain asymptomatic children infected with HIV (see HIV infection). Children with impaired humoral immunity may be immunized.

Immunodeficiency should be excluded before immunization in children with a family history of hereditary immunodeficiency. The presence of an immunodeficient or HIV-seropositive family member does not contraindicate vaccine use in other family members.

Acute lymphocytic leukemia. Although the current vaccine is not licensed for routine use in children with malignant neoplasms, immunization should be considered when a child with ALL has been in continuous remission for at least 1 year and has a lymphocyte count greater than 700/µL (0.7×10^9/L) and a platelet count greater than 100×10^3/µL (100×10^9/L). Immunization has been demonstrated to be safe, immunogenic, and effective in these children, and the vaccine may be obtained free for use in a research protocol. This protocol requires approval by the appropriate institutional review board, as well as monitoring for safety.*

HIV infection. Routine screening for HIV is not indicated before routine varicella immunization. Children known to be infected with HIV may be at increased risk of morbidity from varicella and herpes zoster compared with healthy children. Limited data on immunization of HIV-infected children in CDC Class 1 with a CD4+ T-lymphocyte percentage of 25% or greater indicate that the vaccine is safe, immunogenic, and effective. Therefore, after weighing potential risks and benefits, varicella vaccine should be considered for HIV-infected children in CDC Class 1 with a CD4+ T-lymphocyte percentage of 25% or greater. Eligible children should receive 2 doses of varicella vaccine with a 3-month interval between doses and return for evaluation if they experience a postimmunization varicella-like rash. With the increased use of varicella vaccine and the resulting decrease in incidence of varicella in the community, exposure of immunocompromised hosts to VZV will decrease. As the risk of exposure decreases and more data are generated on the use of varicella vaccine in high-risk populations, the risk vs benefit of varicella immunization in HIV-infected children will need to be reassessed.

Children receiving corticosteroids. Varicella vaccine should not be administered to persons who are receiving high doses of systemic corticosteroids (2 mg/kg per day or more of prednisone or its equivalent or 20 mg/d of prednisone if their weight is >10 kg) for 14 days or more. If these doses are given for 14 days or more, the recom-

* To immunize a child with ALL, contact: The Varivax Coordinating Center, IBAH Inc, 4 Valley Square, 512 Township Line Rd, Blue Bell, PA 19422 (215-283-0897).

mended interval between discontinuation of therapy and immunization with varicella vaccine is at least 1 month. Other recommendations about varicella vaccine use in children receiving corticosteroids can be found in Immunocompromised Children, p 633.

Households with potential contact with immunocompromised persons. Transmission of vaccine-type VZV from healthy persons has been documented, albeit rarely (see Adverse Events, p 56). Even in families with immunocompromised persons, including persons with HIV infection, no precautions are needed after immunization of healthy children in whom a rash does not develop. Immunized persons in whom a rash develops should avoid direct contact with immunocompromised susceptible hosts for the duration of the rash. If contact inadvertently occurs, the routine use of VZIG is not recommended currently because transmission is rare, and disease, if it develops, would be expected to be mild. However, some experts recommend that immunocompromised persons in whom skin lesions develop, possibly related to vaccine virus, should receive acyclovir treatment. In contrast, varicella due to wild virus in immunocompromised persons and pregnant women can be severe or fatal. Hence, the benefits of immunizing household contacts of high-risk persons, reducing the spread of wild virus, outweigh the potential risks.

Pregnancy and Lactation. Varicella vaccine should not be administered to pregnant women, since the possible effects on fetal development are unknown.* When postpubertal females are immunized, pregnancy should be avoided for at least 1 month after immunization. A pregnant mother or other pregnant household member is not a contraindication for immunization of the child. Transmission of vaccine virus is rare; more than 95% of adults are immune, and immunization of the child likely will protect the susceptible mother from exposure to wild VZV.

Whether vaccine-acquired VZV is secreted in human milk and the infectiousness of vaccine virus in human milk to infants are unknown. Varicella vaccine may be considered for a susceptible nursing mother, if risk of exposure to natural VZV is high.

Immune Globulin. Whether immune globulin (IG) can interfere with varicella vaccine–induced immunity is unknown, although IG can interfere with immunity induced by measles vaccine. Pending additional data, varicella vaccine should be withheld for the same intervals after receipt of any form of IG or other blood product as measles vaccine (see Measles, p 385). In addition, IG should be withheld for at least 2 weeks after receipt of varicella vaccine. Transplacental antibodies to VZV do not interfere with the immunogenicity of varicella vaccine administered at 12 months of age or older.

Salicylates. Whether Reye syndrome results from administration of salicylates after immunization for varicella in children is unknown. No cases have been reported. The vaccine manufacturer, however, recommends that salicylates not be administered for 6 weeks after the varicella vaccine has been given because of the association between Reye syndrome, natural varicella infection, and salicylates. Physicians need to weigh the theoretical risks associated with varicella vaccine

---

* The manufacturer, in collaboration with the CDC, has established the VARIVAX Pregnancy Registry to monitor the maternal and fetal outcomes of women who inadvertently are given varicella vaccine 3 months before or at any time during pregnancy. Reporting cases is encouraged and may be done by telephone (800-986-8999).

against the known risks of the wild type virus in children receiving long-term salicylate therapy.

Allergy to Vaccine Components. Varicella vaccine should not be administered to persons who have had an anaphylactic-type reaction to any component of the vaccine, including gelatin and neomycin. Most persons with allergy to neomycin have contact dermatitis, which is not a contraindication to immunization. The vaccine does not contain preservatives or egg protein.

VIBRIO INFECTIONS

Cholera

(Vibrio cholerae)

CLINICAL MANIFESTATIONS: Cholera is characterized by painless voluminous diarrhea without abdominal cramps or fever. Dehydration, hypokalemia, metabolic acidosis, and, occasionally, hypovolemic shock can occur in 4 to 12 hours if fluid losses are not replaced. Coma, seizures, and hypoglycemia also can occur, particularly in children. Stools are colorless, with small flecks of mucus ("rice-water"), and contain high concentrations of sodium, potassium, chloride, and bicarbonate. However, most infected persons with toxigenic *Vibrio cholerae* O1 have no symptoms, and some have only mild-to-moderate diarrhea, whereas fewer than 5% have severe watery diarrhea, vomiting, and dehydration *(cholera gravis)*.

ETIOLOGY: *Vibrio cholerae* is a gram-negative, curved, motile bacillus with many serogroups. Until recently, only enterotoxin-producing organisms of serogroup O1 have caused epidemics. *Vibrio cholerae* O1 is divided into 2 serotypes, Inaba and Ogawa, and 2 biotypes, classical and El Tor. The predominant biotype is El Tor. In 1992, a cholera epidemic due to toxigenic *V cholerae* serogroup O139 Bengal (a non-O1 toxigenic strain) caused epidemic cholera in the Indian subcontinent and southeast Asia. Serogroups of *V cholerae* other than O1 and O139 Bengal and nontoxicogenic strains of *V cholerae* O1 can cause sporadic diarrheal illness, but they do not cause epidemics.

EPIDEMIOLOGY: During the last 3 decades, *V cholerae* O1, biotype El Tor, has spread from India and Southeast Asia to Africa, the Middle East, Southern Europe, and the Western Pacific Islands (Oceania). In 1991, epidemic cholera caused by toxigenic *V cholerae* O1, serotype Inaba, biotype El Tor, appeared in Peru and has spread to most countries in South and North America. In the United States, cases resulting from travel to Latin America or Asia and due to ingestion of contaminated food transported from Latin America or Asia have been reported. In addition, the Gulf Coast of Louisiana and Texas has an endemic focus of a unique strain of toxigenic *V cholerae* O1. Most cases of disease from this strain have resulted from consumption of raw or undercooked shellfish. Humans are the only documented natural host, but free-living *V cholerae* organisms can exist in the aquatic environment. The usual mode of infection is ingestion of contaminated water or food (particularly raw or undercooked shellfish), moist grains held at ambient temperature, and raw or partially dried fish. The boiling of water or treating it with chlorine or iodine and adequate cooking of food kills the organism. Direct person-to-person spread by contact has not been documented. Persons with low gastric acidity are at increased risk for cholera infection. The period of communicability is unknown but presumably is related to duration of carriage.

The **incubation period** is usually 1 to 3 days, with a range of a few hours to 5 days.

DIAGNOSTIC TESTS: *Vibrio cholerae* can be cultured from fecal specimens or vomitus plated on appropriate selective media. Suspect colonies are confirmed serologically by agglutination with specific antisera. Because most laboratories in the United States do not culture routinely for *V cholerae* or other vibrios, clinicians should request appropriate cultures for clinically suspected cases. Isolates of *V cholerae* should be sent to a state health department laboratory for serogrouping; those of serogroup O1 or O139 Bengal are then sent to the Centers for Disease Control and Prevention for testing for production of cholera toxin. A 4-fold rise in vibriocidal antibody titers between acute and convalescent serum samples or a 4-fold decline in vibriocidal titers between early and late convalescent (more than a 2-month interval) serum samples can confirm the diagnosis retrospectively.

TREATMENT: Oral or parenteral rehydration therapy to correct dehydration and electrolyte abnormalities is the most important modality of therapy and should be initiated as soon as the diagnosis is suspected.* Oral rehydration with the World Health Organization Oral Rehydration Solution or its equivalent is preferred unless the patient is in shock, is obtunded, or has intestinal ileus.

Antimicrobial therapy results in prompt eradication of vibrios, reduces the duration of diarrhea, and reduces requirements for fluid replacement. It should be considered for persons who are moderately to severely ill. Oral tetracycline (50 mg/kg per day, maximum 2 g/d, in 4 divided doses) for 3 days or doxycycline (6 mg/kg, maximum 300 mg, as a single dose) are the drugs of choice for cholera due to *V cholerae* O1 and O139 Bengal. The use of tetracyclines generally is not recommended for children younger than 8 years of age, but in cases of severe cholera, the benefits may offset the risk of staining of developing teeth (see Antimicrobial Agents and Related Therapy, p 646). If strains are resistant to tetracyclines, trimethoprim-sulfamethoxazole (8 mg/kg per day of trimethoprim and 40 mg/kg per day of sulfamethoxazole), erythromycin (40 mg/kg per day, maximum 1000 mg), or furazolidone (5 to 8 mg/kg per day, maximum 400 mg) may be used. *Vibrio cholerae* O139 Bengal strains typically are not susceptible to trimethoprim-sulfamethoxazole or furazolidone. Ciprofloxacin or ofloxacin are effective therapeutic agents for infection due to *V cholerae* O1 and O139 Bengal but generally should be used only for persons at least 18 years old (see Antimicrobial Agents and Related Therapy, p 645). Antimicrobial susceptibilities of newly isolated organisms should be determined.

---

* American Academy of Pediatrics Committee on Quality Improvement, Subcommittee on Acute Gastroenteritis. Practice parameter: the management of acute gastroenteritis in young children. *Pediatrics*. 1996;97:424–435

ISOLATION OF THE HOSPITALIZED PATIENT: In addition to standard precautions, contact precautions are indicated for diapered or incontinent children for the duration of illness.

CONTROL MEASURES:

Hygiene. Because cholera spreads by contaminated food or water, and infection frequently requires ingestion of large numbers of organisms, disinfection or boiling of water prevents transmission. Thoroughly cooking crabs, oysters, and other shellfish from the Gulf Coast before eating also is recommended to reduce the likelihood of transmission. Foods such as fish, rice, or grain gruels should be refrigerated promptly after use. Appropriate hand washing after defecating and before preparing or eating food is important for preventing transmission.

Treatment of Contacts. The administration of tetracycline, doxycycline, or trimethoprim-sulfamethoxazole within 24 hours of identification of the index case may effectively prevent coprimary and secondary cases of cholera among household contacts if the household secondary rate is high. The use of tetracyclines generally is not recommended for children younger than 8 years of age (see Antimicrobial Agents and Related Therapy, p 646). Chemoprophylaxis is not recommended in the United States, since secondary spread is rare, unless unusual sanitary and hygienic conditions indicate that the rate of secondary transmission could be high.

Vaccine. The only available vaccine in the United States is of limited value. It protects approximately 50% of those immunized for only 3 to 6 months, does not prevent excretion of or inapparent infection with *Vibrio* organisms, and is unrelated serologically to serotype O139 Bengal and does not protect against this strain (see Etiology, p 638). Furthermore, travelers using appropriate precautions are at a low risk of infection in countries with cholera. Cholera immunization is not required for travelers entering the United States from cholera-affected areas, and the World Health Organization no longer recommends immunization for travel to or from cholera-infected areas. No country requires cholera vaccine for entry. The vaccine should not be administered to contacts of patients with cholera or used to control the spread of infection, and it is not recommended generally for international travelers. Several recently developed, orally administered vaccines with fewer side effects than the parenteral vaccine are being evaluated to assess efficacy in travelers.

Reporting. Confirmed cases of cholera must be reported to health authorities in any country in which they occur or were contracted. State health departments should be notified immediately of presumed or known cases of cholera due to *V cholerae* O1 or O139 Bengal.

Other *Vibrio* Infections

CLINICAL MANIFESTATIONS: *Vibrio* species are associated with the following 3 major syndromes: diarrhea, septicemia, and wound infection. Diarrhea is most frequent, characterized by acute onset of watery stools and crampy abdominal pain. Approximately half of those afflicted will have low-grade fever, headache, and chills;

about 30% will have vomiting. Spontaneous recovery follows in 2 to 5 days. Bacteremia is rare.

Infection can develop in contaminated wounds. Skin infections in immunocompromised persons can cause extensive and rapid tissue necrosis. Patients with immunodeficiency or liver disease are susceptible to septicemia from bowel or skin infections, often resulting in shock, bullous or necrotic skin lesions, and death.

ETIOLOGY: Vibrios are facultatively anaerobic, motile, gram-negative bacilli that are tolerant of salt. The most important noncholera *Vibrio* species associated with diarrhea are *Vibrio parahaemolyticus, V cholerae* non-O1, *Vibrio mimicus, Vibrio hollisae, Vibrio fluvialis,* and *Vibrio furnissii. Vibrio vulnificus* causes septicemia and wound infections in immunocompromised patients, especially those with liver disease. *Vibrio parahaemolyticus, Vibrio damsela,* and *Vibrio alginolyticus* also are associated with wound infections. *Vibrio alginolyticus* has been associated with otitis externa.

EPIDEMIOLOGY: Noncholera vibrios commonly are found in seawater, increasing quantitatively during the summer. Most infections occur during the summer and fall. Enteritis usually is acquired from seafood that is eaten raw or undercooked, especially oysters, crabs, and shrimp. The disease probably is not communicable from person to person. Wound infections commonly result from exposure of abrasions to contaminated seawater or from punctures resulting from handling of contaminated shellfish. Persons with increased susceptibility to infection with *Vibrio* species include those with liver disease, low gastric acidity, and immunodeficiency, including persons with human immunodeficiency virus infection.

The median **incubation period** of enteritis is 23 hours, with a range of 5 to 92 hours.

DIAGNOSTIC TESTS: *Vibrio* organisms can be isolated from stool or vomitus of patients with diarrhea, from blood, and from wound exudates. Because identification of the organism requires special techniques, laboratory personnel should be notified when infection with *Vibrio* species is suspected.

TREATMENT: Most episodes of diarrhea are mild and self-limited and do not require treatment other than oral rehydration. Antibiotic therapy may benefit those with severe diarrhea or wound infections. Most organisms are susceptible to tetracycline (which usually should not be given to patients younger than 8 years of age), cefotaxime, gentamicin, and chloramphenicol.

ISOLATION OF THE HOSPITALIZED PATIENT: In addition to standard precautions, contact precautions are recommended for diapered or incontinent children.

CONTROL MEASURES: Seafood should be cooked adequately, and, if not ingested immediately, it should be refrigerated. Uncooked mollusks and crustaceans should be handled with care. Abrasions suffered by ocean bathers should be rinsed with clean fresh water. All children, including children with liver disease or immunodeficiency, should be warned to avoid eating raw oysters or clams.

Yersinia enterocolitica and *Yersinia pseudotuberculosis* Infections

(Enteritis and Other Illnesses)

CLINICAL MANIFESTATIONS: *Yersinia enterocolitica* and *Yersinia pseudotuberculosis* cause several age-specific syndromes and a variety of uncommon presentations. The most common manifestation of infection with *Y enterocolitica* is enterocolitis with fever and diarrhea; stool often contains leukocytes, blood, and mucus. This syndrome occurs most often in young children. A pseudoappendicitis syndrome (fever, abdominal pain, tenderness in the right lower quadrant of the abdomen, and leukocytosis) occurs primarily in older children and young adults. Focal infections, abscess formation (such as hepatic and splenic), and bacteremia occur most often in patients with predisposing conditions, such as excessive iron storage. Other manifestations of infection are uncommon and include pharyngitis, meningitis, osteomyelitis, pyomyositis, conjunctivitis, pneumonia, acute proliferative glomerulonephritis, peritonitis, and primary cutaneous infection. Postinfectious sequelae observed with *Y enterocolitica* include erythema nodosum and reactive arthritis and occur most often in adults.

The major triad of infection caused by *Y pseudotuberculosis* is fever, rash, and abdominal symptoms. The rash usually is scarlatiniform. Acute abdominal pain syndromes are most common, resulting from mesenteric adenitis, appendicitis, or terminal ileitis. Other findings include diarrhea, erythema nodosum, septicemia, and sterile pleural and joint effusions. Clinical features can mimic those of Kawasaki disease.

ETIOLOGY: *Yersinia enterocolitica* and *Y pseudotuberculosis* are gram-negative bacilli; 34 serotypes of *Y enterocolitica* and 5 serotypes of *Y pseudotuberculosis* are recognized. Differences in virulence exist among various serotypes of *Y enterocolitica*; O:3 and O:9 are the most common causes of diarrhea.

EPIDEMIOLOGY: The reservoirs of the organisms are animals, including rodents and many bird species *(Y pseudotuberculosis)* and swine *(Y enterocolitica)*. Infection is believed to be transmitted by ingestion of contaminated food, especially uncooked pork products and unpasteurized milk, or contaminated water; by direct or indirect contact with animals; by transfusion with packed red blood cells; and possibly by fecal-oral, person-to-person transmission. Bottle-fed infants can be infected if their caregivers simultaneously are handling raw pork intestines (chitterlings). *Yersinia enterocolitica* is isolated more frequently in cooler climates and more frequently in winter than in summer. Patients with excessive iron storage syndromes (eg, ß-thalassemia), as well as patients receiving deferoxamine for iron overload, have unusual susceptibility to *Yersinia* bacteremia. The period of communicability is unknown; it is probably for the duration of excretion of the specific organisms, which averages 6 weeks after diagnosis.

The **incubation period** typically is 4 to 6 days, varying from 1 to 14 days.

DIAGNOSTIC TESTS: *Yersinia enterocolitica* and *Y pseudotuberculosis* can be recovered from throat swabs, mesenteric lymph nodes, peritoneal fluid, and blood. Stool cultures generally are positive during the first 2 weeks of illness, regardless of the nature of the gastrointestinal tract manifestations. *Yersinia enterocolitica* also has been isolated from synovial fluid, bile, urine, cerebrospinal fluid, sputum, and wounds. Because of the relatively low incidence of *Yersinia* infection and because laboratory identification of organisms from stool requires specific techniques, laboratory personnel should be notified that *Yersinia* infection is suspected. Pathogenic strains of *Y enterocolitica* usually are pyrazinamidase-negative. Infection can be confirmed by demonstrating increases in the serum antibody titer after infection, but these tests generally are available only in reference or research laboratories. Cross-reactions of these antibodies with *Brucella, Vibrio, Salmonella,* and *Rickettsia* species and *Escherichia coli* lead to false-positive *Y enterocolitica* and *Y pseudotuberculosis* titers. In patients with thyroid disease, persistently elevated *Y enterocolitica* antibody titers can result from antigenic similarity of the organism with antigens of the thyroid epithelial cell membrane.

TREATMENT: *Yersinia enterocolitica* and *Y pseudotuberculosis* are susceptible to aminoglycosides, cefotaxime, tetracycline (which usually should not be given to children younger than 8 years of age), chloramphenicol, and trimethoprim-sulfamethoxazole. *Yersinia enterocolitica* isolates typically are resistant to first-generation cephalosporins and to most penicillins. Patients with septicemia or sites of infection other than the gastrointestinal tract and immunocompromised hosts with enterocolitis should receive antibiotic therapy. Benefit from antibiotic therapy for patients with enterocolitis, the pseudoappendicitis syndrome, or mesenteric adenitis, other than reduced duration of excretion of the organism in stool, has not been established.

ISOLATION OF THE HOSPITALIZED PATIENT: In addition to standard precautions, contact precautions are indicated for diapered and incontinent children with enterocolitis for the duration of illness.

CONTROL MEASURES: Ingestion of uncooked meat, contaminated water, or unpasteurized milk should be avoided. Persons handling pork intestines should wash their hands after contact.

Antimicrobial Agents and Related Therapy

INTRODUCTION

In some instances, drugs are recommended for specific indications other than those in the product label (package insert) approved by the Food and Drug Administration (FDA). An FDA-approved indication means that adequate and well-controlled studies were conducted and then reviewed by the FDA. However, accepted medical practice often includes drug use that is not reflected in approved drug labeling. Lack of approval does not necessarily mean lack of effectiveness, but indicates that the appropriate studies have not been performed or data have not been submitted to the FDA for approval for that indication. Unapproved use does not imply improper use, provided that reasonable medical evidence justifies doing so and that use of the drug is deemed in the best interest of the patient. The decision to prescribe a drug rests with the physician who must weigh the risks and benefits of using the drug, regardless of whether the drug has received FDA approval for the specific indication and age of the patient.

Some antimicrobial agents with proven therapeutic benefit in humans are not approved by the FDA for use in pediatric patients or are considered contraindicated in children because of possible toxicity. Some of these drugs, however, such as the fluoroquinolones and tetracyclines (in children younger than 8 years of age), may be used in special circumstances after careful assessment of the risks and benefits. Obtaining informed consent before use is prudent. The following information delineates general principles for the use of these classes of drugs.

Fluoroquinolones

Use of fluoroquinolones (for example, ciprofloxacin, ofloxacin, norfloxacin, enoxacin, levofloxacin, lomefloxacin, sparfloxacin, and trovafloxacin) generally is contraindicated, according to FDA-approved product labeling, in children and adolescents younger than 18 years of age because the fluoroquinolones have been shown to cause cartilage damage in every juvenile animal model tested at doses that approximate those needed to be therapeutic. The mechanism for this is unknown. Pefloxacin, a fluoroquinolone that had been used extensively in France, causes arthropathy in children and adults. Furthermore, recent data suggest that alatrofloxacin and trovofloxacin can cause acute liver failure that has resulted in a number of deaths.

To date ciprofloxacin is the fluoroquinolone that has been used most extensively in children. This drug appears to be well tolerated, does not appear to cause arthropathy, and is effective as an oral agent for treating a number of diseases that would otherwise require parenteral therapy. Accordingly, in special circumstances after careful assessment of the risks and benefits for the individual patient, use of a fluoroquinolone can be justified. Circumstances in which fluoroquinolones may be useful include those in which (1) no other oral agent is available, necessitating an alternative drug given parenterally and (2) infection is caused by multidrug-resistant, gram-negative, enteric, and other pathogens, such as certain *Pseudomonas* and *Mycobacterium* strains. Possible uses, accordingly, include the following:

- Urinary tract infection caused by *Pseudomonas aeruginosa* or other multidrug-resistant gram-negative bacteria
- Chronic suppurative otitis media or malignant otitis externa
- Chronic osteomyelitis
- Exacerbation of cystic fibrosis
- Mycobacterial infections
- Other gram-negative bacterial infections in immunocompromised hosts in which prolonged oral therapy is desired

Food and Drug Administratrion approval of one or more fluoroquinolones for use in children, and with limited indications, may occur. Until then, however, if use of a fluoroquinolone is recommended for a patient younger than 18 years of age, the risks and benefits should be explained to the patients and parents.

Tetracyclines

Use of tetracyclines has been limited because they can cause permanent dental discoloration in children younger than 8 years of age. Published studies have documented that tetracyclines and their colored degradation products that are bound to teeth are observed in the dentin and incorporated diffusely in the enamel. The period of odontogenesis to completion of the formation of enamel in permanent teeth appears to be the critical time for the effects of these drugs and is virtually complete by 8 years of age, at which time the drug can be given without concern for dental staining. The degree of staining appears to depend on dosage and duration of therapy, with the total dosage received being the most important factor. In addition to dental discoloration, tetracyclines also may cause enamel hypoplasia and reversible delay in rate of bone growth.

These possible adverse events have resulted in the use of alternative, equally effective antimicrobial agents in most circumstances in young children in which tetracyclines are likely to be effective. However, in some cases the benefits of therapy with a tetracycline can exceed the risks, particularly if alternative drugs are associated with significant adverse effects or may be less effective. In these cases, the use of tetracyclines in young children is justified. Examples include life-threatening rickettsial infections such as Rocky Mountain spotted fever (see p 491) and ehrlichiosis (see p 234). Doxycycline is usually the agent of choice in such children because the risk of dental staining is less with this product than that with other tetracyclines. In addition, the drug is given twice a day in contrast to the more frequent dosing regimen of other tetracyclines.

JUDICIOUS USE OF ANTIMICROBIAL AGENTS

The spread of antimicrobial resistance is an issue of increasing concern to patients as well as health care professionals. Rarely, highly resistant pathogens such as *Burkholderia cepacia* or *Enterococcus faecium* are not treatable with available agents. More commonly, the presence of resistant pathogens complicates therapy, increases expense, and makes treatment failure more likely. Resistant foodborne pathogens, such as fluoroquinolone-resistant *Campylobacter jejuni;* community-acquired pathogens, such as drug-resistant *Streptococcus pneumoniae;* and hospital-acquired pathogens, such as vancomycin-resistant enterococci, have unique epidemiologic features and require specific control measures. The control of antimicrobial resistance among foodborne pathogens has focused on measures such as irradiating food products prior to consumption and reducing the addition of antimicrobial agents to animal feed. Among community-acquired and hospital-acquired pathogens, the overuse of antimicrobial agents in humans is largely responsible for the increase in resistance. The following principles for the judicious use of antimicrobial agents have become a central focus of public health control measures.

Principles of Judicious Use for Upper Respiratory Tract Infections

Approximately three fourths of all outpatient prescriptions for children are given for the following 5 conditions: otitis media, sinusitis, cough illness/bronchitis, pharyngitis, and nonspecific upper respiratory tract infection (the common cold). Physicians report that many patients and parents try to pressure them into dispensing unnecessary antimicrobial agents. Children treated with an antimicrobial agent are at increased risk of becoming carriers of resistant bacteria, including *S pneumoniae* and *Haemophilus influenzae.* Carriers of a resistant strain who develop illness from that strain are more likely to fail antimicrobial therapy. In some conditions, therefore, such as otitis media with effusion, observation without antimicrobial therapy is the preferable option, while in other conditions such as the common cold or cough, antimicrobial therapy is not indicated. The following principles, with detailed supporting evidence, were published by the American Academy of Pediatrics, American Academy of Family Physicians, and Centers for Disease Control and Prevention to identify areas where antimicrobial therapy might be curtailed without compromising patient care.*

OTITIS MEDIA

- Episodes of otitis media should be classified as acute otitis media (AOM) or otitis media with effusion (OME).

* Dowell SF, Schwartz B, Phillips WR, Gerber MA, Schwartz B. Principles of judicious use of antimicrobial agents for pediatric upper respiratory infections. *Pediatrics.* 1998;101:s163–s184, and Dowell SF, Schwartz B, Phillips WR. Appropriate use of antibiotics for URIs in children: part II. cough, pharyngitis, and the common cold. The Pediatric URI Consensus Team. *Am Fam Phys.* 1998;58:1335–1342, 1345

- Antimicrobial agents are indicated for treatment of AOM; however, diagnosis requires documented middle ear effusion *and* signs or symptoms of acute local or systemic illness.
- Acute otitis media can be treated with a 5- to 7-day course of antimicrobial agents in certain children 2 years of age or older. Younger children and children with underlying medical conditions, craniofacial abnormalities, chronic or recurrent otitis media, or perforation of the tympanic membrane, should be treated with a standard 10-day course.
- Persistent middle ear effusion (OME) for 2 to 3 months after therapy for AOM is expected and does not require retreatment.
- Antimicrobial agents are not indicated for initial treatment of OME; treatment may be indicated if effusions persist for 3 months or more.
- Antimicrobial prophylaxis should be reserved for control of recurrent AOM, defined as 3 or more distinct and well-documented episodes per 6 months or 4 or more episodes per 12 months.

ACUTE SINUSITIS

- Clinical diagnosis of bacterial sinusitis requires the following: nasal discharge and daytime cough without improvement for 10 to 14 days, or more severe signs and symptoms of acute sinusitis (ie, temperature of 39°C (102°F) or higher, facial swelling, facial pain).
- The common cold is a rhinosinusitis that often includes radiologic evidence of sinus involvement; radiographs, therefore, should be used only in selected circumstances and should be interpreted with caution. Radiographs may be indicated when episodes of sinusitis are recurrent, when complications are suspected, or when the diagnosis is unclear.
- Initial antimicrobial treatment of acute sinusitis should be with the agent with the narrowest spectrum that is active against the likely pathogens.

COUGH ILLNESS/BRONCHITIS

- Nonspecific cough illness/bronchitis in children, regardless of duration, rarely warrants antimicrobial treatment.
- Antimicrobial treatment for prolonged cough (>10 to 14 days) may be indicated in certain conditions including *Bordetella pertussis* and *Mycoplasma pneumoniae* infections, and appropriate diagnostic studies for these infections should be obtained. Pertussis should be treated according to established recommendations (see Pertussis, p 345). *Mycoplasma pneumoniae* can cause bronchitis or pneumonia and prolonged cough, usually in children older than 5 years of age; a macrolide agent (or tetracycline for children 8 years of age or older) can be used for treatment (see *M pneumoniae,* p 408). Children with underlying chronic pulmonary disease other than asthma may benefit from antimicrobial therapy for acute exacerbations.

PHARYNGITIS

(see Group A Streptococcal Infections, p 526)

- Diagnosis of group A streptococcal pharyngitis should be made based on results of appropriate laboratory tests in conjunction with clinical and epidemiologic findings.
- Antimicrobial therapy should not be given to a child with pharyngitis in the absence of identified group A streptococci or another bacterial pathogen known to cause pharyngitis. If presumptive therapy is given for group A streptococcal pharyngitis, it should be discontinued if the pharyngeal culture is negative for this organism.
- A penicillin remains the drug of choice for treating group A streptococcal pharyngitis.

THE COMMON COLD

- Antimicrobial agents should not be given for the common cold.
- Mucopurulent rhinitis (thick, opaque, or discolored nasal discharge) frequently accompanies the common cold and is not an indication for antimicrobial treatment unless it persists for 10–14 days, suggesting possible sinusitis.

Principles of Judicious Use of Vancomycin*

During the past decade, vancomycin-resistant enterococci have emerged rapidly as nosocomial pathogens at hospitals throughout the United States. Most recently, strains of *Staphylococcus aureus* with intermediate resistance to vancomycin and other glycopeptides also have been reported. The major risk factor for emergence of both vancomycin-resistant enterococci and *S aureus* with reduced susceptibility to vancomycin has been the increased use of vancomycin, particularly among patients on the hematology-oncology, neonatology, cardiac surgery, and neurosurgery services. Prevention of further emergence of vancomycin resistance will depend on more appropriate use of vancomycin.

Situations in which the use of vancomycin is appropriate include the following:

- Treatment of serious infections due to ß-lactam–resistant gram-positive organisms.
- Treatment of infections due to gram-positive microorganisms in patients with serious allergy to ß-lactam agents.
- When antibiotic-associated colitis fails to respond to metronidazole therapy or if it is severe and potentially life-threatening (see *Clostridium difficile,* p 214).
- Prophylaxis, as recommended by the American Heart Association, for endocarditis following certain procedures in patients at high risk for endocarditis (see Prevention of Bacterial Endocarditis, p 735).
- Prophylaxis for major surgical procedures involving implantation of prosthetic materials or devices at institutions with a high rate of infections due to methicillin-resistant *S aureus* or methicillin-resistant coagulase-negative staphylococci.

* Recommendations for preventing the spread of vancomycin resistance recommendations of the Hospital Infection Control Practices Advisory Committee. *MMWR Morb Mortal Wkly Rep.* 1995;44(RR-12):1–13

Situations in which the use of vancomycin should be discouraged:

- Routine prophylaxis in any of the following situations:
  - Surgical patients, other than in a patient with a life-threatening allergy to ß-lactam antibiotics.
  - Very low-birth-weight infants.
  - Patients receiving continuous ambulatory peritoneal dialysis or hemodialysis.
  - To prevent infection or colonization of indwelling central or peripheral intravascular catheters (either systemic or antibiotic lock)
- Empiric antimicrobial therapy for a febrile neutropenic patient, unless strong evidence indicates an infection due to gram-positive microorganisms and the prevalence of infections due to methicillin-resistant *S aureus* in the hospital is substantial.
- Treatment in response to a single blood culture positive for coagulase-negative staphylococcus, if other blood cultures obtained in the same period are negative.
- Continued empiric use for presumed infections in patients whose cultures are negative for ß-lactam–resistant gram-positive microorganisms.
- Selective decontamination of the digestive tract.
- Eradication of methicillin-resistant *S aureus* colonization.
- Primary treatment of antibiotic-associated colitis (see *Clostridium difficile,* p 214).
- Treatment of infections due to ß-lactam–susceptible gram-positive microorganisms including vancomycin given for dosing convenience in patients with renal failure.
- Topical application or irrigation.

TABLES OF ANTIBACTERIAL DRUG DOSAGES

The recommended dosages for antimicrobial agents commonly used for newborn infants (see Table 4.1, p 651) and for older infants and children (see Table 4.2, p 653) are given separately because of the physiologic immaturity of the newborn infant and resulting different pharmacokinetics. The table for newborn infants is divided by postnatal age and birth weight because all infections in this age group are considered potentially severe.

The recommended dosages are not absolute and are intended only as a guide. Clinical judgment about the disease, alterations in renal or hepatic function, coadministration of other drugs, and other factors affecting pharmacokinetics, patient response, and laboratory results may dictate modifications of these recommendations in an individual patient. In some cases, monitoring of serum drug concentrations is recommended to avoid toxicity and to ensure therapeutic efficacy.

Product label information should be consulted for details such as the diluent for reconstitution of injectable preparations, measures to be taken to avoid incompatibilities, drug interactions, and other precautions.

Table 4.1 **Antibacterial Drugs for Newborn Infants: Dose* (mg/kg or Units [U]/kg) and Frequency of Administration†**

Drug	Route	Infants 0–4 wk	Infants <1 wk old		Infants ≥1 wk old	
		BW <1200 g	BW ≤1200–2000 g	BW >2000 g	BW ≤2000–2000 g	BW >2000 g
Aminoglycosides‡§						
Amikacin	IV, IM	7.5 every 18–24 h	7.5 every 12 h	7.5–10 every 12 h	7.5–10 every 8 or 12 h	10 every 8 h
Gentamicin	IV, IM	2.5 every 18–24 h	2.5 every 12 h	2.5 every 12 h	2.5 every 8 or 12 h	2.5 every 8 h
Neomycin	PO only	...	25 every 6 h	25 every 6 h	25 every 6 h	25 every 6 h
Tobramycin	IV, IM	2.5 every 18–24 h	2.5 every 12 h	2.5 every 12 h	2.5 every 8 or 12 h	2.5 every 8 h
Antistaphylococcal penicillins‖						
Methicillin	IV, IM	25 every 12 h	25–50 every 12 h	25–50 every 8 h	25-50 every 8 h	25–50 every 6 h
Nafcillin	IV, IM	25 every 12 h	25 every 12 h	25 every 8 h	25 every 8 h	25–35 every 6 h
Oxacillin	IV, IM	25 every 12 h	25–50 every 12 h	25–50 every 8 h	25–50 every 8 h	25–50 every 6 h
Aztreonam	IV, IM	30 every 12 h	30 every 12 h	30 every 8 h	30 every 8 h	30 every 6 h
Carbapenicillins¶						
Imipenem/cilastatin	IV	25 every 12 h	25 every 12 h	25 every 12 h	25 every 8 h	25 every 8 h
Cephalosporins						
Cefotaxime	IV, IM	50 every 12 h	50 every 12 h	50 every 8 or 12 h	50 every 8 h	50 every 6 or 8 h
Ceftazidime	IV, IM	50 every 12 h	50 every 12 h	50 every 8 or 12 h	50 every 8 h	50 every 8 h
Ceftriaxone#	IV, IM	50 every 24 h	50 every 24 h	50 every 24 h	50 every 24 h	50–75 every 24 h
Clindamycin	IV, IM, PO	5 every 12 h	5every 12 h	5 every 8 h	5 every 8 h	5–7.5 every 6 h
Erythromycin	PO	10 every 12 h	10 every 12 h	10 every 12 h	10 every 8 h	10 every 6 or 8 h
Metronidazole¶	IV, PO	7.5 every 48 h	7.5 every 24 h	7.5 every 12 h	7.5 every 12 h	15 every 12 h

*Table 4.1 **Antibacterial Drugs for Newborn Infants: Dose* (mg/kg or Units [U]/kg) and Frequency of Administration,† continued**

		Infants 0–4 wk	Infants <1 wk old		Infants ≥1 wk old	
Drug	Route	BW <1200 g	BW ≤1200–2000 g	BW >2000 g	BW ≤2000–2000 g	BW >2000 g
Penicillins						
Ampicillin[‖**]	IV, IM	25–50 every 12 h	25–50 every 12 h	25–50 every 8 h	25-50 every 8 h	25–50 every 6 h
Penicillin G,[‖**] aqueous	IV, IM	25 000–50 000 U every 12 h	25 000–50 000 U every 12 h	25 000–50 000 U every 8 h	25 000–50 000 U every 8 h	25 000–50 000 U every 6 h
Penicillin G, procaine	IM	…	50 000 U every 24 h	50 000 U every 24 h	50 000 U every 24 h	50 000 U every 24 h
Ticarcillin	IV, IM	75 every 12 h	75 every 12 h	75 every 8 h	75 every 8 h	75 every 6 h
Vancomycin[‖‡]	IV	15 every 24 h	10–15 every 12–18 h	10–15 every 8–12 h	10–15 every 8–12 h	10–15 every 6 or 8 h

* Unless otherwise listed, dosages are given as mg/kg.
† BW indicates body weight; IV, intravenous; IM, intramuscular; PO, oral.
‡ Optimal dosage should be based on determination of serum concentrations, especially in low-birth-weight (<1500 g) infants. In very low-birth-weight infants (<1200 g) every 18 to 24 hour dosing may be appropriate in the first week of life.
§ Dosages for the aminoglycosides may differ from those recommended by the manufacturer in the package insert.
‖ For meningitis, the larger dosage is recommended.
¶ Safety in infants and children has not been established.
\# Drug should not be administered to hyperbilirubinemic neonates, especially those born prematurely.
** Higher doses are recommended for the treatment of group B streptococcal meningitis (see Group B Streptococcal Infections, p 537).

Table 4.2. **Antibacterial Drugs for Pediatric Patients Beyond the Newborn Period**

Drug, Generic (Trade Name)	Route	Dosage per kg/d: Mild to Moderate Infections	Dosage per kg/d: Severe Infections	Comments
Aminoglycosides*				
Amikacin (Amikin)	IV, IM	Inappropriate	15–22.5 mg in 3 doses (daily adult dose, 15 mg/kg; maximum, 1.5 g)	30 mg in 3 doses is recommended by some consultants
Gentamicin (Garamycin)	IV, IM	Inappropriate	3–7.5 mg in 3 doses (daily adult dose is the same)	Once daily dosing (5–6 mg/kg every 24 h) is investigational in children
Kanamycin (Kantrex)	IV, IM	Inappropriate	15–22.5 mg in 3 doses (daily adult dose, 1–1.5 g)	30 mg in 3 doses is recommended by some consultants
Neomycin (numerous types)	PO only	100 mg in 4 doses	100 mg in 4 doses	For some enteric infections
Netilmicin (Netromycin)	IV, IM	Inappropriate	3–7.5 mg in 3 doses (daily adult dose is the same)	...
Paromomycin (Humatin)	PO	30 mg in 3 doses (maximum daily adult dose, 4 g)	Inappropriate	...
Tobramycin (Nebcin)	IV, IM	Inappropriate	3–7.5 mg in 3 doses (daily adult dose, 3–5 mg in 3 doses)	Once daily dosing (5–6 mg/kg every 24 h) is investigational in children
Aztreonam[†] (Azactam)	IV, IM	90 mg in 3 doses (daily adult dose, 3 g)	120 mg in 4 doses (maximum daily adult dose, 8 g)	...
Cephalosporins[†]				
Cefaclor (Ceclor)	PO	20–40 mg in 2 or 3 doses (daily adult dose, 750 mg–1.5 g)	Inappropriate	A twice daily regimen has been demonstrated to be effective for treatment of acute otitis media
Cefadroxil (Duricef, Utracef)	PO	30 mg in 2 doses (maximum daily adult dose, 2 g)	Inappropriate	...

Table 4.2. **Antibacterial Drugs for Pediatric Patients Beyond the Newborn Period, continued**

Drug, Generic (Trade Name)	Route	Dosage per kg/d: Mild to Moderate Infections	Dosage per kg/d: Severe Infections	Comments
Cefazolin (Kefzol, Ancef)	IV, IM	25–50 mg in 3 doses (daily adult dose, 750 mg–2 g)	50–100 mg in 3 doses (maximum adult dose 4–6 g)	...
Cefdinir (Omnicef)	PO	14 mg in 1 or 2 doses (maximum 600 mg/d)	Inappropriate	Inadequate activity against resistant pneumococcus
Cefepime (Maxipime)	IV, IM	100–150 mg in 3 doses (daily adult dose, 1–2 g)	150 mg in 3 doses (daily adult dose, 2–4 g)	Not approved for therapy of meningitis
Cefixime (Suprax)	PO	8 mg in 1 or 2 doses (daily adult dose, 400 mg)	Inappropriate	Diarrhea occurs in 10%–15% of patients; inadequate activity against penicillin nonsusceptible pneumococci
Cefonicid (Monocid)	IV, IM	20–40 mg in 1 dose (maximum daily adult dose, 2 g)	No data available	Not approved for children
Cefoperazone (Cefobid)	IV, IM	100–150 mg in 2 or 3 doses (maximum daily adult dose, 4 g)	No data available	Not approved for children
Cefotaxime (Claforan)	IV, IM	75–100 mg in 3 or 4 doses (daily adult dose, 4–6 g)	150–200 mg in 3 or 4 doses (daily adult dose, 8–10 g)	A regimen of 300 mg in 3 or 4 doses can be used for therapy of meningitis
Cefotetan (Cefotan)	IV, IM	Inappropriate	40-80 mg in 2 doses (maximum daily adult dose, 6 g)	Not approved for children
Cefoxitin (Mefoxin)	IV, IM	80–100 mg in 3–4 doses (daily adult dose, 3–4 g)	80–160 mg in 4–6 doses (daily adult dose, 6–12 g)	...
Cefpodoxime proxetil (Vantin)	PO	10 mg in 2 doses (maximum daily adult dose, 800 mg)	Inappropriate	...
Cefprozil (Cefzil)	PO	15–30 mg in 2 doses (maximum daily adult dose, 1 g)	Inappropriate	30-mg dosage recommended for treatment of acute otitis media
Ceftazidime (Fortaz, Tazicef, Tazidime)	IV, IM	75–100 mg in 3 doses (daily adult dose, 3 g)	125–150 mg in 3 doses (daily adult dose, 6 g)	Only cephalosporin with anti-*Pseudomonas* activity that has been approved for use in children

Table 4.2. **Antibacterial Drugs for Pediatric Patients Beyond the Newborn Period, continued**

Drug, Generic (Trade Name)	Route	Dosage per kg/d: Mild to Moderate Infections	Dosage per kg/d: Severe Infections	Comments
Ceftibuten (Cedax)	PO	9 mg in 1 dose (maximum daily adult dose: see package insert)	Inappropriate	Inadequate activity against intermediate and resistant pneumococci
Ceftizoxime (Cefizox)	IV, IM	100–150 mg in 3 doses (daily adult dose, 3–4 g)	150–200 mg in 3 or 4 doses (daily adult dose, 4–6 g)	...
Ceftriaxone (Rocephin)	IV, IM	50–75 mg in 1 or 2 doses (daily adult dose, 2 g)	80–100 mg in 1 or 2 doses (daily adult dose, 4 g)	Larger dosage appropriate for penicillin-resistant pneumococcal meningitis
Cefuroxime (Zinacef)	IV, IM	75–100 mg in 3 doses (daily adult dose, 2–4 g)	100–150 mg in 3 doses (daily adult dose, 4–6 g)	...
Cefuroxime axetil (Ceftin)	PO	20–30 mg in 2 doses (daily adult dose, 1–2 g)	Inappropriate	The higher dosage recommended for treatment of otitis media
Cephalexin (Keflex)	PO	25–50 mg in 3–4 doses (daily adult dose, 1–4 g)	Inappropriate	...
Cephalothin (Keflin)	IV, IM	80–100 mg in 4 doses (daily adult dose, 2–4 g)	100–150 mg in 4–6 doses (daily adult dose, 8–12 g)	...
Cephradine				
(Anspor)	PO	25–50 mg in 2–4 doses (daily adult dose, 1–4 g)	Inappropriate	...
(Velosef)	IV, IM	50–100 mg in 4 doses (daily adult dose, 2–8 g)	100 mg in 4 doses (daily adult dose, 6–8 g)	...
Loracarbef (Lorabid)	PO	30 mg for otitis media and 15 mg for other indications in 2 doses (maximum daily adult dose, 800 mg)	Inappropriate	...

Table 4.2. **Antibacterial Drugs for Pediatric Patients Beyond the Newborn Period, continued**

Drug, Generic (Trade Name)	Route	Dosage per kg/d: Mild to Moderate Infections	Dosage per kg/d: Severe Infections	Comments
Chloramphenicol (Chloromycetin)				
Chloramphenicol palmitate	PO (not available in the United States)	Inappropriate	50–100 mg in 4 doses (daily adult dose, 1–2 g)	Optimal dosage is determined by measurement of serum concentrations with resulting modifications to achieve therapeutic concentrations
Chloramphenicol succinate	IV	Inappropriate	50–100 mg in 4 doses (daily adult dose, 2–4 g)	Use only for serious infections because of the rare occurrence of aplastic anemia after administration
Clindamycin (Cleocin)	IM, IV	15–25 mg in 3–4 doses (daily adult dose, 600 mg–3.6 g)	25–40 mg in 3–4 doses (daily adult dose, 1.2–2.7 g)	Active against anaerobes, especially *Bacteroides* species; active against many multidrug-resistant pneumococci
	PO	10–20 mg in 3–4 doses (daily adult dose, 600 mg–1.8 g)	Inappropriate	Effective for otitis media caused by many multidrug-resistant pneumococci
Fluoroquinolones‡				
Ciprofloxacin (Cipro)	PO	20–30 mg in 2 doses (daily adult dose, 0.5–1.5 mg)	30 mg in 2 doses (daily adult dose, 1.0–1.5 g)	Not approved for use in persons younger than 18 years of age‡; however, drug has selective indications in children and adolescents (see p 645)
	IV	Inappropriate	20-30 mg in 2 doses (daily adult dose, 400–800 mg in 2 doses)	

Table 4.2. **Antibacterial Drugs for Pediatric Patients Beyond the Newborn Period, continued**

Drug, Generic (Trade Name)	Route	Dosage per kg/d: Mild to Moderate Infections	Dosage per kg/d: Severe Infections	Comments
Carbapenems				
Imipenem[†§] (Primaxin)	IV, IM	40–60 mg in 4 doses (daily adult dose, 1–2 g)	60 mg in 4 doses (daily adult dose, 2–4 g)	Caution in use for therapy of meningitis because of possible seizures
Meropenem[†§] (Merrem)	IV	60 mg in 3 doses (daily adult dose, 4 g)	60–120 mg in 3 doses (daily adult dose, 4–6 g)	Larger dosage is used for therapy of meningitis
Macrolides				
Erythromycins (numerous types)	PO	30–50 mg in 2–4 doses (daily adult dose, 1–2 g)	Inappropriate	Available in base, stearate, ethyl succinate, and estolate preparations
	IV	Inappropriate	15–50 mg in 4 doses (daily adult dose, 1–4 g)	Administer in a continuous drip or by slow infusion over 60 min or longer; may cause cardiac arrhythmia
Azithromycin (Zithromax)	PO	5–12 mg/kg once daily (maximum daily adult dose, 600 mg)	Inappropriate	Otitis: 10 mg/kg on first day, 5 mg/kg per day for an additional 4 d Pharyngitis: 12 mg/kg per day for 5 days
Clarithromycin (Biaxin)	PO	7.5 mg in 2 doses (maximum daily adult dose, 1 g)	Inappropriate	
Methenamine mandelate (Mandelamine)	PO	50–75 mg in 3–4 doses (daily adult dose, 2–4 g)	Inappropriate	Should not be used for infants; urine pH must be adjusted to 5–5.5
Metronidazole (Flagyl)	PO	15–35 mg in 3 doses (maximum daily adult dose, 1–2 g)	Inappropriate	Safety in infants and children has not been established
Nitrofurantoin (Furadantin)	PO	5–7 mg in 4 doses (daily adult dose, 200–400 mg)	Inappropriate	Should not be used for young infants; prophylactic dose is 1–2 mg/kg per day in 1 dose

Table 4.2. **Antibacterial Drugs for Pediatric Patients Beyond the Newborn Period, continued**

Drug, Generic (Trade Name)	Route	Dosage per kg/d: Mild to Moderate Infections	Dosage per kg/d: Severe Infections	Comments
PENICILLINS†				
Broad–spectrum penicillins				
Ampicillin (numerous types) adult dose, 2–4 g)	IV, IM	100–150 mg in 4 doses (daily adult dose, 2–4 g)	200–400 mg in 4 doses (daily adult dose, 6–12 g)	Larger dosage recommended for treatment of meningitis
	PO	50–100 mg in 4 doses (daily adult dose, 2–4 g)	Inappropriate	Diarrhea occurs in approximately 20% of recipients
Ampicillin-sulbactam (Unasyn)‖	IV	100–150 mg of ampicillin in 4 doses	200–400 mg of ampicillin in 4 doses (daily adult dose, 6–12 g)	Not approved for infants and children
Amoxicillin (numerous types)	PO	25–50 mg in 3 doses (daily adult dose, 750 mg–1.5 g)	Inappropriate	Larger dosage (80–90 mg in 2 doses) for otitis media caused by penicillin-resistant pneumococci
Amoxicillin-clavulanate (7:1 formulation) (Augmentin)	PO	45 mg of amoxicillin in 2–3 doses	Inappropriate	A 14:1 amoxicillin:clavulanate formulation awaiting Food and Drug Administration approval Dosage: 90 mg in 2 doses for multidrug-resistant pneumococcal otitis media
Mezlocillin (Mezlin)	IV, IM	100–150 mg in 4 doses (daily adult dose, 6–8 g)	200–300 mg in 4–6 doses (daily adult dose, 12–18 g)	…
Piperacillin‖ (Pipracil)	IV, IM	100–150 mg in 4 doses (daily adult dose, 6–8 g)	200–300 mg in 4–6 doses (daily adult dose, 12–18 g)	…
Piperacillin/tazobactam‖ (Zosyn)	IV	Inappropriate	240 mg of piperacillin in 3 doses	Not approved for children

Table 4.2. **Antibacterial Drugs for Pediatric Patients Beyond the Newborn Period, continued**

Drug, Generic (Trade Name)	Route	Dosage per kg/d: Mild to Moderate Infections	Dosage per kg/d: Severe Infections	Comments
Ticarcillin (Ticar)	IV, IM	100–200 mg in 4 doses (daily adult dose, 4–6 g)	200–300 mg in 4–6 doses (daily adult dose, 12–24 g)	Contains 5.2 mEq of Na per gram
Ticarcillin-clavulanate (Timentin)	IV, IM	100–200 mg of ticarcillin in 4 doses (4–6 g)	200–300 mg of ticarcillin in 4 doses (12–24 g)	…
Penicillin G and V[†‖]				
Penicillin G, crystalline K or Na (numerous types)	IV, IM	25 000–50 000 U in 4 doses	250 000–400 000 U in 4–6 doses	Larger dosage appropriate for central nervous system infections
Penicillin G, procaine (numerous types)	IM	25 000–50 000 U in 1–2 doses	Inappropriate	Contraindicated in procaine allergy
Penicillin G, benzathine (Bicillin, Permapen)	IM	<27.3 kg (60 lb): 600 000 U ≥27.3 kg: 1 200 000 U	Inappropriate	Major use is prevention of rheumatic fever by treatment and prophylaxis of streptococcal infections
Penicillin G, potassium oral (numerous types)	PO	25 000–50 000 U in 3 or 4 doses	Inappropriate	Variable absorption; optimal to administer unbuffered penicillin G at least 1 h before, or 2 h after meals
Penicillin V (numerous types)	PO	25 000–50 000 U in 3 or 4 doses	Inappropriate	Optimal to administer on an empty stomach

Table 4.2. **Antibacterial Drugs for Pediatric Patients Beyond the Newborn Period, continued**

Drug, Generic (Trade Name)	Route	Dosage per kg/d: Mild to Moderate Infections	Dosage per kg/d: Severe Infections	Comments
Penicillinase-resistant penicillins†				Methicillin (oxacillin)-resistant staphylococci are usually resistant to all other semisynthetic antistaphylococcal cephalosporins
Methicillin (Staphcillin)	IV, IM	100–150 mg in 4 doses (daily adult dose, 4–8 g)	150–200 mg in 4–6 doses (daily adult dose, 4–12 g)	Interstitial nephritis (ie, hematuria) occurs in 0%–4% of patients
Oxacillin (Prostaphlin, Bactocill)	IV, IM	100–150 mg in 4 doses (daily adult dose, 2–4 g)	150–200 mg in 4–6 doses (daily adult dose, 4–12 g)	…
Nafcillin (Unipen, Nafcil)	IV, IM	50–100 mg in 4 doses (daily adult dose, 2–4 g)	100–150 mg in 4 doses (daily adult dose, 4–12 g)	Serum concentrations after oral administration are low compared with those after other orally administered antistaphylococcal drugs
Cloxacillin (Tegopen, Cloxapen)	PO	50–100 mg in 4 doses (daily adult dose, 2–4 g)	Inappropriate	…
Dicloxacillin (Dynapen, Pathocil)	PO	25–50 mg in 4 doses (daily adult dose, 1–2 g)	Inappropriate	Excellent serum concentrations after oral administration
Rifampin (numerous types)	PO	10–20 mg in 1–2 doses (daily adult dose, 600 mg)	20 mg in 2 doses	Should not be used as monotherapy except when given for prophylaxis
	IV	10–20 mg in 1–2 doses (daily adult dose, 600 mg)	20 mg in 2 doses	…

Table 4.2. **Antibacterial Drugs for Pediatric Patients Beyond the Newborn Period, continued**

Drug, Generic (Trade Name)	Route	Dosage per kg/d: Mild to Moderate Infections	Dosage per kg/d: Severe Infections	Comments
Sulfonamides				
Sulfadiazine	PO	100–150 mg in 4 doses	120–150 mg in 4–6 doses	...
Sulfisoxazole (Gantrisin)	PO	120–150 mg in 4–6 doses	120–150 mg in 4–6 doses	...
Triple sulfonamides (numerous types)	PO	120–150 mg in 4 doses	120–150 mg in 4 doses	...
Trimethoprim–sulfamethoxazole (Bactrim, Septra)	PO	8–12 mg trimethoprim—40–60 mg sulfamethoxazole in 2 doses (daily adult dose, 320 mg trimethoprim and 1.6 g sulfamethoxazole)	20 mg trimethoprim—100 mg sulfamethoxazole in 4 doses (for use only in *Pneumocystis carinii* pneumonia)	For prophylaxis in immunocompromised patients, recommended daily dose is 5 mg trimethoprim—25 mg sulfamethoxazole per kg/d in 2 doses
	IV	Inappropriate	8–12 mg trimethoprim—40–60 mg sulfamethoxazole in 4 doses	Use intravenous formulation when oral formulation cannot be administered
			OR	
			20 mg trimethoprim—100 mg sulfamethoxazole in 4 doses (for treatment of *Pneumocystis* infection)	...
Tetracyclines (numerous types)	IV	Inappropriate	10–25 mg in 2–4 doses (daily adult dose, 1–2 g)	Responsible for staining of developing teeth; use only in children 8 years of age or older except in circumstances in which the benefits of therapy exceed the risks and alternative drugs are less effective or more toxic (see p 646)

Table 4.2. **Antibacterial Drugs for Pediatric Patients Beyond the Newborn Period, continued**

Drug, Generic (Trade Name)	Route	Dosage per kg/d: Mild to Moderate Infections	Dosage per kg/d: Severe Infections	Comments
Tetracyclines (numerous types), continued	PO	20–50 mg in 4 doses (daily adult dose, 1–2 g)	Inappropriate	...
Doxycycline (numerous types)	PO, IV	2–4 mg in 1–2 doses (daily adult dose, 100–200 mg)	Inappropriate	Side effects similar to those of other tetracycline products except that risk of dental staining in children younger than 8 years of age is less
Vancomycin (Vancocin, Vancoled, Vancor)	IV	40 mg in 3–4 doses (daily adult dose,¶ 1–2 g)	40–60 mg in 4 doses (daily adult dose,¶ 2–4 g)	In meningitis, 60 mg/kg dose should be given during at least 60 min; routine monitoring of serum concentrations is unnecessary

* Dosages for the aminoglycosides may differ from those recommended by the manufacturers (see package insert).

† In patients with history of allergy to penicillin or one of its many congeners, alternative drugs are recommended. In some circumstances, a cephalosporin or other ß-lactam class drug may be acceptable. However, these drugs should not be used in patients with an immediate hypersensitivity (anaphylaxis) to penicillin because approximately 5% to 15% of penicillin-allergic patients will also be allergic to the cephalosporins.

‡ Not approved for use in patients younger than 18 years old. Some fluoroquinolones currently are being studied in selected children and adolescents (see Fluoroquinolones, p 645).

§ Not approved for use in patients younger than 12 years old.

‖ Patients with a history of allergy to penicillin G or V should be considered for subsequent skin testing. Many such patients can be treated safely with penicillin, since only 10% of children with such history are proven allergic when skin-tested.

¶ In adults, daily dose is given in 2 to 4 divided doses.

SEXUALLY TRANSMITTED DISEASES

Table 4.3. **Guidelines for Treatment of Sexually Transmitted Diseases in Children and Adolescents According to Syndrome** Preferred regimens are listed. For further information concerning other acceptable regimens and diseases not included, see specific recommendations in disease-specific chapters in Section 3. In addition, revised recommendations on the treatment of sexually transmitted diseases have been issued by the Centers for Disease Control and Prevention in 1998.*

Syndrome	Organism(s)/Diagnoses	Treatment of Adolescent	Treatment of Infant/Child
Urethritis and cervicitis Urethritis: Inflammation of urethra with mucoid, mucopurulent, or purulent discharge Cervicitis: Inflammation of cervix with mucopurulent or purulent cervical discharge; cervicitis occurs rarely in prepubertal girls (see Prepubertal vaginitis below)	*Neisseria gonorrhoeae, Chlamydia trachomatis* Other causes of urethritis and cervicitis include *Ureaplasma urealyticum,* possibly *Mycoplasma genitalium,* and sometimes *Trichomonas vaginalis* and herpes simplex virus (HSV)	Cefixime, 400 mg orally in a single dose **OR** Ceftriaxone, 125 mg IM in a single dose **OR** Ciprofloxacin, 500 mg orally in a single dose† **OR** Ofloxacin, 400 mg orally in a single dose† **PLUS** Azithromycin, 1 g orally in a single dose **OR** Doxycycline, 100 mg orally twice a day for 7 d	Ceftriaxone, 125 mg IM in a single dose **OR** Spectinomycin, 40 mg/kg (maximum 2 g) IM in a single dose **PLUS** Erythromycin base, 50 mg/kg per day orally, in 4 divided doses (maximum 2 g/d) for 10–14 d **OR** Azithromycin, 10 mg/kg orally in a single dose (maximum 1 g)
Prepubertal vaginitis (STD-related):	*N gonorrhoeae*	...	Ceftriaxone, 125 mg in a single dose
	C trachomatis	...	Erythromycin base, 50 mg/kg per day orally, in 4 divided doses (maximum 2 g/d) for 10–14 d
	T vaginalis	...	Metronidazole, 15 mg/kg per day orally in 3 divided doses (maximum 2 g/d) for 7 d

Table 4.3. **Guidelines for Treatment of Sexually Transmitted Diseases in Children and Adolescents According to Syndrome, continued**

Syndrome	Organism(s)/Diagnoses	Treatment of Adolescent	Treatment of Infant/Child
Prepubertal vaginitis (STD-related), continued:	Bacterial vaginosis	...	Metronidazole, 15 mg/kg per day orally in 2 divided doses (maximum 1 g/d) for 7 d
	HSV — primary infection	...	Acyclovir, 80 mg/kg per day orally in 3–4 divided doses (maximum 1.2 g/d) for 7–10 d
Adolescent vulvo-vaginitis	*T vaginalis*	Metronidazole, 2 g orally in a single dose **OR** Metronidazole, 500 mg twice daily for 7 d	...
	Bacterial vaginosis	Metronidazole, 500 mg twice daily for 7 d **OR** Clindamycin cream 2%, 1 full applicator (5 g) intravaginally at bed time for 7 d **OR** Metronidazole gel 0.75%, 1 full applicator (5 g) intravaginally twice a day for 5 d **OR** Metronidazole, 2 g orally in a single dose **OR** Clindamycin 300 mg orally twice a day for 7 d	...
	Candida species	See Table 4.4, Recommended regimens for vulvovaginal candidiasis, p 667	...
	HSV — primary infection	Acyclovir, 1000–1200 mg/d orally in 3–5 divided doses for 7–10 d	...

Table 4.3. **Guidelines for Treatment of Sexually Transmitted Diseases in Children and Adolescents According to Syndrome, continued**

Syndrome	Organism(s)/Diagnoses	Treatment of Adolescent	Treatment of Infant/Child
Pelvic inflammatory disease (PID)	*N gonorrhoeae, C trachomatis,* anaerobes, coliform bacteria, and *Streptococcus* species	See Pelvic Inflammatory Disease (Table 3.42, p 434)	PID occurs rarely, if at all, in prepubertal girls
Syphilis	*Treponema pallidum*	See Syphilis, p 547	Same as for congenital syphilis (see p 553, Table 3.56, p 555)
Genital ulcer disease	*T pallidum*	Same as for syphilis	Same as for congenital syphilis (see p 553, Table 3.56, p 555
	HSV — primary infection	Acyclovir, 1000–1200 mg/d orally in 3–5 divided doses for 7–10 d	Acyclovir, 80 mg/kg per day orally in 3–4 divided doses (maximum 1.0 g/d) for 7–10 d
	Haemophilus ducreyi (chancroid)	Azithromycin, 1 g orally in a single dose **OR** Ceftriaxone, 250 mg IM in a single dose **OR** Ciprofloxacin, 500 mg orally twice a day for 3 d[†] **OR** Erythromycin base, 500 mg orally 4 times a day for 7 d	Ceftriaxone, 50 mg/kg IM in a single dose **OR** Azithromycin, 20 mg/kg orally in a single dose (maximum 1 g)
Sexually acquired epididymitis	*C trachomatis, N gonorrhoeae,* gram-negative enteric organisms[‡]	Ceftriaxone, 250 mg IM in a single dose **OR** Cefixime, 400 mg orally in a single dose **PLUS** Doxycycline, 100 mg orally twice a day for 10 d	…

Table 4.3. **Guidelines for Treatment of Sexually Transmitted Diseases in Children and Adolescents According to Syndrome, continued**

Syndrome	Organism(s)/Diagnoses	Treatment of Adolescent	Treatment for Infant/Child
Anogenital warts	Human papillomavirus	*Patient-applied:* Podofilox, 0.5% solution or gel[§] **OR** Imiquimod, 5% cream *Provider-administered:* Cryotherapy **OR** Podophyllin resin 10%-25%[§] **OR** Trichloroacetic acid **OR** Bichloroacetic acid **OR** Surgical removal	Same as for adolescents

* For additional information and recommendations, see the following: Centers for Disease Control and Prevention. 1998 guidelines for treatment of sexually transmitted diseases. *MMWR Morb Mortal Wkly Rep*. 1998;47(RR-1):1—116. IM indicates intramuscularly; STD, sexually transmitted disease; some regimens are not indicated for pregnant adolescents.

† Ciprofloxacin and ofloxacin are contraindicated for pregnant and lactating women and for persons younger than 18 years of age.

‡ For epididymitis most likely caused by enteric organisms or persons allergic to cephalosporins or tetracyclines: ofloxacin 300 mg twice a day for 10 days.

§ Not tested for safety in children and contraindicated in pregnancy.

Table 4.4. **Recommended Regimens for Vulvovaginal Candidiasis**

Intravaginal agents:

Butoconazole, 2% cream, 5 g intravaginally for 3 d,*†

OR

Clotrimazole, 1% cream, 5 g intravaginally for 7–14 d,*†

OR

Clotrimazole, 100-mg vaginal tablet for 7 d,*

OR

Clotrimazole, 100-mg vaginal tablet, 2 tablets for 3 d,*

OR

Clotrimazole, 500-mg vaginal tablet, 1 tablet in a single application,*

OR

Miconazole, 2% cream, 5 g intravaginally for 7 d,*†

OR

Miconazole, 200-mg vaginal suppository, 1 suppository for 3 d,*†

OR

Miconazole, 100-mg vaginal suppository, 1 suppository for 7 d,*†

OR

Nystatin, 100 000-unit vaginal tablet, 1 tablet for 14 d,

OR

Tioconazole, 6.5% ointment, 5 g intravaginally in a single application,*†

OR

Terconazole, 0.4% cream, 5 g intravaginally for 7 d,*

OR

Terconazole, 0.8% cream, 5 g intravaginally for 3 d,*

OR

Terconazole, 80-mg vaginal suppository, 1 suppository for 3 d.*

Oral agent:

Fluconazole 150-mg oral tablet, 1 tablet in single dose.

* These creams and suppositories are oil-based and might weaken latex condoms and diaphragms. Refer to condom product labeling for additional information.

† Over-the-counter preparations.

Antifungal Drugs for Systemic Fungal Infections

Polyenes: Amphotericin B deoxycholate or conventional amphotericin B is the drug of choice for most progressive, potentially life-threatening fungal infections. Amphotericin B is fungicidal against a broad array of fungal species excluding *Fusarium* and *Pseudallescheria boydii.* It may cause adverse reactions, particularly renal toxic effects, that limit its use in certain patients.

Amphotericin B is administered in 5% dextrose in water at a concentration of 0.1 mg/mL for delivery through a central or peripheral venous catheter (see Table 4.5, p 670). Amphotericin B is administered intravenously in a single daily dose of 0.5–1.5 mg/kg per day. Prolonged infusions were once recommended to avoid toxicity, but in adults and older children an infusion time of 1 hour is often well tolerated and theoretically increases blood-to-tissue gradient, thereby improving drug delivery. After completing 1 week of daily therapy, adequate serum concentrations of the drug usually can be maintained by administering double the daily dose (maximum, 1.5 mg/kg) on alternate days. The duration of therapy depends on the type and extent of the specific fungal infection.

Amphotericin B is eliminated by a renal mechanism for weeks after therapy is discontinued. No adjustment in dose is required for neonates or for children with impaired renal function because the serum concentration is not significantly increased in these patients. Hemodialysis and peritoneal dialysis do not significantly lower serum concentrations of the drug.

Infusion-related reactions to amphotericin B include fever, chills, and sometimes nausea, vomiting, headache, generalized malaise, hypotension, and arrhythmias. Onset usually is within 1 to 3 hours after starting the infusion; duration typically is less than an hour. Hypotension and arrhythmias are idiosyncratic reactions that are unlikely to occur if not observed after the initial dose, but also occur in association with rapid infusion. Multiple regimens have been used to attempt to prevent infusion-related reactions, but few have been studied in controlled clinical trials. Pretreatment with acetaminophen, alone or combined with diphenhydramine, may alleviate febrile reactions, although these reactions appear to be less common in children than in adults. Hydrocortisone (25 to 50 mg in adults and older children) also can be added to the infusion to reduce febrile and other systemic reactions. Tolerance to the febrile reactions develops with time, allowing tapering and eventual discontinuation of the hydrocortisone and often antipyretics.

Meperidine and ibuprofen have been effective in preventing or treating fever and chills in the occasional patient who is refractory to the conventional premedication regimen. Toxicity from amphotericin B may include nephrotoxicity, hepatotoxicity, thrombophlebitis, anemia, and neurotoxicity. Nephrotoxicity is secondary to decreased renal blood flow and can be prevented or ameliorated by hydration, saline-loading (0.9% saline over 30 minutes) before infusion of amphotericin B, and avoiding diuretic drugs. Hypokalemia is common and can be exacerbated by sodium loading. Renal tubular acidosis can occur but usually is mild. Permanent nephrotoxicity is related to cumulative dose. Nephrotoxicity can be enhanced by concomitant administration of amphotericin B and aminoglycosides, cyclosporine, tacrolimus, cisplatin, nitrogen mustard compounds, and acetazolamide. Anemia is secondary to inhibition of erythropoietin production. Neurotoxicity occurs rarely, and can be manifested as confusion, delirium, obtundation, psychotic behavior, seizures, blurred vision, or hearing loss.

Lipid formulations of amphotericin B have a role in some children who are intolerant of or refractory to amphotericin B deoxycholate (see Table 4.5, p 670). None of these formulations have been demonstrated to have efficacy that is superior to that of conventional amphotericin B. Amphotericin B lipid complex (Abelcet) is approved by the Food and Drug Administration for treatment of invasive fungal infections in children and adults who are refractory to or intolerant of conventional amphotericin B therapy, which is defined as (1) renal dysfunction with a serum creatinine level of 1.5 mg/dL or greater that develops during therapy or (2) disease progression after a total dose of amphotericin B of at least 10 mg/kg. Amphotericin B cholesteryl sulfate complex (Amphotec) is a colloidal complex that is approved by the Food and Drug Administration for treatment of invasive aspergillosis in adults who cannot tolerate or fail to respond to amphotericin B deoxycholate. The liposomal formulation of amphotericin B (AmBisome) is approved for adults who cannot tolerate or fail to respond to conventional amphotericin B therapy for aspergillosis, candidiasis, cryptococcosis, or febrile neutropenia. In recommended doses, these lipid formulations cost 10 to 65 times more per day than amphotericin B. These lipid formulations currently are undergoing clinical evaluation for treatment of other fungal infections and for use in children.

Pyrimidines: Among pyrimidine antifungal agents, only flucytosine (5-fluorocytosine) is approved for use in children. This drug has a limited spectrum of activity against fungi, a potential for toxicity (see Table 4.5, p 670), and when used as a single agent resistance often emerges. Flucytosine is used in combination with amphotericin B for cryptococcal meningitis and some life-threatening *Candida* infections such as meningitis.

Azoles: Three oral azoles—ketoconazole, and especially fluconazole and itraconazole—have a relatively broad spectrum of activity against common fungi and can be alternatives to amphotericin B therapy in certain patients (see Table 4.5, p 670). Limited data are available regarding the safety and efficacy of the azoles in pediatric patients, and trials comparing these agents to amphotericin B have not been conducted. The azoles are easy to administer and have little toxicity, but their use can be limited by the frequency of their interactions with certain coadministered drugs. These drug-drug interactions may result in decreased serum concentrations of the azole (ie, poor therapeutic activity) or unexpected toxicity from the coadministered drug (ie, increased serum concentrations of the coadministered drug by altering cytochrome P-450 system). When considering the use of azoles, the physician should carefully review the patient's concurrent medications to avoid potential adverse clinical outcomes. Another potential limitation of the azoles is the emergence of resistance to fungi, especially of *Candida* species to fluconazole. Use of fluconazole for therapy or prophylaxis has resulted in an increased frequency of non-*albicans Candida* species as a cause of bloodstream infections. Table 4.6 (see p 672) provides recommendations for treatment of serious fungal infections with amphotericin B, flucytosine, the azoles, and other antifungal agents. Table 4.6 (see p 672) provides information regarding dosage, route of administration, and adverse reactions.

RECOMMENDED DOSES OF PARENTERAL AND ORAL ANTIFUNGAL DRUGS

Table 4.5. **Recommended Doses of Parenteral and Oral Antifungal Drugs**

Drug	Route*	Dose (per day)	Adverse Reactions[†‡]
Amphotericin B (see Antifungal Drugs for Systemic Fungal Infections, p 668, for detailed information)	IV	0.25–0.5 mg/kg initially, increase as tolerated to 0.5–1.5 mg/kg; infuse as single dose over 2–3 h; 0.5–1.0 mg/kg weekly for suppressive therapy in HIV-infected patients with cryptococcosis or histoplasmosis	Fever, chills, gastrointestinal tract symptoms, headache, hypotension, renal dysfunction, hypokalemia, anemia, cardiac arrhythmias, neurotoxicity, anaphylaxis
	IT	0.025 mg, increase to 0.5 mg twice a week	Headache, gastrointestinal tract symptoms, arachnoiditis/radiculitis
Amphotericin B Lipid Complex (ABLC)[§‖]	IV	5 mg/kg infused over 2 h	Fever, chills, other reactions associated with amphotericin B, but less nephrotoxicity; hepatotoxicity
Amphotericin B cholesteryl sulfate complex (ABCD)[§‖]	IV	3–6 mg/kg infused at a rate of 1 mg/kg per hour	Fever, chills, other reactions associated with amphotericin B, but less nephrotoxicity; hepatotoxicity
Liposomal Amphotericin B Lipid Complex (AmBisome)[§‖]	IV	5 mg/kg infused over 1–2 h	Fever, chills, other reactions associated with amphotericin B, but less nephrotoxicity; hepatotoxicity
Clotrimazole	PO	10-mg tablet 5 times a day (dissolved slowly in the mouth)	Gastrointestinal tract symptoms, hepatotoxicity
Fluconazole[‖]	IV PO	Children: 3–6 mg/kg per day, single dose Adults: 200 mg once, followed by 100 mg/d for oropharyngeal, esophageal candidiasis; 400–800 mg/d for other invasive fungal infections; 200 mg/d for suppressive therapy in HIV-infected patients with cryptococcal meningitis	Rash, gastrointestinal tract symptoms, hepatotoxicity, Stevens-Johnson syndrome, anaphylaxis

Table 4.5. **Recommended Doses of Parenteral and Oral Antifungal Drugs, continued**

Drug	Route*	Dose (per day)	Adverse Reactions
Flucytosine	PO	50 to 150 mg/kg per day in 4 doses at 6-h intervals (adjust dose if renal dysfunction)	Bone marrow suppression, renal dysfunction, gastrointestinal tract symptoms, rash, neuropathy, hepatotoxicity, confusion, hallucinations
Griseofulvin	PO	Ultramicrosize: 5–10 mg/kg, single dose; maximum dose, 750 mg Microsize: 10–20 mg/kg per day divided in 2 doses; maximum dose, 1000 mg	Rash, paresthesias, leukopenia, gastrointestinal symptoms, proteinuria, hepatotoxicity, mental confusion, headache
Itraconazole[‖‡]	PO	Children: 5–10 mg/kg per day as a single dose or divided into 2 doses Adults: 100–200 mg/d once or twice a day; 200 mg once or twice a day for suppressive therapy in HIV-infected patients with histoplasmosis	Gastrointestinal tract symptoms, rash, edema, headache, hypokalemia, hepatotoxicity, thrombocytopenia, leukopenia; cardiac toxicity is possible in patients also taking terfenadine or astemizole
Ketoconazole[‡]	PO	Children[¶]: 3.3–6.6 mg/kg per day, single dose Adults: 200-400 mg once or twice a day	Hepatotoxicity, gastrointestinal tract symptoms, rash, anaphylaxis, thrombocytopenia, hemolytic anemia, gynecomastia, adrenal insufficiency; cardiac toxicity is possible in patients also taking terfenadine or astemizole
Nystatin	PO	Infants: 200 000 U, 4 times a day, after meals Children and adults: 400 000–600 000 U, 3 times a day, after meals	Gastrointestinal tract symptoms, rash

* IV indicates intravenous; IT, intrathecal; PO, oral; HIV, human immunodeficiency virus.
† See package insert or listing in current edition of the *Physicians' Desk Reference.* Montvale, NJ: Medical Economics.
‡ Interactions with other drugs are common. Consult the *Physicians' Desk Reference,* a drug interaction reference or database, or a pharmacist before prescribing these medications.
§ Experience with drug in children is limited.
‖ Limited or no information about use in newborn infants is available.
¶ For children 2 years old and younger, the daily dose has not been established.

DRUGS FOR INVASIVE AND OTHER SERIOUS FUNGAL INFECTIONS IN CHILDREN

Table 4.6. **Drugs for Invasive and Other Serious Fungal Infections***

	Intravenous	Oral, Absorbable		Intravenous or Oral	
Disease	Amphotericin B	Flucytosine	Ketoconazole†	Itraconazole	Fluconazole
Aspergillosis	P,S	...	...	A,M,S	...
Blastomycosis	P	...	A,M	A,M,(P)	A,M
Candidiasis:					
Chronic, mucocutaneous	A	...	A	A	P
Oropharyngeal, gastrointestinal	A (Severe cases)	...	A	A	P
Systemic	P,S	S	...	...	A,M
Coccidioidomycosis	P	...	A,M	A,M	(P),A,M
Cryptococcosis	C	C	...	A,M	A
Histoplasmosis	P	..	A,M	(P),A	A,M
Mucormycosis	P	...	...	...	...
Paracoccidioidomycosis (South American blastomycosis)	P‡ (Severe cases)	...	(P),M	(P),M	...
Pseudallescheriasis	...	...	P	...	(P)
Sporotrichosis	P	...	...	P	A,M

* P indicates preferred treatment in most cases (parentheses indicate drug is considered preferred treatment by some experts); M, for mild and moderately severe cases; A, efficacy less well established or alternative drug; C, combination recommended; S, combination recommended if infection is severe or central nervous system is involved.

† Efficacy and safety have not been established for children.

‡ Usually in combination with itraconazole.

TOPICAL DRUGS FOR SUPERFICIAL FUNGAL INFECTIONS

Table 4.7. **Topical Drugs for Superficial Fungal Infections**

Drug	Strength	Formulation*	Trade Name(s) (Examples)†	Application(s) (per day)	Adverse Reactions/Notes
Amphotericin B	3%	C, O	Fungizone	2–4	Irritant dermatitis‡; more effective topical preparations are now available
Butenafine	1%	C	Mentax	1	Irritant dermatitis
Ciclopirox	1%	C, L	Loprox	2	Irritant dermatitis
Clotrimazole	1%	C, L, S, Su	Desenex,§ Lotrimin,§ Mycelex,§ Fungoid§	2	Irritant dermatitis; hives
Econazole	1%	C	Spectazole	1	Irritant dermatitis
Haloprogin	1%	C, S	Halotex	2	Irritant dermatitis
Ketoconazole	2%	C, Sh	Nizoral	2	Irritant dermatitis
Miconazole	2%	C, P, S, Su	Desenex,§ Lotramin,§ Fungoid,§ Micatin,§ Monistat-Derm, Monistat-3 2	2	Irritant dermatitis
Naftifine	1%	C, gel	Naftin	2	Irritant dermatitis; fungicidal agent
Nystatin	100 000 U/mL or 100 000 U/g	C, L, P, O, Su	Mycolog,§ Mycostatin,§ Mytrex, Nilstat, Nystatin, Nystex	2–3	Rare adverse reactions; effective against yeast only
Oxiconazole	1%	C, L	Oxistat	1–2	Irritant dermatitis
Sulconazole	1%	C, S	Exelderm	1–2	Irritant dermatitis
Terbinafine	1%	C	Lamisil	2	Irritant dermatitis

Table 4.7. **Topical Drugs for Superficial Fungal Infections**

Drug	Strength	Formulation*	Trade Name(s) (Examples)†	Application(s) (per day)	Adverse Reactions/Notes
Tolnaftate	1%	C, P, S	Tinactin,§ Ting,§ Tolfinate§	2	Rare adverse reactions
Triacetin	% varies	C, O	Fungoid§	3	Irritant dermatitis
Undecylenate	10%–25%	P, C, O, L	Caldesene,§ Cruex,§ Desenex§	2–3	Irritant dermatitis
Other Remedies					
Gentian violet	1%–2%	S	...	2	Staining
Selenium sulfide	2.5%	L, Sh	Exsel§	1	For tinea capitis,‖¶ tinea versicolor
	1%	Sh	Head & Shoulders,§ Selsun Blue§	1	For tinea capitis,‖¶ tinea versicolor¶
Sodium thiosulfate	25%	L	Tinver§	1–2	For tinea versicolor

* C indicates cream; L, lotion; O, ointment; P, powder; S, solution; Sh, shampoo; Su, suppositories.

† Not all inclusive. Some are duplicated for different "active" antifungals, with different "suffixes" for different active antifungals.

‡ Symptoms of irritant dermatitis include itching, burning, or stinging with erythema and edema that results in the skin becoming shiny; scaling is a secondary change. In some cases true allergic contact dermatitis can result, with more pronounced findings, such as vesicles or blisters. Unlike irritant dermatitis, allergic contact dermatitis spreads beyond the skin to which medication is applied. Either adverse reaction can be due to any component ingredient of a preparation and not to the active ingredient.

§ Nonprescription drug.

‖ Reduces transmission only; primary therapy is oral griseofulvin. For further information, see Tinea Capitis, p 569.

¶ 1% shampoo may be used as a lotion for treatment. For further information, see Tinea Versicolor, p 574.

Antiviral Drugs for Non-Human Immunodeficiency Virus Infections

Table 4.8. **Antiviral Drugs for Non–Human Immunodeficiency Virus Infections**

Generic (Trade Name)	Indication	Route	Usually Recommended Dosage
Acyclovir*† (Zovirax)	Genital herpes simplex virus (HSV) infection; first episode	Oral	1000–1200 mg/d in 3–5 divided doses for 5–10 d Oral pediatric dose: 40-80 mg/kg per day divided in 3–4 doses for 5–10 days (maximum 1.0 g/d)
		IV	15 mg/kg per day in 3 divided doses for 5–7 d
	Genital HSV infection: recurrence	Oral	1000–1200 mg/d in 3-5 divided doses for 5 d
	Recurrent genital and cutaneous (ocular) HSV episodes in patient with frequent recurrences, chronic suppressive therapy	Oral	400–1200 mg/d in 2–3 divided doses for as long as 12 continuous months
	HSV in immunocompromised host (localized, progressive, or disseminated)	IV	15–30 mg/kg per day in 3 divided doses for 7–14 d
		Oral	1000 mg/d in 3–5 divided doses for 7–14 d
	Prophylaxis of HSV in immunocompromised host	Oral	600–1000 mg/d in 3–5 divided doses during period of risk
	HSV-seropositive patients	IV	15 mg/kg in 3 divided doses during period of risk
	HSV encephalitis	IV	30 mg/kg per day in 3 divided doses for a minimum of 14–21 d
	Neonatal HSV	IV	60 mg/kg per day in 3 divided doses for 14–21 d
	Varicella in immunocompromised host	IV	For children <1 year of age: 30 mg/kg per day in 3 divided doses for 7–10 d; some experts also recommend this dose for children ≥1 year of age
		IV	For children ≥1 year of age: 1500 mg/M^2 per day in 3 divided doses for 7–10 d
	Zoster in immunocompetent host	IV	Same as for varicella in immunocompromised host
		Oral	4000 mg/d in 5 divided doses for 5–7 d for patients ≥12 years of age
	Varicella in immunocompetent host‡	Oral	80 mg/kg per day in 4 divided doses for 5 d; maximum dose, 3200 mg/d

Table 4.8. **Antiviral Drugs for Non–Human Immunodeficiency Virus Infections, continued**

Generic (Trade Name)	Indication	Route	Usually Recommended Dosage
Amantadine (Symmetrel)	Influenza A: treatment and prophylaxis	Oral	100 mg twice a day if ≥40 kg; see Influenza (p 351), including Table 3.32 (p 355)
Cidofovir	Cytomegalovirus (CMV) retinitis	IV	Induction: 5 mg/kg once with probenecid with hydration Weekly maintenance: 3 mg/kg once with probenecid and hydration
Famciclovir	Genital HSV infection	Oral	For adolescents, 750 mg/d in 3 divided doses for 7–10 d
	Episodic recurrent genital HSV infection	Oral	For adolescents, 250 mg/d in 2 divided doses for 5 d
	Daily suppressive therapy	Oral	For adolescents, 250–500 mg/d in 2 divided doses for 1 y, then reassess for recurrence of HSV infection
Formvirisen	CMV retinitis	IO	1 vial (330 μg) injected into the vitreous, then repeated every 2–4 wk
Foscarnet* (Foscavir)	CMV retinitis in patients with acquired immunodeficiency syndrome	IV	180 mg/kg per day in 3 divided doses for 14–21 d, then 90–120 mg/kg once a day as maintenance dose
	HSV infection resistant to acyclovir in immunocompromised host	IV	80–120 mg/kg per day in 2–3 divided doses until infection resolves
Ganciclovir* (Cytovene)	Acquired CMV retinitis in immunocompromised host§	IV	10 mg/kg per day in 2 divided doses for 14–21 d; for long-term suppression, 5 mg/kg per day for 5–7 d/wk
	Prophylaxis of CMV in high-risk host	IV	10 mg/kg per day in 2 divided doses for 1 wk, then 5 mg/kg per day in 1 dose for 100 d
		PO	1 g orally 3 times per day
Oseltamivir phosphate (Tamiflu)	Influenza A and B: treatment	PO	For persons ≥18 years of age; 75 mg twice a day for 5 d
Ribavirin (Virazole)	Treatment of respiratory syncytial virus infection	Aerosol	Given by a small-particle generator, in a solution of 6 g in 300 mL sterile water (20 mg/mL), delivered for 18 h per day for 3–7 d or 6 g in 100 mL of sterile water for 2 h, 3 times per day; longer treatment may be necessary in some patients

Table 4.8. **Antiviral Drugs for Non–Human Immunodeficiency Virus Infections, continued**

Generic (Trade Name)	Indication	Route	Usually Recommended Dosage
Rimantadine (Flumadine)	Influenza A: treatment and prophylaxis	Oral	100 mg twice a day if ≥40 kg; see Influenza (p 351), including Table 3.32 (p 355)
Valaciclovir	Genital HSV infection	Oral	For adolescents 2 g/d in 2 divided doses for 7–10 d
	Episodic recurrent genital HSV infection	Oral	For adolescents, 1 g/d in 2 divided doses for 5 d
	Daily suppressive therapy for (HSV) infection	Oral	For adolescents, 500–1000 mg once daily for 1 y, then reassess for recurrences
Zanamivir	Influenza A and B: treatment	Inhalation	For persons ≥12 years of age, 10 mg inhaled twice a day for 5 d with a special breath-activated plastic inhaler

* Dose should be decreased in patients with impaired renal function.

† Oral dosage of acyclovir in children should not exceed 80 mg/kg per day.

‡ Selective indications; see Varicella-Zoster Infections (p 624).

§ Some experts use ganciclovir in immunocompromised host with CMV gastrointestinal tract disease and CMV pneumonitis (with or without CMV Immune Globulin Intravenous).

Antiretroviral Therapy

Table 4.9. **Characteristics of Antiretroviral Drugs*: Nucleoside Analogue Reverse Transcriptase Inhibitors**

Drug (Abbreviation)/ Trade Name	Dosage	Major Toxic Effects	Drug Interactions	Special Instructions
Abacavir (formerly 1592U89) (ABC)/ Ziagen *Preparations:* Pediatric oral solution: 20 mg/mL Tablets: 300 mg	*Neonatal:* Not approved for infants younger than 3 mo of age. For infants between 1 and 3 mo of age, a dosage of 8 mg/kg of body weight twice daily is under study. *Pediatric and adolescent:* 8 mg/kg of body weight twice daily; maximum dosage 300 mg twice daily *Adult:* 300 mg twice daily	*Most frequent:* Nausea, vomiting, headache, fever, rash, anorexia, and fatigue. *Unusual (more severe):* Approximately 5% of adults and children develop a potentially fatal hypersensitivity reaction. Symptoms include fever, fatigue, malaise, nausea, vomiting, diarrhea, and abdominal pain. Physical findings include lymphadenopathy, ulceration of mucous membranes, and maculopapular or urticarial skin rash. A hypersensitivity reaction can occur without a rash. Laboratory abnormalities include elevated liver function test results, elevated creatine phosphokinase and creatinine levels, and lymphopenia. This reaction generally occurs in the first 6 weeks of therapy. For patients suspected of having a hypersensitivity reaction, ABC should be stopped and not restarted since hypotension and death have occurred on rechallenge.	No significant interactions between ABC, zidovudine (ZDV), and lamivudine (3TC). Abacavir does not inhibit and is not metabolized by hepatic cytochrome P-450 enzymes. Thus, it should not cause changes in drug levels or clearance of agents metabolized through these pathways, such as protease inhibitors and NNRTIs.	. . .

Table 4.9. **Characteristics of Antiretroviral Drugs*: Nucleoside Analogue Reverse Transcriptase Inhibitors, continued**

Drug (Abbreviation)/ Trade Name	Dosage	Major Toxic Effects	Drug Interactions	Special Instructions
Didanosine (ddl)/ Videx *Preparations*: Pediatric powder for oral solution (must be mixed with antacid): 10 mg/mL Chewable tablets with buffers: 25, 50, 100, and 150 mg Buffered powder for oral solution: 100, 167, and 250 mg	*Usual pediatric:* In combination with other antiretrovirals: 90 mg/m^2 q 12 h *Pediatric range:* 90 to 150 mg/m^2 q 12 h (Note: May need higher dosage for patients with central nervous system disease). *Neonatal (<90 d of age):* Based on pharmacokinetic data from PACTG 239: 50 mg/m^2 q 12 h *Adolescent and adult:* Weight, >60 kg: 200 mg bid. Weight, <60 kg: 125 mg bid	*Most frequent:* Diarrhea, abdominal pain, nausea, vomiting *Unusual (more severe):* Peripheral neuropathy (dose-related), electrolyte abnormalities, hyperuricemia *Uncommon:* Pancreatitis (dose-related) seems less common in children than adults; increased liver enzyme levels, retinal depigmentation (asymptomatic, reported with pediatric administration)	Possible decrease in absorption of ketoconazole, itraconazole, tetracycline; administer at least 2 h before or 2 h after ddl. Ciprofloxacin absorption significantly decreased (chelation of drug by antacid); administer 2 h before or 6 h after ddl. Concomitant administration of ddl and delavirdine may decrease the absorption of these drugs; separate dosing by at least 2 h. Ganciclovir may increase the AUC and peak levels of ddl and predispose to toxic effects. Administration with protease inhibitors: indinavir should be administered at least 1 h apart from ddl on an empty stomach. Ritonavir should be administered at least 2.5 h apart from ddl.	ddl formulation contains buffering agents or antacids. Food decreases absorption; administer ddl on an empty stomach (1 h before or 2 h after meal). Further evaluation in children regarding administration with meals is under study. For oral solution: Shake well, and keep refrigerated; admixture stable for 30 d.
Lamivudine (3TC)/ Epivir *Preparations*: Solution: 10 mg/ mL	*Pediatric:* 4 mg/kg q 12 h *Neonatal (<30 d of age):* Under study in clinical trials:	*Most frequent:* Headache, fatigue, nausea, diarrhea, skin rash, abdominal pain *Unusual (more severe):* Pancreatitis (primarily seen in children with	TMP-SMX increases 3TC blood levels (possibly competes for renal tubular secretion); unknown significance.	Can be administered with food. For oral solution: Store at room temperature. Decrease dosage for

Table 4.9. **Characteristics of Antiretroviral Drugs*: Nucleoside Analogue Reverse Transcriptase Inhibitors, continued**

Drug (Abbreviation)/ Trade Name	Dosage	Major Toxic Effects	Drug Interactions	Special Instructions
Lamivudine (3TC)/ Epivir, continued Tablets: 150 mg	2 mg/kg q 12 h *Adolescent and adult:* 150 mg bid	advanced HIV infection receiving multiple other medications), decreased neutrophil count, increased liver enzyme levels	When used with ZDV may prevent emergence of resistance, and for ZDV-resistant virus, revision to phenotypic ZDV sensitivity may be observed.	patients with impaired renal function.
Stavudine (d4T)/ Zerit *Preparations*: Solution: 1 mg/mL Capsules: 15, 20, 30, and 40 mg	*Pediatric:* 1 mg/kg q 12 h (up to weight of 30 kg) *Neonatal:* Under evaluation in PACTG 332 *Adolescent and adult:* Weight, >60 kg: 40 mg bid. Weight, 30–60 kg: 30 mg bid	*Most frequent:* Headache, GI disturbances, skin rashes *Uncommon (more severe):* Peripheral neuropathy, pancreatitis *Other:* Increased liver enzyme levels	Drugs that decrease renal function could decrease clearance. Should not be administered in combination with ZDV (poor antiretroviral effect).	Can be administered with food. Decrease dosage for patients with renal impairment. For oral solution: Shake well and keep refrigerated; solution stable for 30 days.
Zalcitabine (ddC)/ Hivid *Preparations:* Syrup: mg/mL (investigational) Tablets: 0.375 mg and 0.75 mg	*Usual pediatric:* 0.01 mg/kg q 8 h *Pediatric range:* 0.005 to 0.01 mg/kg q 8 h *Neonatal:* Unknown	*Most frequent:* Headache, malaise *Unusual (more severe):* Peripheral neuropathy, pancreatitis, hepatic toxic effects, skin rashes, oral ulcers, esophageal ulcers, hematologic toxic effects	Cimetidine, amphotericin, foscarnet and aminoglycosides may decrease renal clearance of zalcitabine. Antacids decrease absorption. Concomitant use with ddI is not recommended because of the increased risk of peripheral neuropathy.	Administer on an empty stomach (1 h before or 2 h after a meal). Decrease dosage in patients with impaired renal function.

Table 4.9. **Characteristics of Antiretroviral Drugs*: Nucleoside Analogue Reverse Transcriptase Inhibitors, continued**

Drug (Abbreviation)/ Trade Name	Dosage	Major Toxic Effects	Drug Interactions	Special Instructions
Zalcitabine (ddC)/ Hivid, continued	*Adolescent and adult:* 0.75 mg tid		Intravenous pentamidine increases the risk of pancreatitis (do not use concurrently).	
Zidovudine (ZDV, AZT)/Retrovir *Preparations:* Syrup: 10 mg/mL syrup Capsules: 100 mg Tablets: 300 mg Concentrate for injection/for IV infusion: 10 mg/mL	*Usual pediatric:* Oral: 160 mg/m^2 q 8 h IV (intermittent infusion): 1–2 mg/kg q 4 h IV (continuous infusion): 20 mg/m^2 per hour *Pediatric range:* 90 mg/m^2 to 180 mg/m^2 q 6–8 h *Neonatal:* Oral: 2 mg/kg q 6 h IV: 1.5 mg/kg q 6 h *Premature infants:* (Standard neonatal dose may be excessive for premature infants)	*Most frequent:* Hematologic toxic effects, including granulocytopenia and anemia, headache *Unusual:* Myopathy, myositis, hepatic toxic effects	Increased toxic effects may be observed with concomitant administration of the following drugs (therefore, more intensive monitoring for toxic effects may be warranted): ganciclovir, interferon ∝, TMP-SMX, acyclovir. The following drugs may increase ZDV concentration (and therefore potential toxic effects): probenecid, atovaquone, methadone, valproic acid. Decreased renal clearance may be observed with coadministration of cimetidine (may be significant in patients with renal impairment). Fluconazole interferes with metabolism and clearance of	Can be administered with food (although the manufacturer recommends administration 30 min before or 1 h after a meal). Decrease dosage for patients with severe renal impairment. Significant granulocytopenia or anemia may necessitate interruption of therapy until marrow recovery is observed; use of erythropoietin or reduced ZDV dosage may be necessary for some patients. Reduced dosage may be indicated for patients with significant hepatic dysfunction. Infuse loading doses and IV doses over 1 h. Dilute with

Table 4.9. **Characteristics of Antiretroviral Drugs*: Nucleoside Analogue Reverse Transcriptase Inhibitors, continued**

Drug (Abbreviation)/ Trade Name	Dosage	Major Toxic Effects	Drug Interactions	Special Instructions
Zidovudine (ZDV, AZT)/Retrovir, continued	Under study in PACTG 331:1.5 mg/kg q 12 h from birth to 2 wk of age; then increase to 2 mg/kg q 8 h after 2 wk of age *Adolescent and adult:* 200 mg tid or 300 mg bid		ZDV (increases ZDV AUC). ZDV metabolism may be increased with coadministration of rifampin and rifabutin; clarithromycin decreases concentrations of ZDV probably by interfering with absorption (administer 4 h apart). Ribavirin decreases the intracellular phosphorylation of ZDV (conversion to active metabolite). Phenytoin concentrations may increase or decrease. Should not be administered in combination with stavudine (poor antiretroviral effect).	D_5W to concentration of ≤4 mg/mL. For IV solution: Refrigerated diluted solution stable for 24 h. Some experts use a dosage of 180 mg/m^2 q 12 h when used in combination with other antiretroviral compounds, but data on this dosing in children are limited.

* Adolescent dosing by Tanner Stage: adolescents in early puberty (Tanner I–II) should be dosed using pediatric schedules, while those in late puberty (Tanner stage V) should be dosed using adult schedules. Youth who are in the midst of their growth spurt (Tanner III females and Tanner IV males) should be closely monitored for medication efficacy and toxic effects when choosing adult or pediatric dosing guidelines. NNRTI indicates nonnucleoside reverse transcriptase inhibitor; q, every; bid, twice a day; AUC, area under the curve; HIV, human immunodeficiency virus; TMP-SMX, trimethoprim-sulfamethoxazole; GI, gastrointestinal; IV, intravenous; D_5W, dextrose 5% in water; and tid, three times a day.

Table 4.10. **Characteristics of Antiretroviral Drugs: Nonnucleoside Reverse Transcriptase Inhibitors**

Drug (Abbreviation)/ Trade Name	Dosage	Major Toxic Effects	Drug Interactions	Special Instructions
Delavirdine (DLV)/ Rescriptor *Preparations:* Tablets: 100 mg	*Pediatric:* Unknown *Neonatal:* Unknown *Adolescent and adult:* 400 mg tid	*Most frequent:* Headache, fatigue, gastrointestinal complaints, rash (may be severe).	Metabolized in part by hepatic cytochrome P-450 3A; potential for multiple drug interactions (see Note).* Before administration, the patient's medication profile should be reviewed carefully for potential drug interactions. Not recommended for concurrent use (DLV decreases the drug's metabolism, resulting in increased drug levels): antihistamines (astemizole, terfenadine); sedative-hypnotics (alprazolam, midazolam, triazolam); calcium channel blockers (nifedipine); ergot alkaloid derivatives; amphetamines; cisapride; warfarin; rifabutin or rifampin (also increase clearance of DLV); anticonvulsants (phenytoin, carbamazepine, phenobarbital; also increase clearance of DLV). Decreased absorption of delavirdine if given with antacids, $histamine_2$-receptor antagonists. Increased trough concentrations of delavirdine if given with ketoconazole, fluoxetine (increases trough by ~50%); increased levels of both drugs if delavirdine given with clarithromycin. DLV also increases levels of dapsone, quinidine. Administration with protease inhibitors: decreases metabolism of saquinavir and indinavir, resulting in a significant increase in saquinavir and indinavir concentrations and a slight decrease in DLV concentrations.	Can be administered with food. Should be taken 1 h before or 1 h after ddI or antacids. Tablets can be dissolved in water and the resulting dispersion taken promptly.

Table 4.10. **Characteristics of Antiretroviral Drugs: Nonnucleoside Reverse Transcriptase Inhibitors, continued**

Drug (Abbreviation)/ Trade Name	Dosage	Major Toxic Effects	Drug Interactions	Special Instructions
Efavirenz (formerly DMP 266)/ Sustiva *Preparations:* Capsules: 50, 100, and 200 mg	*Pediatric:* Administered once daily. Body weight 10 to <15 kg: 200 mg; 15 to <20 kg: 250 mg; 20 to <25 kg: 300 mg; 25 to <32.5 kg: 350 mg; 2.5 to <40 kg: 400 mg; ≥40 kg: 600 mg. Currently no data are available on the appropriate dosage for children younger than 3 y of age. *Adolescent and adult:* 600 mg once daily	*Most frequent:* Skin rash, central nervous system (somnolence, insomnia, abnormal dreams, confusion, abnormal thinking, impaired concentration, amnesia, agitation, depersonalization, hallucinations, euphoria), primarily reported in adults; increased aminotransferase levels, teratogenic in primates (use in pregnancy should be avoided, and women of childbearing potential should undergo pregnancy testing before initiating therapy).	Mixed inducer/inhibitor of cytochrome P-450 3A4 enzymes; concentrations of concomitant drugs can be increased or decreased depending on specific enzyme pathway involved. Not recommended for concurrent use; antihistamines (astemizole or terfenadine), sedative-hypnotics (midazolam or triazolam), cisapride, or ergot alkaloid derivatives. Drug interactions requiring careful monitoring if coadministered: warfarin levels potentially increased; while of uncertain clinical significance, a reliable method of barrier contraception should be used in addition to oral contraceptives. Enzyme inducers such as rifampin, rifabutin, phenobarbital, and phenytoin may decrease efavirenz concentrations; clinical significance unknown. Efavirenz is highly plasma-protein bound, and has the potential for drug interactions with other highly protein-bound drugs (eg, phenobarbital and phenytoin). Clarithromycin levels are decreased, while the levels of its metabolite are increased; alternatives to clarithromycin, such as azithromycin, should be considered.	Efavirenz can be taken with and without food. The relative bioavailability of efavirenz was increased by 50% (range 11%–128%) following a high fat meal (1070 kcal, 82 g fat, 62% of calories from fat). Because there is no information on safety of efavirenz in dosages higher than recommended, administration with a high-fat meal should be avoided because of the potential for increased absorption. Capsules may be opened and added to liquids or foods, but efavirenz has a peppery taste; grape jelly has been used to disguise the taste.

Table 4.10. **Characteristics of Antiretroviral Drugs: Nonnucleoside Reverse Transcriptase Inhibitors, continued**

Drug (Abbreviation)/ Trade Name	Dosage	Major Toxic Effects	Drug Interactions	Special Instructions
Efavirenz (formerly DMP 266)/Sustiva, continued			Other macrolide antibiotics have not been studied in combination with efavirenz. Administration with protease inhibitors: coadministration decreases levels of saquinavir (AUC decreased by 50%) and indinavir (AUC decreased by 31%). Coadministration of saquinavir as a sole protease inhibitor is not recommended; indinavir dose should be increased if given with efavirenz (for adults, from 800 mg to 1000 mg every 8 h). Coadministration increases levels of both ritonavir and efavirenz (AUC increased by 20% for both) and is associated with a higher frequency of adverse clinical and laboratory findings; monitoring of liver enzyme levels is recommended if coadministered. Coadministration increases levels of nelfinavir (AUC increased by 20%), but no dose adjustment is needed.	Bedtime dosing is recommended; particularly during the first 2–4 wk of therapy, to improve tolerability of central nervous system side effects.
Nevirapine (NVP)/ Viramune *Preparations:*	*Pediatric:* 120 to 200 mg/m^2 q 12 h Note: Initiate therapy	*Most frequent:* Skin rash (some severe), sedative effect,	Induces hepatic cytochrome P-450 3A; autoinduction of metabolism occurs in 2–4 wk with a 1.5–2 times increase in	Can be administered with food. May be administered concurrently with ddI.

Table 4.10. **Characteristics of Antiretroviral Drugs: Nonnucleoside Reverse Transcriptase Inhibitors, continued**

Drug (Abbreviation)/ Trade Name	Dosage	Major Toxic Effects	Drug Interactions	Special Instructions
Nevirapine (NVP)/ Viramune, continued Suspension: 10 mg/mL (investigational) Tablets: 200 mg	with 120 mg/m^2 given once daily for 14 d. Increase to full dose administered q 12 h if no rash or other untoward effects. *Neonatal (through 3 mo of age):* Under study in PACTG 356: 5 mg/kg once daily for 14 d, followed by 120 mg/m^2 q 12 h for 14 d, followed by 200 mg/m^2 q 12 h *Adolescent and adult:* 200 mg q 12 h. Note: Initiate therapy at half dose for the first 14 d. Increase to full dose if no rash or other untoward effects.	headache, diarrhea, nausea *Unusual:* Elevated liver enzyme levels, rarely hepatitis	clearance. Potential for multiple drug interactions (see Note).* Before administration, the patient's medication profile should be reviewed carefully for potential drug interactions. Drugs having suspected interactions should be used only with careful monitoring: rifampin and rifabutin; oral contraceptives (alternative or additional methods of birth control should be used if coadministering with hormonal methods of birth control); sedative-hypnotics (triazolam, midazolam); oral anticoagulants; digoxin; phenytoin; theophylline. Administration with protease inhibitors: decreases indinavir and saquinavir concentrations significantly; may also decrease ritonavir concentration. Not known if increased doses of protease inhibitors are needed.	For investigational suspension: Must be shaken well; store at room temperature.

* Note: Drugs metabolized by the hepatic cytochrome P-450 3A (CYP 3A) enzyme system have the potential for significant interactions with multiple drugs, some of which may be life-threatening. These interactions are outlined in detail in the guidelines for use of antiretroviral agents in HIV-infected adults and adolescents (Centers for Disease Control and Prevention. Report of the NIH Panel to Define Principles of Therapy of HIV Infection and guidelines for the use of antiretroviral agents in HIV-infected adults and adolescents. *MMWR Morb Mortal Wkly Rep.* 1998;47(RR-5):1–82) and in prescribing information available from the drug companies. These interactions will not be reiterated in this document, and the health care professional should review those documents for detailed information. Before therapy with these drugs is initiated, the patient's medication profile should be reviewed carefully for potential drug interactions.

Table 4.11. **Characteristics of Antiretroviral Drugs: Protease Inhibitors***

Drug (Abbreviation)/ Trade Name	Dosage	Major Toxic Effects	Drug Interactions	Special Instructions
Indinavir/Crixivan *Preparations:* Capsules: 200 and 400 mg	*Pediatric:* Under study in clinical trials: 350–500 mg/m^2 q 8 h *Neonatal:* Unknown Because of adverse effect of hyperbilirubinemia, should not be given to neonates until further information available *Adolescent and adult:* 800 mg q 8 h	*Most frequent:* Nausea, abdominal pain, headache, asymptomatic hyperbilirubinemia (10%) *Unusual (more severe):* Nephrolithiasis (4%) *Rare:* Spontaneous bleeding episodes in patients with hemophilia; hyperglycemia; diabetes mellitus	Cytochrome P-450 3A4 responsible for metabolism. Potential for multiple drug interactions (see Note).[†] Before administration, the patient's medication profile should be reviewed carefully for potential drug interactions. Not recommended for concurrent use (indinavir decreases the drug's metabolism, resulting in increased drug levels): antihistamines (astemizole, terfenadine); cisapride; ergot alkaloid derivatives; sedative-hypnotics (triazolam, midazolam); rifampin (greatly reduces indinavir levels). Rifabutin concentrations are increased, and a dose reduction of rifabutin to half the usual daily dose is recommended. Ketoconazole and itraconazole cause an increase in indinavir concentrations (consider reduction of adolescent and adult indinavir dosage to 600 mg q 8 h). Clarithromycin coadministration increases serum concentration of both drugs. Nevirapine coadministration may decrease indinavir serum concentration. Administration with other protease inhibitors: ritonavir decreases the metabolism of indinavir and results in greatly increased indinavir concentrations.	Administer on an empty stomach 1 h before or 2 h after a meal (or can take with a light meal). Adequate hydration required to minimize risk of nephrolithiasis. If coadministered with ddl, give at least 1 h apart on an empty stomach. Grapefruit juice decreases serum levels of indinavir (by about 26%). Decrease dosage for patients with cirrhosis. Capsules are sensitive to moisture and should be stored in original container with desiccant.

Table 4.11. **Characteristics of Antiretroviral Drugs: Protease Inhibitors,* continued**

Drug (Abbreviation)/ Trade Name	Dosage	Major Toxic Effects	Drug Interactions	Special Instructions
Nelfinavir/Viracept *Preparations:* Powder for oral suspension: 50 mg per one level scoop (200 mg per one level teaspoon) Tablets: 250 mg tablet	*Pediatric:* 30 mg/kg tid *Neonatal:* Under study in PACTG 353: 10 mg/kg tid (Note: no preliminary data available, investigational) *Adolescent and adult:* 750 mg tid	*Most frequent:* Diarrhea *Less common:* Asthenia, abdominal pain, rash *Rare:* Hyperglycemia and diabetes mellitus	Nelfinavir is in part metabolized by cytochrome P-450 3A4. Potential for multiple drug interactions (see Note).† Before administration, the patient's medication profile should be reviewed carefully for potential drug interactions. Not recommended for concurrent use (nelfinavir decreases the drug's metabolism, resulting in increased drug levels): antihistamine (astemizole, terfenadine); cisapride; ergot alkaloid derivatives; sedative-hypnotics (triazolam, midazolam); rifampin (greatly reduces nelfinavir levels). Rifabutin causes less decline in nelfinavir concentrations; if coadministered with nelfinavir, rifabutin should be reduced to one half the usual dose. Oral contraceptives: estradiol levels are reduced by nelfinavir, and alternative or additional methods of birth control should be used if coadministering with hormonal methods of birth control. Administration with other protease inhibitors: nelfinavir increases levels of saquinavir and indinavir.	Administer with meal or light snack. For oral solution: Powder may be mixed with water, milk, pudding, ice cream, or formula (for up to 6 h). Do not mix with acidic food or juice because of resulting poor taste. Do not add water to bottles of oral powder; a special scoop is provided with oral powder for measuring. Tablets readily dissolve in water and produce a dispersion that can be mixed with milk, chocolate milk; tablets also can be crushed and administered with pudding.

Table 4.11. **Characteristics of Antiretroviral Drugs: Protease Inhibitors,* continued**

Drug (Abbreviation)/ Trade Name	Dosage	Major Toxic Effects	Drug Interactions	Special Instructions
Ritonavir/Norvir *Preparations:* Oral solution: 80 mg/mL Capsules: 100 mg	*Pediatric:* 400 mg/m^2 q 12 h To minimize nausea and vomiting, initiate therapy starting at 250 mg/m^2 q 12 h and increase stepwise to full dose over 5 d as tolerated. *Pediatric range:* 350 to 400 mg/m^2 q 12 h *Neonatal:* Under study in PACTG 354 (single-dose pharmacokinetics) *Adolescent and adult:* 600 mg q 12 h	*Most frequent:* Nausea, vomiting, diarrhea, headache, abdominal pain, anorexia *Less common:* Circumoral paresthesias, increased liver enzyme levels *Rare:* Spontaneous bleeding episodes in patients with hemophilia; pancreatitis; increased triglycerides and cholesterol levels; hyperglycemia; and diabetes mellitus	Ritonavir is metabolized extensively in the liver by the cytochrome P-450 enzyme 3A (CYP3A). Potential for multiple drug interactions (see Note).[†] Before administration, the patient's medication profile should be reviewed carefully for potential drug interactions. Not recommended for concurrent use: analgesics (meperidine, piroxicam, propoxyphene); antihistamines (astemizole, terfenadine); certain cardiac drugs (amiodarone, bepridil, encainide, flecainide, propafenone, quinidine); ergot alkaloid derivatives; cisapride; sedative hypnotics (clorazepate, diazepam, estazolam, flurazepam, midazolam, triazolam, zolpidem); certain psychotropic drugs (bupropion, clozapine); rifabutin. Oral contraceptives: estradiol levels are reduced by ritonavir, and alternative or additional methods of birth control should be used if coadministering with hormonal methods of birth control. Ritonavir decreases levels of sulfamethoxazole; theophylline (levels should be monitored, and dosage may need to be increased); zidovudine.	Administration with food increases absorption. If administered with ddl, should be administered 2.5 h apart. Oral capsules must be kept refrigerated. For oral solution: Must be kept refrigerated and stored in original container; can be kept at room temperature if used within 30 d. To minimize nausea, therapy should be initiated at a low dose and increased to full dose over 5 d as tolerated. Techniques to increase tolerance by children: Mixing oral solution with milk, chocolate milk, vanilla or chocolate pudding, or ice cream; dulling the taste buds before administration by chewing ice, giving Popsicles or spoonfuls of partially frozen orange or grape juice concentrates;

Table 4.11. **Characteristics of Antiretroviral Drugs: Protease Inhibitors,* continued**

Drug (Abbreviation)/ Trade Name	Dosage	Major Toxic Effects	Drug Interactions	Special Instructions
Ritonavir/Norvir, continued			Ritonavir increases levels of clarithromycin (dosage adjustment may be necessary for patients with impaired renal function); desipramine; warfarin (monitoring of anticoagulant effect necessary). Ritonavir may increase or decrease digoxin levels (monitoring of levels is recommended). Drugs that increase CYP3A activity, such as carbamazepine, dexamethasone, phenobarbital, and phenytoin (anticonvulsant levels should be monitored as ritonavir can affect the metabolism of these drugs as well), can lead to increased clearance and, therefore, lower levels of ritonavir. Administration with other protease inhibitors: decreases the metabolism of indinavir and saquinavir and results in greatly increased concentrations of these drugs.	Coating the mouth by giving peanut butter to eat before the dose. Administration of strong-tasting foods, such as maple syrup or cheese or strong-flavored chewing gum immediately after dose.
Saquinavir/ Fortovase *Preparations:* Soft gel capsules: 200 mg	*Pediatric:* Under study in clinical trials: 50 mg/ kg tid *Neonatal:* Unknown *Adolescent and adult:* 1200 mg tid	*Most frequent:* Diarrhea, abdominal discomfort, headache, and nausea *Rare:* Spontaneous bleeding episodes in patients with hemophilia; hyperglycemia; diabetes mellitus	Saquinavir is metabolized by the cytochrome P-450 3A system in the liver, and there are numerous potential drug interactions. Before administration, the patient's medication profile should be reviewed carefully for potential drug interactions. Not recommended for concurrent use (saquinavir decreases the drug's metabolism, resulting in increased drug levels):	Administer within 2 h of a full meal to increase absorption. Concurrent administration of grapefruit juice increases saquinavir concentration. Sun exposure can cause photosensitivity reactions; sunscreen or protective clothing is recommended.

Table 4.11. **Characteristics of Antiretroviral Drugs: Protease Inhibitors,* continued**

Drug (Abbreviation)/ Trade Name	Dosage	Major Toxic Effects	Drug Interactions	Special Instructions
Saquinavir/ Fortovase, continued			antihistamines (astemizole, terfenadine); cisapride; ergot alkaloid derivatives; rifampin and rifabutin (decrease saquinavir levels by 80% and 40%, respectively). Saquinavir levels are decreased by carbamazepine, dexamethasone, phenobarbital, and phenytoin. Saquinavir levels are increased by DLV, ketoconazole. Saquinavir may increase levels of calcium channel blockers, dapsone, quinidine, triazolam. Administration with other protease inhibitors: coadministration of ritonavir decreases the metabolism of saquinavir and results in greatly increased saquinavir concentrations.	

* Data for children are limited, and doses may change as more information is obtained about the pharmacokinetics of these drugs in children.

† Note: Drugs metabolized by the hepatic cytochrome P-450 3A (CYP 3A) enzyme system have the potential for significant interactions with multiple drugs, some of which may be life-threatening. These interactions are outlined in detail in the guidelines for use of antiretroviral agents in HIV-infected adults and adolescents (Centers for Disease Control and Prevention. Report of the NIH Panel to Define Principles of Therapy of HIV Infection and guidelines for the use of antiretroviral agents in HIV-infected adults and adolescents. *MMWR Morb Mortal Wkly Rep.* 1998;47(RR-5):1–82) and in prescribing information available from the drug companies. These interactions will not be reiterated in this document, and the health care professional should review those documents for detailed information. Before therapy with these drugs is initiated, the patient's medication profile should be reviewed carefully for potential drug interactions.

Table 4.12. **Considerations for Changing Antiretroviral Therapy**

Virologic Considerations*

1. Less than a minimally acceptable virologic response after 8 to 12 weeks of therapy. For children receiving antiretroviral therapy with 2 NRTIs and a protease inhibitor, this is defined as less than a 10-fold (1.0 $\log_{10}$) decrease from baseline HIV RNA levels. For children who are receiving less potent antiretroviral therapy (ie, dual NRTI combinations), this is defined as less than a 5-fold (0.7 $\log_{10}$) decrease in HIV RNA levels from baseline.
2. Lack of suppression of HIV RNA levels to undetectable after 4 to 6 months of antiretroviral therapy.[†]
3. Repeated detection of HIV RNA in children who had initially responded to antiretroviral therapy with undetectable levels.[‡]
4. For children who have had a significant HIV RNA response, but still have low levels of detectable HIV RNA, a reproducible increase in copy number, defined as a persistent 3-fold or greater ($\geq 0.5 \log_{10}$) increase in copy number from the nadir reached after initiation of a new therapeutic regimen. In children under 2 years of age, biologic variability may be greater, and it may be desirable to use a 5-fold or greater increase ($\geq 0.7 \log_{10}$) to define a significant rise.

Immunologic Considerations*

1. Change in immunologic classification (Table 3.24, p 327)[§]
2. For children with a CD4 percentage <15% (immunologic category 3), a persistent decline of 5 percentiles or more in CD4+ cell percentage (eg, from 15% to 10%).
3. A rapid and extensive decrease in absolute CD4+ lymphocyte count decrease (eg, >30% in <6 mo).

Clinical Considerations

1. Progressive neurodevelopmental deterioration.
2. Growth failure defined as persistent decline in weight-growth velocity despite adequate nutritional support and without other explanation.
3. Disease progression, as defined by advancement from one pediatric clinical category to another (Table 3.24, p 327)[‖]

* At least 2 measurements (1 wk apart) should be performed before considering a change. NRTI, nucleoside analogue reverse transcriptase inhibitor; HIV, human immunodeficiency virus.

† Most experts also would take into consideration the initial HIV RNA level of the child at the start of therapy and the level achieved with therapy when contemplating potential drug changes. For example, an immediate change in therapy may not necessarily be warranted if there is a sustained 1.5 to 2.0 $\log_{10}$ fall in HIV RNA copy number, even if this results in RNA levels of about 10 000 copies per milliliter. Problems with adherence or drug bioavailability also should be assessed.

‡ Close observation should be considered if the extent of HIV RNA increase is limited (eg, if using an HIV RNA assay with a lower limit of detection of 1000 copies per milliliter, a $\leq 0.7 \log_{10}$ increase from undetectable to ~5000 copies per milliliter occurs). If inconsistent adherence to therapy is identified, renewed efforts to educate the caregivers and patients and closer follow-up from supportive members of a multidisciplinary care team may improve adherence.

§ Small changes in CD4+ percentile that may result in immunologic category change (eg, from 26% to 24%, or 16% to 14%) may not be as concerning as a major rapid large change in CD4+ percentile within the same immunologic category (eg, a drop from 35% to 25% in a short period).

‖ For patients with stable immunologic and virologic parameters, progression from one clinical category to another may not in itself represent an indication to change therapy. Thus, for patients whose disease progression is not related to neurologic deterioration or growth failure, virologic and immunologic considerations are important when deciding whether to change therapy.

DRUGS FOR PARASITIC INFECTIONS

The following tables (4.13, 4.14, and 4.15) are reproduced from *The Medical Letter*.* They provide recommendations that are likely to be consistent in many cases with those of the Committee on Infectious Diseases, as given in the chapters on specific diseases in Section 3. However, because *The Medical Letter* recommendations are developed independently, these recommendations occasionally may differ from those of the Committee. Accordingly, both should be consulted. The Committee thanks *The Medical Letter* for their courtesy in allowing this information to be reprinted.

In Table 4.13 (p 694), first-choice and alternative drugs with recommended adult and pediatric dosages for most parasitic infections are given. In each case, the need for treatment must be weighed against the toxic effects of the drug. A decision to withhold therapy often may be correct, particularly when the drugs can cause severe adverse effects. When the first-choice drug is initially ineffective and the alternative is more hazardous, a second course of treatment with the first drug before giving the alternative may be prudent. Adverse effects of some antiparasitic drugs are listed in Table 4.15 (p 720).

Several drugs recommended in Table 4.13 have not been approved by the Food and Drug Administration and, thus, are investigational (see footnotes). When prescribing an unapproved drug, the physician should inform the patient of the investigational status and adverse effects of the drug.

These recommendations are periodically (usually every other year) updated by *The Medical Letter* and, thus, are likely to be superseded by new ones before the next edition of the *Red Book* is published (www.medletter.com).

* Reprinted with permission from *The Medical Letter.*

Table 4.13. **Drugs for Treatment of Parasitic Infections**

Infection	Drug	Adult Dosage	Pediatric Dosage
Acanthamoeba keratitis			
Drug of choice:	See footnote 1		
AMEBIASIS *(Entamoeba histolytica)*			
asymptomatic			
Drug of choice:	Iodoquinol	650 mg tid × 20d	30–40 mg/kg/d (max. 2g) in 3 doses × 20d
OR	Paromomycin	25–35 mg/kg/d in 3 doses × 7d	25–35 mg/kg/d in 3 doses × 7d
Alternative:	Diloxanide furoate*	500 mg tid × 10d	20 mg/kg/d in 3 doses × 10d
mild to moderate intestinal disease [2]			
Drug of choice:	Metronidazole	500–750 mg tid × 10d	35–50 mg/kg/d in 3 doses × 10d
OR	Tinidazole[3]*	2 grams/d divided tid × 3d	50 mg/kg (max. 2g) qd × 3d
severe intestinal and extraintestinal disease			
Drug of choice:[2]	Metronidazole	750 mg tid × 7d	35–50 mg/kg/d in 3 doses × 7d
OR	Tinidazole[3]*	600 mg bid to 800 mg tid × 5d	50–60 mg/kg/d (max. 2 g) × 5d

* Availability problems. See table on page 718.

1. For treatment of keratitis caused by *Acanthamoeba*, concurrent topical use of 0.1% propamidine isethionate *(Brolene)* plus neomycin-polymyxin B-gramicidin ophthalmic solution has been successful (SL Hargrave et al, Ophthalmology, 106:952, 1999). In addition, 0.02% topical polyhexamethylene biguanide (PHMB) and/or chlorhexadine has been used successfully in a large number of patients (CF Radford et al, Br J Ophthalmol, 82:1387, 1998). PHMB is available as *Baquacil* (ICI America), a swimming pool disinfectant (E Yee and TK Winarko, Am J Hosp Pharm, 50:2523, 1993).
2. Treatment should be followed by a course of iodoquinol or paromomycin in the dosage used to treat asymptomatic amebiasis.
3. A nitro-imidazole similar to metronidazole, but not marketed in the USA, tinidazole appears to be at least as effective as metronidazole and better tolerated. Ornidazole, a similar drug, is also used outside the USA. Higher dosage is for hepatic abscess.

Table 4.13. **Drugs for Treatment of Parasitic Infections, continued**

Infection	Drug	Adult Dosage	Pediatric Dosage
AMEBIC MENINGOENCEPHALITIS, PRIMARY			
Naegleria			
Drug of choice:	Amphotericin B[4,5]	1 mg/kg/d IV, uncertain duration	1 mg/kg/d IV, uncertain duration
Acanthamoeba			
Drug of choice:	See footnote 6		
Balamuthia mandrillaris			
Drug of choice:	See footnote 7		
ANCYLOSTOMA caninum (Eosinophilic enterocolitis)			
Drug of choice:	Albendazole[5]	400 mg once	400 mg once
OR	Mebendazole	100 mg bid × 3d	100 mg bid × 3d
OR	Pyrantel pamoate[5]	11 mg/kg (max. 1g) × 3d	11 mg/kg (max. 1g) × 3d
Ancylostoma duodenale, see Hookworm			

4. A *Naegleria* infection was treated successfully with intravenous and intrathecal use of both amphotericin B and miconazole, plus rifampin (J Seidel et al, N Engl J Med, 306:346, 1982). Other reports of successful therapy are questionable.
5. An approved drug, but considered investigational for this condition by the U.S. Food and Drug Administration
6. Strains of *Acanthamoeba* isolated from fatal granulomatous amebic encephalitis are usually susceptible *in vitro* to pentamidine, ketoconazole *(Nizoral)*, flucytosine *(Ancobon)* and (less so) to amphotericin B. One patient with disseminated cutaneous infection was treated successfully with intravenous pentamidine isethionate, topical chlorhexidine and 2% ketoconazole cream, followed by oral itraconazole (CA Slater et al, N Engl J Med, 331:85, 1994).
7. A recently described free-living leptomyxid ameba that causes subacute to chronic granulomatous disease of the CNS. *In vitro* pentamidine isethionate 10 µg/ml is amebastatic (CF Denney et al, Clin Infect Dis, 25:1354, 1997). One patient, according to Medical Letter consultants, was successfully treated with clarithromycin *(Biaxin)* 500 mg t.i.d., fluconazole *(Diflucan)* 400 mg once daily, sulfadiazine 1.5 g q6h and flucytosine *(Ancobon)* 1.5 g q6h.

Table 4.13. **Drugs for Treatment of Parasitic Infections, continued**

Infection	Drug	Adult Dosage	Pediatric Dosage
ANGIOSTRONGYLIASIS			
Angiostrongylus cantonensis			
Drug of choice:[8]	Mebendazole[5]	100 mg bid × 5d	100 mg bid × 5d
Angiostrongylus costaricensis			
Drug of choice:	Mebendazole[5]	200–400 mg tid × 10d	200–400 mg tid × 10d
Alternative:	Thiabendazole[5]	75 mg/kg/d in 3 doses × 3d (max. 3 grams/d)[9]	75 mg/kg/d in 3 doses × 3d (max. 3 grams/d)[9]
ANISAKIASIS *(Anisakis)*			
Treatment of choice:	Surgical or endoscopic removal		
ASCARIASIS *(Ascaris lumbricoides,* roundworm)			
Drug of choice:	Albendazole[5]	400 mg once	400 mg once
OR	Mebendazole	100 mg bid × 3d or 500 mg once	100 mg bid × 3d or 500 mg once
OR	Pyrantel pamoate[5]	11 mg/kg once (max. 1 gram)	11 mg/kg once (max. 1 gram)
BABESIOSIS *(Babesia microti)*			
Drugs of choice:[10]	Clindamycin[5]	1.2 grams bid IV or 600 mg tid PO × 7d	20–40 mg/kg/d PO in 3 doses × 7d
	plus quinine	650 mg tid PO × 7d	25 mg/kg/d PO in 3 doses × 7d
OR	Atovaquone[5]	750 mg bid PO × 7–10d	20 mg/kg bid PO × 7–10d
	plus azithromycin[5]	1000 mg daily PO × 3d, then 500 mg daily × 7d	12 mg/kg daily PO × 7–10d

* Availability problems. See table on p 718.

8. Antiparasitic drugs can provoke neurologic symptoms, and most patients recover spontaneously without them. Analgesics, corticosteroids, and careful removal of CSF at frequent intervals can relieve symptoms (FD Pien and BC Pien, Int J Infect Dis, 3:161, 1999). Albendazole, levamisole *(Ergamisol),* or ivermectin have been used successfully in animals.
9. This dose is likely to be toxic and may have to be decreased.
10. Exchange transfusion has been used in severely ill patients with high (>10%) parasitemia (MR Boustani and JA Gelfard, Clin Infect Dis, 22:611, 1996). Combination therapy with atovaquone and azithromycin may be better tolerated (PJ Krause et al, American Society of Tropical Medicine and Hygiene Annual Meeting, 46:247, 1997, abstract 430). Concurrent use of pentamidine and trimethoprim-sulfamethoxazole has been reported to cure an infection with *B. divergens* (D Raoult et al, Ann Intern Med, 107:944, 1987).

Table 4.13. **Drugs for Treatment of Parasitic Infections, continued**

Infection	Drug	Adult Dosage	Pediatric Dosage
Balamuthia mardrillaris, see AMEBIC MENINGOENCEPHALITIS, PRIMARY			
BALANTIDIASIS *(Balantidium coli)*			
Drug of choice:	Tetracycline[5,11]	500 mg qid × 10d	40 mg/kg/d (max. 2 g) in 4 doses × 10d
Alternatives:	Iodoquinol[5]	650 mg tid × 20d	40 mg/kg/d in 3 doses × 20d
	Metronidazole[5]	750 mg tid × 5d	35–50 mg/kg/d in 3 doses × 5d
BAYLISASCARIASIS *(Baylisascaris procyonis)*			
Drug of choice:	See footnote 12		
BLASTOCYSTIS *hominis* infection			
Drug of choice:	See footnote 13		
CAPILLARIASIS *(Capillaria philippinensis)*			
Drug of choice:	Mebendazole[5]	200 mg bid × 20d	200 mg bid × 20d
Alternatives:	Albendazole[5]	400 mg daily × 10d	400 mg daily × 10d
Chagas' disease, see TRYPANOSOMIASIS			
Clonorchis sinensis, see FLUKE infection			

11. Use of tetracyclines is contraindicated in pregnancy and in children less than 8 years old.
12. No drugs have been demonstrated to be effective. However, albendazole, mebendazole, thiabendazole, levamisole *(Ergamisol)* and ivermectin could be tried. Steroid therapy may be helpful, especially in eye and CNS infections. Ocular baylisascariasis has been treated successfully using laser photocoagulation therapy to destroy the intraretinal larvae.
13. Clinical significance of these organisms is controversial, but metronidazole 750 mg tid × 10d or iodoquinol 650 mg tid × 20d has been reported to be effective (DJ Stenzel and PFL Borenam, Clin Microbiol Rev, 9:563, 1996). Metronidazole resistance may be common (K Haresh et al, Trop Med Int Health, 4:274, 1999). Trimethoprim-sulfamethoxazole is an alternative regimen (UZ Ok et al, Am J Gastroenterol, 94:3245, 1999).

Table 4.13. **Drugs for Treatment of Parasitic Infections, continued**

Infection	Drug	Adult Dosage	Pediatric Dosage
CRYPTOSPORIDIOSIS *(Cryptosporidium)*			
Drug of choice:[14]	Paromomycin[5]	25–35 mg/kg/d in 2 or 4 doses	25–35 mg/kg/d in 2 or 4 doses
CUTANEOUS LARVA MIGRANS (creeping eruption, dog and cat hookworm)			
Drug of choice:	Albendazole[5]	400 mg daily × 3d	400 mg daily × 3d
OR	Ivermectin[5]	200 µg/kg daily × 1–2d	200 µg/kg daily × 1–2d
OR	Thiabendazole[15]	Topically	Topically
CYCLOSPORA infection			
Drug of choice:	Trimethoprim-sulfamethoxazole[5,16]	TMP 160 mg, SMX 800 mg bid × 7d	TMP 5 mg/kg, SMX 25 mg/kg bid × 7d
CYSTICERCOSIS, see TAPEWORM infection			
DIENTAMOEBA *fragilis* infection			
Drug of choice:	Iodoquinol	650 mg tid × 20d	30–40 mg/kg/d (max. 2g) in 3 doses × 20d
OR	Paromomycin[5]	25–35 mg/kg/d in 3 doses × 7d	25–30 mg/kg/d in 3 doses × 7d
OR	Tetracycline[5,11]	500 mg qid × 10d	40 mg/kg/d (max. 2g) in 4 doses × 10d
Diphyllobothrium latum, see TAPEWORM infection			

14. Treatment is not curative in immunocompromised patients and infection is self-limited in immunocompetent patients. Combination therapy with azithromycin 600 mg daily has been effective in some patients (NH Smith et al, J Infect Dis, 178:900, 1998). Nitazoxanide (an investigational drug in the USA manufactured by Romark Laboratories, Tampa, Florida, 813-282-8544, www.romarklaboratories.com) 500-1000 PO bid may be used as an alternative (J-F Rossignol et al, Trans R Soc Trop Med Hyg, 92:663, 1998). Duration of therapy is uncertain.
15. HD Davis et al, Arch Dermatol, 129:588, 1993.
16. HIV infected patients may need higher dosage and long-term maintenance.

Table 4.13. **Drugs for Treatment of Parasitic Infections, continued**

Infection	Drug	Adult Dosage	Pediatric Dosage
DRACUNCULUS *medinensis* (guinea worm) infection			
Drug of choice:	Metronidazole[5,17]	250 mg tid × 10d	25 mg/kg/d (max. 750 mg) in 3 doses × 10d
Echinococcus, see TAPEWORM infection			
Entamoeba histolytica, see AMEBIASIS			
ENTAMOEBA *polecki* infection			
Drug of choice:	Metronidazole[5]	750 mg tid × 10d	35–50 mg/kg/d in 3 doses × 10d
ENTEROBIUS *vermicularis* (pinworm) infection			
Drug of choice:	Pyrantel pamoate	11 mg/kg base once (max. 1 gram); repeat in 2 weeks	11 mg/kg once (max. 1 gram); repeat in 2 weeks
OR	Mebendazole	100 mg once; repeat in 2 weeks	100 mg once; repeat in 2 weeks
OR	Albendazole[5]	400 mg once; repeat in 2 weeks	400 mg once; repeat in 2 weeks
Fasciola hepatica, see FLUKE infection			
FILARIASIS			
Wuchereria bancrofti, Brugia malayi			
Drug of choice:[18,19]	Diethylcarbamazine[20]*	Day 1: 50 mg, p.c. Day 2: 50 mg tid Day 3: 100 mg tid Days 4 through 14: 6 mg/kg/d in 3 doses	Day 1: 1 mg/kg p.c. Day 2: 1 mg/kg tid Day 3: 1–2 mg/kg tid Days 4 through 14: 6 mg/kg/d in 3 doses

* Availability problems. See table on p 718.

17. Not curative, but decreases inflammation and facilitates removing the worm. Mebendazole 400–800 mg/d for 6d has been reported to kill the worm directly.
18. A single dose of ivermectin, 200 µg/kg, is effective for treatment of microfilaremia but does not kill the adult worm. In a limited study, single-dose diethylcarbamazine (6 mg/kg) was as macrofilaricidal as a multi-dose regimen against *W. bancrofti* (J Norões et al, Trans R Soc Trop Med Hyg, 91:78, 1997).
19. Antihistamines or corticosteroids may be required to decrease allergic reactions due to disintegration of microfilariae in treatment of filarial infections, especially those caused by *Loa loa.*
20. For patients with no microfilariae in the blood, full doses can be given from day one.

Table 4.13. **Drugs for Treatment of Parasitic Infections, continued**

Infection	Drug	Adult Dosage	Pediatric Dosage
Loa loa			
Drug of choice:[19,21]	Diethylcarbamazine[20]*	Day 1: 50 mg p.c. Day 2: 50 mg tid Day 3: 100 mg tid Days 4 through 21: 9 mg/kg/d in 3 doses	Day 1: 1 mg/kg p.c. Day 2: 1 mg/kg tid Day 3: 1–2 mg/kg tid Days 4 through 21: 9 mg/kg/d in 3 doses
Mansonella ozzardi			
Drug of choice:	See footnote 22		
Mansonella perstans			
Drug of choice:	Mebendazole[5]	100 mg bid × 30d	100 mg bid × 30d
OR	Albendazole[5]	400 mg bid × 10d	400 mg bid × 10d
Mansonella streptocerca			
Drug of choice:[23]	Diethylcarbamazine*	6 mg/kg/d × 14d	6 mg/kg/d × 14d
	Ivermectin[5]	150 μg/kg once	150 μg/kg once
Tropical Pulmonary Eosinophilia (TPE)			
Drug of choice:	Diethylcarbamazine*	6 mg/kg/d in 3 doses × 14d	6 mg/kg/d in 3 doses × 14d
Onchocerca volvulus (River blindness)			
Drug of choice:	Ivermectin[24]	150 μg/kg once, repeated every 6 to 12 months until asymptomatic	150 μg/kg once, repeated every 6 to 12 months until asymptomatic

21. In heavy infections with *Loa loa,* rapid killing of microfilariae can provoke an encephalopathy. Apheresis has been reported to be effective in lowering microfilarial counts in patients heavily infected with *Loa loa* (EA Ottesen, Infect Dis Clin North Am, 7:619, 1993). Albendazole or ivermectin have also been used to reduce microfilaremia but because of slower onset of action, albendazole is preferred (AD Klion et al, J Infect Dis, 168:202, 1993; M Kombila et al, Am J Trop Med Hyg, 58:458, 1998). Albendazole may be useful for treatment of loiasis when diethylcarbamazine is ineffective or cannot be used but repeated courses may be necessary (AD Klion et al, Clin Infect Dis, 29:680, 1999). Diethylcarbamazine, 300 mg once weekly, has been recommended for prevention of loiasis (TB Nutman et al, N Engl J Med, 319:752, 1988).
22. Diethylcarbamazine has no effect. Ivermectin, 200 μg/kg once, has been effective.
23. Diethylcarbamazine is potentially curative due to activity against both adult worms and microfilariae, but is not available in the US for this indication from the CDC. Ivermectin is only active against microfilariae.
24. Annual treatment with ivermectin 150 μg/kg can prevent blindness due to ocular onchocerciasis (D Mabey et al, Ophthalmology, 103:1001, 1996).

Table 4.13. **Drugs for Treatment of Parasitic Infections, continued**

Infection	Drug	Adult Dosage	Pediatric Dosage
FLUKE, hermaphroditic, infection			
Clonorchis sinensis **(Chinese liver fluke)**			
Drug of choice:	Praziquantel	75 mg/kg/d in 3 doses × 1d	75 mg/kg/d in 3 doses × 1d
OR	Albendazole[5]	10 mg/kg × 7d	10 mg/kg × 7d
Fasciola hepatica **(sheep liver fluke)**			
Drug of choice:[25]	Triclabendazole*	10 mg/kg once	10 mg/kg once
Alternative:	Bithionol*	30–50 mg/kg on alternate days × 10–15 doses	30–50 mg/kg on alternate days × 10–15 doses
Fasciolopsis buski, Heterophyes heterophyes, Metagonimus yokogawai **(intestinal flukes)**			
Drug of choice:	Praziquantel[5]	75 mg/kg/d in 3 doses × 1d	75 mg/kg/d in 3 doses × 1d
Metorchis conjunctus **(North American liver fluke)[26]**			
Drug of choice:	Praziquantel[5]	75 mg/kg/d in 3 doses × 1d	75 mg/kg/d in 3 doses × 1d
Nanophyetus salmincola			
Drug of choice:	Praziquantel[5]	60 mg/kg/d in 3 doses × 1d	60 mg/kg/d in 3 doses × 1d
Opisthorchis viverrini **(Southeast Asian liver fluke)**			
Drug of choice:	Praziquantel	75 mg/kg/d in 3 doses × 1d	75 mg/kg/d in 3 doses × 1d
Paragonimus westermani **(lung fluke)**			
Drug of choice:	Praziquantel[5]	75 mg/kg/d in 3 doses × 2d	75 mg/kg/d in 3 doses × 2d
Alternative:[27]	Bithionol*	30–50 mg/kg on alternate days × 10–15 doses	30–50 mg/kg on alternate days × 10–15 doses

* Availability problems. See table on p 718.

25. Unlike infections with other flukes, *Fasciola hepatica* infections may not respond to praziquantel. Triclabendazole (*Fasinex* — Novartis), a veterinary fasciolide, may be safe and effective but data are limited (R López-Vélez et al, Eur J Clin Microbiol, 18:525, 1999). It should be given with food for better absorption.
26. JD MacLean et al, Lancet, 347:154, 1996.
27. Triclabendazole may be effective in a dosage of 5 mg/kg once daily for 3 days or 10 mg/kg twice in one day (M Calvopiña et al, Trans R Soc Trop Med Hyg, 92:566, 1998).

Table 4.13. **Drugs for Treatment of Parasitic Infections, continued**

Infection	Drug	Adult Dosage	Pediatric Dosage
GIARDIASIS *(Giardia lamblia)*			
Drug of choice:	Metronidazole[5]	250 mg tid × 5d	15 mg/kg/d in 3 doses × 5d
Alternatives:[28]	Quinacrine[29]	100 mg PO tid × 5d (max. 300 mg/d)	2 mg/kg PO tid × 5d (max. 300 mg/d)
	Tinidazole[2*]	2 grams once	50 mg/kg once (max. 2 g)
	Furazolidone	100 mg qid × 7–10d	6 mg/kg/d in 4 doses × 7–10d
	Paromomycin[5,30]	25–35 mg/kg/d in 3 doses × 7d	25–35 mg/kg/d in 3 doses × 7d
GNATHOSTOMIASIS *(Gnathostoma spinigerum)*			
Treatment of choice:[31]	Surgical removal		
OR	Albendazole[5]	400 mg bid × 21d	
GONGYLONEMIASIS *(Gongylonema sp.)*			
Treatment of choice:[32]	Surgical removal		
OR	Albendazole[5]	10 mg/kg/d × 3 d	10 mg/kg/d × 3 d
HOOKWORM infection *(Ancylostoma duodenale, Necator americanus)*			
Drug of choice:	Albendazole[5]	400 mg once	400 mg once
OR	Mebendazole	100 mg bid × 3d or 500 mg once	100 mg bid × 3d or 500 mg once
OR	Pyrantel pamoate[5]	11 mg/kg (max. 1g) × 3d	11 mg/kg (max. 1g) × 3d
Hydatid cyst, see TAPEWORM infection			

28. Albendazole 400 mg daily × 5d may be effective (A Hall and Q Nahar, Trans R Soc Trop Med Hyg, 87:84, 1993). Bacitracin zinc or bacitracin 120,000 U bid for 10 days may also be effective (BJ Andrews et al, Am J Trop Med Hyg, 52:318, 1995).
29. Quinacrine is not available commercially, but as a service can be compounded by Medical Center Pharmacy, New Haven, CT (203-785-6818) or Panorama Compounding Pharmacy 6744 Balboa Blvd, Van Nuys, CA 91406 (800-247-9767).
30. Not absorbed; may be useful for treatment of giardiasis in pregnancy.
31. Ivermectin has been reported to be effective in animals but there are few data in humans (MT Anantaphruti et al, Trop Med Parasitol, 43:65, 1992; R Ruiz-Maldonado and MA Mosqueda-Cabrera, Int J Dermatol, 38:52, 1999).
32. M Eberhard et al, Am J Trop Med Hyg, 61:51, 1999

Table 4.13. **Drugs for Treatment of Parasitic Infections, continued**

Infection	Drug	Adult Dosage	Pediatric Dosage
Hymenolepis nana, see TAPEWORM infection			
ISOSPORIASIS *(Isospora belli)*			
Drug of choice:	Trimethoprim-sulfamethoxazole[5,33]	160 mg TMP, 800 mg SMX qid × 10d, then bid × 3 wks	
LEISHMANIASIS (Cutaneous due to *L. mexicana, L. tropica, L. major, L. braziliensis;* mucocutaneous mostly due to *L. braziliensis;* visceral due to *L. donovani* [Kala-azar], *L. infantum, L. chagasi)*			
Drug of choice:[34]	Sodium stibogluconate*	20 mg Sb/kg/d IV or IM × 20–28d[35]	20 mg Sb/kg/d IV or IM × 20–28d[35]
OR	Meglumine antimonate*	20 mg Sb/kg/d IV or IM × 20–28d[35]	20 mg Sb/kg/d IV or IM × 20–28d[35]
OR	Amphotericin B[5]	0.5 to 1 mg/kg IV daily or every 2d for up to 8 wks	0.5 to 1 mg/kg IV daily or every 2d for up to 8 wks
OR	Liposomal Amphotericin B[36]	3 mg/kg/d (days 1–5) and 3 mg/kg/d days 14, 21[37]	3 mg/kg/d (days 1–5) and 3 mg/kg/d days 14, 21[37]

* Availability problems. See table on p 718.

33. In sulfonamide-sensitive patients, pyrimethamine 50–75 mg daily in divided doses has been effective (JP Ackers, Semin Gastrointest Dis, 8:33, 1997).
34. For treatment of kala-azar, oral miltefosine 100–150 mg daily for 4 weeks was 97% effective after 6 months. Gastrointestinal adverse effects are common and the drug is contraindicated in pregnancy (TK Jha et al, N Engl J Med, 341:1795, 1999).
35. May be repeated or continued. A longer duration may be needed for some forms of visceral leishmaniasis (BL Herwaldt, Lancet, 354:1191, 1999).
36. Three preparations of lipid-encapsulated amphotericin B have been used for treatment of visceral leishmaniasis. Largely based on clinical trials in patients infected with *L. infantum,* the FDA approved liposomal amphotericin B *(AmBisome)* for treatment of visceral leishmaniasis (A Meyerhoff, Clin Infect Dis, 28:42, 1999; JD Berman, Clin Infect Dis, 28:49, 1999). Amphotericin B lipid complex *(Abelcet)* and amphotericin B cholesteryl sulfate *(Amphotec)* have also been used with good results. Some studies indicate that *L. donovani* resistant to pentavalent antimonial agents may respond to lipid-encapsulated amphotericin B (S Sundar et al, Ann Trop Med Parasitol, 92:755, 1998).
37. The dose for immunocompromised patients with HIV is 4 mg/kg/d (days 1–5) and 4 mg/kg/d on days 10, 17, 24, 31, 38. The relapse rate is high, suggesting that maintenance therapy may be indicated.

Table 4.13. **Drugs for Treatment of Parasitic Infections, continued**

Infection	Drug	Adult Dosage	Pediatric Dosage
LEISHMANIASIS, continued			
Alternatives:	Pentamidine	2–4 mg/kg daily or every 2d IV or IM for up to 15 doses[38]	2–4 mg/kg daily or every 2d IV or IM for up to 15 doses[38]
OR	Paromomycin [39]*	Topically twice daily × 10–20d	
LICE infestation *(Pediculus humanus, P. capitis, Phthirus pubis)*[40]			
Drug of choice:	1% Permethrin[41]	Topically	Topically
OR	0.5% Malathion[42]	Topically	Topically
Alternative:	Pyrethrins with piperonyl butoxide[41]	Topically	Topically
OR	Ivermectin 5,[43]	200 µg/kg once	200 µg/kg once
Loa loa, see FILARIASIS			

38. 4 mg/kg qod x 15 doses for *L. donovani;* 2 mg/kg qod × 7 or 3 mg/kg qod × 4 doses for cutaneous disease.
39. Two preparations of paromomycin have been studied. The first, a formulation of 15% paromomycin and 12% methylbenzethonium chloride in soft white paraffin for topical use, has been reported to be effective in some patients against cutaneous leishmaniasis due to *L. major* (O Ozgoztasi and I Baydar, Int J Dermatol, 36:61, 1997). The second, injectable paromomycin (aminosidine, not available in the USA), has been used successfully for the treatment of kala-azar in India where antimony resistance is common (TK Jha et al, BMJ, 316:1200, 1998).
40. For infestation of eyelashes with crab lice, use petrolatum. For pubic lice, treat with 5% permethrin or ivermectin as for scabies.
41. A second application is recommended one week later to kill hatching progeny. Some lice are resistant to pyrethrins and permethrin (RO Pollach, Arch Pediatr Adolesc Med, 153:969, 1999).
42. Medical Letter, 41:73, 1999.
43. Ivermectin is effective against adult lice but has no effect on nits (TA Bell, Pediatr Infect Dis J, 17:923, 1998).

Table 4.13. **Drugs for Treatment of Parasitic Infections, continued**

Infection	Drug	Adult Dosage	Pediatric Dosage
MALARIA, Treatment of *(Plasmodium falciparum, P. ovale, P. vivax,* and *P. malariae)*			
Chloroquine-resistant *P. falciparum*[44]			
ORAL			
Drugs of choice:	Quinine sulfate	650 mg q8h × 3–7d 45	25mg/kg/d in 3 doses × 3–7d[45]
	plus doxycycline[5,11]	100 mg bid × 7d	2 mg/kg/d × 7d
	or plus tetracycline[5,11]	250 mg qid × 7d	6.25 mg/kg qid × 7d
	or plus pyrimethamine-sulfadoxine[46]	3 tablets at once on last day of quinine	<1 yr: ¼ tablet 1–3 yrs: ½ tablet 4–8 yrs: 1 tablet 9–14 yrs: 2 tablets
	or plus clindamycin[5,47]	900 mg tid × 5d	20–40 mg/kg/d in 3 doses × 5d
Alternatives:[48]	Mefloquine[49,50]	750 mg followed by 500 mg 12 hrs later	15 mg/kg PO followed by 10 mg/kg PO 8–12 hours later (<45 kg)

44. Chloroquine-resistant *P. falciparum* occur in all malarious areas except Central America west of the Panama Canal Zone, Mexico, Haiti, the Dominican Republic, and most of the Middle East (chloroquine resistance has been reported in Yemen, Oman, Saudi Arabia and Iran).
45. In Southeast Asia, relative resistance to quinine has increased and the treatment should be continued for seven days.
46. *Fansidar* tablets contain 25 mg of pyrimethamine and 500 mg of sulfadoxine. Resistance to pyrimethamine-sulfadoxine has been reported from Southeast Asia, the Amazon basin, sub-Saharan Africa, Bangladesh and Oceania.
47. For use in pregnancy.
48. For treatment of multiple-drug-resistant *P. falciparum* in Southeast Asia, especially Thailand, where resistance to mefloquine and halofantrine is frequent, a 7-day course of quinine and tetracycline is recommended (G Watt et al, Am J Trop Med Hyg, 47:108, 1992). Artesunate plus mefloquine (C Luxemburger et al, Trans R Soc Trop Med Hyg, 88:213, 1994), artemether plus mefloquine (J Karbwang et al, Trans R Soc Trop Med Hyg, 89:296, 1995) or mefloquine plus doxycycline are also used to treat multiple-drug-resistant *P. falciparum.*
49. At this dosage, adverse effects including nausea, vomiting, diarrhea, dizziness, disturbed sense of balance, toxic psychosis and seizures can occur. Mefloquine is teratogenic in animals and should not be used for treatment of malaria in pregnancy. It should not be given together with quinine, quinidine or halofantrine, and caution is required in using quinine, quinidine or halofantrine to treat patients with malaria who have taken mefloquine for prophylaxis. The pediatric dosage has not been approved by the FDA. Resistance to mefloquine has been reported in some areas, such as the Thailand-Myanmar and Cambodia borders and in the Amazon, where 25 mg/kg should be used.
50. In the USA, a 250-mg tablet of mefloquine contains 228 mg mefloquine base. Outside the USA, each 275-mg tablet contains 250 mg base.

Table 4.13. **Drugs for Treatment of Parasitic Infections, continued**

Infection	Drug	Adult Dosage	Pediatric Dosage
MALARIA, continued			
Chloroquine-resistant *P. falciparum*			
ORAL, continued			
Alternatives, continued	Halofantrine[51]*	500 mg q6h × 3 doses; repeat in 1 week[52]	8 mg/kg q6h × 3 doses (<40 kg); repeat in 1 week[52]
	Atovaquone[53]	500 mg bid × 3d	11–20 kg: 125 mg bid × 3d 21–30 kg: 250 mg bid × 3d 31–40 kg: 375 mg bid × 3d
	plus proguanil	200 mg bid × 3d	11–20 kg: 50 mg bid x 3d 21–30 kg: 100 mg bid x 3d 31–40 kg: 150 mg bid x 3d
	or plus doxycycline[5,11]	100 mg bid × 3d	2 mg/kg/d × 3d
	Artesunate*	4 mg/kg/d × 3d	
	plus mefloquine[49,50]	750 mg followed by 500 mg 12 hrs later	15 mg/kg followed 8–12 hrs later by 10 mg/kg

* Availability problems. See table on page 718.

51. May be effective in multiple-drug-resistant *P. falciparum* malaria, but treatment failures and resistance have been reported, and the drug has caused lengthening of the PR and QTc intervals and fatal cardiac arrhythmias. It should not be used for patients with cardiac conduction defects or with other drugs that may affect the QT interval, such as quinine, quinidine and mefloquine. Cardiac monitoring is recommended. Variability in absorption is a problem; halofantrine should not be taken one hour before to two hours after meals because food increases its absorption. It should not be used in pregnancy.
52. A single 250-mg dose can be used for repeat treatment in mild to moderate infections (JE Touze et al, Lancet, 349:255, 1997).
53. Atovaquone plus proguanil is marketed as a combination tablet in many countries and will soon be available in the United States (250 mg atovaquone/100 mg proguanil as *Malarone* – Glaxo Wellcome and 62.5 mg atovaquone/25 mg proguanil as *Malarone Pediatric*). The combination should be used only for acute uncomplicated malaria caused by *P. falciparum.* The dose of *Malarone* for 3-day treatment of malaria is 4 tablets daily in adults; 3 adult tablets daily for children 31–40 kg; 2 adult tablets daily for children 21-30 kg; and 1 adult tablet daily for children 11–20 kg. To enhance absorption, it should be taken within 45 minutes after eating (S Looareesuwan et al, Am J Trop Med Hyg, 60:533, 1999). Although approved for once daily dosing, to decrease nausea and vomiting the dose can be divided in two.

Table 4.13. **Drugs for Treatment of Parasitic Infections, continued**

Infection	Drug	Adult Dosage	Pediatric Dosage
MALARIA, continued			
Chloroquine-resistant *P. vivax*[54]			
Drug of choice:	Quinine sulfate	650 mg q8h × 3–7d[45]	25 mg/kg/d in 3 doses × 3–7d[45]
	plus		
	doxycycline[5,11]	100 mg bid × 7d	2 mg/kg/d × 7d
	or plus		
	pyrimethamine-sulfadoxine[46]	3 tablets at once on last day of quinine	<1 yr: ¼ tablet 1–3 yrs: ½ tablet 4–8 yrs: 1 tablet 9–14 yrs: 2 tablets
OR	Mefloquine	750 mg followed by 500 mg 12 hr later	15 mg/kg followed 8–12 hrs later by 10 mg/kg
Alternatives:	Halofantrine[51,55]*	500 mg q6h × 3 doses	8 mg/kg q6h × 3 doses
	Chloroquine	25 mg base/kg in 3 doses over 48 hrs	
	plus		
	primaquine[56]	2.5 mg base/kg in 3 doses over 48 hrs	
All *Plasmodium* except Chloroquine-resistant *P. falciparum*[44] and Chloroquine-resistant *P. vivax*[54]			
ORAL			
Drug of choice:	Chloroquine phosphate[57]	1 gram (600 mg base), then 500 mg (300 mg base) 6 hrs later, then 500 mg (300 mg base) at 24 and 48 hrs	10 mg base/kg (max. 600 mg base), then 5 mg base/kg 6 hrs later, then 5 mg base/kg at 24 and 48 hrs

54. *P. vivax* with decreased susceptibility to chloroquine is a significant problem in Papua-New Guinea and Indonesia. There are also a few reports of resistance from Myanmar, India, Thailand, the Solomon Islands, Vanuatu, Guyana, Brazil and Peru.
55. JK Baird el al, J Infect Dis, 171:1678, 1995
56. Primaquine phosphate can cause hemolytic anemia, especially in patients whose red cells are deficient in glucose-6-phosphate dehydrogenase. This deficiency is most common in African, Asian, and Mediterranean peoples. Patients should be screened for G-6-PD deficiency before treatment. Primaquine should not be used during pregnancy.
57. If chloroquine phosphate is not available, hydroxychloroquine sulfate is as effective; 400 mg of hydroxychloroquine sulfate is equivalent to 500 mg of chloroquine phosphate.

Table 4.13. **Drugs for Treatment of Parasitic Infections, continued**

Infection	Drug	Adult Dosage	Pediatric Dosage
MALARIA, continued			
All *Plasmodium*			
PARENTERAL			
Drug of choice:[58]	Quinidine gluconate[59,60]	10 mg/kg loading dose (max. 600 mg) in normal saline slowly over 1 to 2 hrs, followed by continuous infusion of 0.02 mg/kg/min until oral therapy can be started	Same as adult dose
OR	Quinine dihydrochloride[59,60]	20 mg/kg loading dose IV in 5% dextrose over 4 hrs, followed by 10 mg/kg over 2–4 hrs q8h (max. 1800 mg/d) until oral therapy can be started	Same as adult dose
Alternative:	Artemether[61]*	3.2 mg/kg IM, then 1.6 mg/kg daily × 5–7d	Same as adult dose
Prevention of relapses: *P. vivax* and *P. ovale* only			
Drug of choice:	Primaquine phosphate[56,62]	26.3 mg (15 mg base)/d × 14d or 79 mg (45 mg base)/wk × 8 wks	0.3 mg base/kg/d × 14d

* Availability problems. See table on p 718.

58. Exchange transfusion has been helpful for some patients with high-density (>10%) parasitemia, altered mental status, pulmonary edema or renal complications (KD Miller et al, N Engl J Med, 321:65, 1989).
59. Continuous EKG, blood pressure and glucose monitoring are recommended, especially in pregnant women and young children.
60. Quinidine may have greater antimalarial activity than quinine. The loading dose should be decreased or omitted in those patients who have received quinine or mefloquine. If more than 48 hours of parenteral treatment is required, the quinine or quinidine dose should be reduced by ⅓ to ½.
61. NJ White, N Engl J Med, 335:800, 1996. Not available in the United States.
62. Relapses have been reported with this regimen, and should be treated with a second 14-day course of 30 mg base/day.

Table 4.13. **Drugs for Treatment of Parasitic Infections, continued**

Infection	Drug	Adult Dosage	Pediatric Dosage
MALARIA, Prevention of[63]			
Chloroquine-sensitive areas[44]			
Drug of choice:	Chloroquine phosphate[64,65]	500 mg (300 mg base), once/week[66]	5 mg/kg base once/week, up to adult dose of 300 mg base[66]
Chloroquine-resistant areas[44]			
Drug of choice:	Mefloquine[50,65,67]	250 mg once/week[66]	<15 kg: 5 mg/kg[66] 15–19 kg: ¼ tablet[66] 20–30 kg: ½ tablet[66] 31–45 kg: ¾ tablet[66] >45 kg: 1 tablet[66]
OR	Doxycycline[5,65]	100 mg daily[68]	2 mg/kg/d, up to 100 mg/day[68]
OR	Atovaquone/Proguanil[53]	250 mg/100 mg (1 tablet) daily[69]	11–20 kg: 62.5 mg/25 mg[69] 21–30 kg: 125 mg/50 mg[69] 31–40 kg: 187.5 mg/75 mg[69]

63. No drug regimen guarantees protection against malaria. If fever develops within a year (particularly within the first two months) after travel to malarious areas, travelers should be advised to seek medical attention. Insect repellents, insecticide-impregnated bed nets and proper clothing are important adjuncts for malaria prophylaxis.
64. In pregnancy, chloroquine prophylaxis has been used extensively and safely.
65. For prevention of attack after departure from areas where *P. vivax* and *P. ovale* are endemic, which includes almost all areas where malaria is found (except Haiti), some experts prescribe in addition primaquine phosphate 15 mg base (26.3 mg)/d or, for children, 0.3 mg base/kg/d during the last two weeks of prophylaxis. Others prefer to avoid the toxicity of primaquine and rely on surveillance to detect cases when they occur, particularly when exposure was limited or doubtful. See also footnotes 56 and 62.
66. Beginning one to two weeks before travel and continuing weekly for the duration of stay and for four weeks after leaving.
67. The pediatric dosage has not been approved by the FDA, and the drug has not been approved for use during pregnancy. However, it has been reported to be safe for prophylactic use during the second or third trimester of pregnancy and possibly during early pregnancy as well (CDC Health Information for International Travel, 1999-2000, page 120; BL Smoak et al, J Infect Dis, 176:831, 1997). Mefloquine is not recommended for patients with cardiac conduction abnormalities. Patients with a history of seizures or psychiatric disorders should avoid mefloquine (Medical Letter, 32:13, 1990). Resistance to mefloquine has been reported in some areas, such as Thailand; in these areas, doxycycline should be used for prophylaxis. In children less than eight years old, proguanil plus sulfisoxazole has been used (KN Suh and JS Keystone, Infect Dis Clin Pract, 5:541, 1996).
68. Beginning 1-2 days before travel and continuing for the duration of stay and for 4 weeks after leaving. Use of tetracyclines is contraindicated in pregnancy and in children less than eight years old. Doxycycline can cause gastrointestinal disturbances, vaginal moniliasis and photosensitivity reactions.
69. GE Shanks et al, Clin Infect Dis, 27:494, 1998; B Lell et al, Lancet, 351:709, 1998. Beginning 1 to 2 days before travel and continuing for the duration of stay and for 1 week after leaving.

Table 4.13. **Drugs for Treatment of Parasitic Infections, continued**

Infection	Drug	Adult Dosage	Pediatric Dosage
MALARIA, Prevention of (continued)			
Chloroquine-resistant areas[44]			
Alternative:	Primaquine[5,56,70]	30 mg base daily	0.5 mg/kg base daily
	Chloroquine phosphate[65]	Same as above	Same as above
	plus pyrimethamine-sulfadoxine[46] for presumptive treatment[71]	Carry a single dose (3 tablets) for self-treatment of febrile illness when medical care is not immediately available	<1 yr: ¼ tablet 1–3 yrs: ½ tablet 4–8 yrs: 1 tablet 9–14 yrs: 2 tablets
	or plus proguanil[72]	200 mg daily	<2 yrs: 50 mg daily 2–6 yrs: 100 mg 7–10 yrs: 150 mg >10 yrs: 200 mg
MICROSPORIDIOSIS			
Ocular *(Encephalitozoon hellem, Encephalitozoon cuniculi, Vittaforma corneae [Nosema corneum])*			
Drug of choice:	Albendazole[5]	400 mg bid	
	plus fumagillin[73]		

70. Several studies have shown that daily primaquine beginning one day before departure and continued until two days after leaving the malaria area provides effective prophylaxis against chloroquine-resistant *P. falciparum* (E Schwartz and G Regev-Yochay, Clin Infect Dis, 29:1502, 1999). Some studies have shown less efficacy against *P. vivax.*
71. In areas with strains resistant to pyrimethamine-sulfadoxine, atovaquone/proguanil or atovaquone plus doxycycline can also be used for presumptive treatment. See page 114 for dosage.
72. Proguanil (*Paludrine* — Wyeth Ayerst, Canada; Zeneca, United Kingdom), which is not available alone in the USA but is widely available in Canada and overseas, is recommended mainly for use in Africa south of the Sahara. Prophylaxis is recommended during exposure and for four weeks afterwards. Proguanil has been used in pregnancy without evidence of toxicity (PA Phillips-Howard and D Wood, Drug Saf, 14:131, 1996).
73. Ocular lesions due to *E. hellem* in HIV-infected patients have responded to fumagillin eyedrops prepared from *Fumidil-B*, a commercial product (Mid-Continent Agrimarketing, Inc., Olathe, Kansas, 1-800-547-1392) used to control a microsporidial disease of honey bees (MC Diesenhouse, Am J Ophthalmol, 115:293, 1993). For lesions due to *V. corneae,* topical therapy is generally not effective and keratoplasty may be required (RM Davis et al, Ophthalmology, 97:953, 1990).

Table 4.13. **Drugs for Treatment of Parasitic Infections, continued**

Infection	Drug	Adult Dosage	Pediatric Dosage
MICROSPORIDIOSIS, continued			
Intestinal *(Enterocytozoon bieneusi, Encephalitozoon [Septata] intestinalis)*			
Drug of choice:[74]	Albendazole[5]	400 mg bid	
Disseminated *(E. hellem, E. cuniculi, E. intestinalis, Pleistophora sp., Trachipleistophora sp.* and *Brachiola vesicularum)*			
Drug of choice:[75]	Albendazole[5]	400 mg bid	
Mites, see SCABIES			
MONILIFORMIS *moniliformis* infection			
Drug of choice:	Pyrantel pamoate[5]	11 mg/kg once, repeat twice, 2 wks apart	11 mg/kg once, repeat twice, 2 wks apart
***Naegleria* species,** see AMEBIC MENINGOENCEPHALITIS, PRIMARY			
Necator americanus, see HOOKWORM infection			
OESOPHAGOSTOMUM *bifurcum*			
Drug of choice:	See footnote 76		
Onchocerca volvulus, see FILARIASIS			
Opisthorchis viverrini, see FLUKE infection			
Paragonimus westermani, see FLUKE infection			
Pediculus capitis, humanus, Phthirus pubis, see LICE			

74. Octreotide *(Sandostatin)* has provided symptomatic relief in some patients with large volume diarrhea. Oral fumagillin (see footnote 73) has been effective in treating *E. bieneu-si* (J-M Molina et al, AIDS, 11:1603, 1997), but has been associated with thrombocytopenia. Highly active antiretroviral therapy may lead to microbiologic and clinical response in HIV-infected patients with microsporidial diarrhea (NA Foudraine et al, AIDS, 12:35, 1998; A Carr et al, Lancet, 351:256, 1998).
75. J-M Molina et al, J Infect Dis, 171:245, 1995. There is no established treatment for *Pleistophora.*
76. Albendazole or pyrantel pamoate may be effective (HP Krepel et al, Trans R Soc Trop Med Hyg, 87:87, 1993).

Table 4.13. **Drugs for Treatment of Parasitic Infections, continued**

Infection	Drug	Adult Dosage	Pediatric Dosage
Pinworm, see ENTEROBIUS			
***PNEUMOCYSTIS** carinii* pneumonia (PCP)[77]			
Drug of choice:	Trimethoprim-sulfamethoxazole	TMP 15 mg/kg/d, SMX 75 mg/kg/d, oral or IV in 3 or 4 doses × 14–21d	Same as adult dose
Alternatives:	Pentamidine	3–4 mg/kg IV daily × 14–21 days	Same as adult dose
OR	Trimetrexate	45 mg/m² IV daily × 21 days	
	plus folinic acid	20 mg/m² PO or IV q6h × 24 days	
OR	Trimethoprim[5]	5 mg/kg PO tid × 21 days	
	plus dapsone[5]	100 mg PO daily × 21 days	
OR	Atovaquone	750 mg bid PO × 21d	
OR	Primaquine[5,56]	30 mg base PO daily × 21 days	
	plus clindamycin[5]	600 mg IV q6h × 21 days, or 300–450 mg PO q6h × 21 days	
Primary and secondary prophylaxis			
Drug of Choice:	Trimethoprim-sulfamethoxazole	1 tab (single or double strength) PO daily or 1 DS tab 3x/week	TMP 150 mg/m², SMX 750 mg/m² in 2 doses PO on 3 consecutive days per week
Alternatives:[78]	Dapsone[5]	50 mg PO bid, or 100 mg PO daily	2 mg/kg (max. 100 mg) PO daily
OR	Dapsone[5]	50 mg PO daily or 200 mg each week	
	plus pyrimethamine[79]	50 mg or 75 mg PO each week	
OR	Pentamidine aerosol	300 mg inhaled monthly via *Respirgard II* nebulizer	>5 yrs: same as adult dose
OR	Atovaquone[5]	1500 mg daily PO	

77. In severe disease with room air $PO_2 \leq 70$ mmHg or Aa gradient ≥35 mmHg, prednisone should also be used (S Gagnon et al, N Engl J Med, 323:1444, 1990; E Caumes et al, Clin Infect Dis, 18:319, 1994).
78. Weekly therapy with sulfadoxine 500 mg/pyrimethamine 25 mg/leucovorin 25 mg was effective PCP prophylaxis in liver transplant patients (J Torre-Cisneros et al, Clin Infect Dis, 29:771, 1999).

Table 4.13. **Drugs for Treatment of Parasitic Infections, continued**

Infection	Drug	Adult Dosage	Pediatric Dosage
Roundworm, see ASCARIASIS			
SCABIES *(Sarcoptes scabiei)*			
Drug of choice:	5% Permethrin	Topically	Topically
Alternatives:	Ivermectin[5,80]	200 µg/kg PO once	200 µg/kg PO once
	10% Crotamiton	Topically	Topically
SCHISTOSOMIASIS *(Bilharziasis)*			
S. haematobium			
Drug of choice:	Praziquantel	40 mg/kg/d in 2 doses × 1d	40 mg/kg/d in 2 doses × 1d
S. japonicum			
Drug of choice:	Praziquantel	60 mg/kg/d in 3 doses × 1d	60 mg/kg/d in 3 doses × 1d
S. mansoni			
Drug of choice:	Praziquantel	40 mg/kg/d in 2 doses × 1d	40 mg/kg/d in 2 doses × 1d
Alternative:	Oxamniquine[81]	15 mg/kg once[82]	20 mg/kg/d in 2 doses × 1d[82]
S. mekongi			
Drug of choice:	Praziquantel	60 mg/kg/d in 3 doses × 1d	60 mg/kg/d in 3 doses × 1d
Sleeping sickness, see TRYPANOSOMIASIS			
STRONGYLOIDIASIS *(Strongyloides stercoralis)*			
Drug of choice:[83]	Ivermectin	200 µg/kg/d × 1–2d	200 µg/kg/d × 1–2d
Alternative:	Thiabendazole	50 mg/kg/d in 2 doses (max. 3 grams/d) × 2d[9]	50 mg/kg/d in 2 doses (max. 3 g/d) × 2d[9]

79. Plus leucovorin 25 mg with each dose of pyrimethamine.
80. Effective for crusted scabies in immunocompromised patients (M Larralde et al, Pediatr Dermatol, 16:69, 1999; A Patel et al, Australas J Dermatol, 40:37, 1999).
81. Oxamniquine has been effective in some areas in which praziquantel is less effective (FF Stelma et al, J Infect Dis, 176:304, 1997). Oxamniquine is contraindicated in pregnancy.
82. In East Africa, the dose should be increased to 30 mg/kg, and in Egypt and South Africa, 30 mg/kg/d × 2d. Some experts recommend 40–60 mg/kg over 2–3 days in all of Africa (KC Shekhar, Drugs, 42:379, 1991).
83. In immunocompromised patients or disseminated disease, it may be necessary to prolong or repeat therapy or use other agents. A veterinary parenteral formulation of ivermectin was used in one patient (PL Chiodini et al, Lancet, 355:43, 2000).

Table 4.13. **Drugs for Treatment of Parasitic Infections, continued**

Infection	Drug	Adult Dosage	Pediatric Dosage
TAPEWORM infection —			
Adult (intestinal stage)			
Diphyllobothrium latum **(fish),** ***Taenia saginata*** **(beef),** ***Taenia solium*** **(pork),** ***Dipylidium caninum*** **(dog)**			
Drug of choice:	Praziquantel[5]	5–10 mg/kg once	5–10 mg/kg once
Alternative:	Niclosamide	2 gm once	50 mg/kg once
Hymenolepis nana **(dwarf tapeworm)**			
Drug of choice:	Praziquantel[5]	25 mg/kg once	25 mg/kg once
Larval (tissue stage)			
Echinococcus granulosus **(hydatid cyst)**			
Drug of choice:[84]	Albendazole	400 mg bid × 1–6 months	15 mg/kg/d (max. 800 mg) × 1–6 months
Echinococcus multilocularis			
Treatment of choice:	See footnote[85]		
Cysticercus cellulosae **(cysticercosis)**			
Treatment of choice:	See footnote 86		
Alternative:	Albendazole	400 mg bid × 8–30d; can be repeated as necessary	15 mg/kg/d (max. 800 mg) in 2 doses × 8–30d; can be repeated as necessary
OR	Praziquantel[5]	50–100 mg/kg/d in 3 doses × 30d	50–100 mg/kg/d in 3 doses × 30d
Toxocariasis, see VISCERAL LARVA MIGRANS			

84. Patients may benefit from or require surgical resection of cysts. Praziquantel is useful preoperatively or in case of spill during surgery. Percutaneous drainage with ultrasound guidance plus albendazole therapy has been effective for management of hepatic hydatid cyst disease (MS Khuroo et al, N Engl J Med, 337:881, 1997).
85. Surgical excision is the only reliable means of treatment. Some reports have suggested use of albendazole or mebendazole (W Hao et al, Trans R Soc Trop Med Hyg, 88:340, 1994; WHO Group, Bull WHO, 74:231, 1996).
86. Initial therapy of parenchymal disease with seizures should focus on symptomatic treatment with anticonvulsant drugs. Treatment of parenchymal disease with albendazole and praziquantel is controversial and randomized trials have not shown a benefit. Obstructive hydrocephalus is treated with surgical removal of the obstructing cyst or CSF diversion. Prednisone 40 mg PO may be given in conjunction with surgery. Arachnoiditis, vasculitis or cerebral edema is treated with prednisone 60 mg daily or dexamethasone 4–16 mg/d combined with albendazole or praziquantel (AC White, Jr, Annu Rev Med, 51:187, 2000). Any cysticercocidal drug may cause irreparable damage when used to treat ocular or spinal cysts, even when corticosteroids are used. An ophthalmic exam should always be done before treatment to rule out intraocular cysts.

Table 4.13. **Drugs for Treatment of Parasitic Infections, continued**

Infection	Drug	Adult Dosage	Pediatric Dosage
TOXOPLASMOSIS *(Toxoplasma gondii)*[87]			
Drug of choice:[88]	Pyrimethamine[89]	25–100 mg/d × 3–4 wks	2 mg/kg/d x 3d, then 1 mg/kg/d (max. 25 mg/d) x 4 wks[90]
	plus sulfadiazine	1–1.5 grams qid × 3-4 wks	100–200 mg/kg/d × 3–4 wks
Alternative:[91]	Spiramycin*	3–4 grams/d × 3–4 wks	50–100 mg/kg/d × 3–4 wks
TRICHINOSIS *(Trichinella spiralis)*			
Drugs of choice:	Steroids for severe symptoms		
	plus mebendazole[5]	200–400 mg tid × 3d, then 400–500 mg tid × 10d	200-400 mg tid × 3d, then 400–500 mg tid × 10d
Alternative:	Albendazole[5]	400 mg PO bid × 8–14d	400 mg PO bid × 8–14d
TRICHOMONIASIS *(Trichomonas vaginalis)*			
Drug of choice:[92]	Metronidazole	2 grams once; or 250 mg tid or 375 mg bid PO × 7d	15 mg/kg/d orally in 3 doses × 7d
OR	Tinidazole[3]*	2 grams once	50 mg/kg once (max. 2 g)

87. In ocular toxoplasmosis with macular involvement, corticosteroids are recommended for an anti-inflammatory effect on the eyes.
88. To treat CNS toxoplasmosis in HIV-infected patients, some clinicians have used pyrimethamine 50 to 100 mg daily (after a loading dose of 200 mg) with a sulfonamide and, when sulfonamide sensitivity developed, have given clindamycin 1.8 to 2.4 g/d in divided doses instead of the sulfonamide (JS Remington et al, Lancet, 338:1142, 1991; BJ Luft et al, N Engl J Med, 329:995, 1993). Atovaquone plus pyrimethamine appears to be an effective alternative in sulfa-intolerant patients (JA Kovacs et al, Lancet, 340:637, 1992). Treatment is followed by chronic suppression with lower dosage regimens of the same drugs. For primary prophylaxis in HIV patients with <100 CD4 cells, either trimethoprim-sulfamethoxazole, pyrimethamine with dapsone or atovaquone with or without pyrimethamine can be used (USPHS/IDSA, MMWR, Morbid Mortal Weekly Report, 48, RR-10:41, 1999). See also footnote 89.
89. Plus leucovorin 10 to 25 mg with each dose of pyrimethamine.
90. Congenitally infected newborns should be treated with pyrimethamine every two or three days and a sulfonamide daily for about one year (JS Remington and G Desmonts in JS Remington and JO Klein, eds, *Infectious Disease of the Fetus and Newborn Infant,* 4th ed, Philadelphia: Saunders, 1995, page 140).
91. For prophylactic use during pregnancy. If it is determined that transmission has occurred *in utero,* therapy with pyrimethamine and sulfadiazine should be started.
92. Sexual partners should be treated simultaneously. Metronidazole-resistant strains have been reported and should be treated with metronidazole 2–4 g/d × 7–14d. Desensitization has been recommended for patients allergic to metronidazole (MD Pearlman et al, Am J Obstet Gynecol, 174:934, 1996).

Table 4.13. **Drugs for Treatment of Parasitic Infections, continued**

Infection	Drug	Adult Dosage	Pediatric Dosage
TRICHOSTRONGYLUS infection			
Drug of choice:	Pyrantel pamoate[5]	11 mg/kg base once (max. 1 g)	11 mg/kg once (max. 1 gram)
Alternative:	Mebendazole[5]	100 mg bid × 3d	100 mg bid × 3d
OR	Albendazole[5]	400 mg once	400 mg once
TRICHURIASIS (*Trichuris trichiura,* whipworm)			
Drug of choice:	Mebendazole	100 mg bid × 3d or 500 mg once	100 mg bid × 3d or 500 mg once
Alternative:	Albendazole[5]	400 mg once[93]	400 mg once[93]
TRYPANOSOMIASIS			
T. cruzi **(American trypanosomiasis, Chagas' disease)**			
Drug of choice:	Benznidazole*	5–7 mg/kg/d in 2 divided doses × 30–90d	Up to 12 yrs: 10 mg/kg/d in 2 doses × 30–90d
OR	Nifurtimox[94]*	8–10 mg/kg/d in 3–4 doses × 90–120d	1–10 yrs: 15–20 mg/kg/d in 4 doses × 90d; 11–16 yrs: 12.5–15 mg/kg/d in 4 doses × 90d
T. brucei gambiense **(West African trypanosomiasis, sleeping sickness) hemolymphatic stage**			
Drug of choice:[95]	Pentamidine isethionate[5]	4 mg/kg/d IM × 10d	4 mg/kg/d IM × 10d
Alternative:	Suramin*	100–200 mg (test dose) IV, then 1 gram IV on days 1,3,7,14, and 21	20 mg/kg on days 1,3,7,14, and 21
OR	Eflornithine*	See footnote 96	

* Availability problems. See table on p 718.

93. In heavy infection, it may be necessary to extend therapy to 3 days.

94. No longer manufactured, but available from CDC in selected cases. The addition of gamma interferon to nifurtimox for 20 days in a limited number of patients and in experimental animals appears to have shortened the acute phase of Chagas' disease (RE McCabe et al, J Infect Dis, 163:912, 1991).

95. Suramin is the drug of choice for treatment of *T.b. rhodesiense.* For treatment of T.b. gambiense, pentamidine and suramin have equal efficacy but pentamidine is better tolerated.

96. Eflornithine is highly effective in *T.b. gambiense* and variably effective in *T. b. rhodesiense* infections. It is available in limited supply only from the WHO, and is given 400 mg/kg/d IV in 4 divided doses for 14 days.

Table 4.13. **Drugs for Treatment of Parasitic Infections, continued**

Infection	Drug	Adult dosage	Pediatric dosage
TRYPANOSOMIASIS, continued			
T. b. rhodesiense **(East African trypanosomiasis, sleeping sickness)**			
hemolymphatic stage			
Drug of choice:	Suramin*	100–200 mg (test dose) IV, then 1 gram IV on days 1, 3, 7, 14, and 21	20 mg/kg on days 1, 3, 7, 14, and 21
OR	Eflornithine*	See footnote 96	
late disease with CNS involvement *(T.b. gambiense or T.b. rhodesiense)*			
Drug of choice:	Melarsoprol[97]*	2–3.6 mg/kg/d IV × 3 d; after 1 wk 3.6 mg/kg per day IV × 3d; repeat again after 10–21 days	18–25 mg/kg total over 1 month; initial dose of 0.36 mg/kg IV, increasing gradually to max. 3.6 mg/kg at intervals of 1–5d for total of 9–10 doses
OR	Eflornithine	See footnote 96	
VISCERAL LARVA MIGRANS[98] (Toxocariasis)			
Drug of choice:	Albendazole[5]	400 mg bid × 5d	400 mg bid × 5d
	Mebendazole[5]	100–200 mg bid × 5d	100-200 mg bid × 5d
Whipworm, see TRICHURIASIS			
Wuchereria bancrofti, see FILARIASIS			

* Availability problems. See table on p 718.

97. In frail patients, begin with as little as 18 mg and increase the dose progressively. Pretreatment with suramin has been advocated for debilitated patients. Corticosteroids have been used to prevent arsenical encephalopathy (J Pepin et al, Trans R Soc Trop Med Hyg, 89:92, 1995). Up to 20% of patients fail to respond to melarsoprol (MP Barrett, Lancet, 353:1113, 1999).

98. For severe symptoms or eye involvement, corticosteroids can be used in addition.

Table 4.14. **Manufacturers of Some Antiparasitic Drugs**

albendazole —*Albenza* (SmithKline Beecham)
§ aminosidine, see paromomycin
§ artemether—*Artenam* (Arenco, Belgium)
§ artesunate—(Guilin No. 1 Factory, People's Republic of China)
atovaquone —*Mepron* (Glaxo-Wellcome)
atovaquone/proguanil — *Malarone* (Glaxo-Wellcome)
bacitracin—many manufacturers
§ bacitracin-zinc—(Apothekernes Laboratorium A.S., Oslo, Norway)
§ benznidazole—*Rochagan* (Roche, Brazil)
† bithionol—*Bitin* (Tanabe, Japan)
chloroquine HCl and chloroquine phosphate—*Aralen* (Sanofi), others
crotamiton—*Eurax* (Westwood-Squibb)
dapsone—(Jacobus)
† diethylcarbamazine citrate USP—(University of Iowa School of Pharmacy)
§ diloxanide furoate—*Furamide* (Boots, United Kingdom)
§ eflornithine (Difluoromethylornithine, DFMO)—*Ornidyl* (Ilex-Oncology, Inc)
furazolidone—*Furoxone* (Roberts)
§ halofantrine —*Halfan* (SmithKline Beecham)
iodoquinol—*Yodoxin* (Glenwood), others
ivermectin—*Stromectol* (Merck)
malathion—*Ovide* (Medicis)
mebendazole—*Vermox* (McNeil)
mefloquine—*Lariam* (Roche)
§ meglumine antimonate—*Glucantime* (Rhône-Poulenc Rorer, France)
§ melarsoprol—*Arsobal* (Rhône-Poulenc Rorer)
metronidazole—*Flagyl* (Searle), others
§ miltefosine—(Asta Medica, Germany)
§ niclosamide—*Yomesan* (Bayer, Germany)
† nifurtimox—*Lampit* (Bayer, Germany)
§ nitazoxanide—*Cryptaz* (Romark)
§ ornidazole—*Tiberal* (Hoffman-LaRoche, Switzerland)
oxamniquine—*Vansil* (Pfizer)
paromomycin—*Humatin* (Parke-Davis); aminosidine (topical and parenteral formulations not available in USA)
pentamidine isethionate—*Pentam 300, NebuPent* (Fujisawa)
permethrin—*Nix* (Glaxo-Wellcome), *Elimite* (Allergan), *Lyclear* (Canada)
praziquantel—*Biltricide* (Bayer)
primaquine phosphate USP
§ proguanil—*Paludrine* (Wyeth Ayerst, Canada; Zeneca, United Kingdom)
§ propamidine isethionate—*Brolene* (Rhône-Poulenc Rorer, Canada)
pyrantel pamoate—*Antiminth* (Pfizer)
pyrethrins and piperonyl butoxide—RID (Pfizer), others

Table 4.14. Manufacturers of Some Antiparasitic Drugs, continued

pyrimethamine USP—*Daraprim* (Glaxo-Wellcome)
quinine sulfate—many manufacturers
§ quinine dihydrochloride
† sodium stibogluconate —*Pentostam* (Glaxo-Wellcome, United Kingdom)
* spiramycin—*Rovamycine* (Rhône-Poulenc Rorer)
† suramin sodium—(Bayer, Germany)
thiabendazole—*Mintezol* (Merck)
§ tinidazole—*Fasigyn* (Pfizer)
§ triclabendazole—*Fasinex* (Novartis Agri-business)
trimetrexate—*Neutrexin* (US Bioscience)

* Available in the USA only from the manufacturer.
§ Not available in the USA.
† Available under an Investigational New Drug (IND) protocol from the CDC Drug Service, Centers for Disease Control and Prevention, Atlanta, Georgia 30333; 404-639-3670 (evenings, weekends, or holidays: 404-639-2888).

Table 4.15. **Principal Adverse Effects of Some Antiparasitic Drugs***

ALBENDAZOLE *(Albenza)*

Occasional: abdominal pain; reversible alopecia; increased serum transaminase activity; migration of ascaris through mouth and nose

Rare: leukopenia; rash; renal toxicity

AMPHOTERICIN B (*Fungizone*, others)

Frequent: renal damage; hypokalemia; thrombophlebitis at site of peripheral vein infusion; anorexia; headache; nausea; weight loss; bone marrow suppression with reversible decline in hematocrit; chills, fever, vomiting during infusion, possibly with delirium, hypotension or hypertension, wheezing, and hypoxemia, especially in cardiac or pulmonary disease

Occasional: hypomagnesemia; normocytic, normochromic anemia

Rare: hemorrhagic gastroenteritis; blood dyscrasias; rash; blurred vision; peripheral neuropathy; convulsions; anaphylaxis; arrhythmias; acute liver failure; reversible nephrogenic diabetes insipidus; hearing loss; acute pulmonary edema; spinal cord damage with intrathecal use

ARTEMETHER *(Artenam)*

Occasional: neurological toxicity; possible increase in length of coma; increased convulsions; prolongation of QTc interval

ARTESUNATE

Occasional: ataxia; slurred speech; neurological toxicity; possible increase in length of coma; increased convulsions; prolongation of QTc interval

ATOVAQUONE (*Mepron, Malarone* [with proguanil])

Frequent: rash; nausea

Occasional: diarrhea; increased aminotransferase activity; cholestasis

BENZNIDAZOLE *(Rochagan)*

Frequent: allergic rash; dose-dependent polyneuropathy; gastrointestinal disturbances; psychic disturbances

BIOTHIONOL *(Bitin)*

Frequent: photosensitivity reactions, vomiting; diarrhea; abdominal pain; urticaria

Rare: leukopenia; toxic hepatitis

CHLOROQUINE HCL and **CHLOROQUINE PHOSPHATE** (*Aralen*, and others)

Occasional: pruritus; vomiting; headache; confusion; depigmentation of hair; skin eruptions; corneal opacity; weight loss; partial alopecia; extraocular muscle palsies; exacerbation of psoriasis, eczema, and other exfoliative dermatoses; myalgias; photophobia

Rare: irreversible retinal injury (especially when total dosage exceeds 100 grams); discoloration of nails and mucous membranes; nerve-type deafness; peripheral neuropathy and myopathy; heart block; blood dyscrasias; hematemesis

CLINDAMYCIN (*Cleocin,* others)

Frequent: diarrhea; allergic reactions

Occasional: pseudomembranous colitis, sometimes severe, can occur even with topical use

Rare: blood dyscrasias; esophageal ulceration; hepatotoxicity; arrhythmia due to QTC prolongation

Table 4.15. **Principal Adverse Effects of Some Antiparasitic Drugs,* continued**

CROTAMITON *(Eurax)*
Occasional: rash

DAPSONE
Frequent: rash; transient headache; GI irritation; anorexia; infectious mononucleosis-like syndrome
Occasional: cyanosis due to methemoglobinemia and sulfhemoglobinemia; other blood dyscrasias, including hemolytic anemia; nephrotic syndrome; liver damage; peripheral neuropathy; hypersensitivity reactions; increased risk of lepra reactions; insomnia; irritability; uncoordinated speech; agitation; acute psychosis
Rare: renal papillary necrosis; severe hypoalbuminemia; epidermal necrolysis; optic atrophy; agranulocytosis; neonatal hyperbilirubinemia after use in pregnancy

DIETHYLCARBAMAZINE CITRATE *(Hetrazan)*
Frequent: severe allergic or febrile reactions in patients with microfilaria in the blood or the skin; GI disturbances
Rare: encephalopathy

DILOXANIDE FUROATE *(Furamide)*
Frequent: flatulence
Occasional: nausea; vomiting; diarrhea
Rare: diplopia; dizziness; urticaria; pruritus

DOXYCYCLINE — See Tetracyclines

EFLORNITHINE (Difluoromethylornithine, DFMO, *Ornidyl*)
Frequent: anemia; leukopenia
Occasional: diarrhea; thrombocytopenia; seizures
Rare: hearing loss

FURAZOLIDONE *(Furoxone)*
Frequent: nausea; vomiting
Occasional: allergic reactions, including pulmonary infiltration; hypotension; urticaria; fever; vesicular rash; hypoglycemia; headache
Rare: hemolytic anemia in G-6-PD deficiency and neonates; disulfiram-like reaction with alcohol; MAO-inhibitor interactions; polyneuritis

HALOFANTRINE *(Halfan)*
Occasional: diarrhea; abdominal pain; pruritus; prolongation of QTc and PR interval

IODOQUINOL (*Yodoxin,* others)
Occasional: rash; acne; slight enlargement of the thyroid gland; nausea; diarrhea; cramps; anal pruritus
Rare: optic neuritis; optic atrophy; loss of vision; peripheral neuropathy after prolonged use in high dosage (for months); iodine sensitivity

IVERMECTIN *(Stromectol)*
Occasional: Mazzotti-type reaction seen in onchocerciasis, including fever, pruritus, tender lymph nodes, headache, and joint and bone pain
Rare: hypotension

MALATHION *(Ovide)*
Occasional: local irritation

Table 4.15. **Principal Adverse Effects of Some Antiparasitic Drugs,* continued**

MEBENDAZOLE *(Vermox)*
Occasional: diarrhea; abdominal pain; migration of ascaris through mouth and nose
Rare: leukopenia; agranulocytosis; hypospermia

MEFLOQUINE *(Lariam)*
Frequent: vertigo; lightheadedness; nausea; other gastrointestinal disturbances; nightmares; visual disturbances; headache; insomnia
Occasional: confusion
Rare: psychosis; hypotension; convulsions; coma; paresthesias

MEGLUMINE ANTIMONATE *(Glucantime)* — Similar to sodium stibogluconate

MELARSOPROL *(Arsobal)*
Frequent: myocardial damage; albuminuria; hypertension; colic; Herxheimer-type reaction; encephalopathy; vomiting; peripheral neuropathy
Rare: shock

METRONIDAZOLE (*Flagyl,* others)
Frequent: nausea; headache; anorexia; metallic taste
Occasional: vomiting; diarrhea; insomnia; weakness; dry mouth; stomatitis; vertigo; tinnitus; paresthesia; rash; dark urine; urethral burning; disulfiram-like reaction with alcohol; candidiasis
Rare: seizures; pseudomembranous colitis; ataxia; leukopenia; peripheral neuropathy; pancreatitis; encephalopathy

NICLOSAMIDE *(Niclocide)*
Occasional: nausea; abdominal pain

NIFURTIMOX *(Lampit)*
Frequent: anorexia; vomiting; weight loss; loss of memory; sleep disorders; tremor; paresthesias; weakness; polyneuritis
Rare: convulsions; fever; pulmonary infiltrates and pleural effusion

ORNIDAZOLE *(Tiberal)*
Occasional: dizziness; headache; gastrointestinal disturbances
Rare: reversible peripheral neuropathy

OXAMNIQUINE *(Vansil)*
Occasional: headache; fever; dizziness; somnolence and insomnia; nausea; diarrhea; rash; hepatic enzyme changes; ECG changes; EEG changes; orange-red discoloration of urine
Rare: seizures; neuropsychiatric disturbances

PAROMOMYCIN (aminosidine; *Humatin*)
Frequent: GI disturbances with oral use
Rare: eighth-nerve damage (mainly auditory) and renal damage when aminosidine is given IV; vertigo; pancreatitis

PENTAMIDINE ISETHIONATE (*Pentam 300, NebuPent,* others)
Frequent: hypotension; hypoglycemia often followed by diabetes mellitus; vomiting; blood dyscrasias; renal damage; pain at injection site; GI disturbances
Occasional: may aggravate diabetes; shock; hypocalcemia; liver damage; cardiotoxicity; delirium; rash
Rare: Herxheimer-type reaction; anaphylaxis; acute pancreatitis; hyperkalemia and vomiting with amoxicillin/clavulanic acid in children

Table 4.15. **Principal Adverse Effects of Some Antiparasitic Drugs,* continued**

PERMETHRIN (*Nix* others)
Occasional: burning; stinging; numbness; increased pruritus; pain; edema; erythema; rash

PRAZIQUANTEL *(Biltricide)*
Frequent: abdominal pain; diarrhea; malaise; headache; dizziness
Occasional: sedation; fever; sweating; nausea; eosinophilia
Rare: pruritus; rash; edema; hiccups

PRIMAQUINE PHOSPHATE
Frequent: hemolytic anemia in G-6-PD deficiency
Occasional: neutropenia; GI disturbances; methemoglobinemia
Rare: CNS symptoms; hypertension; arrhythmias

PROGUANIL (*Paludrine; Malarone* [with atovaquone])
Occasional: oral ulceration; hair loss; scaling of palms and soles; urticaria
Rare: hematuria (with large doses); vomiting; abdominal pain; diarrhea (with large doses); thrombocytopenia

PYRANTEL PAMOATE (*Antiminth,* others)
Occasional: GI disturbances; headache; dizziness; rash; fever

PYRETHRINS with **PIPERONYL BUTOXIDE** (*RID,* others)
Occasional: allergic reactions

PYRIMETHAMINE *(Daraprim)*
Occasional: blood dyscrasias; folic acid deficiency
Rare: rash; vomiting; convulsions; shock; possibly pulmonary eosinophilia; fatal cutaneous reactions with **pyrimethamine-sulfadoxine** *(Fansidar)*

QUININE SULFATE — many manufacturers

QUININE DIHYDROCHLORIDE
Frequent: cinchonism (tinnitus, headache, nausea, abdominal pain, visual disturbance)
Occasional: deafness; hemolytic anemia; other blood dyscrasias; photosensitivity reactions; hypoglycemia; arrhythmias; hypotension; drug fever
Rare: blindness; sudden death if injected too rapidly

SODIUM STIBOGLUCONATE *(Pentostam)*
Frequent: muscle and joint pain; fatigue; nausea; increased aminotransferase activity; T-wave flattening or inversion; pancreatitis
Occasional: weakness; abdominal pain; liver damage; bradycardia; leukopenia; thrombocytopenia; rash; vomiting
Rare: diarrhea; pruritus; myocardial damage; hemolytic anemia; renal damage; shock; sudden death

SPIRAMYCIN *(Rovamycine)*
Occasional: GI disturbances
Rare: allergic reactions

Table 4.15. **Principal Adverse Effects of Some Antiparasitic Drugs,* continued**

SULFONAMIDES

Frequent: allergic reactions (rash, photosensitivity, drug fever)

Occasional: kernicterus in newborn; renal damage; liver damage; Stevens-Johnson syndrome (particularly with long-acting sulfonamides); hemolytic anemia; other blood dyscrasias; vasculitis

Rare: transient acute myopia; pseudomembranous colitis; reversible infertility in men with sulfasalazine; CNS toxicity with trimethoprim-sulfamethoxazole in patients with AIDS

SURAMIN SODIUM

Frequent: vomiting; pruritus; urticaria; paresthesias; hyperesthesia of hands and feet; photophobia; peripheral neuropathy

Occasional: kidney damage; blood dyscrasias; shock; optic atrophy

TETRACYCLINES (demeclocycline — *Declomycin;* doxycycline — *Vibramycin,* others; minocycline — *Minocin,* others; oxytetracycline —*Terramycin,* others; tetracycline hydrochloride — *Sumycin,* others)

Frequent: GI disturbance; bone lesions and staining and deformity of teeth in children up to 8 years old, and in the newborn when given to pregnant women after the fourth month of pregnancy

Occasional: malabsorption; enterocolitis; photosensitivity reactions (most frequent with demeclocycline); vestibular toxicity with minocycline; increased azotemia with renal insufficiency (except doxycycline, but exacerbation of renal failure with doxycycline has been reported); renal insufficiency with demeclocycline in cirrhotic patients; hepatic injury; parenteral doses may cause serious liver damage, especially in pregnant women and patients with renal disease receiving 1 gram or more daily; esophageal ulcerations; cutaneous and mucosal hyperpigmentation, tooth discoloration with minocycline

Rare: allergic reactions, including serum sickness and anaphylaxis; pseudomembranous colitis; blood dyscrasias; drug-induced lupus with minocycline; autoimmune hepatitis increased intracranial pressure; fixed-drug eruptions; diabetes insipidus with demeclocycline; transient acute myopia; blurred vision, diplopia, papilledema; photoonycholysis and onycholysis; acute interstitial nephritis with minocycline; aggravation of myasthenic symptoms with IV injection, reversed with calcium; possibly transient neuropathy; hemolytic anemia

THIABENDAZOLE *(Mintezol)*

Frequent: nausea; vomiting; vertigo; headache; drowsiness, pruritus

Occasional: leukopenia; crystalluria; rash; hallucinations and other psychiatric reactions; visual and olfactory disturbance; erythema multiforme

Rare: shock; tinnitus; intrahepatic cholestasis; convulsions; angioneurotic edema; Stevens-Johnson syndrome

TINIDAZOLE *(Fasigyn)*

Occasional: metallic taste; nausea; vomiting; rash

TRIMETHOPRIM (*Proloprim,* others)

Frequent: nausea, vomiting with high doses

Occasional: megaloblastic anemia; thrombocytopenia; neutropenia; rash; fixed drug eruption

Rare: pancytopenia; hyperkalemia

Table 4.15. **Principal Adverse Effects of Some Antiparasitic Drugs,* continued**

TRIMETHOPRIM-SULFAMETHOXAZOLE (*Bactrim, Septra,* others)
Frequent: rash; fever; nausea and vomiting
Occasional: hemolysis in G-6-PD deficiency; acute megaloblastic anemia; granulocytopenia; thrombocytopenia; pseudomembranous colitis; kernicterus in newborn; hyperkalemia
Rare: agranulocytosis; aplastic anemia; hepatotoxicity; Stevens-Johnson syndrome; aseptic meningitis; fever; confusion; depression; hallucinations; deterioration in renal disease; intrahepatic cholestasis; methemoglobinemia; pancreatitis; ataxia; CNS toxicity in patients with AIDS; renal tubular acidosis; hyperkalemia

TRIMETREXATE (*Neutrexin;* with "leucovorin rescue")
Occasional: rash; peripheral neuropathy; bone marrow depression; increased serum aminotransferase activity

*Drug interactions are generally not included here; see the current edition of *The Medical Letter Handbook of Adverse Drug Interactions.*

MEDWATCH — THE FDA MEDICAL PRODUCTS REPORTING PROGRAM

MEDWATCH, the Food and Drug Administration (FDA) Medical Products Reporting Program, is an educational and promotional initiative to enhance the effectiveness of postmarking surveillance of all medical products regulated by the FDA, including drugs and biologics as well as medical devices and special nutritional products including medical foods, dietary supplements, and infant formulas. Physicians and other health care professionals are in the best position to recognize problems and deficiencies arising from the use of medical products. The FDA and the manufacturer are most dependent on clinicians to monitor for and report adverse events and other problems with medical products, which is why the FDA strongly encourages such reporting in the interest of public health. The only human medical product exception is vaccines. Adverse events and problems associated with vaccines should be reported to the Vaccine Adverse Events Reporting System (VAERS) (see Reporting of Adverse Events, p 31).

The program, MEDWATCH, has 4 general goals: (1) to increase awareness of medical product-induced disease; (2) to clarify what should (and should not) be reported to the agency; (3) to make reporting easier, and (4) to provide regular feedback to the health care community about safety issues involving medical products.

Reporting is facilitated by a 1-page, postage-paid, voluntary form (see Fig 4.1, p 727) that enables health care professionals and consumers to report directly to the agency and/or the manufacturer. A 24-hour toll-free number (800-FDA-1088) also is available for health care professionals to report by telephone. This number can be used by health care professionals and consumers to request forms either via fax or mail, or to obtain a copy of the *FDA Desk Guide to Adverse Event and Product Problem Reporting,* which includes examples of events to report, completed sample forms, and also blank forms with instructions. Reports also can be transmitted to MEDWATCH by fax (800-FDA-0178) or by using the interactive form on the MEDWATCH Web site (www.fda.gov/medwatch).

Fig 4.1. MedWatch reporting form.

Form Approved: OMB No. 0910-0291 Expires: 11/30/98
See OMB statement on reverse

MEDWATCH
THE FDA MEDICAL PRODUCTS REPORTING PROGRAM

For use by user-facilities, distributors and manufacturers for MANDATORY reporting

Page ___ of ___

Mfr report #
UF/Dist report #
FDA Use Only

PLEASE TYPE OR USE BLACK INK

A. Patient information

1. Patient identifier — In confidence
2. Age at time of event: or Date of birth:
3. Sex — female / male
4. Weight — lbs or kgs

B. Adverse event or product problem

1. Adverse event and/or Product problem (e.g., defects/malfunctions)
2. Outcomes attributed to adverse event (check all that apply)
   - death (mo/day/yr)
   - life-threatening
   - hospitalization – initial or prolonged
   - disability
   - congenital anomaly
   - required intervention to prevent permanent impairment/damage
   - other:
3. Date of event (mo/day/yr)
4. Date of this report (mo/day/yr)
5. Describe event or problem
6. Relevant tests/laboratory data, including dates
7. Other relevant history, including preexisting medical conditions (e.g., allergies, race, pregnancy, smoking and alcohol use, hepatic/renal dysfunction, etc.)

C. Suspect medication(s)

1. Name (give labeled strength & mfr/labeler, if known) #1 #2
2. Dose, frequency & route used #1 #2
3. Therapy dates (if unknown, give duration) from/to (or best estimate) #1 #2
4. Diagnosis for use (indication) #1 #2
5. Event abated after use stopped or dose reduced — #1 yes no doesn't apply; #2 yes no doesn't apply
6. Lot # (if known) #1 #2
7. Exp. date (if known) #1 #2
8. Event reappeared after reintroduction — #1 yes no doesn't apply; #2 yes no doesn't apply
9. NDC # – for product problems only (if known) - -
10. Concomitant medical products and therapy dates (exclude treatment of event)

D. Suspect medical device

1. Brand name
2. Type of device
3. Manufacturer name & address
4. Operator of device — health professional / lay user/patient / other:
5. Expiration date (mo/day/yr)
6. model # / catalog # / serial # / lot # / other #
7. If implanted, give date (mo/day/yr)
8. If explanted, give date (mo/day/yr)
9. Device available for evaluation? (Do not send to FDA) yes no returned to manufacturer on (mo/day/yr)
10. Concomitant medical products and therapy dates (exclude treatment of event)

E. Initial reporter

1. Name & address — phone #
2. Health professional? yes no
3. Occupation
4. Initial reporter also sent report to FDA — yes no unk

FDA

FDA Form 3500A

Submission of a report does not constitute an admission that medical personnel, user facility, distributor, manufacturer or product caused or contributed to the event.

The MEDWATCH form contains 2 pages. Contact the FDA for both pages of this form.

Antimicrobial Prophylaxis

ANTIMICROBIAL PROPHYLAXIS

Antimicrobial agents commonly are prescribed to prevent infections in infants and children. The efficacy of the prophylactic use of these agents has been documented for some conditions but is unsubstantiated for most. Chemoprophylaxis is directed at different, but not mutually exclusive, targets: specific pathogens, infection-prone body sites, and vulnerable hosts. Effective prophylaxis is achieved more readily with specific pathogens and certain body sites. In any situation in which prophylactic antimicrobial therapy is being considered, the risk of emergence of resistant organisms must be weighed against the potential benefits. Prophylactic agents should have as narrow a spectrum of antimicrobial activity as possible and should be used for as brief a period of time as possible.

Specific Pathogens

Prophylaxis is feasible if the physician can recognize situations associated with an increased risk of serious infection with a specific pathogen and select an antimicrobial agent that will eliminate the pathogen from persons at risk with minimal adverse effects. For some pathogens that initially colonize the upper respiratory tract, elimination of the carrier state can be difficult. It may require the use of an antimicrobial agent, such as rifampin, that achieves effective concentrations in nasopharyngeal secretions, a property often lacking among antimicrobial agents ordinarily used to treat infections caused by such pathogens. In cases in which prophylaxis is recommended, the regimen is described in the disease-specific chapter in Section 3.

Infection-Prone Body Sites

Prevention of infection of vulnerable body sites may be possible if (1) the period of risk is defined and brief, (2) the expected pathogens have predictable antimicrobial susceptibility, and (3) the site is accessible to antimicrobial agents. Discussion of the prevention of surgical wound infection and neonatal ophthalmia is given in this section.

Otitis media recurs less frequently in otitis-prone children treated prophylactically with antimicrobial agents. Studies have demonstrated that either amoxicillin or sulfisoxazole is effective. However, antimicrobial prophylaxis may alter the nasopharyngeal flora and foster colonization with resistant organisms, compromising long-term efficacy of the prophylactic drug. Antimicrobial prophylaxis should be reserved for control of recurrent acute otitis media, defined by 3 or more distinct and well-documented episodes during a period of 6 months or 4 or more episodes during a period of 12 months.

Protection afforded the urinary tract by chemoprophylaxis depends on the rate of emergence of antimicrobial resistance in the gastrointestinal tract flora, the usual source of bacteria that invade the urinary tract. The long-term effectiveness of nitrofurantoin and trimethoprim-sulfamethoxazole is explained by the minimal effect of these drugs on development of resistant flora. Both drugs are concentrated in urine, and adequate inhibitory activity can be obtained with less than the usual therapeutic dose. Use of a single dose at bedtime has been successful.

Chemoprophylaxis of human and animal bite wounds has become common practice even though dog bites, the most common wound, become infected in only 5% of cases (see Bite Wounds, p 155, for recommendations).

Vulnerable Hosts

Most attempts to prevent bacterial infections in vulnerable patients with antimicrobial prophylaxis have been unsuccessful because of the rapid emergence of bacteria resistant to those antimicrobials. Recommendations for prevention of opportunistic infections in persons infected with human immunodeficiency virus are available.*

ANTIMICROBIAL PROPHYLAXIS IN PEDIATRIC SURGICAL PATIENTS

A major use of antimicrobial agents in hospitalized children is for prophylaxis against postoperative wound infections. In view of this frequent use and the emerging consensus on recommendations for prevention of surgical wound infections, guidelines for surgical antimicrobial prophylaxis in children have been developed. *Prophylaxis* is defined as the use of antimicrobial drugs in the absence of suspected or documented infection to reduce the incidence of infection.

Frequency of Antimicrobial Prophylaxis

In hospitalized patients, antimicrobial drugs commonly are initiated for prophylaxis of wound infection after surgery or an invasive procedure, such as cystoscopy or cardiac catheterization. The frequency and reasons for antimicrobial use have been studied primarily in general hospitals, but the patterns of use in children are similar to those in adults. Two studies have demonstrated that prophylaxis accounts for approximately 75% of antibiotic use on pediatric surgical services. The efficacy of antimicrobial agents in lowering the incidence of postoperative infection after certain types of surgery has been amply demonstrated in controlled clinical trials. These and earlier studies in experimental animals have delineated the principles for effective use of antimicrobial agents in prophylaxis of wound infections, including choice of drugs, optimal time of administration, and duration of prophylaxis.

* Centers for Disease Control and Prevention. 1999 USPHS/IDSA guidelines for the prevention of opportunistic infections in persons infected with human immunodeficiency virus. US Public Health Service and Infectious Diseases Society of America. *MMWR Morb Mortal Wkly Rep.* 1999;48(RR-10):1–66

Inappropriate Antimicrobial Prophylaxis

Prophylaxis has been identified as a major cause of inappropriate use of antimicrobial agents in both adults and children. In a study of children younger than 6 years of age undergoing surgery in which appropriateness of use was assessed on the basis of commonly accepted guidelines, prophylactic antimicrobial agents were administered inappropriately to 42% of children receiving preoperative antimicrobial agents, 67% receiving intraoperative antimicrobial agents, and 55% receiving postoperative antimicrobial agents. Similarly, in a large teaching hospital, 66% of antimicrobial use in children on surgical services was considered inappropriate for reasons of wrong drug, dose, time of initiation, duration, or lack of indication. These studies suggest that the use of antimicrobial agents in children undergoing surgery and other invasive procedures should be subject to periodic review. The consequences of inappropriate or excessive use of prophylactic antimicrobial agents include increased costs through unnecessary drug use, potential emergence of resistant organisms, and adverse events.

Guidelines for Appropriate Use

Studies documenting that systemic prophylaxis reduces the incidence of surgical wound infections have been performed primarily in adults. Because the pathogenesis of these infections is the same in children, the principles of surgical prophylaxis in children should be similar. In the absence of studies in children, guidelines recommended by *The Medical Letter,** the American College of Surgeons, the Surgical Infection Society,† and the Hospital Infections program of the Centers for Disease Control and Prevention‡ provide standards for use of systemic prophylactic antibiotics in pediatric surgical patients. The following general principles are recommended as guidelines, with the understanding that studies in children may result in changes and that factors unique to infants and children, such as prematurity or certain immunodeficiencies, may justify exceptions.

Indications for Prophylaxis

Systemic prophylaxis is indicated when the benefits of preventing wound infection outweigh the risks of potential toxic or allergic drug reactions and the emergence of resistant bacteria. The latter poses a potential risk not only to the recipient, but also to other hospitalized patients in whom a nosocomial infection caused by antibiotic-resistant organisms may develop. Procedures in which the benefits justify the risks incurred in antimicrobial prophylaxis are those associated with a significant incidence of postoperative infection and those in which the likelihood of infection may not be great but the consequences of infection are extreme morbidity or mortality, such as with prosthetic materials.

* Antimicrobial prophylaxis in surgery. *Med Lett Drugs Ther.* 1999;41:75–80

† Page CP, Bohnen JMA, Fletcher JR, McManus AT, Solomkin JS, Wittmann DH. Antimicrobial prophylaxis for surgical wounds: guidelines for clinical care [published correction appears in *Arch Surg.* 1993;128:410]. *Arch Surg.* 1993;128:79–88

‡ Mangram AJ, Horan TC, Pearson ML, Silver LC, Jarvis WR. Guideline for prevention of surgical site infection, 1999. *Infect Control Hosp Epidemiol.* 1999;20:247–278

A major determinant of the probability of surgical wound infection is the number of microorganisms in the wound at the completion of the procedure. This fact allows the classification of surgical procedures (see the Addendum, p 734) based on an estimation of bacterial contamination and the risk of subsequent infection, into the 4 following categories: (1) clean wounds, (2) clean-contaminated wounds, (3) contaminated wounds, and (4) dirty and infected wounds. As evidenced by the wide variation in infection rates within these categories, however, wound classification is not the only factor in the risk of wound infection. Significant additive risk factors include the site of operation, the duration of the procedure, and the patient's health status. The use of a patient risk index, which in addition to classifying wounds as contaminated or dirty and infected also considers the American Society of Anesthesiologists preoperative assessment score and the duration of the operation, has been demonstrated to be a better predictor of postoperative wound infection than wound classification alone.*

CLEAN WOUNDS

Conventional use of antibiotic prophylaxis primarily involves clean-contaminated and selected contaminated wounds. The benefits of systemic antimicrobial prophylaxis may not justify the potential risks associated with antimicrobial use in most clean wound procedures. Several exceptions exist in which the consequences of infection may be major and life-threatening. Examples are implantation of a prosthetic foreign body (eg, insertion of a prosthetic heart valve), open-heart surgery for repair of structural defects, compromised immune status (such as patients receiving high doses of corticosteroids or chemotherapy for a malignant neoplasm or persons with prior splenectomy), and body cavity exploration in neonates. Prophylaxis has been given in these circumstances, although studies establishing efficacy have not been performed. Prophylaxis may be justified for patients with 2 or more of the risk factors previously listed. Systemic antimicrobial agents also have been recommended empirically for clean procedures in patients with infection at another site.

CLEAN-CONTAMINATED WOUNDS

In clean-contaminated wound procedures, the degree of contamination is variable, and prophylaxis is limited to procedures with significant risk of wound contamination and infection. Based on data from adults, indications for prophylaxis for pediatric patients include the following: (1) many alimentary tract procedures, (2) selected biliary tract operations (eg, with common duct stones), and (3) urinary tract surgery or instrumentation in the presence of bacteriuria or obstructive uropathy.

CONTAMINATED WOUNDS AND DIRTY AND INFECTED WOUNDS

In contaminated wound procedures, antibiotic prophylaxis against postoperative wound infections is appropriate for selected cases involving acute nonpurulent inflammation isolated to and contained within an inflamed viscus (such as acute appendicitis or cholecystitis). In contaminated wounds resulting from other causes,

* Culver DH, Horan TC, Gaynes RP, et al. Surgical wound infection rates by wound class, operative procedure, and patient risk index: National Nosocomial Infections Surveillance System. *Am J Med.* 1991;91(suppl 3B):152S–157S

however, antimicrobial therapy should be considered treatment rather than prophylaxis.

In dirty and infected wound procedures, such as those for a perforated abdominal viscus, a compound fracture, or a laceration due to an animal or human bite, or if a major break in sterile technique has occurred, antimicrobial agents are given as treatment rather than prophylaxis.

When Should Prophylactic Antibiotics Be Given?

Prophylaxis of infection requires effective drug concentrations in tissues during surgical procedures because bacterial contamination occurs intraoperatively. Antimicrobial administration within 2 hours before surgery has been demonstrated to reduce the risk of wound infection. Accordingly, administration is recommended 30 minutes before the surgical incision to ensure adequate tissue concentration throughout the operation. The exception is for patients undergoing cesarean section, in whom the drug should be given after the umbilical cord is clamped.

Duration of Administration of Antimicrobial Agents

A single antimicrobial dose that provides adequate tissue concentration throughout the procedure usually is sufficient. When surgery is prolonged (more than 4 hours) or major blood loss occurs, or an antimicrobial agent with a short half-life is used, one or more doses is advisable during the procedure. While published studies of antimicrobial prophylaxis often use 1 or 2 doses postoperatively in addition to 1 preoperative dose, most surgeons believe that postoperative doses of prophylactic drugs are unnecessary. These recommendations are based on studies in adults and may not apply to all pediatric patients, particularly neonates. However, inasmuch as the pathogenesis of wound infection does not differ with age, the recommendation for brief duration of prophylaxis probably is applicable to patients of all ages.

Which Antibiotics Should Be Given?

The choice of an antimicrobial agent is based on knowledge of the common bacteria causing infectious complications after the specific procedure, bacterial susceptibility to the drug, proven efficacy of the drug selected, and the safety of the drug. New, costly antimicrobial agents generally should not be used unless prophylactic efficacy has been proven superior to that of drugs of established benefit. The drugs should be active against the most likely pathogens. They do not have to be active against every potential organism, since effective prophylaxis seems to correlate with a decrease in the total number of pathogens rather than eradication of all organisms. Routine use of vancomycin and extended-spectrum cephalosporins for surgical prophylaxis is not indicated. Recommended doses and route of administration are based on the need to achieve therapeutic blood and tissue concentrations throughout the procedure; parenteral (usually intravenous) administration usually is necessary. Antimicrobial prophylaxis for most surgical procedures (including gastric, biliary, thoracic [noncardiac], vascular, neurosurgical, and orthopedic operations) can be achieved effectively using an agent such as a first-generation cephalosporin (eg, cefazolin). For colorectal surgery and appendectomy, effective prophylaxis requires antimicrobial agents that are active against intestinal anaerobes and gram-negative anaerobes, such as cefoxitin. Optimal prophylaxis against wound infection after colon surgery involves a combination of mechanical bowel cleansing, oral neomycin-erythromycin, and appropriate parenteral antibiotics.

Physicians should be aware of potential interactions and adverse effects associated with prophylactic antimicrobial agents and other medications that the patient is receiving.

Conclusions

These guidelines for antimicrobial prophylaxis of surgical wound infections in children were developed originally by the Committee on Infectious Diseases in collaboration with the Committee on Drugs and the Section on Surgery of the American Academy of Pediatrics in 1984.* They have been modified in accordance with recent data and recommendations. Because the benefit of systemic antimicrobial prophylaxis in many pediatric surgical procedures has not been established, additional studies in commonly performed surgical procedures in children (eg, insertion of neurosurgical shunts and orthopedic procedures) are needed. Pediatricians, pediatric surgeons, and surgical subspecialists should review the prophylactic use of antimicrobial agents as part of the monitoring of antibiotic use in their hospitals, and they should use the guidelines given here to develop standards for antimicrobial use to reduce the incidence of postoperative wound infections and the expenses and adverse reactions caused by inappropriate or excessive antibiotic use.

Addendum

Definitions of surgical wounds in the classification scheme are as follows:

CLEAN WOUNDS

Clean wounds are uninfected operative wounds in which no inflammation is encountered, and the respiratory, alimentary, and genitourinary tracts and oropharyngeal cavity are not entered. The operative procedures are elective, and the wounds are closed primarily and, if necessary, drained with closed drainage. No break in technique occurs. Operative incisional wounds that follow nonpenetrating (blunt) abdominal trauma should be included in this category, provided that the surgical procedure does not entail entry into the gastrointestinal or genitourinary tracts.

CLEAN-CONTAMINATED WOUNDS

In clean-contaminated operative wounds, the respiratory, alimentary, or genitourinary tract is entered under controlled conditions and without unusual contamination. Operations involving the biliary tract, appendix, vagina, and oropharynx and urgent or emergency surgery in an otherwise clean procedure are included in this category, provided that no evidence of infection is encountered and no major break in technique occurs.

* See American Academy of Pediatrics Committee on Infectious Diseases, Committee on Drugs, and Section on Surgery. Antimicrobial prophylaxis in pediatric surgical patients. *Pediatrics*. 1984;74:437–439

CONTAMINATED WOUNDS

Contaminated wounds include open, fresh, accidental wounds; operative wounds in the setting of major breaks in sterile technique or gross spillage from the gastrointestinal tract; penetrating trauma less than 4 hours before; and incisions in which acute nonpurulent inflammation is encountered.

DIRTY AND INFECTED WOUNDS

Dirty and infected wounds include penetrating traumatic wounds of more than 4 hours' duration, those with retained devitalized tissue, and wounds involving existing clinical infection or perforated viscera. This definition suggests that the organisms causing postoperative infection were present in the operative field before surgery.

PREVENTION OF BACTERIAL ENDOCARDITIS

The Committee on Rheumatic Fever, Endocarditis, and Kawasaki Disease of the American Heart Association issues detailed recommendations on the rationale, indications, and antibiotic regimens for the prevention of bacterial endocarditis for persons at increased risk. The most recent recommendations were published in 1997.* The cardiac conditions associated with endocarditis, the procedures for which endocarditis prophylaxis is recommended for persons with cardiac conditions that put them at risk, and the specific prophylactic regimens are presented in Tables 5.1 through 5.5 (pp 736–740). Health care professionals should consult the published recommendations for further details.

PREVENTION OF NEONATAL OPHTHALMIA

Ophthalmia neonatorum, defined as conjunctivitis occurring within the first 4 weeks of life, occurs in 1% to 12% of neonates. The prevalence of infection with *Chlamydia trachomatis* and *Neisseria gonorrhoeae* is related directly to the prevalence of infection among pregnant women and whether pregnant women are screened and treated or newborn infants are given ophthalmia prophylaxis. The major causes of ophthalmia neonatorum are presented in Table 5.6, p 742.

Screening of all pregnant women for chlamydia and gonorrhea infection followed by appropriate treatment and follow-up of all infected women and their partner(s) can minimize the risk of perinatal transmission (see Chlamydial Infections, p 205, and Gonococcal Infections, p 254).

Gonococcal Ophthalmia

For newborn infants, topical 1% silver nitrate solution, 0.5% erythromycin ointment, and 1% tetracycline ointment are considered equally effective for prophylaxis

* Dajani AS, Taubert KA, Wilson W, et al. Prevention of bacterial endocarditis: recommendations by the American Heart Association. *JAMA*. 1997;277:1794–1801

Table 5.1. **Cardiac Conditions Associated With Endocarditis**

Endocarditis Prophylaxis		
Recommended		**Not Recommended**
HIGH RISK	*MODERATE RISK*	*NEGLIGIBLE RISK**
Prosthetic cardiac valves, including bioprosthetic and homograft valves	Most other congenital cardiac malformations (other than those in the high-risk and negligible-risk categories)	Isolated secundum atrial septal defect
Previous bacterial endocarditis	Acquired valvular dysfunction (eg, rheumatic heart disease)	Surgical repair of atrial septal defect, ventricular septal defect, or patent ductus arteriosus (without residua and beyond 6 mo of age)
Complex cyanotic congenital heart disease (eg, single ventricle states, transposition of the great arteries, tetralogy of Fallot)	Hypertrophic cardiomyopathy	Previous coronary artery bypass graft surgery
Surgically constructed systemic pulmonary shunts or conduits	Mitral valve prolapse with valvular regurgitation and/or thickened leaflets†	Mitral valve prolapse without valvular regurgitation†
		Physiologic, functional, or innocent heart murmurs†
		Previous Kawasaki disease without valvular dysfunction
		Previous rheumatic fever without valvular dysfunction
		Cardiac pacemakers (intravascular and epicardial) and implanted defibrillators

* No greater risk than the general population.

† For further details, see Dajani AS, Taubert KA, Wilson W, et al. Prevention of bacterial endocarditis: recommendations by the American Heart Association. *JAMA.* 1997;277:1794–1801

Table 5.2. **Dental Procedures and Endocarditis Prophylaxis**

Endocarditis Prophylaxis	
Recommended*	**Not Recommended**
Dental extractions	Restorative dentistry† (operative and prosthodontic) with or without retraction cord‡
Periodontal procedures, including surgery, scaling and root planing, probing, and routine maintenance	Local anesthetic injections (nonintraligamentary)
Dental implant placement and reimplantation of avulsed teeth	Intracanal endodontic treatment; postplacement and buildup
Endodontic (root canal) instrumentation or surgery only beyond the apex	Placement of rubber dams
Subgingival placement of antibiotic fibers or strips	Postoperative suture removal
Initial placement of orthodontic bands but not brackets	Placement of removable prosthodontic or orthodontic appliances
Intraligamentary local anesthetic injections	Taking of oral impressions
Prophylactic cleaning of teeth or implants during which bleeding is anticipated	Fluoride treatments
	Taking of oral radiographs
	Orthodontic appliance adjustment
	Shedding of primary teeth

* Prophylaxis is recommended for patients with high- and moderate-risk cardiac conditions.

† This includes restoration of decayed teeth (filling cavities) and replacement of missing teeth.

‡ Clinical judgment may indicate antibiotic use in selected circumstances that may create significant bleeding.

Table 5.3. **Other Procedures and Endocarditis Prophylaxis**

	Endocarditis Prophylaxis	
	Recommended	**Not Recommended**
Respiratory tract	Tonsillectomy, adenoidectomy, or both Surgical operations that involve respiratory mucosa Bronchoscopy with a rigid bronchoscope	Endotracheal intubation Bronchoscopy with a flexible bronchoscope, with or without biopsy* Tympanostomy tube insertion
Gastrointestinal tract†	Sclerotherapy for esophageal varices Esophageal stricture dilation Endoscopic retrograde cholangiography with biliary obstruction Biliary tract surgery Surgical operations that involve intestinal mucosa	Transesophageal echocardiography* Endoscopy with or without gastrointestinal biopsy*
Genitourinary tract	Prostatic surgery Cystoscopy Urethral dilation	Vaginal hysterectomy* Vaginal delivery* Cesarean section In uninfected tissue: Urethral catheterization Uterine dilatation and curettage Therapeutic abortion Sterilization procedures Insertion or removal of intrauterine devices
Other		Cardiac catheterization, including balloon angioplasty Implanted cardiac pacemakers, implanted defibrillators, and coronary stents Incision or biopsy of surgically scrubbed skin Circumcision

* Prophylaxis is optional for high-risk patients.
† Prophylaxis is recommended for high-risk patients; optional for medium-risk patients.

Table 5.4. **Prophylactic Regimens for Dental, Oral, Respiratory Tract, or Esophageal Procedures**

Situation	Agent	Regimen*
Standard general prophylaxis	Amoxicillin	Adults: 2.0 g; children: 50 mg/kg orally 1 h before procedure
Unable to take oral medications	Ampicillin	Adults: 2.0 g intramuscularly (IM) or intravenously (IV); children: 50 mg/kg IM or IV within 30 min before procedure
Allergic to penicillin	Clindamycin	Adults: 600 mg; children: 20 mg/kg orally 1 h before procedure
	OR	
	Cephalexin† or cefadroxil†	Adults: 2.0 g; children: 50 mg/kg orally 1 h before procedure
	OR	
	Azithromycin or clarithromycin	Adults: 500 mg; children: 15 mg/kg orally 1 h before procedure
Allergic to penicillin and unable to take oral medications	Clindamycin	Adults: 600 mg; children: 20 mg/kg IV within 30 min before procedure
	OR	
	Cefazolin†	Adults: 1.0 g; children: 25 mg/kg IM or IV within 30 min before procedure

* Total children's dose should not exceed adult dose.

† Cephalosporins should not be used for persons with immediate-type hypersensitivity reaction (urticaria, angioedema, or anaphylaxis) to penicillins.

Table 5.5. **Prophylactic Regimens for Genitourinary and Gastrointestinal Tract (Excluding Esophageal) Procedures**

Situation	Agents*	Regimen†
High-risk patients	Ampicillin **PLUS** Gentamicin	Adults: ampicillin 2.0 g intramuscularly (IM) or intravenously (IV) plus gentamicin 1.5 mg/kg (not to exceed 120 mg) within 30 min of starting the procedure; 6 h later, ampicillin 1 g IM or IV or amoxicillin 1 g orally Children: ampicillin 50 mg/kg IM or IV (not to exceed 2.0 g) plus gentamicin 1.5 mg/kg within 30 min of starting the procedure; 6 h later, ampicillin 25 mg/kg IM or IV or amoxicillin 25 mg/kg orally
High-risk patients allergic to ampicillin or amoxicillin	Vancomycin **PLUS** Gentamicin	Adults: vancomycin 1.0 g IV over 1–2 h plus gentamicin 1.5 mg/kg IV or IM (not to exceed 120 mg); complete injection/infusion within 30 min of starting the procedure Children: vancomycin 20 mg/kg IV over 1–2 h plus gentamicin 1.5 mg/kg IV or IM; complete injection or infusion within 30 min of starting the procedure
Moderate-risk patients	Amoxicillin **OR** Ampicillin	Adults: amoxicillin 2.0 g orally 1 h before procedure, or ampicillin 2.0 g IM or IV within 30 min of starting the procedure Children: amoxicillin 50 mg/kg orally 1 h before procedure, or ampicillin 50 mg/kg IM or IV within 30 min of starting the procedure
Moderate-risk patients allergic to ampicillin or amoxicillin	Vancomycin	Adults: vancomycin 1.0 g IV over 1–2 h; complete infusion within 30 min of starting the procedure Children: vancomycin 20 mg/kg IV over 1–2 h; complete infusion within 30 min of starting the procedure

* Total children's dose should not exceed adult dose.

† No second dose of vancomycin or gentamicin is recommended.

of ocular gonorrheal infection. Each is available in single-dose tubes. Povidone-iodine in a 2.5% solution also might be useful for preventing gonococcal ophthalmia, but more studies are required, and a product for this purpose currently is not available in the United States. Silver nitrate causes more chemical conjunctivitis than other agents but is recommended in areas where the incidence of penicillinase-producing *Neisseria gonorrhoeae* (PPNG) is appreciable. The efficacy of erythromycin or povidone-iodine prophylaxis against PPNG is not known; 1 study has demonstrated tetracycline to be effective for prophylaxis of PPNG infections. Infants born to women with untreated gonococcal infection should receive 1 dose of ceftriaxone (25-50 mg/kg) or cefotaxime (100 mg/kg), as well as topical prophylaxis. Infants who have gonococcal ophthalmia should be hospitalized and evaluated for signs of disseminated infection (see Gonococcal Infections, p 254).

Chlamydial Ophthalmia

Neonatal ophthalmia due to *Chlamydia trachomatis,* although not as severe as gonococcal conjunctivitis, is common in the United States. Results of studies on the clinical efficacy of erythromycin and of tetracycline ointment for prophylaxis of chlamydial conjunctivitis have been conflicting. Topical antibiotics and silver nitrate do not have proven efficacy in preventing conjunctivitis or nasopharyngeal colonization. One study has shown that 2.5% povidone-iodine is likely to be more effective than either topical erythromycin or silver nitrate for preventing chlamydial conjunctivitis but does not prevent nasopharyngeal colonization and subsequent risk of pneumonia. Infants with ophthalmia neonatorum caused by *C trachomatis* should be evaluated and treated (see Chlamydial Infections, p 205).

Nongonococcal Nonchlamydial Ophthalmia

Silver nitrate, povidone-iodine, and, probably, erythromycin are effective for preventing nongonococcal nonchlamydial conjunctivitis during the first 2 weeks of life.

Administration of Neonatal Ophthalmic Prophylaxis for Gonorrhea. Before administering local prophylaxis, each eyelid should be wiped gently with sterile cotton. Two drops of a 1% silver nitrate solution or a 1-cm ribbon of antibiotic ointment (0.5% erythromycin or 1% tetracycline) are placed in each lower conjunctival sac. The eyelids should then be massaged gently to spread the solution or ointment. After 1 minute, excess solution or ointment may be wiped away with sterile cotton. None of the prophylactic agents should be flushed from the eyes after instillation since flushing may reduce the efficacy of prophylaxis.

Infants born by cesarean section should receive prophylaxis against neonatal gonococcal ophthalmia. Although gonococcal and chlamydial infections usually are transmitted to the infant during passage through the birth canal, infection by the ascending route also occurs.

Prophylaxis should be given shortly after birth. Some experts suggest that prophylaxis may be administered more effectively in the nursery than in the delivery room. Delaying prophylaxis for as long as 1 hour after birth to facilitate parent-infant bonding is unlikely to influence efficacy. Longer delays have not been studied for efficacy. Hospitals should establish a system to ensure that all infants are treated.

Table 5.6. **Major and Minor Pathogens in Ophthalmia Neonatorum**

Etiology of Ophthalmia Neonatorum	Percentage of Cases	Incubation Period (d)	Severity of Conjunctivitis*	Associated Problems
Chlamydia trachomatis	2–40	5–14	+	Pneumonitis 3 wk to 3 mo (see Chlamydial Infections, p 205)
Neisseria gonorrhoeae	<1	2–7	+++	Disseminated infection (see Gonococcal Infections, p 254)
Other bacterial microbes†	30–50	5–14	+	Variable
Herpes simplex virus	<1	6–14	+	Disseminated infection (see Herpes Simplex, p 309); keratitis and ulceration also possible
Chemical	Varies with silver nitrate use	1	+	...

* + indicates mild; +++, severe.

† *Staphylococcus* species; *Streptococcus pneumoniae; Haemophilus influenzae,* nontypeable; *Streptococcus mitis;* group A and B streptococci; *Neisseria cinerea; Corynebacterium* species; *Moraxella catarrhalis; Escherichia coli; Klebsiella pneumoniae; Pseudomonas aeruginosa.*

APPENDIX I.

Directory of Resources

Organizations	Telephone/ Fax numbers	Web sites*
American Academy of Pediatrics (AAP) 141 Northwest Point Blvd Elk Grove Village, IL 60007-1098	USA 1-847-228-5005 1-847-228-5097 (Fax)	http://www.aap.org/
AIDS Clinical Trials Information Service (ACTIS) PO Box 6421 Rockville, MD 20849-6421	USA 1-800-Trials-A (1-800-874-2572) TTY: 1-888-480-3739 1-301-519-0459 (International) 1-301-519-6616 (Fax)	http://www.actis.org/
AIDS/HIV Treatment Information Service (ATIS) PO Box 6303 Rockville, MD 20849-6303 USA	1-800-HIV-0440 (1-800-448-0440) (USA & Canada) 1-301-519-0459 (International) 1-301-519-6616 (Fax)	http://www.hivatis.org/
Canadian Paediatric Society (CPS) 2204 Walkley Rd, Ste 100 Ottawa, Ontario K1G 4G8 Canada	1-613-526-9397 1-613-526-3332 (Fax)	http://www.cps.ca/
Centers for Disease Control and Prevention (CDC) 1600 Clifton Rd Atlanta, GA 30333 USA	1-404-639-3311	http://www.cdc.gov/
• 24-Hour Service	1-404-332-4555	
• ABCs of Safe and Healthy Child Care		http://www.cdc.gov/ncidod/hip/abc/contents.htm

* Internet addresses and phone/fax numbers are current at the time of publication.

Directory of Resources, continued

Organizations	Telephone/ Fax numbers	Web sites*
Centers for Disease Control and Prevention (CDC) (continued)	1-404-639-3311	http://www.cdc.gov
• Division of Bacterial and Mycotic Diseases	1-404-639-1603	http://www.cdc.gov/ncidod/dbmd/
• Division of Parasitic Diseases	1-770-488-7775 OR 1-770-488-7760	http://www.cdc.gov/ncidod/dpd/aboutdpd.default.htm/
• Division of Tuberculosis Control	1-404-639-8120	http://www.cdc.gov/niosh/tb.html/
• Division of Viral & Rickettsial Diseases	1-404-639-3574	http://www.cdc.gov/ncidod/dvrd/default.htm/
• Drug Service (weekdays, 8 am to 4:30 pm ET)	1-404-639-3670	http://www.cdc.gov/ncidod/srp/drugservice/index.htm/
• Drug Service (weekends, nights, holidays)	1-404-639-2888	http://www.cdc.gov/ncidod/srp/drugservice/index.htm/
• Voice/Fax Information Service (including international travel and immunization)	1-404-332-4555 (Voice) 1-404-332-4565 (Fax)	http://www.cdc.gov/epo/mmwr/preview/mmwrhtml/00033199.htm/
• Hepatitis Branch	1-404-639-2709	http://www.cdc.gov/ncidod/diseases/hepatitis/
• Immunization, Infectious Diseases, and Other Health Information—Voice Information System	1-800-232-SHOT (1-800-232-7468)	
• International Traveler's Hotline and Fax	1-404-332-4559 1-888-232-3299 (Fax)	http://www.cdc.gov/travel/index.htm/
• National Center for Infectious Diseases	1-404-639-3401	http://www.cdc.gov/ncidod/
• National HIV and AIDS Hotline	1-800-342-AIDS (1-800-342-2437)	http://www.ashastd.org/nah/nah.html/

* Internet addresses and phone/fax numbers are current at the time of publication.

Directory of Resources, continued

Organizations	Telephone/ Fax numbers	Web sites*
Centers for Disease Control and Prevention (CDC) (continued)	1-404-639-3311	http://www.cdc.gov
• National Immunization Program	1-404-639-8200	http://www.cdc.gov/nip/
• National Prevention Information Network		http://www.cdc.gov/hiv/hivinfo/npin.htm
• National Vaccine Injury Compensation Program (for information on filing claims)	1-800-338-2382	http://www.cdc.gov/nip/vacsafe/ qvcipqa2.htm/
• National Vaccine Program Office (NVPO)	1-404-639-4450	http://www.cdc.gov/od/nvpo/
• Public Inquiries	1-404-639-3534	
• Publications	1-404-639-8828 (Fax)	http://www.cdc.gov/publications. htm#pubs/
• Software		http://www.cdc.gov/publications.htm#soft/
• Vector-Borne Infectious Diseases	1-970-221-6400	http://www.cdc.gov/ncidod/ dvbid/dvbid.htm/
Food and Drug Administration (FDA) 5600 Fishers Ln Rockville, MD 20857 USA	1-888-463-6332	http://www.fda.gov/
• Center for Biologics Evaluation and Research	1-301-827-2000 OR 1-800-835-4709	http://www.fda.gov/cber/
• Center for Drug Evaluation and Research	1-301-594-6740	http://www.fda.gov/cder/
• Division of Special Pathogen and Immunologic Drug Products	1-301-827-2127 1-301-927-2475 (Fax)	
• HIV/AIDS Office of Special Health Issues		http://www.fda.gov/oashi/aids/hiv.html/
• Kids' Vaccinations		http://www.fda.gov/opacom/catalog/ vaccine.html/

* Internet addresses and phone/fax numbers are current at the time of publication.

Directory of Resources, continued

Organizations	Telephone/ Fax numbers	Web sites*
Food and Drug Administration (FDA) (continued)		
• MEDWATCH	1-800-FDA-1088 (1-800-332-1088)	http://www.fda.gov/medwatch/
• Vaccine Adverse Events Reporting System (VAERS)	1-800-822-7967	http://www.fda.gov/cber/vaers/new.htm/
Immunization Action Coalition (IAC) 1573 Selby Ave St Paul, MN 55104 USA	1-651-647-9009 1-651- 647-9131 (Fax)	http://www.immunize.org/
Infectious Diseases Society of America (IDSA) 99 Canal Center Plaza, Ste 210 Alexandria, VA 22314 USA	1-703-299-0200 1-703-299-0204 (Fax)	http://www.idsociety.org/
Institute of Medicine (IOM) 2101 Constitution Ave, NW Washington, DC 20418 USA	1-202-334-3300	http://www.iom.edu/
National Network for Immunization Information (NNII) 99 Canal Center Plaza, Ste 210 Alexandria, VA 22314 USA		http://www.idsociety.org/vaccine/index.html/

* Internet addresses and phone/fax numbers are current at the time of publication.

Directory of Resources, continued

Organizations	Telephone/ Fax numbers	Web sites*
National Institutes of Health (NIH) Bethesda, Maryland 20892 USA		http://www.nih.gov/
• National Institute of Allergy and Infectious Diseases (NIAID)		http://www.niaid.nih.gov/
• NIAID Collaborative Antiviral Study Group	1-205-939-9594	http://www.peds.uab.edu/casg/
• U.S. National Library of Medicine 8600 Rockville Pike Bethesda, MD 20894 USA	1-888-346-3656	http://www.nlm.nih.gov/
National Pediatric & Family HIV Resource Center (NPHRC) University of Medicine & Dentistry of New Jersey 30 Bergen St, ADMC #4 Newark, NJ 07103 USA	1-800-362-0071 1-973-972-0399 (Fax)	http://www.pedhivaids.org/
Pediatric AIDS Drug Trials—Information:		
• Pediatric Branch, National Cancer Institute	1-301-402-0696	
• Pediatric Clinical Trials Group (NIAID-sponsored)	1-800-TRIALS-A (1-800-874-2572)	
Pediatric Infectious Diseases Society 99 Canal Center Plaza, Ste 210 Alexandria, VA 22314 USA	1-703-299-6764 1-703-299-0204 (Fax)	http://www.pids.org/
World Health Organization (WHO) Avenue Appia 20 1211 Geneva 27 Switzerland	(+41 22) 791 21 11 (+00 41 22) 791 0746 (Fax)	http://www.who.int/

* Internet addresses and phone/fax numbers are current at the time of publication.

APPENDIX II.

Standards for Pediatric Immunization Practices*

Recommended by the
National Vaccine Advisory Committee (1992)
Approved by the
United States Public Health Service
Endorsed by the
American Academy of Pediatrics

The Standards represent the consensus of the National Vaccine Advisory Committee (NVAC) and of a broad group of medical and public health experts about what constitute the most desirable immunization practices. While not all of the current immunization practices of public and private providers (health care professionals) are in compliance with the Standards, they should be useful as a means of helping providers to identify needed changes, to obtain resources if necessary, and to actually implement the desirable immunization practices in the future.

STANDARDS FOR PEDIATRIC IMMUNIZATION PRACTICES

Preamble

Ideally, immunizations should be given as part of comprehensive child health care. This is the ultimate goal toward which the nation must strive if all of America's children are to benefit from the best primary disease prevention our health care system has to offer.

Overall improvement in our primary care delivery system requires intensive effort and will take time. However, we should not wait for changes in this system before providing immunizations more effectively to our children. Current health care policies and practices in all settings result in the failure to deliver vaccines on schedule to many of our vulnerable preschool-aged children. This failure is due primarily to barriers that impede vaccine delivery and to missed opportunities during clinic visits. Changes in policies and practices can immediately improve coverage. The present system should be geared to "user-friendly," family-centered, culturally sensitive, and comprehensive primary health care that can provide rapid, efficient, and consumer-oriented services to the users, ie, children and their parents. The failure to do so is evidenced by the recent resurgence of measles and measles-related childhood mortality, which may be an omen of other vaccine-preventable disease outbreaks.

Present childhood immunization practices must be changed if we wish to protect the nation's children and immunize 90% of 2-year-olds by the year 2010.

* Modified from *Standards for Pediatric Immunization Practices.* Atlanta, Ga: US Dept of Health and Human Services, Public Health Services, Centers for Disease Control and Prevention; 1993. The major change is an update in the list of vaccine contraindications and precautions to be consistent with current recommendations.

The following standards for pediatric immunization practices address these issues. These standards are recommended for use by **all** health professionals in the public and private sector who administer vaccines to or manage immunization services for infants and children. These **Standards** represent the most desirable immunization practices that health care providers should strive to achieve to the extent possible. By adopting these Standards, providers can begin to enhance and change their own policies and practices. While not all providers will have the funds necessary to fully implement the Standards immediately, those providers and programs lacking the resources to implement the Standards fully should find them a useful tool for better delineating immunization needs and for obtaining additional resources in the future to achieve the Healthy People 2010 immunization objectives.

Standards

Standard 1. Immunization services are **readily available.**
Standard 2. **No barriers** or **unnecessary prerequisites** to the receipt of vaccines exist.
Standard 3. Immunization services are available **free** or for a minimal fee.
Standard 4. Providers use all clinical encounters to **screen** and, when indicated, **immunize** children.
Standard 5. Providers **educate** parents and guardians about immunization in general terms.
Standard 6. Providers **question** parents or guardians about **contraindications** and, before immunizing a child, **inform** them in specific terms about the risks and benefits of the immunizations their child is to receive.
Standard 7. Providers follow only true **contraindications.**
Standard 8. Providers administer **simultaneously** all vaccine doses for which a child is eligible at the time of each visit.
Standard 9. Providers use accurate and complete **recording procedures.**
Standard 10. Providers **coschedule** immunization appointments in conjunction with appointments for other child health services.
Standard 11. Providers **report adverse events** after immunization promptly, accurately, and completely.
Standard 12. Providers operate a **tracking system.**
Standard 13. Providers adhere to appropriate procedures for **vaccine management.**
Standard 14. Providers conduct semiannual **audits** to assess immunization coverage levels and to review immunization records in the patient populations they serve.
Standard 15. Providers maintain up-to-date, easily retrievable **medical protocols** at all locations where vaccines are administered.
Standard 16. Providers operate with **patient-oriented** and **community-based** approaches.
Standard 17. Vaccines are administered by **properly trained** individuals.
Standard 18. Providers receive **ongoing education** and **training** on current immunization recommendations.

Discussion

1. **Immunization services are *readily available.***
Immunization services should be responsive to the needs of patients. For example, in large urban areas, public immunization clinic services should be available daily, 8 hours per day. In smaller cities and rural areas, clinics may operate less frequently. To be fully responsive, providers in many locations should consider offering immunization services each working day, as well as during some off hours (eg, weekends, evenings, early mornings, or lunch hours). Immunization services should be considered for all days and at all hours that other child health services in the same site are offered (eg, Special Supplemental Food Program for Women, Infants, and Children [WIC]). Private providers who offer primary care to infants and children always should include immunization services as a routine part of that care.
Ready availability of immunization services also requires that the supply of vaccines be adequate at all times.
2. ***No barriers* or *unnecessary prerequisites* to the receipt of vaccines exist.**
Appointment-only systems often serve as barriers to immunization in both public and private settings. Thus, immunization services also should be available on a walk-in basis at all times for both routine and new enrollee visits. Waiting time should be minimized and generally not exceed 30 minutes. Furthermore, administration of needed vaccines should not be contingent on enrollment in a well-baby program unless enrollment is immediately available. Children presenting only for immunizations should be rapidly and efficiently screened without requiring other comprehensive health services. However, children receiving immunizations in such an "express lane" fashion and found not to have a primary care physician should be referred to one.
Physical examinations and temperature measurements before immunization should not be required if they delay or impede the timely receipt of immunizations (eg, appointments for physical examination in some facilities may take weeks to months). A reliable decision to vaccinate can be based exclusively on the information elicited from a parent or guardian and on the provider's observations and judgment about the child's wellness at the time of vaccination. At a minimum, children should have preimmunization assessments, including the following: (a) observing the child's general state of health, (b) asking the parent or guardian if the child is well, and (c) questioning the parent or guardian about potential contraindications (see Table, p 755).
In public clinic settings, the administration of vaccines should not be dependent on individual written orders or on a referral from a primary care physician. Rather, standing orders should be developed and implemented.
3. **Immunization services are available *free* or for a minimal fee.**
In the public sector, immunizations should be free of charge. If fees must be collected, they should be kept to a minimum. In the private sector, charges should include the cost of the vaccine and a reasonable administration fee. Affordable vaccinations will limit the fragmentation of care and help assure the immunization of the greatest number of children. Public and private providers

charging a fee to administer vaccines obtained through a consolidated federal contract should prominently display a state-approved sign indicating that no one will be denied immunization services because of inability to pay the fee.

4. **Providers use all clinical encounters to *screen* for needed vaccines and, when indicated, *immunize* children.**
Each encounter with a health care provider, including an emergency room visit or hospitalization, is an opportunity to screen the immunization status and, if indicated, administer needed vaccines. Before discharge from the hospital, children should receive immunizations for which they are eligible by age or health status. The child's regular health care provider should be informed about the immunizations administered. Implementation of this standard minimizes the number of missed opportunities to vaccinate.
In addition, children accompanying parents or siblings who are seeking any service should also be screened and, when indicated, given needed vaccines.
Providers in subspecialty clinics (eg, oncology) who care for children should pay particular attention to the immunization status of their patients and vaccinate or refer them to immunization services or primary health care providers as appropriate.
Providers in other specialties also should note the immunization status of children and refer or immunize as appropriate.

5. **Providers *educate* parents and guardians about immunization in general terms.**
Providers should educate parents and guardians in a culturally sensitive way, preferably in their own language, about the importance of immunizations, the diseases they prevent, the recommended immunization schedules, the need to receive immunizations at recommended ages, and the importance of bringing their child's immunization record to each visit. Parents should be encouraged to take responsibility for ensuring that their child completes the full series. Providers should answer all questions parents and guardians may have and provide appropriate educational materials at suitable reading levels in pertinent languages.

6. **Providers *question* parents or guardians about *contraindications* and, before immunizing a child, *inform* them in specific terms about the risks and benefits of the immunizations their child is to receive.**
Minimal acceptable screening procedures for precautions and contraindications include asking questions to elicit a possible history of adverse events after prior immunizations and determining any existing precautions or contraindications (see Table, p 755).
The Vaccine Information Statements required by federal regulation to be used universally for measles, mumps, rubella, diphtheria, tetanus, pertussis, *Haemophilus influenzae* type B, hepatitis B, hepatitis A, and polio by all providers administering vaccine, including those who purchase their own vaccines, should be provided and reviewed with parents or guardians at each visit when administering one or more of these vaccines. Providers should ensure that information materials are current and available in appropriate languages. Providers should ask parents or guardians if they have questions about what they have read and should ensure that they receive satisfactory answers to their questions.

Providers should explain where and how to obtain medical care during day- and night-time hours in case of an adverse event following vaccination.

7. **Providers follow only true *contraindications.***
Accepting conditions that are not true contraindications as being true contraindications (see Table, p 755) often results in the needless deferment of indicated immunizations. The table of true contraindications is based on the recommendations of the Advisory Committee on Immunization Practices (ACIP) and the recommendations of the Committee on Infectious Diseases of the American Academy of Pediatrics (AAP). Sometimes these recommendations may vary from those contained in the manufacturer's package inserts. For more detailed information, providers should consult the published recommendations of the ACIP, the AAP, the American Academy of Family Physicians (AAFP), and the manufacturer's package inserts.
8. **Providers administer *simultaneously* all vaccine doses for which a child is eligible at the time of each visit.**
Available evidence suggests that the simultaneous administration of childhood immunizations is safe and effective. In addition, evidence suggests that the simultaneous administration of multiple needed vaccines potentially can raise immunization coverage by 9% to 17%. If providers elect not to administer a needed vaccine simultaneously with others (based either on their judgment that this action will not compromise the timely immunization of the child or on a request by the parent or guardian), they should document such actions and the reasons the vaccine was not administered. The record should be flagged with an automatic recall for an appointment to receive the needed vaccine(s). This next appointment should be discussed with the parent or guardian of the child.
Measles, mumps, rubella (MMR) vaccine should always be used in combined form when providing routine childhood immunizations.
9. **Providers use accurate and complete *recording procedures.***
Providers are required by statute to record what vaccine was given, the date the vaccine was given (month, day, year), the name of the manufacturer of the vaccine, the lot number, the signature and title of the person who gave the vaccine, and the address where the vaccine was given. In addition, providers should record on the child's personal immunization record card (preferably the official state version) what vaccine was given, the date the vaccine was given, and the name of the provider. Providers should encourage parents or guardians to maintain a copy of their child's personal immunization record card. This card should be updated at each visit for immunizations. If a parent fails to bring their child's card, a new one should be issued containing all previous immunizations and designated as a replacement record card. When accepting immunization record data from parents, providers should confirm that prior doses of vaccines actually have been administered, either by reviewing immunization record cards or by contacting former providers and entering this verified information into their records. When a provider who does not routinely vaccinate or care for a child administers a vaccine to that child, the regular provider should be informed.
Providers with manual record-keeping systems should maintain separate or easily retrievable files of the immunization records of preschoolers to facilitate assessment of coverage and the identification and recall of children who miss

appointments. In addition, preschooler immunization files should be sorted periodically, with inactive records placed into a separate file. Providers should indicate in their records, or in an appropriately identified place, all primary care services that each child receives to facilitate coscheduling with other services.

10. **Providers *coschedule* immunization appointments in conjunction with appointments for other child health services.**
Providers of immunization-only services that require an appointment should co-schedule immunization appointments with other needed health care services such as WIC, dental examinations, or developmental screening, provided such scheduling does not create a barrier by delaying needed immunizations.

11. **Providers *report adverse events* after immunization promptly, accurately, and completely.**
Providers should encourage parents or legal guardians to inform them of adverse events after immunization. Providers should report all such clinically significant events, including those required by law, to the Vaccine Adverse Event Reporting System, regardless of whether they believe the events are caused by the vaccines. Report forms and assistance are available by calling 800-822-7967. Providers should document fully the adverse event in the medical record at the time of the event or as soon as possible thereafter.

12. **Providers operate a *tracking system.***
A tracking system should produce reminders of upcoming immunizations, as well as recalls for children who are overdue for immunizations. A system may be automated or manual and may include mailed or telephone messages. In the public sector, health department staff also may make home visits. All providers should identify, for additional intensive tracking efforts, children considered at high risk of failing to complete the immunization series on schedule (eg, children who start their series late).

13. **Providers adhere to appropriate procedures for *vaccine management.***
Vaccines should be handled and stored as recommended in the manufacturer's package inserts. The temperatures at which vaccines are stored and transported should be monitored daily, and the expiration date for each vaccine should be noted.

    Providers using publicly purchased vaccine should periodically report usage, wastage, loss, and inventory as required by state or local public health authorities.

14. **Providers conduct semiannual *audits* to assess immunization coverage levels and to review immunization records in the patient populations they serve.**
In the public and private sectors, the assessment of immunization services for preschool-aged patients should include audits of immunization records or inspection of a random sample of records to (1) determine the immunization coverage level (ie, the percentage of children that are up-to-date by their second birthday), (2) identify how frequently opportunities for simultaneous immunization are missed, and (3) assess the quality of documentation. The results of such assessments should be discussed by providers as part of their ongoing quality assurance reviews and used to develop solutions to the problems identified.

15. Providers maintain up-to-date, easily retrievable *medical protocols* at all locations where vaccines are administered.
Providers administering vaccines should maintain a protocol that, at a minimum, discusses the appropriate vaccine dosage, vaccine contraindications, the recommended sites and techniques for vaccine administration, and possible adverse events and their emergency management. Such protocols should specify the necessary emergency medical equipment, drugs (including dosage), and personnel to safely and competently deal with any medical emergency that may arise after the administration of a vaccine. All providers should be familiar with the content of these protocols, their location, and how to follow them. Vaccines can be administered in any setting (eg, schools, churches) where providers can adhere to these protocols.

16. Providers practice *patient-oriented* and *community-based* approaches.
Public providers routinely should seek the input of their patients on specific approaches to better serve their immunization needs and implement the changes necessary to provide more user-friendly services.

Public providers should adopt a community-based approach to the provision of immunization services that calls for reaching high coverage levels in their catchment area populations and not only in the active patient populations they serve. Such a community-based approach requires all public providers to publicize the availability of their immunization services and to conduct community outreach activities to increase demand for immunization services. Private providers should cooperate with local health officials in their efforts to assure high coverage levels throughout the community. Without high immunization coverage levels, no community is completely protected against vaccine-preventable diseases. All providers share in the responsibility to achieve the highest possible degree of community protection.

17. Vaccines are administered by *properly trained* individuals.
Only properly trained individuals should administer vaccines. However, the task of administering vaccines need not be assigned exclusively to physicians and nurses. With appropriate training, including the management of emergency situations, and under professional supervision, other personnel can skillfully and safely administer vaccines. In some jurisdictions, statutory requirements may limit the administration of vaccines to licensed physicians and/or nurses, which could, therefore, create barriers to immunization. If so, legal opinion should be sought locally to determine the necessary steps to overcome this barrier.

18. Providers receive *ongoing education* and *training* on current immunization recommendations.
Providers include all individuals who are involved in the administration of vaccines, the management of immunization clinics, or the support of these functions. Training and education should cover current guidelines and recommendations of the ACIP, AAP, and the AAFP, as well as the Standards for Pediatric Immunization Practices and other immunization information sources, such as the manufacturer's package inserts. Providers also should receive information about ongoing national efforts to reach the year 2010 goal of 90% series complete immunization by the second birthday.

Table. Guide to Contraindications and Precautions to Immunizations, January 2000[a]

This information is based on the recommendations of the Advisory Committee on Immunization Practices (ACIP) and of the Committee on Infectious Diseases of the American Academy of Pediatrics (AAP). Sometimes these recommendations vary from those in the manufacturers' product label. For more detailed information, providers should consult the published recommendations of the ACIP, AAP, and the manufacturers' package inserts. These guidelines, originally issued in 1993, have been updated to give current recommendations as of 2000 (based on information available as of December 1999).

Vaccine	Contraindications	Precautions[b]	Not Contraindications (Vaccines May Be Given)
General for all vaccines (DTaP/DTP,[c] IPV, OPV, MMR, Hib, HBV, Var)	Anaphylactic reaction to a vaccine contraindicates further doses of that vaccine Anaphylactic reaction to a vaccine constituent contraindicates the use of vaccines containing that substance	Moderate or severe illnesses with or without a fever	Mild to moderate local reaction (soreness, redness, swelling) following a dose of an injectable antigen Low-grade or moderate fever following a prior vaccine dose Mild acute illness with or without low-grade fever Current antimicrobial therapy Convalescent phase of illnesses Prematurity (same dosage and indications as for healthy, full-term infants) Recent exposure to an infectious disease History of penicillin or other nonspecific allergies or fact that relatives have such allergies Pregnancy of mother or household contact Unimmunized household contact
DTaP/DTP[c]	Encephalopathy within 7 days of administration of previous dose of DTaP/DTP	Temperature of 40.5°C (104.8°F) within 48 hours after vaccination with a prior dose of DTaP/DTP	Family history of seizures[d] Family history of sudden infant death syndrome Family history of an adverse event after DTaP/DTP administration

Table. **Guide to Contraindications and Precautions to Immunizations, January 2000[a], continued**

Vaccine	Contraindications	Precautions[b]	Not Contraindications (Vaccines May Be Given)
DTaP/DTP[c], continued		Collapse or shock-like state (hypotonic-hyporesponsive episode) within 48 hours of receiving a prior dose of DTaP/DTP Seizures within 3 days of receiving a prior dose of DTaP/DTP[d] Persistent inconsolable crying lasting 3 hours, within 48 hours of receiving a prior dose of DTaP/DTP GBS within 6 weeks after a dose[e]	
IPV	Anaphylactic reactions to neomycin or streptomycin	Pregnancy	...
OPV[f,g]	Infection with HIV or a household contact with HIV Known altered immunodeficiency (hematologic and solid tumors, congenital immunodeficiency, and long-term immunosuppressive therapy) Immunodeficient household contact	Pregnancy	Breastfeeding Current antimicrobial therapy Mild diarrhea

Table. **Guide to Contraindications and Precautions to Immunizations, January 2000[a], continued**

Vaccine	Contraindications	Precautions[b]	Not Contraindications (Vaccines May Be Given)
MMR	Pregnancy Anaphylactic reaction to neomycin Anaphylactic reaction to gelatin Known altered immunodeficiency (hematologic and solid tumors, congenital immunodeficiency, severe HIV infection, and long-term immunosuppressive therapy)	Recent (within 3 to 11 months, depending on product and dose) immune globulin administration[h] Thrombocytopenia or history of thrombocytopenic purpura[h,i]	Tuberculosis or positive PPD Simultaneous tuberculin skin testing[j] Breastfeeding Pregnancy of mother of recipient Immunodeficient family member or household contact Infection with HIV Nonanaphylactic reactions to eggs or neomycin
Hib	None	...	...
Hepatitis B	Anaphylactic reaction to baker's yeast	...	Pregnancy
Varicella	Pregnancy Anaphylactic reaction to neomycin Anaphylactic reaction to gelatin Infection with HIV Known altered immunodeficiency (hematologic and solid tumors, congenital immunodeficiency, and long-term immunosuppressive therapy)	Recent immune globulin administration Family history of immunodeficiency[k]	Pregnancy in the mother of the recipient Immunodeficiency in a household contact Household contact with HIV

Table. **Guide to Contraindications and Precautions to Immunizations, January 2000[a], continued**

[a] DTaP indicates diphtheria and tetanus toxoids and acellular pertussis; DTP, diphtheria and tetanus toxoids and pertussis; IPV, inactivated poliovirus; OPV, oral poliovirus; MMR, measles-mumps-rubella; Hib, *Haemophilus influenzae* type b; HBV, hepatitis B virus; Var, varicella; GBS, Guillain-Barré syndrome; HIV, human immunodeficiency virus; and PPD, purified protein derivative (tuberculin).

[b] The events or conditions listed as precautions, although not contraindications, should be reviewed carefully. The benefits and risks of administering a specific vaccine to a person under the circumstances should be considered. If the risks are believed to outweigh the benefits, the immunization should be withheld; if the benefits are believed to outweigh the risks (for example, during an outbreak or foreign travel), the immunization should be given. Whether and when to administer DTaP (or DTP) to children with proven or suspected underlying neurologic disorders should be decided on an individual basis.

[c] DTP is no longer recommended in the United States.

[d] Acetaminophen given before administering DTaP (or DTP) and thereafter every 4 hours for 24 hours should be considered for children with a personal or with a family (ie, siblings or parents) history of seizures.

[e] The decision to give additional doses of DTaP (or DTP) should be based on consideration of the benefit of further vaccination vs the risk of recurrence of GBS. For example, completion of the primary series in children is justified.

[f] A theoretical risk exists that the administration of multiple live virus vaccines within 30 days (4 weeks) of one another if not given on the same day will result in suboptimal immune response. No data substantiate this risk, however.

[g] OPV is no longer recommended for routine use in the United States.

[h] An anaphylactic reaction to egg ingestion previously was considered a contraindication unless skin testing and, if indicated, desensitization had been performed. However, skin testing no longer is recommended as of 1997.

[i] The decision to vaccinate should be based on consideration of the benefits of immunity to measles, mumps, and rubella vs the risk of recurrence or exacerbation of thrombocytopenia after vaccination, or from natural infections of measles or rubella. In most instances, the benefits of vaccination will be much greater than the potential risks and justify giving MMR, particularly in view of the even greater risk of thrombocytopenia after measles or rubella disease. However, if a prior episode of thrombocytopenia occurred in temporal proximity to vaccination, not giving a subsequent dose may be prudent.

[j] Measles vaccination may temporarily suppress tuberculin reactivity. MMR vaccine may be given after, or on the same day as, tuberculin testing. If MMR has been given recently, postpone the tuberculin test until 4 to 6 weeks after administration of MMR. If giving MMR simultaneously with the tuberculin skin test, use the Mantoux test and not multiple puncture tests, because the latter require confirmation if positive, which would have to be postponed for 4 to 6 weeks.

[k] Varicella vaccine should not be given to a member of a household with a family history of immunodeficiency until the immune status of the recipient and other children in the family is documented.

APPENDIX III.

National Vaccine Injury Act. Reporting and Compensation Table.

This table includes adverse events that are reportable to the Vaccine Adverse Event Reporting System (VAERS) (see Vaccine Safety and Contraindications, p 30), as well as vaccines covered by the National Vaccine Injury Compensation Program. The intervals from immunization to the onset of an event for reporting to VAERS and for possible compensation by the Vaccine Injury Compensation Program are given.

National Childhood Vaccine Injury Act Reporting and Compensation Table*

Vaccine	Adverse Event	Interval from Vaccination to Onset of Event: For Reporting[†]	For Compensation[‡]
I. Tetanus toxoid–containing vaccines (eg, DTaP, DTP, DTP-Hib; DT; dT, or TT)	A. Anaphylaxis or anaphylactic shock	0–7 d	0–4 h
	B. Brachial neuritis	0–28 d	2–28 d
	C. Any acute complication or sequela (including death) of above events	No limit	No limit
	D. Events described in manufacturer's package insert as contraindications to additional doses of vaccine	No limit	Not applicable
II. Pertussis antigen–containing vaccines (eg, DTaP, DTP, P, DTP-Hib)	A. Anaphylaxis or anaphylactic shock	0–7 d	0–4 h
	B. Encephalopathy (or encephalitis)	0–7 d	0–72 h
	C. Any acute complication or sequela (including death) of above events	No limit	No limit
	D. Events described in manufacturer's package insert as contraindications to additional doses of vaccine	No limit	Not applicable
III. Measles, mumps, and rubella virus–containing vaccines in any combination (eg, MMR, MR, M, R)	A. Anaphylaxis or anaphylactic shock	0–7 d	0–4 h
	B. Encephalopathy (or encephalitis)	0–15 d	5–15 d
	C. Any acute complication or sequela (including death) of above events	No limit	No limit
	D. Events described in manufacturer's package insert as contraindications to additional doses of vaccine	No limit	Not applicable
IV. Rubella virus–containing vaccines (eg, MMR, MR, R)	A. Chronic arthritis	0–42 d	7–42 d
	B. Any acute complication or sequela (including death) of above event	No limit	No limit
	C. Events described in manufacturer's package insert as contraindications to additional doses of vaccine	No limit	Not applicable
V. Measles virus–containing vaccines (eg, MMR, MR, M)	A. Thrombocytopenic purpura	0–30 d	7–30 d
	B. Vaccine-strain measles viral infection in an immunodeficient recipient	0–6 mo	0–6 mo
	C. Any acute complication or sequela (including death) of above events	No limit	No limit
	D. Events described in manufacturer's package insert as contraindications to additional doses of vaccine	No limit	Not applicable

National Childhood Vaccine Injury Act Reporting and Compensation Table,* continued

Vaccine	Adverse Event	Interval from Vaccination to Onset of Event: For Reporting†	For Compensation‡
VI. Live poliovirus-containing vaccines (OPV)	A. Paralytic polio		
	• in a nonimmunodeficient recipient	0–30 d	0–30 d
	• in an immunodeficient recipient	0–6 mo	0–6 mo
	• in a vaccine-associated community case	No limit	No limit
	B. Vaccine-strain polio viral infection		
	• in a nonimmunodeficient recipient	0–30 d	0–30 d
	• in an immunodeficient recipient	0–6 mo	0–6 mo
	• in a vaccine-associated community case	No limit	No limit
	C. Any acute complication or sequela (including death) of above events	No limit	No limit
	D. Events described in manufacturer's package insert as contraindications to additional doses of vaccine	No limit	Not applicable
VII. Polio inactivated	A. Anaphylaxis or anaphylactic shock	0–7 d	0–4 h
	B. Any acute complication or sequela (including death) of above event	No limit	No limit
	C. Events described in manufacturer's package insert as contraindications to additional doses of vaccine	No limit	Not applicable
VIII. Hepatitis B antigen–containing vaccines	A. Anaphylaxis or anaphylactic shock	0–7 d	0–4 h
	B. Any acute complication or sequela (including death) of above event	No limit	No limit
	C. Events described in manufacturer's package insert as contraindications to additional doses of vaccine	No limit	Not applicable
IX. *Haemophilus influenzae* type b polysaccharide vaccines (unconjugated, PRP vaccines)	A. Early-onset Hib disease	0–7 d	0–7 d
	B. Any acute complication or sequela (including death) of above event	No limit	No limit
	C. Events described in manufacturer's package insert as contraindications to additional doses of vaccine	No limit	Not applicable

National Childhood Vaccine Injury Act Reporting and Compensation Table,* continued

Vaccine	Adverse Event	Interval from Vaccination to Onset of Event For Reporting†	For Compensation‡
X. *Haemophilus influenzae* type b polysaccharide conjugate vaccines	A. No condition specified for compensation	Not applicable	Not applicable
	B. Events described in manufacturer's package insert as contraindications to additional doses of vaccine	No limit	Not applicable
XI. Varicella virus–containing vaccine	A. No condition specified for compensation	Not applicable	Not applicable
	B. Events described in manufacturer's package insert as contraindications to additional doses of vaccine	No limit	Not applicable
XII. Any new vaccine recommended by the CDC for routine administration to children, after publication by Secretary, HHS of a notice of coverage	A. No condition specified for compensation		
	B. Events described in manufacturer's package insert as contraindications to additional doses of vaccine		

* Effective date: October 22, 1998. DTaP, diphtheria and tetanus toxoids and acellular pertussis; DTP, diphtheria and tetanus toxoids and pertussis; Hib, *Haemophilus influenzae* type b; DT, diphtheria and tetanus toxoids; dT, adult-type diphtheria and tetanus toxoids; TT, tetanus toxoid vaccine; OPV, oral poliovirus; PRP, polyribosylribitol phosphate polysaccharide; CDC, Centers for Disease Control and Prevention; and HHS, US Department of Health and Human Services.

† Taken from the Reportable Events Table (RET), which lists conditions reportable by law (42 USC §300aa-25) to the Vaccine Adverse Event Reporting System (VAERS), including conditions found in the manufacturer's package insert. In addition, physicians are encouraged to report **ANY** clinically significant or unexpected events (even if you are not certain the vaccine caused the event) for **ANY** vaccine, whether or not it is listed on the RET. Manufacturers also are required by regulation (21 CFR §600.80) to report to the VAERS program all adverse events made known to them for any vaccine. VAERS reporting forms and information can be obtained by calling 1-800-822-7967 or from the Web site (http://www.fda.gov/cber/vaers/report.htm).

‡ Taken from the Vaccine Injury Table (VIT) used in adjudication of claims filed with the National Vaccine Injury Compensation Program. Claims also may be filed for a condition with onset outside the designated time intervals or a condition not included in the VIT. The Qualifications and Aids to Interpretation below define conditions or injuries listed on the VIT. Information on filing a claim can be obtained by calling 1-800-338-2382 or through the Vaccine Injury Compensation Program Web site (http://www.hrsa.gov/bhpr/vicp/).

Qualifications and Aids to Interpretation

(1) *Anaphylaxis and anaphylactic shock* mean an acute, severe, and potentially lethal systemic allergic reaction. Most cases resolve without sequelae. Signs and symptoms begin minutes to a few hours after exposure. Death, if it occurs, usually results from airway obstruction caused by laryngeal edema or bronchospasm and may be associated with cardiovascular collapse. Other significant clinical signs and symptoms include the following: cyanosis, hypotension, bradycardia, tachycardia, arrhythmia, edema of the pharynx and/or trachea and/or larynx with stridor and dyspnea. Autopsy findings may include acute emphysema, which results from lower respiratory tract obstruction, edema of the hypopharynx, epiglottis, larynx, or trachea, and minimal findings of eosinophilia in the liver, spleen, and lungs. When death occurs within minutes of exposure and without signs of respiratory distress, there may not be significant pathologic findings.

(2) *Encephalopathy.* For purposes of the Vaccine Injury Table (VIT), a vaccine recipient shall be considered to have suffered an encephalopathy only if such recipient manifests, within the applicable period, an injury meeting the following description of an acute encephalopathy, and then a chronic encephalopathy persists in such person for more than 6 months beyond the date of vaccination.

(i) An *acute encephalopathy* is one that is sufficiently severe so as to require hospitalization (whether or not hospitalization occurred).

(A) *For children younger than 18 months of age* who present without an associated seizure event, an acute encephalopathy is indicated by a "significantly decreased level of consciousness" (see "D" below) lasting for at least 24 hours. Children younger than 18 months of age who present following a seizure shall be viewed as having an acute encephalopathy if their significantly decreased level of consciousness persists beyond 24 hours and cannot be attributed to a postictal state (seizure) or medication.

(B) *For adults and children 18 months of age or older,* an acute encephalopathy is one that persists for at least 24 hours and is characterized by at least 2 of the following:

(1) A significant change in mental status that is not medication-related, specifically a confusional state, a delirium. or a psychosis;

(2) A significantly decreased level of consciousness, which is independent of a seizure and cannot be attributed to the effects of medication; and

(3) A seizure associated with loss of consciousness

(C) Increased intracranial pressure may be a clinical feature of acute encephalopathy in any age group.

(D) A "significantly decreased level of consciousness" is indicated by the presence of at least one of the following clinical signs for at least 24 hours or greater (see paragraphs (2)(i)(A) and (2)(i)(B) of this section for applicable time frames):

(1) Decreased or absent response to environment (responds, if at all, only to loud voice or painful stimuli);

(2) Decreased or absent eye contact (does not fix gaze on family members or other persons); or

(3) Inconsistent or absent responses to external stimuli (does not recognize familiar people or things).

(E) The following clinical features alone or in combination do not demonstrate an acute encephalopathy or a significant change in either mental status or level of consciousness as described above: sleepiness, irritability (fussiness), high-pitched and unusual screaming, persistent inconsolable crying, and bulging fontanelle. Seizures in themselves are not sufficient to constitute a diagnosis of encephalopathy. In the absence of other evidence of an acute encephalopathy, seizures shall not be viewed as the first symptom or manifestation of the onset of an acute encephalopathy.

(ii) *Chronic encephalopathy* occurs when a change in mental or neurologic status, first manifested during the applicable time period, persists for a period of at least 6 months from the date of vaccination. Persons who return to a normal neurologic state after the acute encephalopathy shall not be presumed to have suffered residual neurologic damage from that event; any subsequent chronic encephalopathy shall not be presumed to be a sequela of the acute encephalopathy. If a preponderance of the evidence indicates that a child's chronic encephalopathy is secondary to genetic, prenatal, or perinatal factors, that chronic encephalopathy shall not be considered to be a condition set forth in the VIT.

(iii) An encephalopathy shall not be considered to be a condition set forth in the VIT if, in a proceeding on a petition, it is shown by a preponderance of the evidence that the encephalopathy was caused by an infection, a toxin, a metabolic disturbance, a structural lesion, a genetic disorder, or trauma (without regard to whether the cause of the infection, toxin, trauma, metabolic disturbance, structural lesion, or genetic disorder is known). If at the time a decision is made on a petition filed under section 2111(b) of the Act for a vaccine-related injury or death it is not possible to determine the cause by a preponderance of the evidence of an encephalopathy, the encephalopathy shall be considered to be a condition set forth in the VIT.

(iv) In determining whether or not an encephalopathy is a condition set forth in the VIT, the Court shall consider the entire medical record.

(3) *Residual seizure disorder.* A petitioner may be considered to have suffered a residual seizure disorder for purposes of the VIT, if the first seizure or convulsion occurred 5 to 15 days (not <5 days and not >15 days) after administration of the vaccine and 2 or more additional distinct seizure or convulsion episodes occurred within 1 year after the administration of the vaccine that were unaccompanied by fever (defined as a rectal temperature equal to or greater than 34.4°C (≥101.0°F) or an oral temperature equal to or greater than 37.8°C (≥100.0°F). A distinct seizure or convulsion episode ordinarily is defined as including all seizure or convulsive activity occurring within a 24-hour period, unless competent and qualified expert neurological testimony is presented to the contrary in a particular case.

For purposes of the VIT, a petitioner shall not be considered to have suffered a residual seizure disorder if the petitioner suffered a seizure or convulsion unaccompanied by fever (as defined above) before the fifth day after the administration of the vaccine involved.

(4) *Seizure and convulsion.* For purposes of paragraphs (2) and (3) of this section, the terms, "seizure" and "convulsion" include myoclonic, generalized tonic-clonic (grand mal), and simple and complex partial seizures. Absence (petit mal) seizures shall not be considered to be a condition set forth in the VIT. Jerking movements or staring episodes alone are not necessarily an indication of seizure activity.

(5) *Sequela.* The term sequela means a condition or event that actually was caused by a condition listed in the VIT.

(6) *Chronic arthritis.* For purposes of the VIT, chronic arthritis may be found in a person with no history in the 3 years before vaccination of arthropathy (joint disease) on the basis of:

(A) Medical documentation, recorded within 30 days after the onset, of objective signs of acute arthritis (joint swelling) that occurred between 7 and 42 days after a rubella vaccination;

(B) Medical documentation (recorded within 3 years after the onset of acute arthritis) of the persistence of objective signs of intermittent or continuous arthritis for more than 6 months after vaccination;

(C) Medical documentation of an antibody response to the rubella virus

For purposes of the VIT, the following shall not be considered as chronic arthritis: Musculoskeletal disorders such as diffuse connective tissue diseases (including but not limited to rheumatoid arthritis, juvenile rheumatoid arthritis, systemic lupus erythematosus, systemic sclerosis, mixed connective tissue disease, polymyositis/dermatomyositis, fibromyalgia, necrotizing vasculitis and vasculopathies and Sjögren syndrome), degenerative joint disease, infectious agents other than rubella (whether by direct invasion or as an immune reaction), metabolic and endocrine diseases, trauma, neoplasms, neuropathic disorders, bone and cartilage disorders, and arthritis associated with ankylosing spondylitis, psoriasis, inflammatory bowel disease, Reiter syndrome, or blood disorders.

Arthralgia (joint pain) or stiffness without joint swelling shall not be viewed as chronic arthritis for purposes of the VIT.

(7) *Brachial neuritis* is defined as dysfunction limited to the upper extremity nerve plexus (ie, its trunks, divisions, or cords) without involvement of other peripheral (eg, nerve roots or a single peripheral nerve) or central (eg, spinal cord) nervous system structures. A deep, steady, often severe aching pain in the shoulder and upper arm usually heralds onset of the condition. The pain is followed in days or weeks by weakness and atrophy in upper extremity muscle groups. Sensory loss may accompany the motor deficits but is generally a less notable clinical feature. The neuritis, or plexopathy, may be present on the same side as or the opposite side of the injection; it is sometimes bilateral, affecting both upper extremities. Weakness is required before the diagnosis can be made. Motor, sensory, and reflex findings on physical examination and the results of nerve conduction and electromyographic studies must be consistent in confirming that dysfunction is attributable to the brachial plexus. The condition should thereby be distinguishable from conditions that may give rise to dysfunction of nerve roots (ie, radiculopathies) and peripheral nerves (ie, including multiple mononeuropathies), as well as other peripheral and central nervous system structures (eg, cranial neuropathies and myelopathies).

(8) *Thrombocytopenic purpura* is defined by a serum platelet count less than $50 \times 10^3/\mu L$ ($50 \times 10^9/L$). Thrombocytopenic purpura does not include cases of thrombocytopenia associated with other causes such as hypersplenism, autoimmune disorders (including alloantibodies from previous transfusions) myelodysplasias, lymphoproliferative disorders, congenital thrombocytopenia, or hemolytic uremic syndrome. This does not include cases of immune (formerly called idiopathic) thrombocytopenic purpura that are mediated, for example, by viral or fungal infections, toxins, or drugs. Thrombocytopenic purpura does not include cases of thrombocytopenia associated with disseminated intravascular coagulation, as observed with bacterial and viral infections. Viral infections include, for example, those infections secondary to Epstein-Barr virus, cytomegalovirus, hepatitis A and B, rhinovirus, human immunodeficiency virus, adenovirus, and dengue virus. An antecedent viral infection may be demonstrated by clinical signs and symptoms and need not be confirmed by culture or serologic testing. Bone marrow examination, if performed, must reveal a normal or an increased number of megakaryocytes in an otherwise normal marrow.

(9) *Vaccine-strain measles viral infection* is defined as a disease caused by the vaccine-strain that should be determined by vaccine-specific monoclonal antibody or polymerase chain reaction tests.

(10) *Vaccine-strain polio viral infection* is defined as a disease caused by poliovirus that is isolated from the affected tissue and should be determined to be the vaccine-strain by oligonucleotide or polymerase chain reaction. Isolation of poliovirus from the stool is not sufficient to establish a tissue specific infection or disease caused by vaccine-strain poliovirus.

(11) *Early-onset Hib disease* is defined as invasive bacterial illness associated with the presence of Hib organism on culture of normally sterile body fluids or tissue or clinical findings consistent with the diagnosis of epiglottitis. Hib pneumonia qualifies as invasive Hib disease when radiographic findings consistent with the diagnosis of pneumonitis are accompanied by a blood culture positive for the Hib organism. Otitis media, in the absence of the above findings, does not qualify as invasive bacterial disease. A child is considered to have suffered this injury only if the vaccine was the first Hib immunization received by the child.

APPENDIX IV.

State Immunization Requirements for School Attendance

All states require immunization of children at the time of entry into school, and most states require immunization for entry into licensed child care. In addition, many states require immunization of older children in upper grades, as well as those entering college. The most up-to-date information about which vaccines are required in a specific state can be obtained from the immunization program manager of each state health department, as well as from a number of local health departments.

The Centers for Disease Control and Prevention collects and publishes data on current school entry laws, child care and Head Start immunization regulations, and college immunization requirements in effect in the various states. This survey of school laws usually is published annually. Copies of the latest survey, "State Immunization Requirements for School Attendance," may be obtained by sending a request for single copies to the Centers for Disease Control and Prevention, National Immunization Program, 1600 Clifton Rd, Mailstop E-52, Atlanta, GA 30333, by calling 1-800-311-3435, or from the Web site (http://www.cdc.gov).

APPENDIX V.

Clinical Syndromes Associated With Foodborne Diseases

Foodborne disease is a major cause of morbidity and mortality in children and adults in developed countries. The epidemiology of foodborne disease is complex and changing because of the number of organisms associated with illness, changes in food production and distribution, rapid international distribution of food, changes in dietary habits, potential for extraintestinal manifestations of disease caused by many food-associated pathogens, and the susceptibility of certain immunocompromised persons to severe and prolonged disease.

The diagnosis of foodborne disease should be considered when 2 or more persons who have shared a meal develop an acute illness characterized by nausea, vomiting, diarrhea, neurologic symptoms, and other extraintestinal manifestations. The diagnosis of the specific causative agent is suggested by the clinical syndrome, incubation period, and epidemiologic clues. To aid in the diagnosis, syndromes of foodborne diseases are categorized by incubation period, causative agent, and foods commonly associated with specific causes. The foods listed in the Table (p 768) are representative and not inclusive. The diagnosis can be confirmed by laboratory testing of stool, emesis, and/or blood, depending on the causative agent. If an outbreak is suspected, local or state public health officials should be notified immediately so they can work with local health care professionals, corroborate other reports, and arrange for special laboratory testing not available at the clinical laboratory.

Table. **Clinical Syndromes Associated With Foodborne Diseases**

Clinical Syndrome	Incubation Period	Causative Agents	Commonly Associated Vehicles
Nausea and vomiting	<1–6 h	*Staphylococcus aureus* (preformed toxins, A, B, C, D, E)	Ham, poultry, cream-filled pastries, potato and egg salads, mushrooms
		Bacillus cereus (emetic toxin)	Fried rice, pork
		Heavy metals (copper, tin, cadmium, iron, zinc)	Acidic beverages
Flushing, dizziness, burning of mouth and throat, headache, gastrointestinal symptoms, urticaria	<1 h	Histamine (scombroid)	Fish (bluefish, bonito, mackerel, mahi-mahi, tuna)
Neurologic, including paresthesias and gastrointestinal symptoms	<1–6 h	Tetrodotoxin	Puffer fish
		Ciguatera	Fish (amberjack, barracuda, grouper, snapper)
		Paralytic shellfish poisoning	Shellfish (clams, mussels, oysters, scallops, other mollusks)
		Neurotoxic shellfish poisoning	Shellfish
		Domoic acid	Mussels
		Monosodium glutamate	Chinese food
Neurologic, including confusion, salivation, hallucinations, and gastrointestinal tract manifestations	0–2 h	Mushroom toxins (early onset)	Mushrooms
Moderate-to-severe abdominal cramps and watery diarrhea, vomiting	6–24 h	*B cereus* enterotoxin	Beef, pork, chicken, vanilla sauce
		Clostridium perfringens enterotoxin	Beef, poultry, gravy, dried or precooked foods
	16–72 h	Caliciviruses, including Norwalk	Shellfish, salads, ice, cookies, water, sandwiches, fruit
	1–4 d	Enterotoxigenic *Escherichia coli*	Fruits, vegetables

Table. **Clinical Syndromes Associated With Foodborne Diseases, continued**

Clinical Syndrome	Incubation Period	Causative Agents	Commonly Associated Vehicles
Moderate-to-severe abdominal cramps and watery diarrhea, vomiting, continued	1–5 d	*Vibrio cholerae* O1 and O139	Shellfish (including crabs and shrimp)
		V cholerae non-O1	Shellfish
	1–14 d	*Cyclospora* species	Raspberries, vegetables
	2–14 d	*Cryptosporidium* species	Vegetables, milk
Diarrhea, fever, abdominal cramps, blood and mucus in stools	16–≥72 h	*Salmonella* species	Poultry, pork, beef, eggs, dairy products, including ice cream, vegetables, fruit, orange juice, alfalfa sprouts
		Shigella	Egg salad, vegetables, scallions
		Campylobacter jejuni	Poultry, raw milk
		Enteroinvasive *E coli*	Vegetables
		Yersinia enterocolitica	Pork chitterlings, tofu, raw milk
		Vibrio parahaemolyticus	Fish, shellfish
Bloody diarrhea, abdominal cramps	72–120 h	Enterohemorrhagic *E coli*	Beef (hamburger), raw milk, roast beef, salami, salad dressings, lettuce, apple cider, alfalfa and radish sprouts
Hepatorenal failure	6–24 h	Mushrooms (late onset)	Mushrooms (especially *Amanita* species)
Gastrointestinal then blurred vision, dry mouth, dysarthria, diplopia, descending paralysis	12–48 h	*Clostridium botulinum*	Home-canned vegetables, fruits and fish, salted fish, meats; bottled garlic; baked potatoes in aluminum foil; cheese sauce
Chronic, urgent diarrhea	Varied	Brainerd diarrhea	Unpasteurized milk, water
Extraintestinal manifestations	Varied	*Brucella* species	Cheese, raw milk
		Group A streptococcus	Egg and potato salads
		Hepatitis A virus	Shellfish, strawberries, lettuce
		Listeria monocytogenes	Cheese, raw milk, hot dogs, cole slaw, cold cuts
		Trichinella spiralis	Pork
		Vibrio vulnificus	Shellfish
		Toxoplasma gondii	Beef, pork, lamb, venison

APPENDIX VI.

Potentially Contaminated Food Products

Foodborne diseases are associated with significant morbidity and mortality in persons of all ages. Children and especially immunocompromised persons are particularly susceptible to illness and complications of illness for many of the organisms associated with foodborne illness. The following preventive measures concerning ingestion of potentially contaminated food can be implemented to reduce the risk of infection and disease.

Unpasteurized milk and cheese. Children should not drink unpasteurized milk or eat unpasteurized cheese. Serious systemic infections due to *Salmonella* species, *Campylobacter* species, and *Escherichia coli* O157:H7 have been attributed to consumption of unpasteurized milk, including certified raw milk. Unpasteurized cheese has been associated with illness due to *Brucella* species and *Listeria monocytogenes.* The American Academy of Pediatrics strongly endorses the use of pasteurized milk and recommends that parents and public health officials be fully informed of the important risks associated with consumption of unpasteurized milk. Interstate sale of raw milk is banned by the US Food and Drug Administration (FDA).

Eggs. Children should not eat raw or undercooked eggs, unpasteurized powdered eggs, or products containing raw eggs. The major vehicles of transmission of *Salmonella* species are foods of animal origin, including eggs. Ingestion of raw or improperly cooked eggs can produce severe *Salmonella* disease. Examples of foods that may contain undercooked eggs include some homemade frostings and homemade mayonnaise, eggs prepared sunny-side up, fresh Caesar salad dressing, Hollandaise sauce, and cookie and cake batter.

Raw and undercooked meat. Children should not eat raw or undercooked meat or meat products. Various raw or undercooked meat products have been associated with disease, such as poultry with *Salmonella* and *Campylobacter* infections; ground beef with *E coli* O157:H7; hot dogs with *Listeria* infections; pork with trichinosis; and wild game with brucellosis, tularemia, and trichinosis. Knives, cutting boards, utensils, and plates used for raw meats should not be used for preparation of fresh fruits or vegetables until the utensils have been cleaned properly. The use of radiant energy (irradiation) to sterilize raw meat is being implemented by meat processing plants in the United States.

Unpasteurized juices. Children should only drink pasteurized juice products unless the fruit is washed and freshly squeezed (ie, orange juice) immediately before consumption. Consumption of packaged fruit and vegetable juices that have not undergone pasteurization or a comparable treatment has been associated with foodborne illness due to *E coli* O157:H7 and *Salmonella* species. The FDA now requires that product labels indicate whether a product has been pasteurized. If a packaged juice has not undergone pasteurization or a comparable treatment, consumers must see a warning statement that the product has not been pasteurized and, therefore, may contain harmful bacteria that can cause serious illness in children, elderly persons, or persons with compromised immune systems.

Alfalfa sprouts. The FDA and the Centers for Disease Control and Prevention have reaffirmed health advisories that persons who are at high risk for severe foodborne disease, including children, persons with compromised immune systems, and elderly persons, should avoid eating raw alfalfa sprouts until intervention methods are implemented to improve the safety of these products.* Raw alfalfa sprouts have been associated with outbreaks of illness due to *Salmonella* species and *E coli* O157:H7.

Fresh fruits and vegetables. Many fresh fruits and vegetables have been associated with disease due to *Cryptosporidium*, *Cyclospora*, caliciviruses, *Giardia*, *E coli* species, and *Shigella* species. All fruits and vegetables should be cleaned before ingestion. Knives, cutting boards, utensils, and plates used for raw meats should not be used for preparation of fresh fruits or vegetables until the utensils have been cleaned properly.

Raw shellfish and fish. Many experts recommend that children should not eat raw shellfish, especially raw oysters. Some experts caution against children ingesting raw fish. Raw shellfish, including mussels, clams, oysters, scallops, and other mollusks, have been associated with many pathogens and toxins (see Appendix V, p 767), and raw fish has been associated with transmission of parasites.

Honey. Children younger than 1 year of age should not be given honey unless the product has been certified to be free of *Clostridium botulinum* spores. Honey has been shown to contain spores of *C botulinum.* Light and dark corn syrup also may contain spores of *C botulinum* and should not be fed to infants.

* For additional information, contact the Food and Drug Administration (FDA) Food Information Line at 1-800-FDA-4010 or the US Department of Agriculture at 1-800-535-4555 or 1-202-720-2791 or at the following web sites: http://www.usda.gov or http://www.foodsafety.gov

APPENDIX VII.

Diseases Transmitted by Animals

The transmission of diseases of animals to humans is of special interest in the care of children who may share a household with pets or unwanted rodents or who are otherwise in contact with animals. Important zoonoses that may be encountered in North America and that are reviewed in the *Red Book* (see disease-specific chapters in Section 3 for further information) are provided in the following table, which also provides primary modes of transmission from animals to humans. These modes of transmission include direct contact, scratch, bite, inhalation, contact with urine or feces, and ingestion of contaminated food, water, or feces, as well as contact with arthropod intermediate hosts. Human-to-human transmission also may occur. For a more complete listing of these diseases, one or more of the following resources may be consulted:

- *The Zoonoses* prepared jointly by the US Department of Health and Human Services, the US Public Health Service, the Centers for Disease Control and Prevention, the Centers for Infectious Diseases, and the Office of Biosafety Atlanta, GA 30333; and the University of Texas, School of Public Health, Science Center, Houston, TX 77025.
- Acha PM, Szyfres B. *Zoonoses and Communicable Diseases Common to Man and Animals.* 2nd ed. Washington, DC: Pan American Health Organization, Pan American Sanitary Bureau, Regional Offices of the World Health Organization; 1987. Scientific publication 503 (525 23rd Street, NW, Washington, DC 20037)
- Beran GW, Steele JH. *Handbook of Zoonoses.* 2nd ed. Boca Raton, FL: CRC Press Inc; 1994.
- Weinberg AN, Weber DJ, eds. Animal associated human infections. *Infect Dis Clin North Am.* 1991;5:1-175, 649–731
- Palmer SR, Lord Soulsby, Simpson DIH, eds. *Zoonoses: Biology, Clinical Practice, and Public Health Control.* New York, NY: Oxford University Press; 1998

Morbidity resulting from selected zoonotic diseases in the United States is reported annually by the Centers for Disease Control and Prevention (see *Summary of Notifiable Diseases*).

Table. **Diseases Transmitted by Animals**

Disease and/or Organism	Common Animal Sources	Vector or Modes of Transmission
Bacterial Diseases		
Aeromonas species	Aquatic animals	Wound infection, ingestion of contaminated food
Bartonella henselae (cat-scratch disease)	Cats, infrequently other animals (<10%)	Scratches, bites
Brucellosis (*Brucella* species)	Cattle, goats, sheep, swine, rarely dogs	Direct contact with birth products, ingestion of contaminated milk, inhalation of aerosols
Campylobacteriosis (*Campylobacter jejuni*)	Poultry, dogs, cats, ferrets	Ingestion of contaminated food, direct contact, (particularly with animals with diarrhea)
Capnocytophaga canimorsus	Dogs, rarely cats	Bites, contact
Erysipelothrix rhusiopathiae	Farm animals, fish, shellfish	Direct contact with animal or contaminated animal product
Hemolytic-uremic syndrome (enterohemorrhagic *Escherichia coli*)	Cattle	Ingestion of contaminated food or water
Leptospirosis (*Leptospira* species)	Dogs, rats, livestock	Contact with urine, particularly in contaminated water
Lyme disease (*Borrelia burgdorferi*)	Wild rodents	Tick bite
Mycobacteriosis (*Mycobacterium marinum*, others)	Fish (and cleaning aquaria)	Wound infection
Pasteurella multocida	Cats, infrequently dogs	Bites, scratches
Plague (*Yersinia pestis*)	Wild rodents, wild rabbits, cats	Bite of rodent fleas, direct contact with infected animals
Rat-bite fever (*Streptobacillus moniliformis, Spirillum minus*)	Rodents (particularly rats)	Bites
Relapsing fever (tick-borne) (*Borrelia* species)	Wild rodents	Tick bite
Salmonellosis (*Salmonella* species)	Poultry, reptiles, dogs, cats, rodents, ferrets, turtles, other wild and domestic animals	Ingestion of contaminated food, direct contact
Streptococcus iniae	Fish grown by aquaculture	Skin injury during handling of fish
Tetanus (*Clostridium tetani*)	Any animal, usually indirect via soil	Wound infection, contaminated bites

Table. **Diseases Transmitted by Animals, continued**

Disease and/or Organism	Common Animal Sources	Vector or Modes of Transmission
Bacterial Diseases, continued		
Tularemia *(Francisella tularensis)*	Wild rabbits, rodents, cats	Tick bites, occasionally deerfly bite, direct contact with infected animal, ingestion of contaminated water, mechanical transmission from claws or teeth (cats)
Vibrio species	Shellfish	Wound infection, ingestion of contaminated food
Yersiniosis *(Yersinia enterocolitica)*	Swine; rarely dogs, cats, rodents	Ingestion of contaminated food or water, rarely direct contact
Fungal Diseases		
Cryptococcosis *(Cryptococcus neoformans)*	Birds, particularly pigeons	Inhalation of aerosols from accumulations of pigeon feces
Histoplasmosis *(Histoplasma capsulatum)*	Bats, birds, particularly starlings	Inhalation of aerosols from accumulations of bat and bird feces
Ringworm (*Microsporum* and *Trichophyton* species)	Cats, dogs, rabbits, rodents	Direct contact
Sporotrichosis *(Sporothrix schenkii)*	Cats	Direct contact
Parasitic Diseases		
Anisakiasis (*Anisakis* species)	Saltwater and anadromous fish	Ingestion of undercooked or raw fish (eg, sushi)
Babesiosis (*Babesia* species)	Wild rodents	Tick bite
Balantidiasis (*Balantidium* coli)	Swine	Ingestion of contaminated food or water
Dwarf tapeworm *(Hymenolepis nana)*	Hamsters, rodents	Ingestion of eggs from feces (contaminated food, water)
Cryptosporidiosis (*Cryptosporidium* species)	Domestic animals, particularly cattle	Ingestion of oocysts shed in feces
Cutaneous larva migrans (*Ancylostoma* species)	Dogs, cats	Penetration of skin by larvae, which develop in soil contaminated with eggs shed in feces

Table. **Diseases Transmitted by Animals, continued**

Disease and/or Organism	Common Animal Sources	Vector or Modes of Transmission
Parasitic Diseases, continued		
Cysticercosis *(Taenia solium)*	Swine (intermediate host)	Ingestion of eggs from fecal-oral contact or contaminated food, water
Dog tapeworm *(Dipylidium caninum)*	Dogs, cats	Ingestion of fleas infected with larvae
Echinococcosis, hydatid disease (*Echinococcus* species)	Dogs, foxes, possibly other carnivores	Ingestion of eggs shed in feces
Fish tapeworm (*Diphyllobothrium latum*)	Saltwater and freshwater fish	Ingestion of larvae in raw or undercooked fish
Giardiasis *(Giardia lamblia)*	Wild and domestic animals, including dogs, cats, beavers	Ingestion of cysts from fecal-oral contact or in contaminated food, water
Beef, pork tapeworm, taeniasis (*Taenia saginata* and *Taenia solium*)	Cattle, swine	Ingestion of larvae in undercooked beef or pork
Toxoplasmosis *(Toxoplasma gondii)*	Cats, livestock	Ingestion of oocysts from infected cat feces, consumption of insufficiently cooked meat, contact with birth products of sheep, goats
Trichinosis *(Trichinella spiralis)*	Swine, bears, possibly other wild carnivores	Ingestion of larvae in raw or undercooked meat
Visceral larva migrans (*Toxocara canis* and *Toxocara cati*)	Dogs, cats	Ingestion of eggs, usually from soil contaminated by feces
Chlamydial and Rickettsial Diseases		
Ehrlichiosis (*Ehrlichia* species)	Possibly deer, dogs, ruminants	Tick bite
Psittacosis *(Chlamydia psittaci)*	Psittacine and domestic birds, farm animals	Inhalation of aerosols from feces
Q fever *(Coxiella burnetii)*	Sheep, other livestock, wild rodents, rabbits	Direct contact and aerosols from birth products, ingestion of contaminated milk, occasionally tick bite
Rickettsialpox *(Rickettsia akari)*	House mouse	Mite bite
Rocky Mountain spotted fever *(Rickettsia rickettsii)*	Dogs, wild rodents, rabbits	Tick bite
Typhus, flea-borne endemic typhus *(Rickettsia typhi)*	Rats, opossums	Flea feces scratched into abrasions

Table. **Diseases Transmitted by Animals, continued**

Disease and/or Organism	Common Animal Sources	Vector or Modes of Transmission
Chlamydial and Rickettsial Diseases, continued		
Typhus, louse-borne* epidemic typhus *(Rickettsia prowazekii)*	Flying squirrels	Contact with squirrels, their nests, or ectoparasites
Viral Diseases		
Colorado tick fever	Wild rodents, particularly squirrels	Tick bite
Encephalitis		
California	Wild rodents	Mosquito bite
Eastern equine	Wild birds, poultry, horses	Mosquito bite
Western equine	Wild birds, poultry, horses	Mosquito bite
St Louis	Wild birds, poultry	Mosquito bite
Venezuelan equine	Horses	Mosquito bite
Powassan	Rodents, rabbits	Tick bite
West Nile	Birds	Mosquito bite
Hantaviruses	Rodents	Inhalation of aerosols of infected secreta and excreta
B virus (formerly herpesvirus simiae)	Macaque monkeys	Bite or exposure to secretions
Lymphocytic choriomeningitis	Rodents, particularly hamsters, mice	Direct contact, inhalation of aerosols, ingestion of contaminated food
Rabies	Dogs, cats, ferrets, bats, skunks, foxes, woodchucks	Bites

* Disease usually is transmitted from person to person (see Epidemic Typhus [Louse-borne Typhus], p 621).

APPENDIX VIII.

Nationally Notifiable Infectious Diseases in the United States

Public health officials at state health departments and the Centers for Disease Control and Prevention (CDC) collaborate in determining which diseases should be nationally notifiable (see Table, p 778). The Council of State and Territorial Epidemiologists, with advice from the CDC, makes recommendations annually for additions and deletions to the list of nationally notifiable diseases. A disease may be added to the list as a new pathogen emerges, or a disease may be deleted as its incidence declines. However, reporting of nationally notifiable diseases to the CDC by the states is voluntary. Reporting currently is mandated (ie, by state legislation or regulation) only by the individual states. The list of diseases that are considered notifiable, therefore, varies slightly by state. Additional and specific requirements should be obtained from the appropriate state health department. All states generally report the diseases that are quarantined internationally (ie, cholera, plague, and yellow fever) in compliance with the World Health Organization's International Health Regulations.

When health care professionals suspect or diagnose a case of a disease considered notifiable in the state, they should report the case by telephone or by mail to the local, county, or state health department. Clinical laboratories also report results consistent with reportable diseases. Staff members in the county or state health department implement disease control measures as needed. The written case report is forwarded to the state health department.

The CDC acts as a common agent for the states and territories for collecting information and reporting of nationally notifiable diseases. Reports of the occurrences of nationally notifiable diseases are transmitted to the CDC each week from the 50 states, 2 cities (Washington, DC, and New York, NY), and 5 territories (American Samoa, Commonwealth of Northern Mariana Islands, Guam, Puerto Rico, and the Virgin Islands). Provisional data are published weekly in the *Morbidity and Mortality Weekly Report;* final data are published each year by the CDC in the annual *Summary of Notifiable Diseases, United States.* The timelines of the provisional weekly reports provide information that the CDC and state or local epidemiologists use to detect and more effectively interrupt outbreaks. Reporting also provides the timely information needed to measure and demonstrate the effect of changed immunization laws or a new therapeutic modality. The finalized annual data also provide information on reported disease incidence that is necessary for the study of epidemiologic trends and the development of disease prevention policies. The CDC is the sole repository for these data, which are used widely by schools of medicine and public health, communications media, and pharmaceutical or other companies producing health-related products, as well as by local, state, and federal health agencies and other agencies or persons concerned with the trends of reportable conditions in the United States.

Table. **Infectious Diseases Designated as Notifiable at the National Level*—United States, 1999**

Acquired immunodeficiency syndrome
Anthrax
Botulism[†]
Brucellosis
Chancroid[†]
Chlamydia trachomatis, genital infections
Cholera
Coccidioidomycosis (regional)[†]
Cryptosporidiosis
Cyclosporiasis
Diphtheria
Ehrlichiosis, human granulocytic
Ehrlichiosis, human monocytic
Encephalitis, California serogroup
Encephalitis, eastern equine
Encephalitis, St Louis
Encephalitis, western equine
Escherichia coli O157:H7
Gonorrhea
Haemophilus influenzae (invasive disease)
Hansen disease (leprosy)
Hantavirus pulmonary syndrome
Hemolytic-uremic syndrome, postdiarrheal[†]
Hepatitis A
Hepatitis B
Hepatitis C/non-A, non-B
Human immunodeficiency virus infection, pediatric
Legionellosis
Lyme disease
Malaria
Measles
Meningococcal disease
Mumps
Pertussis
Plague
Poliomyelitis, paralytic
Psittacosis
Rabies, animal
Rabies, human
Rocky Mountain spotted fever
Rubella
Rubella, congenital syndrome
Salmonellosis[†]
Shigellosis[†]
Streptococcal disease, invasive, group A[†]
Streptococcus pneumoniae, drug-resistant invasive disease[†]
Streptococcal toxic shock syndrome
Syphilis
Syphilis, congenital
Tetanus
Toxic shock syndrome
Trichinosis
Tuberculosis
Typhoid fever
Varicella deaths
Yellow fever[†]

* Although varicella is not a nationally notifiable disease, the Council of State and Territorial Epidemiologists recommends reporting of cases of this disease to the Centers for Disease Control and Prevention.

† Not currently published in the weekly tables.

Appendix IX

Services of the Centers for Disease Control and Prevention (CDC)

The Centers for Disease Control and Prevention (US Public Health Service, Department of Health and Human Services, Atlanta, Ga) is the federal agency charged with protecting the public health of the nation by preventing disease and other disabling conditions. The CDC administers national programs for the prevention and control of the following: (1) infectious diseases, (2) occupational diseases and injury, (3) chronic diseases, and (4) environment-related injury and illness. The CDC also provides consultation to other nations and participates with international agencies in the control of preventable diseases. In addition, the CDC directs and enforces foreign quarantine activities and regulations, and it provides consultation and assistance in upgrading the performance of clinical laboratories.

The CDC provides a number of services related to infectious disease management and control. Although the CDC is principally a resource for state and local health departments, it also offers direct and indirect services to hospitals and practicing physicians. The range of services includes reference laboratory diagnosis and epidemiologic consultation, both usually arranged through state health departments. In addition, the CDC Drug Service supplies some specific prophylactic or therapeutic drugs and biologic agents.

Specific immunobiologic products available include botulinal equine (trivalent, ABE) antitoxin, diphtheria equine antitoxin, Vaccinia Immune Globulin (VIG), botulinus pentavalent toxoid, and vaccinia vaccine.

In addition, several drugs for the treatment of parasitic disease, which are not currently licensed for use in the United States, are handled under an Investigational New Drug permit. These antiparasitic drugs include bithionol, dehydroemetine, diethylcarbamazine citrate, melarsoprol, nifurtimox, sodium stibogluconate, and suramin.

Requests for biologic products, antiparasitic drugs, and related information should be directed to the CDC Drug Service (see Appendix I, Directory of Resources, p 743).

Index

Page numbers followed by "t" indicate a table. Page numbers followed by "f" indicate a figure.

A

C

D

E

F

I

J

K

L

M

N

O

P

Q

R

S

T

U

V

W

X

Y

Z